Integrative Pediatrics

Weil Integrative Medicine Library

Published and Forthcoming Volumes

SERIES EDITOR

ANDREW T. WEIL, MD

Donald I. Abrams and Andrew T. Weil: *Integrative Oncology*
Timothy P. Culbert and Karen Olness: *Integrative Pediatrics*
Gerard Mullin: *Integrative Gastroenterology*
Victoria Maizes and Tieraona Low Dog: *Integrative Women's Health*
Randy Horwitz and Daniel Muller: *Integrative Rheumatology, Allergy, and Immunology*
Bernard Beitman and Daniel A. Monti: *Integrative Psychiatry*
Stephen DeVries and James Dalen: *Integrative Cardiology*

Integrative Pediatrics

EDITED BY

Timothy P. Culbert, MD
Medical Director
Integrative Medicine Program
Children's Hospitals and Clinics of Minnesota
Assistant Professor of Clinical Pediatrics
Department of Pediatrics
University of Minnesota Medical School

Karen Olness, MD
Professor of Pediatrics
Family Medicine and Global Health
Case Western Reserve University

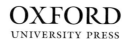

OXFORD
UNIVERSITY PRESS

2010

OXFORD

UNIVERSITY PRESS

Oxford University Press, Inc., publishes works that further
Oxford University's objective of excellence
in research, scholarship, and education.

Oxford New York
Auckland Cape Town Dar es Salaam Hong Kong Karachi
Kuala Lumpur Madrid Melbourne Mexico City Nairobi
New Delhi Shanghai Taipei Toronto

With offices in
Argentina Austria Brazil Chile Czech Republic France Greece
Guatemala Hungary Italy Japan Poland Portugal Singapore
South Korea Switzerland Thailand Turkey Ukraine Vietnam

Copyright © 2010 by Oxford University Press, Inc.

Published by Oxford University Press, Inc.
198 Madison Avenue, New York, New York 10016
www.oup.com

Oxford is a registered trademark of Oxford University Press

Library of Congress Cataloging-in-Publication Data
Integrative pediatrics / [edited by] Timothy P. Culbert, Karen Olness.
p. ; cm.
Includes bibliographical references.
ISBN 978-0-19-538472-7
1. Children—Diseases—Alternative treatment. 2. Integrative
medicine. I. Culbert, Timothy. II. Olness, Karen.
[DNLM: 1. Complementary Therapies—methods. 2. Adolescent.
3. Child. 4. Infant. WB 890 I6086 2009]
RJ53.A48I62 2009
618.92—dc22
2008040390

1 3 5 7 9 8 6 4 2
Printed in the United States of America
on acid-free paper

CONTENTS

Foreword I   ix

Foreword II   xiii

Acknowledgments   xv

Contributors   xvii

I   Foundations of Integrative Pediatric Care

1. Introduction to Integrative Pediatrics   3
   Timothy P. Culbert, Karen Olness, and Sunita Vohra

2. Assessment and Treatment Planning in Integrative Pediatric Practice   13
   Timothy P. Culbert, Victoria Maizes, Tai Mendenhall, and David K. Becker

3. Culture and Spirituality in Integrative Pediatrics   30
   Judson B. Reaney and Gregory A. Plotnikoff

4. Essential Medicine: Self-Care for Pediatric Providers   47
   Danna M. Park

5. Research and Education in Integrative Pediatrics   73
   Sunita Vohra and Trish Dryden

II   Pediatric Perspectives on Specific Therapeutic Approaches

6. A Pediatric Perspective on Acupuncture   103
   Yuan-Chi Lin and Shu-Ming Wang

7. A Pediatric Perspective on Aromatherapy   123
   Maura Fitzgerald and Linda L. Halcón

8. A Pediatric Perspective on Chiropractic   146
   Karen Erickson, Elise G. Hewitt, Amy Lynne Watson,
   Anthony L. Rosner, and Randy L. Hewitt

9. A Pediatric Perspective on Energy Therapies   180
   Mary Jane Ott, Larraine Bossi, and Jeanne Colbath

10. A Pediatric Perspective on Exercise Medicine   204
    Amanda K. Weiss Kelly and Susannah M. Briskin

11. A Pediatric Perspective on Herbals and Supplements   217
Paula Gardiner and Tieraona Lowdog

12. A Pediatric Perspective on Homeopathy   234
David Riley, Menachem Oberbaum, and Shepherd Roee Singer

13. A Pediatric Perspective on Massage   248
Shay Beider, Erin T. O'Callaghan, and Jeffrey I. Gold

14. A Pediatric Perspective on Mind-Body Medicine   267
Daniel P. Kohen

15. A Pediatric Perspective on Naturopathic Medicine   302
Matthew I. Baral, Wendy Weber, and Jessica Mitchell

16. A Pediatric Perspective on Nutritional Therapeutics   314
Benjamin Kligler and Emilie Scott

17. A Pediatric Perspective on Osteopathic Medicine   340
Ali Carine, Miriam Mills, and Viola Frymann

III   Clinical Applications in Integrative Pediatrics

18. Integrative Adolescent Medicine   367
Cora Collette Breuner

19. Integrative Developmental/Behavioral Pediatrics   395
Sanford Newmark

20. Integrative Pediatric Gastroenterology   425
Gerard A. Banez and Rita Steffen

21. Integrative Pediatric Intensive Care   446
David M. Steinhorn and Sheila Wang

22. Integrative Pediatric Mental Health (Assessment and
Treatment Using an Ecological Perspective)   458
Scott M. Shannon

23. Integrative Pediatric Oncology   487
Susan F. Sencer

24. Integrative Pediatric Pain Management   518
Joy A. Weydert and Mark Connelly

25. Integrative Pediatric Palliative Care   569
Stefan J. Friedrichsdorf, Leora Kuttner,
Krista Westendorp, and Ruth McCarty

26. Integrative Pediatric Primary Care   594
Lawrence D. Rosen

27. Integrative Pediatric Pulmonology   621
John D. Mark

IV   The Future of Integrative Pediatrics: Looking Ahead

28. The Future of Integrative Pediatrics   653
Timothy P. Culbert, Kathi J. Kemper, and Lawrence D. Rosen

Index   675

V   Integrative Pediatrics: Additional Chapters—Web-Based Supplement

(www.oup.com/us/integrativepediatrics)

29. Optimal Healing Environments in Pediatrics
Chris Feudtner and Wayne B. Jonas

30. Ethical Perspectives on Integrative Pediatrics
Kathi J. Kemper

31. Designing Integrative Pediatrics Programs: Business and
Administrative Aspects
Lynda Richtsmeier Cyr, Timothy P.Culbert, and Lori Knutson

32. Pediatric Perspectives on Environmental Medicine
Mark D. Miller and Alice C. Brock-Utne

33. A Pediatric Perspective on Creative Arts Therapies
Deforia Lane, Emily Darsie, and Barbara DiScenna

34. A Pediatric Perspective on Yoga
Gurjeet Singh Birdee and Paula Gardiner

35. Global Pediatrics and Health Disparities
Karen Olness and Boris Kalanj

FOREWORD I

Integrative medicine and alternative medicine are not synonymous. Alternative medicine comprises all those therapies not taught in conventional (allopathic) medical schools, based on ideas of variable soundness, ranging from some that are sensible and worth including in mainstream medicine to others that are foolish and a few that are dangerous. The term "alternative medicine" has recently been incorporated into a broader term, "complementary and alternative medicine" or "CAM," used by the US federal government and other institutions; the National Institutes of Health now has a national CAM center (NCCAM).

Neither "alternative" nor "complementary" captures the essence of integrative medicine. The former suggests replacement of conventional therapies by others; the latter adjunctive therapies, added as afterthoughts.

IM does include ideas and practices currently beyond the scope of the conventional, but it neither rejects conventional therapies nor accepts alternative ones uncritically. Most importantly, it emphasizes principles that may or may not be associated with CAM, that is

- *The Natural Healing Power of the Organism*—IM assumes that the body has an innate capacity for healing, for self-diagnosis, self-repair, regeneration, and adaptation to injury or loss. The primary goal of treatment should be to support, facilitate, and augment that innate capacity.
- *Whole Person Medicine*—IM views patients as more than physical bodies. They are also mental/emotional beings, spiritual entities, and members of particular communities and societies. These other dimensions of human life

are relevant to health and to the accurate diagnosis and effective treatment of disease.

- *The Importance of Lifestyle*—Health and disease result from interactions between genes and all aspects of lifestyle, including diet, physical activity, rest and sleep, stress, the quality of relationships, work, and so forth. Lifestyle choices may influence disease risks more than genes and must be a focus of the medical history. Lifestyle medicine, which is one component of IM, gives physicians information and tools to enable them to prevent and treat disease more effectively.

- *The Critical Role of the Doctor–Patient Relationship*—Throughout history people have accorded the doctor–patient relationship special, even sacred, status. When a medically trained person sits with a patient and listens with full attention to his or her story, that alone can initiate healing before any treatment is offered. A great tragedy of contemporary medicine, especially in the USA, is that for-profit, corporate systems have virtually destroyed this core aspect of practice. If practitioners have only a few minutes with each patient—the time limit set by the managed care systems they work for—it is very unlikely they will be able to form the kind of therapeutic relationships that foster health and healing.

Furthermore, this special form of human interaction has been the source of greatest emotional reward for the physician, and its disappearance in our time is a main reason for rising practitioner discontent. IM insists on the paramount importance of the therapeutic relationship and demands that health care systems support and honor it (e.g., by reimbursing physicians for time spent with patients rather than number of patients seen).

In essence, integrative medicine is conservative. It seeks to restore core values of the profession that have eroded in recent times. It honors such ancient precepts as Hippocrates' injunctions on physicians to "first do no harm" and "to value the healing power of nature." It is conservative in practice, favoring less invasive and drastic treatments over more invasive and drastic ones whenever possible, and it is fiscally conservative in relying less on expensive technology and more on simpler methods, *as appropriate to the circumstances of illness.*

How can pediatric medicine benefit from holding to these principles?

The innate healing power of organisms decreases with age. We can observe the workings of the body's healing mechanisms most easily in the young, and we can often support and facilitate them with less invasive, less expensive interventions than those required in adult patients. Homeopathic remedies, osteopathic manipulation, and hypnotherapy, for example, can be remarkably successful in children. By embracing this principle of IM, pediatricians can increase their effectiveness and also decrease costs and risks of treatment.

Some people dismiss the relevance of whole person medicine to the pediatric patient population, believing that the young do not have developed minds and belief systems. But even infants participate in the emotional dynamics of encounters between parents and doctors, and the possibilities for using mind/body interventions in children should never be ignored. Hypnosis and guided imagery can reduce pain and anxiety associated with office visits and procedures. Stress reduction training can reduce the need for medication in many instances.

Lifestyle analysis and counseling should be central in pediatrics, because patterns of behavior that influence long-term health are often set in childhood. Witness the epidemic of childhood obesity in North America, and in its wake, an epidemic of type-2 diabetes (with onset at younger ages than we have ever seen). This calamity is the result of dissonance between genes and lifestyle, in particular the increasing consumption of high-glycemic-load carbohydrates and unhealthy fats in the refined, processed, and manufactured food that has become so prominent in North American diets. A major responsibility of integrative pediatric medicine is to teach parents and children about the health consequences of lifestyle choices and to motivate them to make better ones.

And, of course, the doctor–patient relationship is as important in pediatrics as in any other area of medicine, both for effective practice and for emotional reward. Disruption of continuity of care by profit-driven medicine has made it a rarity for pediatricians to follow patients from infancy to young adulthood, to know them and their families well.

Consumer demand for integrative pediatric medicine is very high. More and more parents are wary of giving kids pharmaceutical drugs for every problem. They question the unprecedented use of psychiatric medication in the young. They ask why more children than ever are developing asthma and allergies. They want to know why the incidence of autism and ADHD is so high. Many even question the safety and value of immunizations. I believe that integrative pediatricians are best trained to listen to these concerns, help parents understand the risks and benefits of treatments, and analyze the nature and causation of disorders that affect children.

Ever since I founded the Program in Integrative Medicine (now the Arizona Center for Integrative Medicine [ACIM]) in 1994, I have worked to make training in IM available to pediatricians and to stimulate research in integrative approaches to pediatric disorders. I served as co-principal investigator (with Dr. Fayez Ghishan) of NCCAM's Center for Pediatric CAM Research at the University of Arizona, helped organize the first conference on integrative pediatric medicine in the US, have treated pediatric patients at the outpatient integrative medicine clinic at the Arizona Health Sciences Center, and have taught pediatricians who have gone through our intensive IM fellowships (see www.integrativemedicine.arizona.edu). My colleagues and I at ACIM are now developing a comprehensive curriculum in IM (in distributed learning format) that we hope will become a required, accredited part of pediatric residency programs.

I do not see any real barriers to this enhancement of training. More than many other practitioners, pediatricians are open to the philosophy of IM. They are also highly motivated to promote health and prevent disease in the young, and eager to learn about low-risk, low-tech, low-cost interventions that not included in their training.

The editors of this volume, Drs. Timothy P. Culbert and Karen Olness, have compiled a great deal of information to help practitioners understand and use IM. I consider it a significant contribution to the emerging field of integrative pediatrics.

Andrew Weil, MD

FOREWORD II

Over the past two decades in the USA; non-traditional approaches (i.e. complementary, alternative, folk or culture-specific non-allopathic practices) to medical care have moved from the fringes of medical care to, if not center stage, at least somewhere on the stage. This is in part because a large percent of people of all ages are using some aspects of these therapies. Even more important in their acceptance, is the scientific approach by many clinicians, who are the authors of this book, to examine their efficacy. Most are not new theories and clinical care modes. Indeed many antedate allopathic medicine by centuries or even millenia. This book will challenge and engage most of us who know little about the many areas covered by this book.

A word about the title given to this field, for awhile "alternative medicine" had some popularity. But most clinicians did not like this term, for clearly there are many conditions for which non-traditional medicine works. We were not happy to discard much of non-traditional medicine. Then "complementary medicine" was in vogue. I liked this term because it implied that these approaches could be added to conventional care. Under the influence of George Engel, I have liked the term "bio-psycho-social" medicine but I have to admit that it has been used primarily by physicians and, while it could include the areas covered in this book, it rarely did. Now the title "integrative medicine" has come into use, as in this book. It is a good term for it puts these many non-traditional therapies on a par with allopathic medicine. An Integrative approach emphasizes the recognition of mind, body, spirit, and sociocultural context as both determinants of illness and treatment foci of care. The challenge for the clinician is to integrate these many therapeutic approaches together in a healing balance, for the best care of the patient.

The authors, each leaders in their fields, have put forward a fine description of the many specific areas of focus within integrative pediatrics. In the book's first section on "Foundations of Integrative Pediatric Care," Vohra discusses the research and educational needs, which are huge since so few pediatricians have received formal education in this area. The next 12 chapters review several of these therapeutic modalities in detail with specific attention to their relevance in pediatric care. The section on "Clinical Applications in Integrative Pediatrics" brings together a number of specific pediatric problems or age groups. I think that this integration of several of the fields described is the real challenge for the clinician. Selecting the most appropriate therapy for the patient and family while balancing risk and benefit with patient preferences is an art and science. It is the challenge taken up in this book. In the final chapter, Culbert et al. conclude with an essay on the future of integrative pediatrics. The goal should be to bring to bear on the patient the most appropriate collection of services in supporting each child and family in a process which facilitates optimal healing and ongoing wellness. This book will go a long way to achieve integrated care for the benefit of our young patients.

Robert Haggerty

ACKNOWLEDGMENTS

I would not have the privilege of editing this volume without my experience in the clinical practice of integrative pediatrics over the past 10 years. My thanks to the staff of the Integrative Medicine Program at Children's Hospitals and Clinics of Minnesota who make this a joyful undertaking, particularly Lynda Richtsmeier-Cyr and Maura Fitzgerald who have been there since the beginning and who participated equally in creating this amazing program. I extend my deep appreciation as well to all of the children and families I have been privileged to serve and learn from along the way.

It is important to recognize the courage and foresight of Julie Morath, former COO of Children's Hospitals and Clinics of Minnesota for her unyielding support as "executive champion" of this program at the leadership level of our organization from the very beginning. I also wish to thank Susan Sencer, MD for co-founding the program in Integrative Medicine at Children's Hospitals and Clinics of Minnesota in 1999, for offering me the chance to join this pioneering effort and for her wise council and positive influence.

I also wish to thank my friends and professional colleagues particularly Sunita Vohra, Kathi Kemper, Larry Rosen, Scott Shannon, Jon Mark, David Steinhorn, Rebecca Kajander, Penny George, Lori Knutson, Gerard Banez, Leora Kuttner, Lonnie Zeltzer, Anthony Galas, Paula Gardiner, Judson Reaney, and Daniel Kohen, who have been a constant source of support and inspiration as I have journeyed down this rewarding path. Thanks as well to the talented, hardworking, and innovative chapter authors for this volume who are defining this new field.

My heartfelt thanks to my co-editor Karen Olness, one of the pioneers of complementary medicine and global pediatrics, who kindled an interest in mind-body skills early on in my career and who has been a great friend and mentor.

Thanks to Andrew Weil, MD for offering me the opportunity to edit this volume and for being a consistent advocate for developing the pediatric area within Integrative Medicine.

With love to Heidi, Sam, Hannah, William, and Joanne Culbert.

Timothy P. Culbert

I dedicate this volume to the many unsung heros and heroines of child health care who have taken good care of children and families integratively in spite of derision, criticism, and lack of reimbursement. My thanks go to the organizations that have facilitated integrative pediatric research, education, and clinical activities in the United States and worldwide. Some of these are Minneapolis Children's, Rainbow Babies and Children's Hospital in Cleveland, the SDBP, ASCH, SCEH, ISH, and others that are also multidisciplinary such as are the AAPB, AHMA, AHNA, IPA, IASP, AAP, SCHIM, and APA. My thanks also go to organizations such as NCCAM and The Bravewell Collaborative that have been willing to "take a chance" in supporting integrative pediatrics education programs and research. To a large extent, this book evolved because they took those chances.

And I thank all those mentors and colleagues on whose shoulders I stand including Erik Wright, Kay Thompson, Bob Pearson, Franz Baumann, Esther Bartlett, Bertha Rodger, Philip Ament, William Kroger, David Merrill, Neal Gault, Arnold Anderson, Robert Good, and Robert Haggerty.

And I especially thank my husband, Hakon, who remains the wind beneath my sails.

Karen Olness

CONTRIBUTORS

Gerard A. Banez, PhD
Program Director, Pediatric Pain
   Rehabilitation Program
Cleveland Clinic Children's Hospital
Cleveland, OH

Matthew I. Baral, ND
Assistant Professor, Medical Director
Hamilton Elementary School Clinic
Southwest College of Naturopathic
   Medicine
Tempe, AZ

David K. Becker, MD, MPH
Director
Pediatric Integrative Pain Clinic
and
Assistant Clinical Professor
UCSF Department of Pediatrics
University of California
San Francisco, CA

Shay Beider, MPH, LMT
Executive Director
Integrative Touch for Kids
Beverly Hills, CA

Gurjeet Singh Birdee, MD, MPH
Clinical Research Fellow
Osher Research Center Harvard Medical
   School
Boston, MA

Larraine Bossi, MS, APRN, BC
Medicine Patient Care Services Project
   Manager
Children's Hospital Boston
Boston, MA

Cora Collette Breuner, MD, MPH
Associate Professor
Department of Pediatrics
Adjunct Associate Professor of
   Orthopedics
Section of Adolescent Medicine and
   Sports Medicine
University of Washington
Seattle Childrens Hospital
Seattle, WA

Susannah M. Briskin, MD, FAAP
Assistant Professor of Pediatrics
Primary Care Sports Medicine
Rainbow Babies and Children's Hospital
University Hospitals Case Medical Center
Cleveland, OH

Alice C. Brock-Utne, MD
Residency Curriculum Project Director
Pediatric Environmental Health Specialty
    Unit
University of California
San Francisco, CA
and
General Pediatrician
Marin Community Clinics
San Rafael, CA

Ali Carine, DO, FACOP, C-NMM/OMM
Clinical Faculty
Ohio University COM
Columbus, OH

**Jeanne Colbath, RN, MSN, APRN, BC,
A-HNC, CHTP**
Coordinator of Cardiac Rehabilitation
Caritas St. Elizabeth's Medical Center
Boston, MA

Mark Connelly, PhD
Assistant Professor of Pediatrics
University of Missouri—Kansas City
    School of Medicine
Children's Mercy Hospitals and Clinics
Kansas City, MO

Timothy P. Culbert, MD
Medical Director
Integrative Medicine Program
Children's Hospitals and Clinics of
    Minnesota
and
Assistant Professor of Clinical Pediatrics
Department of Pediatrics
University of Minnesota Medical School
Minneapolis, MN

Emily Darsie, MA, MT-BC
Music Therapist
Rainbow Babies and Children's Hospital
Cleveland, OH

**Barbara DiScenna, MA, ATR-BC, LSW,
LPC**
Art Therapist
University Hospitals of Cleveland
Cleveland, OH

Tieraona Low Dog, MD
Assistant Professor, Internal Medicine
Director of Education, Program in
    Integrative Medicine
University of Arizona
Tucson, AZ

Trish Dryden, RMT, MEd
Director of Applied Research
Centennial College
Toronto ON
Canada

Karen Erickson, DC
Spokesperson
American Chiropractic Association
    Board of Trustees
New York Chiropractic College
New York, NY

Chris Feudtner, MD, PhD, MPH
Director, Department of Medical Ethics
The Steven D. Handler Endowed
    Chair of Medical Ethics
The Children's Hospital of Philadelphia
and
Assistant Professor of Pediatrics
The University of Pennsylvania School of
    Medicine
Philadelphia, PA

Maura Fitzgerald, RN, MS, MA, CNS
Clinical Nurse Specialist
Integrative Medicine
Children's Hospitals and Clinics of
    Minnesota
Minneapolis, MN

Stefan J. Friedrichsdorf, MD
Pain and Palliative Care Program
Children's Hospitals and Clinics of
    Minnesota
Minneapolis, MN

Viola Frymann, DO, FAAO, FCA
Fellow of the American Academy
    of Osteopathy and Fellow of
    the Cranial Academy
San Diego, CA

Paula Gardiner, MD, MPH
Assistant Professor
Department of Family Medicine
Boston University Medical Center
Boston, MA

Jeffrey I. Gold, PhD
Associate Professor
Anesthesiology & Pediatrics
Keck School of Medicine
University of Southern California
Pediatric Psychologist
Children's Hospital Los Angeles
and
Director
Pediatric Pain Management Clinic
Department of Anesthesiology
Critical Care Medicine Comfort
Pain Management and Palliative Care
    Program
USC University Center for Excellence
Mental Health Childrens Hospital
    Los Angeles
Los Angeles, CA

Linda L. Halcón, PhD, MPH, RN
Associate Professor
School of Nursing
University of Minnesota
Minneapolis, MN

Elise G. Hewitt, DC CST, DICCP, FICC
Board Certified Pediatric Chiropractor
Certified Craniosacral Therapist
President, ACA Council on Chiropractic
    Pediatrics
Board of Directors, Integrative Pediatrics
    Council
Portland Chiropractic Group
Portland, OR

Randy L. Hewitt, DC
Certified Chiropractic Sports Physician
Portland Chiropractic Group
Portland, OR

Wayne B. Jonas, MD
President and CEO
Samueli Institute
Alexandria, VA

Boris Kalanj, MSW, LISW
Director of Health Care Equity and
    Cultural Competence
Children's Hospitals and Clinics of
    Minnesota
Minneapolis, MN

Kathi J. Kemper, MD, MPH
Caryl Guth Chair for Holistic and
    Integrative Medicine
Professor, Pediatrics, Public Health
    Sciences
Wake Forest University School of
    Medicine
Winston-Salem, NC

Benjamin Kligler, MD, MPH
Vice Chair and Research Director
Beth Israel Department of Integrative
  Medicine
Continuum Center for Health and
  Healing
and
Associate Professor of Family and Social
  Medicine
Albert Einstein College of Medicine
New York, NY

Lori Knutson, RN, BSN, HN-BC
Executive Director
Brenden Leadership Chair in Integrative
  Medicine
Penny George Institute for Health and
  Healing
Abbott Northwestern Hospital
Allina Hospital's & Clinic's
Minneapolis, MN

Daniel P. Kohen, MD
Director
Developmental-Behavioral Pediatrics
  Program
and
Professor
Departments of Pediatrics and Family
  Medicine & Community Health
University of Minnesota Medical School
Minneapolis, MN

Leora Kuttner PhD, Reg Psyc
Clinical Professor
Pediatric Deptartment
BC Children's Hospital & University of
  British Columbia
Vancouver, BC
Canada

Deforia Lane, PhD, MT-BC
Director of Music Theraphy
University Hospitals of Cleveland Ireland
  Cancer Center
Cleveland, OH

Yuan-Chi Lin, MD, MPH
Department of Anesthesiology
Peri-operative and Pain Medicine
Children's Hospital Boston
Department of Anaesthesia
Harvard Medical School
Boston, MA

Victoria Maizes, MD
Associate Professor, Internal Medicine
Executive Director, Program in
  Integrative Medicine
University of Arizona
Tucson, AZ

John D. Mark, MD
Clinical Associate Professor of
  Pediatrics
Center of Excellence in Pulmonary
  Biology
Lucile Packard Children's Hospital at
  Stanford
Stanford University
Stanford, CA

Ruth McCarty, MS, LAc
Director of Complementary and
  Alternative Medicine Program
Children's Hospital of Orange County
Orange, CA

Tai Mendenhall, PhD, LMFT, CFT
Assistant Professor
Department of Family Medicine and
   Community Health
University of Minnesota Medical School
Minneapolis, MN
and
Coordinator of Behavioral Medicine
St. John's Family Practice Residency
St. Paul, MA

Mark D. Miller, MD, MPH
Assistant Clinical Professor of Medicine
   and Pediatrics
Director of the Pediatric Environmental
   Health Specialty Unit
University of California
San Francisco, CA
and
Public Health Medical Officer
California Environmental Protection
   Agency
Office of Environmental Health Hazard
   Assessment
Oakland, CA

Miriam V. Mills, MD, FAAP
Clinical Professor and Director of
   Research Division
Department of OMM
Oklahoma State University Center for
   Health Sciences
and
President and Owner
Young People's Clinic
PC, Tulsa, OK

Jessica Mitchell, ND
Fellow, Naturopathic Pediatrics
Southwest College of Naturopathic
   Medicine
Tempe, AZ

Sanford Newmark, MD
Faculty
Arizona Center for Integrative Medicine
University of Arizona
and
Director
Center for Pediatric Integrative Medicine
Tucson, AZ

**Menachem Oberbaum, MD, MFHom
(Lond)**
The Center for Integrative
   Complementary Medicine
Shaare Zedek Medical Center
Jerusalem

Erin T. O'Callaghan, PhD
Postdoctoral Psychology Fellow
Children's Hospital Los Angeles
Los Angeles, CA

Karen Olness, MD
Professor of Pediatrics
Family Medicine and Global Health
Case Western Reserve University
Cleveland, OH

Mary Jane Ott, MN, MA, APRN, BC
Nursing and Patient Care Services
Leonard P. Zakim Center for Integrative
   Therapies
Dana-Farber Cancer Institute
Boston, MA

Danna Park, MD, FAAP
Medical Director
Integrative Healthcare Program
Mission Hospitals System
Asheville, NC

Gregory A. Plotnikoff, MD, MTS, FACP
Medical Director
Institute for Health and Healing
Abbott Northwestern Hospital
Minneapolis, MN

Judson B. Reaney, MD, FAAP
Alexander Center for Child Development
  and Behavior
Park Nicollet Clinic
Saint Louis Park, Minnesota
and Instructor of Pediatrics
University of Minnesota
Minneapolis, MN

Lynda Richtsmeier Cyr, PhD, LP
Program Lead, Integrative Medicine
  Program
Children's Hospitals and Clinics of
  Minnesota
Minneapolis, MN

David Riley, MD
Founder—Integrative Medicine Institute
Clinical Associate Professor, UNM
  Medical School
Santa Fe, NM

Lawrence D. Rosen, MD
Clinical Assistant Professor
New Jersey Medical School
and
Chief
Pediatric Integrative Medicine
Department of Pediatrics
Hackensack University Medical Center
Hackensack, NJ

Anthony L. Rosner, PhD, LL D [Hon.]
Director of Research Initiatives
Parker College of Chiropractic
Brookline, MA

Emilie F. Scott, MD
Assistant Clinical Professor
Department of Family Medicine
University of California
Irvine, CA

Susan F. Sencer, MD
Medical Director
Pediatric Hematology/Oncology
  Department
Children's Hospitals and Clinics of
  Minnesota
Minneapolis, MN

Scott M. Shannon, MD
Assistant Clinical Professor of Child and
  Adolescent Psychiatry
University of Colorado
Children's Hospital
Denver, CO

Shepherd Roee Singer, MD
The Center for Integrative
  Complementary Medicine
Shaare Zedek Medical Center
Jerusalem

Rita Steffen, MD
Staff Physician
Department of Pediatric
  Gastroenterology and Nutrition
and
Medical Director, Pediatric
  Gastroenterology Motility Lab
Children's Hospital
Cleveland Clinic
Cleveland, OH

David M. Steinhorn, MD
Medical Director
Judith Nan Joy Integrative Medicine
 Initiative
Attending Physician, Pediatric Critical
 Care
Children's Memorial Hospital
and
Professor of Pediatrics
Northwestern University Feinberg
 School of Medicine
Chicago, IL

Sunita Vohra, MD, FRCPC, MSc
Director, CARE Program
Department of Pediatrics
Faculty of Medicine
University of Alberta
Edmonton, Alberta
Canada

Sheila Wang, PhD
Director of Research
Judith Nan Joy Integrative Medicine
 Initiative
Children's Memorial Hospital
and
Research Assistant Professor
Northwestern University Feinberg
 School of Medicine
Chicago, IL

Shu-Ming Wang, MD
Department of Anesthesiology
Yale University School of Medicine
New Haven, CT

Amy Lynne Watson, DC
Chiropractor/Owner, Whole Mama
 Whole Child
Founder/Manager, Jyoti Family Wellness
 Center
Founding Member, MotherSource
Secretary, ACA Council on Chiropractic
 Pediatrics
Founder, PIPA: Portland Integrative
 Pediatrics Association
Portland, OR

Wendy Weber, ND, MPH
Research Associate Professor
School of Naturopathic Medicine
Bastyr University
Kenmore, WA

Amanda K. Weiss Kelly, MD, FAAP
Assistant Professor of Pediatrics
Director of Primary Care Sports
 Medicine
Rainbow Babies and Children's Hospital
University Hospitals Case Medical Center
Cleveland, OH

Krista Westendorp, RN
Pain and Palliative Care Program
Children's Hospitals and Clinics of
 Minnesota
Minneapolis, MN

Joy A. Weydert, MD
Assistant Professor of Pediatrics
University of Missouri—Kansas City
 School of Medicine
Children's Mercy Hospitals and Clinics
Kansas City, MO

I

Foundations of Integrative Pediatric Care

1

Introduction to Integrative Pediatrics

TIMOTHY P. CULBERT, KAREN OLNESS, AND SUNITA VOHRA

Reinventing Pediatric Medicine

Health care today is at a crossroads. The way in which we care for our youngest and most vulnerable group—our children—is in need of redesign. Consumers are letting us know this by spending billions of dollars outside of the conventional medical system on themselves and their children. Families are seeking medical service models and providers that espouse and deliver "holistic" care that is congruent with their beliefs about health and disease and which addresses health within the context of mind, body, and spirit. Children, parents, and pediatricians all seem ready for a new, more holistic approach. Like adults, more than 50% of children and teens with chronic illness report the use of a complementary or alternative therapy (Kemper, Vohra, & Walls, 2008)! The evidence for the benefits and safety of complementary and alternative therapies for kids continues to grow (Kemper, Vohra, & Walls, 2008; Plotnikoff, Kemper, & Culbert, 2008). In fact, children are quite capable of engaging in self-care skills such as mind/body therapies (Sussman & Culbert, 1999). Pediatricians are referring more of their patients for complementary therapies (Sikand & Lakensik, 1998), have consistently demanded more continuing medical education options in this area, and are using complementary/alternative medicine (CAM) therapies themselves in significant numbers (Kemper, & O'Connor, 2004). A new model representing a "reinvention" of care, titled "integrative medicine," is the focus of this volume as applied specifically to pediatric healthcare. As described below, integrative pediatrics reflects a "redesign," combining the best available therapies for children from a variety of traditions, in a healing-oriented medicine embracing mind, body, and spirit while balancing safety and efficacy concerns.

Integrative medicine differs from CAM in that the former describes a philosophy of care supported by defining principles (see Table 1-1), whereas the latter merely refers to cares that are "outside the mainstream" of what we tend to designate "conventional" care in the western, allopathic tradition. Of note, what is considered "conventional" in the United States or Canada may well be considered "CAM" in another country/culture. The World Health Organization (WHO) estimates that 80% of the world's population utilizes some form of CAM. As defined by the National Institute of Health's National

Table 1-1. Principles of Pediatric Integrative Medicine

Integrative Pediatrics is a healing-oriented medicine that:

Offers patient and family-centered care that focuses on healing the whole child—mind, body, and spirit—in the context of community and with respect for and celebration of developmental and cultural diversity

Affirms that an optimal balance of mind, body, and spiritual elements is essential to the full attainment of wellness, health, optimal development, and learning

Recognizes that children strive for mastery. An integrative pediatrics approach educates and empowers children to be active participants in their own care, and to take responsibility for their own health and wellness whenever possible and to develop self-care skills they can use throughout their lifetime

Makes use of all appropriate therapeutic approaches and evidence-based global medical modalities to achieve optimal health and healing

Encourages healing partnerships between the provider, patient, and their families as well as other key decision-makers

Supports the individualization of care

Contributes to a culture of wellness with a focus on health promotion, prevention, and the purposeful cultivation of optimal healing environments for all children with a frame of "salutogenesis" rather than "pathogenesis"

Utilizes natural, less invasive interventions before costly, invasive ones whenever possible

Identifies that children have substantial and resilient self-healing capacity. Integrative pediatrics supports approaches that remove barriers to and/or otherwise facilitate the body's natural healing response

Neither rejects conventional medicine nor embraces complementary/alternative therapies uncritically, but which recognizes and differentiates many valid but different "ways of knowing" (hierarchies of evidence)

Source: Adapted from *Best Practices in Integrative Medicine: A Report From the Bravewell Clinical Network.* *Minneapolis*, MN. First Edition. November, 2007. p. 11; Rakel, D. *Integrative Medicine.* 2007. Saunders/Elsevier. Philadelphia. pp. 6–9; Gaudet, T. (1998). The evolution of a new approach to medicine and to medical education. *Integrative Medicine,*1(2), 67–73; Integrative Pediatrics Website. www.integrativepeds.org

Note: These principles were adapted to the pediatric practice of "integrative medicine" from a variety of sources as noted above.

Center for Complementary and Alternative Medicine (NCCAM), there are five major domains of CAM which are commonly described:

1. Mind-body medicine
2. Biologically-based practices
3. Manipulative and body-based practices
4. Energy Medicine
5. Whole medical systems

Integrate
- — combining and coordinating diverse elements into a whole
- — to cause or give equal opportunity of consideration to disparate elements/ideas
- — tending to consolidate

Holism
- — a theory that the universe and especially living nature are correctly seen as interacting "wholes" that are together greater than merely the sum of their parts

Mind-Body
- — taking into account the physiological, psychic, and spiritual connections between the state of the body and that of the mind
- —of, involving, or resulting from the interrelationship between one's physical health and the state of one's mind or spirit

About This Book

Our goals in editing this volume include

- **serving** as an educational resource in the ongoing development and support of clinical care providers in all aspects of integrative pediatric care;
- **increasing** understanding of the value of integrative healthcare among provider organizations, all pediatric healthcare providers, and other healthcare professionals;
- **fostering** respect, understanding, and collaboration among diverse professionals caring for the health of children;
- **encouraging** pediatric providers to learn about clinical approaches derived from other healing traditions.

Our intention in producing this book is to advocate for true integrative pediatrics, including careful, thorough diagnostic interventions and provision of the best and safest treatments for children. We offer information about many complementary/alternative treatments, including honest appraisals about which can be recommended on the basis of solid evidence from carefully conducted clinical trials. We acknowledge that there are numerous interventions for which such evidence does not yet exist. In such cases, we do our best to assess the safety of interventions and the likelihood that they will be validated in ongoing or future clinical trials. Just as has been the case with recent evidence that most conventional cold remedies for children are ineffective, we recognize that some of the interventions described in this volume will be found to be ineffective. All integrative medical practitioners who work with children have obligations to stay up to date with current research related to both conventional and alternative treatments. A useful framework for considering evidence has been provided by Kemper and Cohen and is adapted for Figure 1-1.

This text is divided into four main sections and you will find additional chapters at the website www.oup.com/us/integrativepediatrics

FOUNDATIONS OF INTEGRATIVE PEDIATRIC CARE

Book Chapters: 1–5
Web Chapters: 29–32
This section reflects some broad concepts in pediatric integrative medicine that help to "frame" our approach to the entire field. These important foundational concepts inform

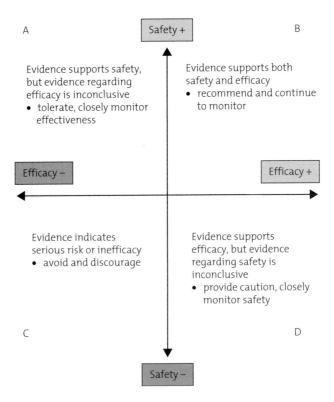

FIGURE 1-1. Balancing Safety and Efficacy Considerations for CAM Therapies. *Source*: Adapted from Cohen and Eisenberg (2002).

a truly "integrative" approach with children taking into account aspects of mind, body, and spirit, in a developmental framework that is essential to pediatric care and which differentiates it from adult health care practice. In addition, we look at the clinical care process through the "lenses" of the family, environmental, and contextual factors, as well as cultural, spiritual, and ethical perspectives. Finally, a key discussion of self-care for practitioners reminds those in direct service provision to "heal thyself" and practice what we preach.

PEDIATRIC PERSPECTIVES ON SPECIFIC THERAPEUTIC APPROACHES

Book Chapters: 6–17
Web Chapters: 33, 34
Although not exhaustive in its scope, this section highlights specific complementary, alternative, and traditional therapeutic approaches that are widely available, popular, and commonly utilized with children and teens. In this section, we review information about safety and evidence (adult and pediatric) with regard to specific modalities, and have asked the authors to share clinical wisdom about potential applications of these therapies in the pediatric setting. Information on training and other professional resources is also provided.

CLINICAL APPLICATIONS IN INTEGRATIVE PEDIATRICS

Book Chapters: 18–27
Web Chapters: None
In this section we ask leading practitioners to offer a sampling of integrative pediatric approaches in several clinical domains within which children/teens are increasingly known to utilize complementary/alternative therapies and for which we have a combination of evidence and solid clinical experience to guide us.

INTEGRATIVE PEDIATRICS: LOOKING AHEAD

Book Chapter: 28
Web Chapter: 35
As we look ahead into the future of pediatrics, the topics, therapies, and approaches delineated in this book will likely play a broader, fully integrated role in pediatric health care globally and become part of standard medical training as well as an area of intensified research.

Complementary/Alternative Medicine in Pediatrics: What Do We Know?

Pediatrics has always been a holistic profession that has included well-child care, *preventive practices* such as immunizations, injury prevention, parenting skills, and consideration of not just the patient but the larger context of the family. An evolution into "integrative pediatrics" is not inconsistent with earlier attempts in pediatric care to broaden the model to include consideration of biopsychosocial factors in assessing and treating pediatric problems. As more children survive with chronic illness and other complex biobehavioral challenges, the limits of what an acute-care, high-tech, allopathic, biomedical reductionistic approach can accomplish becomes more clearly delineated. Parents and children are seeking out less invasive options and are resistant to polypharmacy and its related problems. Thus, CAM options and integrative care models are increasing in popularity.

Research in Pediatric CAM

Child health professionals want to provide children with careful, accurate diagnoses, and safe effective treatments. Increasingly, they have integrated conventional and alternative treatments and have advocated for careful study of both types of treatments. In 1992, the National Institutes of Health created the Office of Alternative Medicine and this was followed by the NIH National Center for Complementary and Alternative Medicine (NCCAM). In the past decade, NCCAM has supported 1500 clinical trials on alternative complementary treatments. Between 2002 and 2007 NCCAM supported 543 clinical research studies, of which 39 included children (7%).

Epidemiological studies support the claim that a large number of children/teens are using CAM, at levels approaching that of adults. Multiple studies of CAM usage in the pediatric population are indicating utilization rates in the 50% range. Some of the key studies for CAM utilization in children and teens include the following:

- A 2002 study found usage rates of 54% that included prayer to specifically improve health and vitamin doses that were more than a once-daily supplement in the past 6 months (MCann, 2006).
- A 2003 study found usage rates of 53% that did not mention prayer and included vitamin and mineral preparations but not iron supplements, vitamin D or K for children under 1 year, or ordinary vitamin tablets (Madsen, 2003).
- A 2003 study that measured how much of CAM has been used in the past 12 months and that has ever been used, and excluded prayer and multivitamins had rates of 49% for ever used (Loman, 2003).
- A 2005 study measuring lifetime use of CAM in adolescents, which included spiritual healing and megavitamin doses, found rates of 68.1% (Braun, 2005).
- A 2007 study measuring CAM use in the past 12 months and over a lifetime that excluded prayer and made no mention of vitamins found usage rates of 54% (Jean, 2007).

The rates of utilization in pediatric subspecialties are often higher than those in the general pediatric population. Rates of utilization in asthma populations have been reported to be as high as 79%–89% (Adams, 2007; Braganza, 2003). Studies of CAM usage rates in pediatric cancer patients have reported rates of between 70% and 84% (Gomez-Martinez, 2007; Kelly, 2000). A 2008 study of utilization patterns, which excluded prayer, found usage rates in patients with IBD of 61% (Gerasimidis, 2008).

Utilization rates vary dramatically depending on how CAM is defined (e.g., inclusion/exclusion of single, megadose, or multivitamins; inclusion/exclusion of prayer), how the question about CAM usage is asked (e.g., definition and examples of CAM provided to the respondents), and even what the period of assessment is (e.g., ever used, past month, past year). Thus pediatric utilization literature has identified rates as low as 2% to as high as 89% (Braganza, 2003; Yussman, 2004).

The quality and amount of scientific studies assessing pediatric CAM is improving as well:

- As of 2001, 47 pediatric CAM systematic review have been conducted (Moher, 2002).
- As of 2001, 1468 pediatric CAM randomized controlled trails have been conducted.
- In one review, the quality of CAM randomized controlled trails was judged to be as good as that of conventional randomized controlled trails (Klassen, 2005).
- A paper examining systematic reviews noted that the quality of CAM systematic review exceeds that of conventional systematic review (Lawson, 2005).

PROGRAMS IN PEDIATRIC INTEGRATIVE MEDICINE

At the time of publication of this book, at least fifteen academic pediatric integrative medicine programs with research, education, and clinical components are identified in the United States; only one at this time in Canada. Of note, 16 of the 41 medical schools belonging to the prestigious Consortium of Academic Health Centers for Integrative Medicine also belong to its pediatric clinical subgroup, suggesting that academic pediatric medicine is growing, including in centers that may not yet have dedicated pediatric initiatives that are comparable to their adult programs.

Pediatric CAM is also growing internationally, with initiatives in the United Kingdom, Israel, Holland, China, Hong Kong, and elsewhere.

Integrative Pediatrics: Supporting Interdisciplinary Collaboration

Integrative pediatrics is about collaboration, communication, and education as well as integration of various care options. In this sense, the practice of integrative pediatrics requires a broader perspective than conventional practice within a single discipline might warrant. This book includes chapters authored by professionals from a wide variety of disciplines and backgrounds, and it is the editor's intent that this diversity of perspectives will serve to cross-pollinate thinking across the various readers who use this book.

We recognize that there are different models and processes in the way integrative pediatrics is practiced:

1. Pediatricians, family physicians, and pediatric nurse practitioners may take training in a few alternative treatment methods (e.g., a physician is board certified in both pediatrics and medical hypnosis, a pediatric nurse practitioner is also licensed in massage, a pediatric anesthesiologist has taken several years of acupuncture training).

2. Alternative medicine practitioners (e.g., naturopaths, homeopaths, chiropractors) may take specific training in pediatric healthcare and then utilize their expertise in various kinds of clinical practice settings (specialty, primary care, wellness).

3. Multidisciplinary collaboration-pediatricians, family physicians and/or pediatric nurse practitioners refer their patients to alternative practitioners such as massage therapists, naturopathic physicians, or acupuncture specialists, OR alternative practitioners refer their child patients to conventional practitioners (e.g., a chiropractor refers a child to a pediatrician for evaluation of a febrile illness) and they communicate about and coordinate care.

4. Integrative practice models-in some places, allopathic and CAM providers work together in the same physical location in an interdisciplinary model offering multimodal assessment and treatment

In all of these examples, it is clear that no single child health professional can be an expert in all of the many treatment options in integrative pediatrics and also that the success of integrative pediatrics depends on close communication and understanding among all who provide healthcare to children in a given community. Ideally, everyone involved needs to maintain humility and a tolerance for uncertainty about our level of knowledge and understanding.

Summary

There are things that are known and things that are unknown and in between there are doors.

Blake

Children are society's most valuable resource and must be nurtured within the context of healthy families, communities, and environments. Seeing to the optimal and vibrant functioning of children in all areas of life is essential to sustaining healthy, self-renewing, evolving societies everywhere. *Integrative pediatrics focuses on the overall goal of defining and delivering "What's Best For Children."*

An "integrative" (or "holistic") approach exemplifies an ideal model of care for all children, and we believe that improving the care of children will ultimately improve the world. As Dr. Kathi Kemper pointed out in 1999, "holistic pediatric care is quite simply, good medicine." In addition, who better to teach about natural, less invasive pathways to wellness than our children—who can then take these skills and tools and apply them across a lifetime.

It is the abiding hope and intention of the authors of this book that for its readers doors of knowledge, insight, and curiosity will be newly opened, informing and aligning all those who care for children in genuine, compassionate, and creative ways. Walking through the door to integrative pediatric practice requires courage and commitment but is truly transformative and worth every step.

REFERENCES

Adams, S. K., Murdock, K. K., & McQuaid, E. L. (2007). Complementary and alternative medication (CAM) use and asthma outcomes in children: An urban perspective. *The Journal of Asthma, 44*(9), 775–782.

Braganza, S., Ozuah, P. O., & Sharif, I. (2003). The use of complementary therapies in inner-city asthmatic children. *The Journal of Asthma, 40*(7), 823–827.

Braun, C. A., Bearinger, L. H., Halcon, L. L., & Pettingell, S. L. (2005). Adolescent use of complementary therapies. *The Journal of Adolescent Health, 37*(1), 76.

Gerasimidis, K., McGrogan, P., Hassan, K., & Edwards, C. A. (2008). Dietary modifications, nutritional supplements and alternative medicine in paediatric patients with inflammatory bowel disease. *Alimentary Pharmacology & Therapeutics, 27,* 155–165.

Gomez-Martinez, R., Tlacuilo-Parra, A., & Garibaldi-Covarrubias, R. (2007). Use of complementary and alternative medicine in children with cancer in occidental, Mexico. *Pediatric Blood and Cancer, 49,* 820–823.

Jean, D., & Cyr, C. (2007). Use of complementary and alternative medicine in a general pediatric clinic. *Pediatrics, 120,* e138–e141.

Kelly, K. M., Jacobson, J. S., Kennedy, D. D., Braudt, S. M., Mallick, M., & Weiner, M. A. (2000). Use of unconventional therapies by children with cancer at an urban medical center. *Journal of Pediatric Hematology/Oncology, 22*(5), 412–416.

Kemper, K., & O'Connor, K. (2004). Pediatricians' recommendations for complementary and alternative medical (CAM) therapies. *Ambulatory Pediatrics, 4*(6), 482–487.

Kemper, K., Vohra, S., & Walls, R. (2008). The task force on complementary medicine and alternative medicine and the provisional section on complementary, holistic and alternative medicine. The use of complementary and alternative medicine in pediatrics. *Pediatrics, 122*(6), 1374–1386.

Klassen, T. P., Pham, B., Lawson M. L., & Moher, D. (2005). For randomized controlled trials, the quality of reports of complementary and alternative medicine was as good as reports of conventional medicine. *Journal of Clinical Epidemiology, 58*(8), 763–768.

Lawson, M. L., Pham, B., Klassen, T. P., & Moher, D. (2005). Systematic reviews involving complementary and alternative medicine interventions had higher quality of reporting than conventional medicine reviews. *Journal of Clinical Epidemiology, 58*(8), 777–784.

Loman, D. G. (2003). The use of complementary and alternative health care practices among children. *Journal of Pediatric Health Care, 17,* 58–63.

Madsen, H., Andersen, S., Nielsen, R. G., Dolmer, B. S., Host, A., & Damkier, A. (2003). Use
of complementary/alternative medicine among paediatric patients. *European Journal of
Pediatrics, 162*(5), 334–341.

McCann, L. J., & Newell, S. J. (2006). Survey of paediatric complementary and alternative medicine use in health and chronic illness. *Archives of Disease in Childhood, 91,* 173–174.

Moher, D., Soeken, K., Sampson, M., Ben-Porat, L., & Berman, B. (2002). Assessing the quality
of reports of systematic reviews in pediatric complementary and alternative medicine. *BMC
Pediatrics, 2,* 3.

Plotnikoff, G., Kemper, K., & Culbert, T. (2008). Complementary and alternative medical therapies. In A. McInerny, K. Campbell, & K. J. Kelleher (Eds.), *American Academy of Pediatrics
Textbook of Pediatric Care.* Elk Grove Village, IL: American Academy of Pediatrics.

Sawni, A., & Thomas, R. (2007). Pediatricians' attitudes, experiences, and referral patterns
regarding complementary/alternative medicine: A national survey. *BMC Complementary and
Alternative Medicine, 7,* 18.

Sikand, A., & Laken, M. (1998). Pediatricians experience with and attitudes toward complemen-
tary/alternative medicine. *Archives of Pediatrics and Adolescent Medicine, 152*(11), 1059–1064.

Sussman, D., & Culbert, T. (1999). Pediatric self-regulation. In M. D. Levine, W. B. Carey, & A. C.
Crocker (Eds.), *Developmental-behavioral pediatrics.* 3rd ed. Philadelphia: Saunders.

Yussman, S., Ryan, S. A., Auinger, P., & Weitzman, M. (2004). Visits to complementary and
alternative medicine providers by children and adolescents in the United States. *Ambulatory
Pediatrics, 4*(5), 429–439.

2

Assessment and Treatment Planning in Integrative Pediatric Practice

TIMOTHY P. CULBERT, VICTORIA MAIZES, TAI MENDENHALL, AND DAVID K. BECKER

KEY CONCEPTS

- The primary purpose of an "integrative" assessment is to intimately understand the child or adolescent who is presenting for care, within a broad context of factors that are likely to have direct or indirect influence on the balance of health, wellness, and illness in their lives, whether this takes place in a primary care clinic or a consultative practice.
- The ability to listen carefully, kindly, and non-judgmentally to a patient's story is a gift you can give to each and every patient and family. Active listening requires effort and undivided attention to what is being said and how it is being said.
- The family is the patient. Research across a broad range of ethnic, cultural, socioeconomic, and geographic diversity has consistently linked the family to its children's physical and mental health.
- Effective integrative treatment plans are often multimodal, requiring collaboration and open communication with parents, pediatric patients, and other caregivers to prioritize, sequence, and track the various therapeutic elements.

Integrative Assessment in Pediatrics: General Considerations

INTRODUCTION

The primary purpose of an "integrative" assessment is to intimately understand the child or adolescent who is presenting for care, within a broad context of factors that are likely to have direct or indirect influence on the balance of health, wellness, and illness (and that may impact any aspect of healing or recovery) in their lives, whether this takes place in a primary care clinic or a consultative practice. Additionally, it is arguable that the assessment component of a clinical encounter can in and of itself, be a therapeutic experience when conducted artfully and patiently. By conveying positive expectation, confidence, compassion, empathy, and warmth, pediatric healthcare providers can immediately begin transforming a clinical situation from an experience of anxiety, discomfort, confusion, or frustration to one of comfort and hope, merely by allowing each person and family to tell their story to a respectful and genuinely interested listener.

With a few directed statements, the clinician can convey their interest in the patient as a full person, beyond physical symptoms including emotions, beliefs, thoughts, and functional changes that accompany their presenting health challenges.

Sample Question

"My goal is to get a sense of who you are as a person, to understand the important relationships and events in your life, in addition to the medical concerns that bring you in today."

Many master clinicians will tell you that for most patients, eliciting a skillful and complete history is far more useful in formulating an accurate diagnosis than myriad laboratory tests and radiologic procedures. Taking a history from parents and children together is a more complex undertaking than interviewing the adult patient. Information from both parent and child/teen (and sometimes teachers and others) must be elicited, corroborated, and then weighed to determine what data are most valid and relevant. A comprehensive, organized approach to assessment for a child or teen ideally will include reviewing medical, developmental, behavioral, environmental, academic, social, personal interest, spiritual, cultural, and family/contextual factors to arrive at a full picture that will then lead to a complete diagnosis. Diagnoses commonly include not only the primary diagnostic question or presenting concern, but also a variety of mediating factors/co-morbid diagnoses that may serve to intensify symptoms, slow recovery, or add to functional impairment. For example, the family of a child with inflammatory bowel disease may be as concerned about the child's academic challenges, social withdrawal, and sleep disturbance as they are with the symptoms of the IBD process per se. In this sense, understanding what the pediatric patient, parent, and other involved caregivers each believe to be the primary focus or need for healing is important and may not always be communicated without directly asking.

Sample Question

"How has this condition impacted your child's life? Your family's life?"

The idea that we should look beyond biological processes and phenomena in considering the etiology, maintenance, and recovery from disease has long been supported in child health. Pediatrics has consistently advocated a biopsychosocial approach for patients with the recognition by pioneers such as Robert Haggerty and Morris Green, that psychological, social, cultural, and broader contextual influences are part and parcel of most disease/illness (Hagan Shaw, & Duncan, 2008). As this chapter suggests, the ideal of a multiaxial assessment is key to the "integrative" model and includes multiple factors that can be reviewed in a structured format.

ACTIVE LISTENING IN PATIENT ENCOUNTERS

Effective assessment begins with careful listening. Good listening is about "presence"- that is to say, presenting oneself in a centered, intentional, calm manner as a provider and partner in the healthcare experience. The ability to listen carefully, kindly, and non-judgmentally to a patient's story is a gift you can give to each and every patient and family. Active listening (Dixon & Stein, 2006) requires effort and undivided attention to what is being said and how it is being said. This requires practice, self-restraint, concentration, and purposefulness in its realization/execution. Listening with intent includes making eye contact, verbal and non-verbal gestures of affirmation and interest, and requires patience. The use of developmentally appropriate language, humor, avoiding technical medical jargon, and a friendly, professional attitude (as opposed to either an authoritarian or overly causal stance) also facilitate the elicitation of complete information.

When done well, active listening goes a long way toward facilitating a "therapeutic relationship," enhancing trust and rapport as it conveys respect and care. With trust and comfort, patients and parents are often more honest, open, and complete in disclosure of information. The use of pauses, silence, and open-ended questions are all helpful tools in this context. The ability to appropriately control one's own emotional responses or judgmental reactions to certain interview content or at times of deep emotional expression by the patient, is also essential.

Being listened to in this generous way is a rare experience in today's fast-paced world. An integrative consultation may be the first time the child's whole story has ever been told. When a story is fully told, new insights may be gained as to the etiology of the illness, supporting factors, and treatment strategies. These insights not only help direct treatment recommendations they affirm the expertise and lived experience of the family.

ELEMENTS OF INTEGRATIVE PEDIATRIC ASSESSMENT

Conventional Elements

History of present illness, additional presenting concerns, functional impairment, past medical history, medication history, family medical history, social and academic history are all typically included in a conventional medical interview.

The "CAM" History

We know that less than 50% of patients reveal their use of complementary/alternative medicine (CAM) to medical providers, fearing judgment, criticism, or negative effects on the therapeutic relationship. Therefore, it is important to ask about the parents' own experience with and ongoing use of CAM, and the patient's use of specific complementary/alternative therapies, perceived benefits of these therapies, length of use or number of treatments, and any adverse effects of CAM therapy. Specifically, it is important to ask about use of vitamins, supplements, herbals, homeopathic remedies, dietary or nutritional approaches, and essential oils explicitly as many persons may not think of these as relevant or even as "complementary." A comprehensive review of CAM therapies will also include specific inquiries about the use of manual therapies such as massage, mind-body practices such as meditation/relaxation, alternative systems such as Chinese Medicine, and other practices including "energy" practices such as Reiki or Healing Touch.

Assessing Development and Behavior

Developmental progress and behavioral differences are important to assess in pediatrics and are a differentiating feature from adult medicine. One may use a variety of formal screening tools (child behavior checklist, behavioral assessment system for children, pediatric symptom checklist), or more focused developmental screening tools for specific issues such as speech/language delay, motor coordination problems, ADHD, Autism, adaptive behavior, etc. Structured interviews can also be used to augment the oral history. These are reviewed in other reference texts in some detail (Glascoe & Dworkin, 2008).

It is important to have some sense of the child's developmental/behavioral functioning in settings outside the home as reported by others—coaches, tutors, teachers, other care providers via standardized questionnaires or structured telephone interviews.

Assessing Lifestyle Factors

Often ignored in the past, lifestyle factors are increasingly recognized as playing an important role in mediating or contributing to the etiology of many pediatric conditions. For example, the chronically sleep deprived child who looks depressed or inattentive, the sedentary child who is obese, the overscheduled child who is experiencing headaches, the child with poor eating habits who experiences constipation. It is very important to elicit good information about these factors including sleep, diet/nutrition, stress management, recreational pursuits and hobbies, exercise, and scheduled activities. Some of this history can be elicited in a health history intake form that is sent out ahead of a scheduled outpatient visit.

Ask your patient to describe a typical day. This will give you a vivid picture of what time the child awakens, what and when he/she eats, how busy or active he/she is, and how well he/she sleeps. A 24-hour diet recall is of great value. Although classically under-reported it still gives an indication of how often fast food is eaten, who prepares

----

Other Useful Questions for Intergative Pediatric Assessment:

What are your favorite foods?
What foods do you least like?
Do you get into arguments with your parents about what you eat?
Do you play any sports? What's your favorite?
What other forms of exercise or activity do you engage in? (biking, running, swimming, skateboarding, etc.)
What stresses you out?
How would someone know you are stressed out?
What do you do to relax?
How many hours of sleep do you get? Do you feel rested on awakening?
What do you do for fun?
Tell me about your friends?
What is the most fun thing that you do together?
What are you good at? What is hard for you?
Do you have a religious or spiritual practice that is important to you?
It is also important to find out what behaviors and habits the parents are modeling. Ask how they manage their own stress, who cooks, whether they take time to relax, and how often they eat out.

----

meals, and the presence (or absence) of vegetables, fruits, fiber, omega-3 fatty acids, and whole grains in the diet.

Spirituality

This area is very relevant to many children and families as they consider the meaning and impact of serious illness, mental health issues, the experience of suffering and beliefs about recovery and locus of control. Inquiring about spirituality, religious beliefs and practices can be uncomfortable for many health care providers but can be facilitated by the use of a structured questionnaire. See Chapter 3 in this book by Reaney and Plotnikoff for an excellent discussion of this topic.

Environmental Factors

Increasingly, environmental exposures of many varieties are being identified as potential causative, or exacerbating factors in a wide variety of pediatric allergic, inflammatory, gastroenterologic, endocrinologic, immune, and neurodevelopmental disorders. An organized approach to this component of the interview—using a mneumonic such as ACHOO—(Etzel & Balk, 2003) is important to uncover all sources of potential exposure for both preventative guidance and also for diagnosis and treatment. We refer the reader to the excellent chapter by M. Miller in this book (Chapter 32).

Environmental Exposures History—ACHOO

Activities: school, day care, church, sports
Community: industrial, agricultural zones, polluted lakes, dump sites, water source
Household: asbestos, lead paint, radon, offgassing of carpets, heating sources, pesticides, tobacco smoke, household cleaners/chemicals
Hobbies: arts, crafts, physical harm/risk, lead, mercury (fishing)
Occupational: parent's occupation, teens-employment site
Oral: Pica or mouthing behaviors, contaminated food sources

Other Helpful Approaches

Questions that get at a patient or family's personal belief system and other idiosyncratic or unrecognized beliefs around illness, disease, and health are important in establishing a common understanding of etiology and appropriate treatment for a given condition. See box below for example questions that can be useful in eliciting this history.

Additional details that are important to consider include the physical layout and positioning of those involved in the interview, and whether parents and children are

---

Questions for a Health Beliefs History

What would you call this problem?
Why do you think you/your child has developed it?
What do you think caused/causes it?
Why do you think it started when it did?
What do you think is happening inside the body?
What are the symptoms that make you know your child has this illness?
What are you most worried about with this illness?
What problems does this illness cause your child?
How do you treat it?
Is the treatment helpful?
What will happen if this problem is not treated?
Do you have any intuition about what needs to happen for this problem to
   go away?
Adapted from Kleinman A, Eisenberg L, and Good B. Culture, Illness and Care:
   Lessons form Anthropologic and Cross-Cultural Research. 1978. *Annals of
   Internal Medicine. 88.* pp. 251–258.

---

interviewed together or individually for at least part of the interview. These issues and related topics are covered well by Dixon and Stein (2006).

Additional "therapeutic interview" approaches/questions for kids include

Setting expectations: "What will be different when you no longer have X
   _____(symptom/condition)"
Validating: "Did you know that lots of other kids have the same problem?"
Demystifying: "What is the worst thing about having this "symptom/condi-
   tion" and what do you worry about the most ?" (dying, permanent injury,
   it will never change, etc)
Giving information and establishing Mind/Body Connections: "Did you know
   that this condition is caused by this (give explanation) and that stress can
   make it worse?"
Shifting From external to internal Locus of Control: "Won't it be great when
   you learn to help yourself and be the boss of your body!? I wonder what
   ways you will choose to do that?"
Reframing: "Is there anything good about having this problem? [or, Has anything good come from having this problem?] Can you think of all things
   you do despite having this symptom/problem?"

Integrative Assessment in Pediatrics: Family Context

Family dynamics and/or dysfunction can play a significant role in pediatric growth, development, health, illness, coping, and wellness. Parents' own experiences with, and beliefs about illness will also of course impact their care choices for their children. The longstanding and aforementioned history of biopsychosocial sensitivity in pediatrics reflects a concomitant awareness of "context" in children's lives and health. Asking about and integrating knowledge about families as key and highly influential environments is, indeed, indicated, insofar as research across a broad range of ethnic, cultural, socioeconomic, and geographic diversity has consistently linked the family to its children's physical and mental health (Alsop-Shields & Dugdale, 2008; Heaton et al., 2005; Oliveira et al., 2007; USDHHS, 2005).

Literature linking family characteristics to child outcomes is well-established, focusing on a myriad of contextual factors ranging from parents' individual and family systems' functioning to role modeling to the structure(s) of the family unit(s). The following is a summary of key knowledge derived from this body of evidence, and represents foci worth consideration in assessment and the provision of care (Alsop-Shields & Dugdale, 2008; Heaton et al., 2005; Oliveira et al., 2007; USDHHS, 2005, 2006).

FAMILY STRUCTURE

Single versus Two-Parent Households

Children tend to fare better in two-parent households. Two-parent households tend to have higher incomes, which represents a major resource (see below) related to child health and well-being. Further, the presence and participation of fathers in childrearing is important for the reason that they are able to play a role in caring for and socializing children alongside the mother.

Family Size

Smaller families are also more likely to maintain higher incomes, or to at least carry fewer expenses. This translates into less crowded and more sanitary living conditions in addition to a variety of other benefits that greater financial resources yield. Parents in smaller families are also better equipped to provide focused-attention and care to their children, and to notice and attend to health-related problems with higher efficiency.

Birth Patterns

Children borne to mothers who carried them in quick succession are more likely to evidence poor outcomes. Not allowing the body adequate time to recover from pregnancy and restore its nutrient levels is linked to low birth weights and higher frequencies of illness episodes. Additionally, children closer in age are more likely to compete for key resources (e.g., parental attention, food, care). Frequent births also mean larger families and greater overall exposure to and spread of potential disease.

FAMILY RESOURCES

Education

Parents' level of education is highly correlated with positive child outcomes. With higher education come higher incomes, improved decision-making ability, increased assertiveness in acquiring and securing care for progeny, and better role-modeling of healthy behaviors and lifestyles (e.g., sensible diet, exercise, not smoking, regular attention to general health). Additionally, parents with high levels of education tend to have fewer children, maintain longer between-birth intervals. They are more likely to represent two-parent households wherein fathers are active and involved.

Income

As outlined above, financial resources within a family are positively correlated with child outcomes across both physical and mental health arenas. With higher incomes come better and more consistent access to health care, better diet and healthy lifestyles, more sanitary living conditions, and ready access to daily living needs (e.g., clothing, medicine, food).

FAMILY ENVIRONMENT

Adaptability

Children's sense of overall security in the home is affected by parents' and families' ability to effectively negotiate change and any variety of stressors that come along with this—whether they be developmentally appropriate (e.g., a child beginning school) or unexpected (e.g., an accident or serious illness). Balancing household members' power structure, respective roles, routines, and rules somewhere between high rigidity and chaotic functioning is key here; maintaining a structure of household hierarchy and routine while at the same time being able to adapt and change in response to stress is positively linked both individuals' health and overall family and relationship satisfaction and functioning (Olson & Gorall, 2003; USDHHS, 2006).

Cohesion

Cohesion, or how emotionally close or bonded family members are to each other, can range from inter-member enmeshment to distant disengagement. As with family adaptability, functioning somewhere in between two extremes of the continuum is better—and this, too, changes over time and maturation of children. Parents and younger children, for example, are likely to be closer and more strongly connected than they are when children are teenagers. Maintaining and changing emotional connections in the family is highly correlated with individuals' health and overall family and relationship satisfaction and functioning (Olson, 1988; Olson & Gorall, 2003).

Communication

Communication in the family is oftentimes seen as a facilitating function of other family environment foci (e.g., adaptability, cohesion). The manner in which parents talk and problem-solve with each other, and with their children, is highly predictive of how well (or not) change is negotiated over time and in the manner that inter-member boundaries and closeness are maintained. Communication that is positive, direct, respectful, and collaborative is highly facilitative of meeting these functions effectively (Olson, 1988; Thomas & Olson, 1993).

FAMILY ASSESSMENT

The manners in which patients and families can be assessed for the above foci are myriad, as the field of family assessment represents an entire discipline unto itself. The following represent a sampling of methods we have found to be useful in practice:

Genograms

While interviewing children and their parents, a good way to facilitate dialogue and information gathering is to complete a genogram together. Families oftentimes get very engaged in sharing with providers their history when it is being visually depicted—as opposed to simply answering a series of questions. Tracking histories and patterns of illness (e.g., diabetes, alcoholism), family size, ages of family members, birth sequences, communication patterns, and relationships (marriages, divorces, cut-offs, etc.) is also an excellent way to join with families and begin establishing trust with them in preparation for the provision of care (McGoldrick, Gerson, & Shellenberger, 1999).

MEASURES OF FAMILY FUNCTIONING AND ADJUSTMENT TO ILLNESS

Family Adaptability and Cohesion Scale (FACES)

The FACES is a 62-item self-report instrument which assesses families' cohesion and family adaptability. It is designed to be administered to families across the life cycle, including those with young and older children. Family communication is also assessed, as this function is seen as an elemental facilitator of adaptability and cohesion continua. Scores are then visually depicted on a circumplex model that makes results easy to visualize and for use in guiding change(s) if indicated (Olson & Gorall, 2003; Place et al., 2005).

Family Assessment Device (FAD)

The FAD is a 53-item self-report instrument that is based on the McMaster Model of Family Functioning (MMFF). In a similar manner to the FACES instrument described above, the FAD assesses for structural and organizational properties of the family and the patterns of transactions between members. The model identifies the following six dimensions of family functioning: Communication, Problem Solving, Roles, Affective Responsiveness, Affective Involvement, and Behavior Control. The FAD also includes a seventh subscale regarding general family functioning (Epstein et al., 1983, 2008; Slattery et al., 2001).

Psychosocial Adjustment to Illness Scale (PAIS)

The PAIS-SR (self-report) is a 46-item semi-structured interview designed to assess the quality of a child or patient's psychosocial adjustment to a current medical illness or the negative sequences associated with a previous illness. Seven primary domains are assessed, including: Health Care Orientation, Vocational Environment, Domestic Environment, Sexual Relationships, Extended Family Relationships, Social Environment, and Psychological Distress. The PAIS can also be modified in format to measure the nature of spouses, parents, or other relatives' adjustment to the identified patient's illness (Derogatis, 1986).

Family Context: A Summary

Children do not live in a vacuum. They live in families, and these systems can play a tremendous role—for better or for worse—in the functioning and health of every one of its members. Through a combination of interviewing and formal assessment measures, we as providers can evaluate families' structure, resources, and environments in a manner that honors the complex biopsychosocial milieus in which the children we care for are positioned.

Treatment Planning in Integrative Pediatrics

Once all of the relevant factors are identified and considered for their contribution to the patient's current medical challenges, a multimodal treatment plan can be developed to address each appropriate domain in the "healing matrix." Even when there is agreement on primary diagnoses and mediating factors as treatment targets, determining the best course of treatment from "evidence-based medicine" alone where the gold standard is the Randomized Controlled Trial, may be limiting. A more integrative approach that takes into account other factors (time, effort, money, patient experience or preference, cultural or religious concerns, and safe complementary therapies) better serves the broad, holistic needs of the patient and family. We attempt to offer some helpful tips for the practicing clinician on successful treatment planning, facilitating lifestyle change, educating patients, and coordinating care in an integrative approach.

Summarizing the Story and Creating a Partnership

Before making recommendations, the integrative provider has an opportunity to summarize the patient's story. This serves two purposes. It shows the patient you have listened carefully, allowing for corrections if something has been misunderstood or missed, and it allows you to list the child's strengths. This then frames the medical problem as one part of the child's experience rather than being the whole or even most important part of the child.

For example, you might say: "You are a drummer and a soccer player who gets mostly As and Bs in school, you have a really good relationship with your parents, and a pretty good relationship with your younger brother, although he sometimes drives you crazy. You are here because your asthma is affecting your soccer game and you want to know what you might do about it besides inhalers. Your parents are particularly curious to know if there may be a dietary link to dairy—but you love pizza and ice cream and are not eager to give them up."

Key Ingredients for Discussion: The Integrative Health Treatment Plan:

Summary of all diagnoses (explained at a developmentally appropriate level)

Clarify patient's and family's goals for treatment (symptom removal versus improved global functioning)

Review recommended and desired priority and sequence of treatments

Identify helpful lifestyle changes (diet, exercise, sleep, schedule)

Teach stress management skills and other self-care approaches

Facilitate parental role as "coach" and role model

Clearly describe details of recommended vitamins, supplements, botanicals (name, best brands, dose, frequency, route, side effects)

Review ongoing, necessary conventional treatments (pharmaceuticals, physician specialists, allied health, rehabilitation therapies, mental health)Describe and provide information about preventative health recommendations

Discuss integrative treatment modalities -explanation of treatments, target symptoms, risks and benefits, anticipated time and cost, provider referral information if appropriate

Provide educational resources (books, websites, articles)

Agree upon a tracking and follow up plan

Through the assessment process we learn that children and their parents may have strong preferences about types of treatments. One may not believe in homeopathy, another may be eager to use it. A child may fear needles and be unwilling to have acupuncture. One child may take supplements with ease, another may hate taking pills. One child may love the use of imagery; while another family may see this as a put-down suggesting that "the problem is all in my child's head." Asking parents about their beliefs and predilections, their intuition about what is needed, and weighing this in with the evidence for different treatments and your own clinical experience is the art of practicing integrative medicine. Ideally these conversations create a partnership between family and physician in service to eliciting a healing response.

Balancing Risks and Benefits: Considering Evidence

With so many options available to consider, and with multiple sources of information easily accessible to consumers, how do we help people make good decisions about treating their most valuable resource—their children—with some sense of safety and validity? Educating parents and pediatric patients (informed consent and assent—see Kemper chapter on Ethics, web based Chapter 30) about options and how they can best weigh those options is at times a daunting task. How do we help people to balance the quality of information available for a given treatment (randomized controlled trials, historical experience, expert opinion, testimonials, personal experience with a therapy) against their own beliefs, biases and preferences while also fulfilling our primary obligations as advocate for children who can be very vulnerable in these situations if competing interests arise?

Identifying reliable websites, journal articles, consumer books, and related resources on CAM for your patients/parents is useful to help them be better consumers of healthcare information and improve health literacy. Information for kids on CAM is important as well and can be viewed at www.childrensintegrativemed.org and www. pedcam.ca Sending a personalized letter detailing the diagnoses and treatment plan to parents and patient is also very helpful.

Making a Referral to a CAM Provider

In some circumstances, referring a pediatric patient to a complementary medicine provider may be appropriate for therapies such as massage, acupuncture, or yoga training, etc. There are several considerations—legal, ethical, and practical—from the standpoint of the pediatric healthcare provider when making such a referral:

Personal knowledge of CAM provider
CAM provider's experience with children/teens
Willingness of CAM provider to communicate openly with other caregivers
CAM provider's philosophy of care: collaborative versus "anti-"conventional
  medicine

Potential risks/benfits of CAM treatment suggested

Costs involved, time involved

Potential interference with other treatments

Your legal liability in making a specific referral

Reasonable evidence for potential efficacy of this treatment for this condition

Parents' willingness to continue necessary evidence-based treatments

Prioritizing and Sequencing Treatments

It is imperative that children receive necessary and/or life-sustaining treatments for serious medical and mental health conditions, particularly when there is clear evidence for safety and efficacy of a specific treatment (e.g., chemotherapy for ALL). An integrative approach attempts to balance conventional with complementary treatments on an individualized basis for each child. Whenever possible, the least invasive, most natural treatment options available are recommended and considerations of safety, cost, and time commitment are also weighed.

> What is "natural?": many claims are made in the name of a 'natural' therapy. Some herbs or supplements are processed to varying degrees, and many pharmaceuticals are purified forms of plants. Mercury is a natural component of our environment, but one that is a well-known toxin. Massage, or other manipulation therapies, may damage sensitive tissue if done inappropriately. On the other hand, aggressive surgical procedures which may be commonly recommended but inappropriate for some conditions (such as certain chronic pain syndromes), should be replaced with appropriate natural approaches (such as meditation or acupuncture) when indicated.

Children and adolescents have a natural developmental drive for mastery and accomplishment. In our experience, enhancing a child's self-efficacy through the use of active, participatory self-management strategies *in which the child is interested and engaged* is a key component of the integrative treatment plan. This may take several forms. It may be helpful to provide all pediatric patients with some form of active, participatory self-management strategy as at least one element in an overall strategy. For example, as opposed to only receiving massage or acupuncture for their headaches, children are also taught relaxation skills and acupressure point stimulation for use at home and school.

When planning integrative, multimodal treatments, consider sequencing individual treatments for a specific time frame (e.g.,12 acupuncture sessions over 6 weeks) for what you might consider an adequate "treatment trial" for that modality and then evaluate specific symptom change and functional impairment over that time frame by tracking a quantifiable outcome/behavior/symptom change over this period—both pre- and post-intervention. It can be as simple as having patient and parent track symptom such as pain, anxiety, or nausea on a visual analogue scale rating "ruler" (0–10) on a daily basis during this time, using a standardized instrument (e.g., ADHD rating scale) or if possible or appropriate, a more specific measurement (CRP, weight gain, change in skin rash). Tracking functional impairment by reviewing school attendance, participation in favorite activities, time spent with friends, physical activity is also very helpful.

Communication amongst all care providers involved with the child is important as CAM interventions may affect the need for certain medications (e.g., less need for pain or sleep medication) and/or could effect other medications (via drug–herb interactions). A specific modality (biofeedback for headache, essential oil of lavender for sleep, acupuncture for nausea) could become the primary or preferred modality for a given symptom, thus necessitating a re-evaluation of the overall approach.

As we offer treatment recommendations across a number of domains, it is important to provide recommendations in writing and to prioritize the most critical, the order in which things are to be added or tried, and identify therapies that are secondary or more "optional. Some recommendations will be less familiar and the rationale may need to be discussed in more detail (i.e., "acupuncture is recommended to help relieve nerve pain" or, "Fish Oils will help reduce inflammation in the body.") In addition, the written plan creates a treatment path that can be reviewed at future visits and is a tangible reminder to the patient and family of the expectation that the problem can be helped.

Counseling Patients and Families about Lifestyle Changes

Helping kids and teens to find the motivation to change diet, sleep, and exercise habits can be challenging and can be strongly influenced by family practices, peer influences, cultural norms and other contextual factors. Yet, these lifestyle issues may play a key role in mediating illness and recovery in conditions such as chronic pain, asthma, cystic fibrosis, diabetes, depression, and constipation, to name a few. Helpful tips for managing lifestyle changes can be found in several chapters in this volume including Chapters 10, 14, and 16.

Summary/Conclusions

The intent of this chapter was to review many of the unique aspects of assessment and treatment planning within the context of an integrative approach in pediatric care. At first glance, it may seem that this holistic approach might add significant time and complexity to both assessment and treatment processes. However, we actually find the opposite. By comprehensively assessing all of the relevant factors contributing to an individual's symptoms/condition/current functional impairment, we avoid the fragmentation of care involved in seeing several different specialists over time as commonly occurs when children/teens are not getting better. This fragmentation also delays needed effective treatments and creates confusion and hopelessness as well as lack of confidence in medical care systems. With a complete understanding of all operative elements from the integrative assessment, one can quickly and powerfully select and direct treatments either sequentially or concurrently, to address the appropriate mind/body/spirit/environmental/contextual factors that are playing key roles and thus support each child's natural healing abilities as they move forward in recovery and onto a state of more optimal health and function.

REFERENCES

Alsop-Sheilds, L., & Dugdale, A. (2008). Influence of families on the growth of children in an Aboriginal community. *Journal of Paediatics and Child Health, 31*, 392–394.

Cohen, M. H., & Kemper, K. J. (2005). Complementary therapies in pediatrics: A legal perspective. *Pediatrics, 115*(3), 774–780.

Derogatis, L. (1986). The Psychosocial Adjustment to Illness Scale (PAIS). *Journal of Psychosomatic Research, 30*, 77–91.

Dixon, S., & Stein, M. (2006). *Encounters with children: Pediatric behavior and development* (4th ed., pp. 2–97). Philadelphia: Mosby/Elsevier.

Epstein, N., Baldwin, L., & Bishop, D.; Subscales of McMaster Family Assessment Device (FAD). (2008). University of California/Los Angeles. Retrieved January 5, 2009, from http://chipts. ucla.edu/assessment/IB/List_Scales/McMaster_Family-Assessment.htm

Epstein, N. B., Bishop, L. M., & Bishop, D. (1983). The McMaster Model view of healthy family functioning. *Journal of Marital and Family Therapy, 9*, 171–180.

Etzel, R., & Balk, S. (2003). *Pediatric environmental health* (2nd ed., pp. 37–50). Elk Grove Village, IL: AAP.

Glascoe, F., & Dworkin, P. (2008). Surveillance and screening for development and behavior. In M. Wolraich, D. Drotar, P. Dworkin, & E. Perrin (Eds.), *Developmental-behavioral pediatrics: Evidence and practice* (pp. 130–144). Philadelphia: Mosby/Elsevier.

Hagan, J., Shaw, J., & Duncan, P. (Eds.). (2008). *Bright futures: Guidelines for health supervision of infants, children, adolescents* (3rd ed., pp. 1–10). Elk Grove Village, IL: AAP.

Heaton, T., Forste, R., Hoffman, J., & Flake, D. (2005). Cross-national variation in family influences on child health. *Social Science & Medicine, 60*, 97–108.

McGoldrick, M., Gerson, R., & Shellenberger, S. (1999). *Genograms: Assessment and intervention* (2nd ed.). New York: W.W. Norton & Company.

Oliveira, A. M., Oliveira, A. C., Almeida, M., Oliveira, N., & Adan, L. (2007). Influence of the family nucleus on obesity in children from northeastern Brazil: A cross sectional study. *BMC Public Health, 7*, 235–239.

Olson, D. (1988). Clinical rating scale (CRS) for the circumplex model of marital and family systems (revised). Saint Paul, MN, University of Minnesota. Ref Type: Pamphlet.

Olson, D., & Gorall, D. (2003). Circumplex model of marital and family systems. In F. Walsh (Ed.), *Normal family processes* (3rd ed., pp. 514–547). New York: Guilford; 2003.

Place, M., Hulsmeier, J., Brownrigg, A., & Soulsby, A. (2005). The Family Adaptability and Cohesion Evaluation Scale (FACES): An instrument worthy of rehabilitation? *Psychological Bulletin, 29*, 215–218.

Slattery, J., Smith, W., Krapf, M., Buchenauer, E., & Bean, T. (2001). Measuring improvement in family therapy using the Family Assessment Device. *Eastern Psychological Association.* Retrieved May 4, 2008, from http://psy1.clarion.edu/rp/archives/research/SlatealEPA01.html

Thomas, V., & Olson, D. (1993). Problem families and the circumplex model: Observational assessment using the clinical rating scale (CRS). *Journal of Marital and Family Therapy, 19*, 159–175.

US Department of Health and Human Services. Family characteristics have more influence on child development than does experience in child care. *National Institutes of Health* 2006. Retrieved May 4, 2008, from http://www.nih.gov/news/pr/oct2006/nichd-03.htm

US Department of Health and Human Services. The health and well-being of children: A portrait of states and the nation. *National Institues for Health* 2005. Retrieved May 4, 2008, from http://mchb.hrsa.gov/thechild/family.htm

3

Culture and Spirituality in Integrative Pediatrics

JUDSON B. REANEY AND GREGORY A. PLOTNIKOFF

KEY CONCEPTS

■ Understanding the cultural and spiritual issues present in every case is necessary for efficient, effective, and person-centered care.
■ Patients and families are experts in their own cultural and spiritual beliefs.
■ All clinicians are powerfully influenced by their own cultural inheritance including the culture of medicine.
■ The most important skill in assessing spirituality needs is listening.
■ Religious and spiritual concerns can be anticipated, assessed, and effectively addressed in clinical practice.

■

Religious and spiritual practices are the most common integrative therapies for health and healing. In contemporary North America, these are commonly misunderstood as personal or individual practices. However, spiritual beliefs and practices are embedded deeply into a culture. Indeed, they form an important part of one's cultural framework. Thus, one cannot talk about spirituality without talking about culture and one cannot address culture without considering its spiritual determinants.

Additionally, all culturally based healing traditions are deeply spiritual and often based in a religious worldview. Readily seen examples in integrative medicine include Native American healing, Ayurveda, Tibetan medicine, and Traditional East Asian Medicine, including that of ancient China, Korea, and Japan (Kampo). Even secular practices such as New Age Healing or TCM (Classical Chinese Medicine as re-worked and promoted by post-1949 China) include strong cultural and spiritual elements. This chapter is included in this textbook because the efficient and effective integrative clinician identifies and works with the cultural and spiritual beliefs of patients and their families.

Every day, in richly pluralistic hospitals and clinics, pediatricians and pediatric nurse practitioners are challenged by new complexities largely unknown to their predecessors. And now, in pediatric care, where communication, understanding, and a working clinician/patient alliance are all crucial to good health outcomes, competence in cultural and spiritual assessment is not optional—it is indispensable.

These three facts are clear. Every patient encounter is a cross-cultural experience. Serious illness is often a spiritual crisis. And every encounter with a child has the potential to be a spiritual experience. How, then, can busy clinicians honor and respond to these dimensions of care? How can they best incorporate cultural and spiritual concerns into their practices? To answer these questions, this chapter will provide the reader with clinically relevant insights and guidance to efficient and effective care. This includes descriptions of five common errors in assessment, five signs of spiritual needs, and five helpful responses to spiritual concerns. The intent is to orient holistically minded practitioners to questions and approaches that can be simply implemented in their practices.

The North American Cultural Context

Pediatricians may be unaware of the extent to which their patients and their families rely on spiritual resources to address and cope with illness. Surveys reveal that 90%–95% of American adolescents believe in a supreme being or God: 30%–50% go to religious services or religious youth activities weekly. Forty-two percent pray alone regularly and 24% read religious scriptures weekly (Gallup, 1999; Smith, 2003).

As for their parents, adult patients in the United States use prayer as a health practice more than twice as often as they use herbal medicines (Barnes, Powell-Griner, McFann, & Nahin, 2004). Eighty-two percent of Americans believe that personal prayer can result in healing (Yankelovich, 1996). Seventy-three percent believe that intercessory prayer for others can cure illness and 77% believe that God sometimes actively intervenes to heal the sick (Yankelovich, 1996). In fact, 56% of adults report that they personally have benefited from prayer in recovering from illness or injury (McNichol, 1996).

"Adult patients in the United States use prayer as a health practice more than twice as often as they use herbal medicines."

Adult patients, and therefore presumably parents, often wish and need to be known by their clinician and to have spiritual needs acknowledged and spiritual practices incorporated into their care. A multi-center survey of adults found that two of every three patients felt their clinician should be aware of their spiritual beliefs. Patient desire for spiritual interaction (prayer) was low for office visits and increased with the severity of the illness setting (MacLean et al., 2003). A 2004 survey of 283 adult primary care patients in Ohio found that 83% of respondents wanted their clinician to inquire about spiritual beliefs in situations like serious illness or the death of a loved one (McCord, Gilchrist, & Grossman, 2002). In spite of the reported desire of patients to have spiritual issues addressed under certain circumstances, patients in a major national survey expressed dissatisfaction with the emotional and spiritual dimensions of the care they were given (Clark, Drain, & Malone, 2003).

Definitions

There is no clear consensus among researchers and scholars about how the terms culture, religion, and spirituality should be used and defined. The concepts overlap but do not completely subsume each other. Religion in modern America variously refers to belief in a divine being, a particular understanding of the natural order of the universe, adherence to certain ethical principals, ritual practices such as prayer or fasting, institutions that sponsor communal events, and/or the traditions of a community that celebrate major life events or holidays (Barnes & Sered, 2005). Spirituality refers to a search for or connection with the source of ultimate meaning. This may be variously experienced through interior processes, nature, a higher power outside oneself, rituals, or relationships with others.

In modern parlance, spirituality is likely to be thought of as a singular construct, though in reality many different "spiritualities" may exist, just as there are many religions. Experts do not agree that there is a universal and metacultural spirituality. There is a growing, post-modern American tendency for many to consider spirituality—an interior, individual process—to be superior to group religious experience. Conversely, some more religiously orthodox individuals view spirituality with suspicion. For them it may appear to be too individualistic and an "anything goes" heterodoxy.

In this chapter, for the sake of clarity and brevity, we have chosen to use the words spirituality and religion at times interchangeably, though we most often use the word spirituality. The reader is advised to not interpret this choice as indicating that religion and spirituality completely overlap one another, that they are totally synonymous, that a judgment has been made by the authors that one is somehow superior to the other, or that there is a singular, universal spirituality.

Culture, Spirituality, and Clinician Self-Awareness

What are the patient's most deeply held beliefs? What meaning do they give to their illness? What spiritual practices promote wholeness and healing for them? What resources do they access in times of health crisis? How does illness or suffering affect their faith? Before seeking answers to such questions, clinicians should develop a keen understanding of their own cultural heritage.

Possession of book knowledge about other cultures and their spiritual traditions does not mean one can communicate well and act correctly in patient relationships. Religious literacy among Americans is woefully inadequate (Prothero, 2007). A fundamental religious literacy provides a good foundation for clinicians. But book knowledge, although helpful, has the potential to create or reinforce stereotypes and may overly simplify reality. The adage "a little knowledge is a dangerous thing" may apply. Without a good dose of humility, the clinician may believe he knows much more than he does and subsequently make rash generalizations. Missing may be acknowledgement of the innumerable differences in culture that exist. Examples of cultural variability include religious practices and beliefs in different geographic regions, sects and subgroups of religions, ethnicity, race, social class, and family of origin. A clinician might assume, for example, that a Hispanic patient is Catholic, but not all are—for example, a growing number belong to The Church of Jesus Christ of Latter Day Saints (Mormon). If, after inquiring, the clinician learned the patient was Catholic, it would also be important to know if they had Curandero beliefs. Macro factors also interplay in individual patients with differences in life experiences based on birth order, gender, gender identity and sexual orientation, traumatic physical and emotional experiences, positive and negative spiritual experiences, and personal epiphanies.

All clinicians are powerfully influenced by their own cultural inheritance including the culture of medicine (Beagan, 2003). To begin to know oneself better, the clinician should address a number of questions. What faith tradition(s) do I come from? What faith tradition(s) does my family come from? What did I accept and what did I reject of my family's faith tradition? Was there conflict in my family about spiritual matters? How was it dealt with? Was spirituality openly discussed and how? Were there any taboo subjects? Did I have any significant formative faith experiences, either positive or negative? What experiences did I have with other traditions? What messages about other faiths did I get when growing up?

Deeper self-knowledge through structured reflection is one of the hallmarks of medical professionalism. Additional questions to consider include, "What is a good death?" "What is good care?" or "What is 'best interest' for a child?" Additionally, "How much and what information is important for my decision-making for my own care?" Even, "What is personalized, patient-centered care?" For such questions, there is no objective, universal answer. This highlights the importance of understanding one's own answers before working with others. While this list of questions is not exhaustive, it provides an important starting point for personal inquiry.

Other means of deepening self-awareness include cultural competency programs through hospitals, clinics, and continuing medical education that use a group process for personal understanding. The group process has the advantages of a structured

---

"Every patient encounter is a cross-cultural experience. Serious illness often is a spiritual crisis. And every encounter with a child has the potential to be a spiritual experience."

---

curriculum and expert facilitation as well as the power of listening to and sharing personal narratives. One particularly useful tool is the cultural genogram that promotes awareness of one's cultural origins (Hardy & Laszloffy, 1995).

The efficient and effective clinician ultimately needs to understand the whole self he or she brings into the exam room or to the bedside. In order to be fully present for the patient, one must bring one's full humanity into the relationship. Unfinished or troubling spiritual issues for the clinician may creep into the patient encounter. For example, a clinician who felt emotionally abused by guilt and shame from her pious parents might have problems talking with a fundamental Christian patient about the importance healing prayer has for them. However, once self-awareness develops, a clinician is much better positioned to deepen their understanding of the uniqueness of the spirituality of a given patient and family or a community of people they regularly serve.

Anticipating Religious and Spiritual Concerns

Any encounter with a child has the potential to be a spiritual experience. Even a seemingly insignificant health issue can have profound meaning. A child may experience wonder at how miraculously the body knows how to heal a cut finger. In a routine physical, a teenager may see their body as a holy place that should not be defiled by tobacco or substances. A child who learns to use their imagination to overcome bedwetting may consider this ability to be a divine gift. The clinician should always keep in mind that each visit with a child holds the possibility for a sacred experience. The very experience of being with a compassionate adult healer who is fully present for them can be very spiritual for the child. Presence and compassion come from the heart. These qualities are universally found in all religious traditions and considered to be attributes of the divine.

The clinician should anticipate that there are certain circumstances where spiritual concerns are more likely to arise. For parents, a particularly vulnerable time is when a child is critically ill or when a child dies. It is unthinkable to parents that they might have a child die before they do. This is even truer in the modern first world where child death due to malnutrition or infectious diseases has become uncommon. Many North American parents have come to expect that medicine will be able to cure their child of life-threatening illnesses. Confronted with the possibility of losing a child to a critical illness or injury, or with the actual loss of a child, parents are bereft and may feel their spiritual foundations crumble. Thus, sacred texts from many traditions contain passages relevant to the grief and lamentation of a parent who has lost a child (see Table 3-1). Parents who learn that a child has a serious chronic illness or disability like mental retardation or autism also experience grief and the loss of dreams they had for their child. This, too, should be anticipated as a possible spiritual struggle. Specific childhood traumas like sexual abuse can also shake a parent's faith and prompt questions such as "How could a loving God let this happen to an innocent child?" In the teenage years, parents may experience a spiritual crisis associated with estrangement from their son or daughter.

There are also predictable times that the clinician should anticipate that a child might have a spiritual concern. It is particularly important that the clinician be aware of significant events in the life of the child. As with adults, loss is a leading trigger for

Table 3-1. Spiritual Resources on Loss of a Child

Scripture

Hebrew Bible

2 Samuel 12:15–23

Psalm 139 (especially lines 13, 14, and 16)

New Testament

Mark 5: 21–24, 35–43

Mark 10: 13–16

Luke 18: 16

Quran

2: 233 (also 185, 195)

31:34

67:2–3

Quranic Hadith

Hadith-al-Tayaalisi

Secular books

"The Dragonfly Door"

A children's story about loss and change intended to be read to a child by an adult.

written by John Adams / illustrated by Barbara L. Gibson ISBN-13: 978-1-934066-12-6 ISBN-10: 1-934066-12-5

Websites

Silentgrief.com (Christian)

Beliefnet.com (multi-faith spiritual resources)

spiritual questions, if not outright crises. Death of a loved one, miscarriage or stillbirth of an anticipated sibling, death of a friend or classmate, death of a pet, or even the death of the parent of a friend can cause a child to question the meaning of life, what happens after death, why there is pain and suffering, and whether they are safe, protected, and loved by a divine being or presence. Profound changes in relationships also create spiritual vulnerability. Examples include parental divorce, family estrangements, a fractured relationship with a good friend, or for teenagers, the end of a significant love relationship.

A child who has significant differences from peers may also have spiritual questions. This might be due to a disability, chronic illness, or mental illness. Sooner or later the child begins to wonder about the meaning of their condition and "Why did this happen to me?" They may experience isolation and despair or possibly anger toward God. Many children are remarkably resilient, but even children without overt disabilities may believe that they are inferior in appearance, are less desirable as a friend, or are lacking in abilities and talents. Children who are the victims of teasing and bullying can have spiritual trauma in addition to the emotional and physical pain they might incur. Teenagers may have an existential crisis when they realize that they might not be able to realistically fulfill their childhood dreams. Lesbian, gay, bisexual, transgender, and questioning youth can have a spiritual struggle about the meaning of their sexual orientation. This can be especially problematic if their sexual orientation conflicts with the religious beliefs and teachings of their family.

The clinician should also anticipate that childhood traumatic events can create spiritual disturbances. This is particularly true for children who are the victims of child abuse. If the abuse is at the hands of a parent, the violation of trust and the perversion of the parent–child relationship can cause a child to lose faith in and mistrust the intentions of a universal loving presence. Child abuse by a father in a family that has an image of God as "God the Father" has the potential to alienate the victim from both her earthly and heavenly fathers. Sexual abuse by clergy is uniquely damaging, in that the clergy can represent the church and God to the child. Children also can experience spiritual wounding from witnessing domestic violence, community violence, or war. Even news accounts of natural disasters, homicides, terrorism like the destruction of the World Trade Center on September 11, 2001, and accounts of war or genocide can spiritually challenge children. Finally, it should be remembered that many children live chronically in poverty, and are hungry, sometimes homeless. The clinician caring for these children needs to remember that poverty can damage not only the body and mind but also the spirit.

Integrative Pediatric Interventions for Cultural and Spiritual Concerns

The primary goal of spiritual inquiry is to understand a given child's and family's personal spiritual beliefs and practices. What are their most deeply held beliefs? What spiritual practices promote wholeness and healing for them? What meaning do they give to the illness? Who provides spiritual care and support for them in time of need? What other cultural or spiritual resources do they access, in times of health crisis? How does illness or suffering affect their faith? The unique answers each family provides are the foundation for patient-centered care and a strong patient alliance.

Pediatricians are not chaplains or clergy and do not need to fulfill such roles. However, pediatricians are increasingly expected by society to identify, assess, and triage spiritual concerns in their patients and their families. Ideally, the pediatrician creates a safe and conducive environment where concerns can be expressed and heard. The simple act of listening deeply and compassionately may itself be therapeutic.

"In North America today, one cannot generalize about any beliefs of any patient at any time based on labels such as ethnicity or religion. The key clinical concern: what does *this* mean for *this* person?"

Assessment of Spirituality

The clinically effective pediatrician or pediatric team understands the patient's beliefs, fears, questions, and uncertainties. This clinical goal can be achieved only by intentional interviewing in the context of a positive relationship with the patient and family. Because religious/spiritual and cultural beliefs can be implicit and unconscious to the patient and family, the use of various spiritual assessment tools can be quite helpful as heuristic means to understand clinically important issues.

Patients and families are experts in their own cultural and spiritual beliefs. From this perspective, clinicians cannot achieve "cultural competence" but should instead express an orientation that might be termed "cultural humility." As in all clinical care, preconceptions, biases, or personal judgments undermine efficacy and must be considered hypotheses and tested. In North America today, one cannot generalize about any beliefs of any patient at any time based on labels such as ethnicity or religion. The key clinical concern: what does *this* mean for *this* person? "Please teach me" is an important approach to personalized care.

The most important skill in assessing spirituality needs is listening. The clinician should be motivated by a desire to truly understand the patient's beliefs, fears, questions, and uncertainties. Judgment and preconceptions or biases have no place in this process. The patient needs to perceive that the clinician is fully present for them and wants to know them as a whole person. They also need to know they can safely and confidentially share intimate interior material. There may be subjects that they have previously never confided to anyone before.

> "The simple act of listening deeply and compassionately may itself be therapeutic."

It is often difficult for clinicians who are trained to provide answers to believe that listening can at times be enough. Bearing witness to doubts, fears, shame, loneliness, and anger can be enough. When assessing spiritual concerns, one must be unhurried and comfortable sitting in silence. Being with a patient in silence can be enough (Miller, 2003).

Clinician questions about cultural and spiritual orientation should be open and honest. This means that they should come without a hidden agenda or value judgment. Their purpose is to identify the values, beliefs, and expected behaviors that are relevant to the patient's and family's care. A good question often is one for which the clinician could not possibly surmise the answer before asking (Palmer, 2004). Examples to understand either cultural or spiritual issues include: "In regards to your child's care, what is most important to you that I know?" Or, "What do you most want me to know about your family?" To access issues of grief, good open-ended questions can include, "Please tell me, in the past few years, have there been any significant changes or losses in your life?" And in all situations where a tough statement or challenge is offered, the simple response, "tell me about it," may open incredibly important subjects as well as establish trust. The clinician's goal is to seek understanding before seeking to be understood.

In introducing such questions, clinicians should confirm that their goal is to understand the patient's and the family's cultural and spiritual beliefs and that such understanding is an important aspect of high-quality healthcare. The clinician should confirm that such questions are routine for all patients, that the questions do not carry judgment, and that they are for understanding the patient as a whole person. Patients also need to know they can safely and confidentially share intimate, interior material. This can be stated verbally but body language and attitude are often much stronger than words.

Several tools have been published to systematically guide assessment of the patient's or family's spiritual perspective and resources. These are brief, easy and easy to remember. They are non-intrusive and fit naturally into the flow of a social history. Easy-to-use mnemonics include the FICA, HOPE, and SPIRIT (Table 3-2) (Anandarajah & Hight, 2003; Maugens, 1996; Puchalski, Larsen, & Post, 2000). These mnemonics offer clinicians rapid recall of key areas to cover. Like a template in an electronic medical record, they reduce variability in medical practice and ensure that vital information is not missed. However, they can be interpreted as all-inclusive leading the clinician to

Table 3-2. SPIRIT

SPIRIT (Maugens, 1996)

S: Spiritual belief system—what is your formal religious affiliation?

P: Personal spirituality—Describe the beliefs and practices of your religion or spiritual system that you personally accept/do not accept.

I: Integration within a spiritual community—Do you belong to a spiritual or religious group or community? What importance does this group have for you?

R: Ritualized practices and restrictions—Are there specific practices that you carry out as part of your religion/spirituality (e.g. prayer and meditation)? What significance do these practices have for you?

I: Implications for medical care—What aspects of your religion/spirituality would you like to keep in mind as I care for you?

T: Terminal events planning—As we plan for your care near the end of life, how does your faith impact on your decisions?

FICA (Puchalski, Larsen, & Post, 2000)

F: Faith or beliefs—What is your faith or belief?

Do you consider yourself spiritual or religious?

What things do you believe in that give meaning to your life?

I: Importance and influence. Is it important in your life?

What influence does it have on how you take care of yourself?

How have your beliefs influenced your behavior during this illness?

What role do your beliefs play in regaining your health?

C: Community—Are you part of a spiritual or religious community?

Is this of support to you and how?

A: Address— How would you like me, your healthcare provider, to address these issues in your healthcare?

HOPE (Anandarajah & Hight, 2001)

H: Hope—What are your sources of hope, meaning, strength, peace, love and connectedness?

O: Organization—Do you consider yourself part of an organized religion?

P: Personal Spirituality and Practices—What aspects of your spirituality or spiritual practices do you find most helpful?

E: Effects—How do your beliefs affect the kind of medical care you would like me to provide?

---

fail to ask other relevant questions. And use of such tools can also feel too *pro forma*, impersonal. They may not always lead to a full understanding of ongoing concerns. Despite their limitations, assessment tools can be a good place for the clinician to start. As comfort with the spiritual assessment grows, one's inquiry is likely to take on a more natural, individualized, and personal quality.

There are no good tools or questionnaires to assess spirituality in children (Barnes, Plotnikoff, Fox, & Pendleton, 2000). Those that exist have been adapted from adult questionnaires and may not be appropriate for children. They also do not take developmental considerations into account. Only a few are culturally sensitive (Greenfield & Cocking, 1994; Hill & Hood, 1999).

Assessment of children must always take into account developmental considerations that necessarily affect the child's experience and understanding of spirituality. The most well-known theory of faith formation and development is that of James Fowler (Fowler, 1981). Drawing upon Erik Erickson's theory of psychosocial development (Erickson, 1980). Kohlberg's theory of moral development (Kohlberg, 1981), and Piaget's theory of cognitive development (Piaget, 1985), Fowler posits that there are stages of human faith development that parallel other aspects of development. Though Fowler did not intend for his stages to represent a hierarchy with spiritual developmental stages progressing from inferior to superior, some have unfortunately interpreted his developmental theory in this way.

For the clinician, it is important to recognize that spiritual formation has developmental dimensions and that psychodynamic and cognitive processes impact upon the child's spiritual understandings and beliefs. The pediatric provider will likely adapt questions in developmentally appropriate ways just as they do for other child interviews. Instead of questions, observation of behavior including play may provide some insight into the child's concerns. The clinician may also deepen understanding via the content of a child's drawings, use of symbols and other natural means of non-verbal expression. In the end, one must sensitively inquire and listen to the individual child.

Five Common Errors in Cultural and Spiritual Assessment

Clinicians are prone to make certain types of mistakes when approaching spiritual issues with patients. There are five common errors that one should be aware of and avoid making.

1. *I have no need to ask; I can presume.* This error may be one of the most common and also one of the most insidious in clinical practice. The clinician makes assumptions about the patient based on limited information often involving stereotypes. These stereotypes may be based on the clinician's own life experiences no matter how limited, incorrect, or biased they may be. They may also be rooted in stereotypes popular in the dominant culture. With a little knowledge, the clinician may presume that all patients with a particular religious background are the same. After all, as Ronald Reagan once stated, "If you've seen one redwood, you've seen them all."

People and their spiritual beliefs and practices are richly diverse. Nevertheless, a clinician may believe that all Muslims have similar beliefs whether Sunni or Shi'as, Arab, African or Indonesian, rural, or urban. Or that all Jewish patients have the same religious observances. Or that all Protestant Christians are similarly pious. And, without asking each family member, the clinician may mistakenly believe that the entire family is on the same page. It could be easy to miss generational differences between a Hmong elder and his second-generation Hmong children. The child or teenage patient may have a different religious perspective than their parents perhaps based on a unique personal belief or perhaps related to developmental considerations. Furthermore, mothers and fathers of pediatric patients often have divergent beliefs that may lie dormant only to awaken when a child is seriously ill. This is one factor that may contribute to the high rate of divorce in parents of children who die or who live with chronic illness.

"Spirituality may be about questions: professional care means support- ing the search for answers and does not mean providing patients with the answers."

Without asking, one cannot know how religious and spiritual differences in a family are discussed (or not), what effect the differences have on family members, and how decisions are ultimately made. Presumption is more likely to be a problem when the clinician talks more than he or she listens for understanding. Many time-pressed clini- cians make assumptions with the best of intentions. However, assumptions only repre- sent hypotheses to be tested. Identifying and testing such hypotheses represents one aspect of person-centered care.

2. *My answers should be your answers.* Some clinicians believe that they have the obli- gation to express, share, or even impose their own beliefs on their patients. Whereas not asking and presuming about cultural and spiritual beliefs might be seen as a "sin of omission," actively attempting to impose one's own beliefs on a patient may be seen as a "sin of commission."

Spirituality is an intensely personal matter. There is a power differential between a clinician and a patient. Great care must always be taken by the clinician to use power and authority for the patient's benefit and to never abuse a patient's dependence and trust. Even when a patient asks the clinician about the clinician's own spiritual beliefs, the clinician should exercise caution and be clear what extent or manner of disclosure is in the best interest of the patient. Spirituality may be about questions: professional care means supporting the search for answers and does not mean providing patients with the answers.

3. *Spiritual issues aren't medically important in pediatric care.* Understanding the cul- tural and spiritual issues present in every case is necessary for efficient, effective, and person-centered care. Failure to understand implicit conflicts between the clinician and the family in treatment priorities, decision making, dietary, and lifestyle prescriptions

guarantees time consuming conflict resolution. Likewise, failure to understand the patient's or family's sources of strength, resilience, or guilt and shame may undermine clinical success.

The most easily understood potential for inefficient and ineffective care is when the legal requirements for pediatric patient advocacy may violate a family's deeply held cultural and spiritual beliefs. Parents may believe that medical decisions that are in the best physiologic interests of the child are not in the best cultural or spiritual interests of the child. Unlike the example of blood transfusions for Jehovah's Witnesses, this conflict may be implicit and unconscious and therefore very hard for parents to articulate. Thus, the burden is on the clinician to interview deeply for cultural and spiritual concerns.

In all cases of potential clinical conflict, the clinician must be clear about what aspects of the case constitute factually supported medical opinion and what aspects represents the personal beliefs of the patient, family, and care team regarding "best interests." The efficient and effective clinician engages in preventive ethics through deep understanding not only of the patient's and family's beliefs, but also of her own. The goal of patient-centered care is to work as much as possible with, rather than against, the patient's beliefs and emotions. Through compassionate listening and the relationship with the patient and family which follows, advance planning for contingencies is much more possible.

Additionally, families may struggle with shameful secrets, challenges to their beliefs or sources of strength, unexpressed guilt or anger, as well as the loss that a child's illness represents. These spiritual concerns represent non-medical risk factors that can fuel frustration and drive conflict in hospital settings. In such instances, the clinician's duty is to consider the differential diagnosis of spiritual, cultural, or psychological issues and make appropriate referrals. Clinical Pastoral Education (CPE) certified chaplains may be in the best position to assess and address the underlying spiritual conflicts.

4. I'm just not comfortable with spiritual issues. Many clinicians may believe that they are not competent to deal with spiritual issues. They might feel that it is better to avoid the topic, since there is little that they have to offer. Clinicians may rightly believe that spiritual leaders, clergy, and chaplains have special abilities and training to address a patient's spiritual needs. These represent great resources and, when appropriate, an

"Exploring spiritual issues does not create problems that do not already exist. Instead it is a step toward understanding the answers and questions, hopes and fears, beliefs and doubts that the patient already has."

opportunity for referrals. However, their availability does not mean that the clinician also does not have an important role to play.

Understanding the spiritual concerns and conflicts of patients does not automatically require provision of an answer or solution. Clinicians are trained to be problem-solvers and the givers of advice and answers for physiologic concerns. However, care of the spirit is more about listening and being present than providing answers. The clinical competency to develop is not the capacity to provide answers to spiritual concerns, but the capacity to be human, to open one's heart, and to be compassionate.

Some clinicians may fear that spiritual issues are a hornet's nest that should not be poked. Exploring spiritual issues does not create problems that do not already exist. Instead it is a step toward understanding the answers and questions, hopes and fears, beliefs and doubts that the patient already has.

5. *If I talk about culture and spirituality, I will offend people.* Surveys confirm that more patients want their clinician to talk about spirituality than those who would rather that the topic not be addressed. Still, the clinician may worry that asking about religious or spiritual concerns could be perceived as proselytizing. How the questions are posed can make a significant difference. Asking respectfully with a genuine desire to understand signals that the clinician's intent is benevolent and not about judgment or evangelizing.

Just as with taking a detailed sexual or chemical use history, clinicians may have certain fears to overcome before asking about cultural or religious matters. This is natural. However, as with other sensitive topics, clinicians can create a safe and respectful atmosphere where such intimate information can be shared.

The clinician may fear that spiritual discussions could be particularly offensive if it involves talking to a child. Spirituality may be perceived to be exclusively in the province of parents. Being clear that the goal is to better understand your patient's beliefs is essential. And once again, approaching the topic with caring and respect will allay most concerns. It may be appropriate to first talk to the parents of a younger child.

Five Common Signs of Unmet Spiritual Needs

In addition to assessing spiritual orientation in pediatrics, the efficient and effective clinician must also look for signs of unmet spiritual needs. This includes needs not only in the patient, but also in other important people in their lives, including their siblings and their parents. We list here five common signs that may indicate the presence of spiritual concerns that need to be addressed:

1. *The patient implies that they are troubled or need assistance.* This would appear to be self-evident and unnecessary to list as a sign of spiritual distress. It is included because patients often verbalize in some way what is bothering them, and their concern goes unanswered. A parent may say. "I feel I have nowhere

to turn. I used to have faith but now I just feel abandoned and alone." A child may say, "I say my prayers, but it doesn't help." Clinicians may ignore the clear signs, however. This may be because they are hurried, because the concern doesn't neatly fit into the interview algorithm, or because the clinician feels inadequate to deal with the issue. Compassionate listening will pick up the possibility of a spiritual need.

2. *The patient asks existential questions.* Sometimes spiritual concerns can be expressed more obliquely and take the form of existential distress. Common questions center on attempts to make cosmic sense of illness and to find meaning in suffering. A child may ask, "Where will I go after I die?" or "Why do I have to have this stupid leukemia? It's not fair." A parent might say, "I don't understand why an innocent child should suffer like this." The meaning of life and suffering are common existential themes. Anger at God or a higher power often accompanies these questions.

3. *The patient feels unloved or unworthy.* Illness can often be accompanied by feelings of despondency. The patient may feel abandoned or alone. Life may not seem worthwhile, and they may feel that no one loves them and further that they are not worthy of being loved. They may consider themselves a burden to others. The astute clinician always monitors for depression in patients who are critically or chronically ill. It is also important to understand that the despair a depressed patient may feel is also a "dark night of the soul."

4. *The patient feels shame or guilt.* In searching for meaning in illness, some patients conclude that they somehow deserve to be afflicted. They may conclude that something they did or did not do resulted in disease. Specifically, they may believe that they are being punished. This may especially be true for younger children who are more concrete and who have little experience or understanding of the scientific explanations for illness and disease. Parents, too, may feel that their transgressions caused their child to fall ill.

5. *The patient abruptly changes spiritual practices or communities.* If a child with a serious or chronic illness or their parent suddenly abandons a spiritual practice or disaffiliates with a previous spiritual community, it may be a sign that they no longer feel sustained by those practices or that group. This may be a thoughtful and deliberate decision. On the other hand, it may be a sign that significant spiritual needs are not being met. It could even mean that the child or family had a negative or traumatic experience in the previous tradition. Other patients may change their spiritual practices by becoming excessively rigid. This may signal that the patient is attempting to overcome the anxiety associated with a loss of control or uncertainty about spiritual questions by imposing rigid solutions.

Five Helpful Responses to Spiritual Concerns

The presence of unmet spiritual needs and ongoing spiritual concerns needs clinician assessment and response. Patients and families may "test" clinicians for their response to challenging issues. They may be asking themselves, "Is this someone I can trust? Is this someone who will listen?" Expressed interest and avoided answer-giving to spiritual concerns make for a strong and positive relationship. Indeed, the clinician's capacity to respond to the patient, rather than to their own concerns, is the hallmark of professional care. Here are five key approaches which enhance the quality of care and which can support one's professional growth and development in integrative care.

1. *Respond simply to the tough questions or statements.* "Tell me about it." Or for a child, ask instead, "Can you draw me a picture about this?"
2. *Seek to understand.* "What now is most important to you?"
3. *Seek to serve.* "What now would be most helpful for you?" Or, "How can I/we be most helpful for you?"
4. *Partner.* Frequently consult the chaplaincy service and/or the patient's/family's preferred spiritual provider.
5. Consider the power of cultural or spiritual rituals.

Conclusion

Culture and spirituality are often implicit and unconscious factors in all experiences of illness. The clinician's challenge is to recognize, understand and respond constructively to these factors which are so important for healing.

The capacity to integrate culture and spirituality into clinical care is important for both children and their parents, as well as for all clinicians. Spiritual practices such as prayer are the most common integrative health practice. And many integrative therapies are actually culturally based healing traditions with a strong spiritual component. The clinical team's support for a patient's or family's cultural and spiritual resources is a significant factor in their comfort and healing.

Spiritual assessment mnemonics can be used to assure that major areas of inquiry are addressed. With sensitive inquiry and generous listening, the clinician can learn about the place that spirituality holds in the lives of children and their families and what they believe is necessary for their caregiver to know and understand.

Spiritual issues may arise in any clinical encounter. Clinicians should be aware of signs that there are unmet spiritual needs and be prepared to address those needs through presence and listening and by making appropriate referrals when necessary. The result is efficient, effective, and compassionate care for patients and their families.

REFERENCES

Anandarajah, G., & Hight, E. (2001). Spirituality and medical practice: Using the HOPE questions as a practical tool for spiritual assessment. *American Family Physician, 63*, 81–88.

Barnes, L,. Plotnikoff, G., Fox, K., & Pendleton, S. (2000). Spirituality, religion, and pediatrics-intersecting worlds of healing. *Pediatrics, 104*, 899–908.

Barnes, L., & Sered, S. (Eds.). (2005). *Religion and healing in America.* New York: Oxford University Press.

Barnes, P. M., Powell-Griner, E., McFann, K., & Nahin, R. L. (2004). Complementary and alternative medicine use among adults in the United States, 2002. *Advance Data, 343*, 1–19.

Beagan, B. (2003). Teaching social and cultural awareness to medical students: "It's all very nice to talk about it in theory, but ultimately it makes no difference." *Academic Medicine, 78*, 605–614.

Clark, P. A., Drain, M., & Malone, M. P. (2003). Addressing patients' emotional and spiritual needs. *Joint Commission Journal on Quality and Safety, 20*, 659–670.

Erickson, E. H. (1980). *Identity and the life cycle.* New York: WW Norton.

Fowler, J .W. (1981). *Stages of faith: The psychology of human development and the quest for meaning.* San Francisco, CA: Harper and Row.

Gallup, G. Jr., & Lindsay, D. M. (1999). *Surveying the religious landscape: Trends in US beliefs.* Harrisburg PA: Morehouse Publishing.

Greenfield, P. M., & Cocking, R. R. (Eds.). (1994). *Cross-cultural roots of minority child development.* Hillside, NJ: Lawrence Erlbaum Associates.

Hardy, K. V., & Laszloffy, T. A. (1995). The cultural genogram: Key to training culturally competent family therapists. *Journal of Marital and Family Therapy, 21*, 227–237.

Hill, P., & Hood, R. (1999). *Measures of religiosity.* Birmingham, AL: Religious Education Press.

Kohlberg, L. (1981). *Essays on moral development.* San Francisco, CA: Harper and Row.

MacLean, C. D., Susi, B., Phifer, N., Schultz, L., Bynum, D., Franco, M., et al. (2003). Patient preference for physician discussion and practice of spirituality. *Journal of General Internal Medicine, 18*, 38–43.

Maugens, T. A. (1996). The SPIRITual history. *Archives of Family Medicine, 5*, 11–16.

McCord, G., Gilchrist, V. J., Grossman, S. G., King, B. D., McCormick, K. E., Oprandi, A. M., et al. (2004). Discussing spirituality with patients: A rational and ethical approach. *Annals of Family Medicine, 2*, 356–361.

McNichol, T. (1996). When religion and medicine meet: The new faith in medicine. *USA Weekend,* April 7, p. 4.

Miller, J. (2003). *The art of listening in a healing way.* Fort Wayne, IN: Willowgreen Publishing.

Palmer, P (2004). *A hidden wholeness: The journey toward an undivided life.* San Francisco, CA: Jossey-Bass.

Piaget, J., (1985). *The equilibration of cognitive structures: The central problem of intellectual development.* Chicago, IL: University of Chicago Press.

Prothero, S. (2007). *Religious literacy: What every American needs to know—and doesn't.* San Francisco, CA: HarperSanFrancisco.

Puchalski, C. M., Larsen, D. B., & Post, S. G. (2000). Physicians and patient spirituality. *Annals of Internal medicine, 133*, 748–749.

Smith, C. (2003). Religious participation and parental moral expectations and supervision of American youth. *Review of Religious Research, 44*, 414–424.

Yankelovich Partners, Inc. Telephone poll for Time/CNN, June 12–13, 1996. *Time,* (June 24), pp. 58–62.

4

Essential Medicine: Self-Care for Pediatric Providers

DANNA M. PARK

You have chosen me to watch over the life and health of your creatures. I am about to apply myself to the duties of my profession...Support me in this great work that it may benefit my fellow creatures...Inspire me with love for my occupation and for your creatures...Preserve my physical and spiritual strength that I may cheerfully be of help to rich and poor, good and bad, friend and foe alike. Let me see only the human being in the sufferer.

—*Physician's Prayer by Moses Maimonides, Physician and Rabbi (1135–1204 AD)*

There is more in us than we know. If we can be made to see it, perhaps for the rest of our lives we will be unwilling to settle for less.

—*Kurt Hahn, Founder of Outward Bound*

KEY CONCEPTS

- Health care provider discontent and stress has negative impacts on all aspects of patient care and satisfaction.
- The new model of optimal, integrative medical care requires a focus on provider self-care.
- Pediatric intensive care specialties are more likely to lead to burnout than is general pediatrics.
- Physician and nurse turnover negatively impacts medical economics.
- Personal health habits of physicians are predictors of whether or not they encourage preventive health habits in their patients.
- Wellness promotion practices include good relationships, spirituality, self care, good work practices, and values as they relate to what constitutes success and/or balance in life.

■

We are reaching a new crossroads in medicine today, one that is taxing every aspect of medical care. No specialty is immune to the changes and challenges inherent in the US healthcare system, and those who care for children have special challenges as they work within a system that is increasingly problematic. Allied healthcare as well as traditional pediatric specialties and subspecialties continue to care well for children despite a system that is overloaded with bureaucracy, documentation requirements, lower reimbursements for services and compressed clinic time. In providing "whole child care," attention is not only on the patient, but also focused on the family unit, financial stressors, access to care, medications and adequate nutrition, and in the case of long-term health issues, the psychosocial milieu inherent in a family that has a child with a chronic illness. In addition, providers must continue to advocate on a local, state, and national level for those who are too young to have a voice in the changes to come. Needless to say, this conglomeration of tasks is challenging all levels of medical practitioners.

It is rare to see a medical text address healthcare provider wellness as a component of patient care. Yet what could be more crucial and critical, especially in today's medical environment? In one 2005 study, the researchers stated it is "impossible to provide the best care to every patient," as it would take 10.6 hours per working day to deliver all recommended care for patients with chronic conditions, plus 7.4 hours per day to provide evidence-based preventive care, to an average panel of 2500 patients (the mean US panel size is 2300) (Ostbye et al., 2005). In addition, the compressed time per visit per patient is making medical practice less effective on a variety of levels. Research shows that it takes a doctor 23 seconds to interrupt a patient's story of the medical issue at hand and that 85% of patients leave the office without fully understanding what their doctor told them. A man will not ask any questions during a medical visit while a woman will ask six questions. Fifty percent of patients leave the office unsure of what they are supposed to do to take care of themselves (Marvel et al., 1999).

The California Medical Association 2001 study, "And Then There Were None: The Coming Physician Supply Problem" showed in graphic detail how provider discontent is translating into a healthcare shortage. Seventy-five percent of physicians reported being less satisfied with their medical practice in the past 5 years and 43% intended to leave practice in the next 3 years. Over one-fourth would not choose medicine as a career if starting over, and two-thirds would not recommend medicine as a career to their children (CMA, 2001).

As providers continue to attempt the impossible on a daily basis, the ongoing healthcare crisis has clearly affected their own abilities to care for themselves, their patients, families, and communities. For providers, there is a conflict between self-care and care for others, and a conflict of not enough time—with patients, with their own families or with themselves. It is an internal conflict between the life of a healer in medicine and the life of a busy practitioner working with insurance demands and financial pressures that are defining the practice of medicine today.

An Integrative Approach to Self-Care

Integrative medicine is defined as healing-oriented medicine that takes account of the whole person (body, mind, and spirit), including all aspects of lifestyle. It emphasizes the therapeutic relationship and makes use of all appropriate therapies, both conventional and alternative (University of Arizona, 2003). An integrative approach to pediatrics, or to any medical specialty for that matter, recognizes that the provider–patient–family triad is a constant back-and-forth, give-and-take, interactive fluctuating relationship. This "relationship-centered care" is defined by the Fetzer Institute/Relationship-Centered Care Network as being "an approach to healthcare and healing that places relationship at the core of the therapeutic process. In this approach, all interactions are based upon a fundamental commitment to mutual respect, self-awareness, humility, openness, and caring" (Fetzer Institute, 2004).

Wellness and relationship-centered care are complex and multifaceted. These concepts recognize that healing extends beyond the physical body, into emotional, spiritual, interprofessional/institutional, and interpersonal spheres. There is a dynamic constant movement and shift between all these realms. When the practitioner recognizes this and chooses to treat "whole patients" and their families, incorporating body, mind, spirit, and relationship-centered care into the treatment plan, it brings a powerful component into practicing medicine. The practitioner–patient relationship itself becomes a tool for healing. The healthcare provider is invited to be an active participant, one who integrates and models wellness in their personal and professional life. From an integrative medicine perspective, this is an essential component of being of service to the patient. To provide this level of integrated care, we as providers need to develop wellness and self-nurturing tools to help sustain and support our physical, emotional, spiritual, and social well-being throughout our medical practice. Developing these tools is an investment in self as well as an investment in exceptional care for patients.

Although this chapter will use data and literature from the physician's point of view, it is no less relevant for other healthcare practitioners. The stressors and issues inherent in the practice of medicine today affect all pediatric healthcare providers—doctors, nurses, nurse practitioners, physician assistants, and allied healthcare professionals alike.

What Is Wellness?

The definition of wellness is inherently personal. What makes one practitioner feel whole, complete, and healthy on a mind/body/spirit level may be vastly different for another. In addition, it is a fluid state—what we need to balance ourselves changes from day to day. Three definitions capture the complexity of these concepts (Table 4-1). The Wellness Definition, from Arizona State University, states "Wellness is an active, lifelong

Table 4-1. Wellness

Components of Wellness	Author/Source
Wellness is an active process Involves making choices for a balanced life	Arizona State University, 2000
Integration of physical, mental, and social well-being	World Health Organization, 1946
Involves deliberate, conscious decision-making Optimal health integrates well-being on mind, body and spirit levels	Ardell/Langdon, 1989

process of becoming aware of choices and making decisions toward a more balanced and fulfilling life." This definition highlights that our choices determine our lifestyle. The World Health Organization's definition of health emphasizes the multidimensional aspects of wellness: "Health is a state of complete physical, mental and social well-being and not merely the absence of disease or infirmity." Ardell and Langdon's definition concentrates on the active role needed to achieve health: "Wellness is a lifestyle approach to personal excellence. It is a deliberate, conscious decision to pursue optimal well-being. It encompasses the body, mind and spirit. It is a positive choice pursued because it is judged to be a richer way to be alive" (Ardell, 1989). These definitions underscore that personal choice, repeated focus on the balance of work/life demands and integration of wellness across mind/body and spirit levels are crucial factors to creating a healthy lifestyle. The idea that health and wellness affects and extends into our relationships (friends, spouse/partner, etc.) is not a new concept, nor is the link between spiritual, emotional, and physical health. The impact of the workplace environment on personal wellness has now been documented as well (the interprofessional/institutional dimension). Most surprising and welcome are studies that show healthcare practitioners' own well being, satisfaction, and health habits have a direct and measurable effect on their patients' health. Literally, taking care of ourselves translates into good medical practice for our patients!

The Model of Medical Practice: Is Transformation Possible?

The culture of medicine is changing. The way medicine was practiced 20 years ago is no longer practical or feasible in today's challenging environment without serious repercussions for personal relationships, work environment (with its "pay for productivity" overlay), financial considerations, or family concerns. The increasing number of women physicians (over 50%) is continuing to change medical practice, incorporating previously unheard-of possibilities such as part-time, job sharing, and childcare at work.

The "old model" of medicine focused on a sense of profession that overrode all other concerns—to be the best practitioner meant completely dedicating one's life to the practice of medicine. Everything else—personal life, family life, personal well-being—was secondary to caring for patients. Through more recent studies, we know that provider self-care is an integral part of providing great medical care to patients, affecting patient well-being, patient satisfaction, and positive patient outcomes. This is the "new model" of medical culture. We know now that healthcare providers' happiness and job satisfaction have a direct impact on patient care and patient satisfaction; however, we rarely focus on the qualities of our medical practice that support our happiness and well-being.

The role of "the old model" of medical culture, plus a group of personality traits that seem to be common among healthcare providers, can ultimately converge to create problems in self-care and well-being (Table 4-2). We are caring, compassionate, perfectionistic, driven, stressed by multiple demands on time and usually sleep deprived (Lipsenthal, 2007).The stressors in the medical practice environment, in combination with the more subtle factors above, can contribute to what is euphemistically called "provider discontent."

There are many studies that show the effects, both on a personal and professional level, of a variety of stressors inherent in medical culture, practice, and training (Table 4-3). Despite studies like these, medical culture continues to support a practitioner's ability to deny his or her own needs (both physical and psychological). In addition, medical training, practice, and culture usually requires delayed gratification (whether subjectively through long training programs or literally through incurred debt), and

Table 4-2. Medical Culture (Lipsenthal, 2007)

The Role of Medical Culture	Personality Traits of Healthcare Providers
Draws out personality traits such as perfectionism and competitiveness	Pressured to succeed
Enhances ability to deny one's needs (physical and psychological)	Rushing against time
Requires delayed gratification	Opinionated
Rewards "workaholic" tendencies (Hard to set appropriate limits, rewards long hours)	Pressured speech
Personal weakness/vulnerability unacceptable	Not trusting others to do the job right
Defense mechanisms make it hard to ask for help when needed	Competitive
"Culture of silence" (Sharing with professional peers about problems, concerns and difficulties not acceptable)	Need to prove self-worth with performance

Table 4-3. Stressors Inherent in Medical Culture, Training, and Practice

Focus of Study	Author	Outcomes
Sleep deprivation	Dawson, 1997; Miller, 2000	Promotes cognitive impairment and emotional fragility Staying awake for 24 hours affects cognitive psychomotor performance as much as a blood alcohol level of 0.1% (0.08% is the drunk driving limit in most states).
Medical errors Compared a traditional "every third night" call schedule (up to 34 continuous hours of work) vs. an "intervention schedule" (up to 16 consecutive hours of work)	Landrigan, 2004	Traditional schedule group had 36% more serious medical errors than intervention schedule group. During traditional schedule, the total rate of serious errors in the critical care units was 22% higher. There were 5.6 times more diagnostic errors made and 21% more serious medication errors made in the traditional versus intervention schedule group.
Stress Job dissatisfaction	Haas, 2001	Stressed and unsatisfied physicians have more health complaints, higher job turnover, earlier retirement and file more disability claims.
Personal medical care	Gross, 2000	34% of physicians had no personal healthcare provider, 28% did not have regular medical care and 7% self-treated.
Burnout	Hendrie, 1990; Schwartz, 1987; Shanafeldt, 2002	Burnout rates among practicing physicians range from 25% to 60%. Burnout is related to self-reporting of suboptimal patient care. Burnout, depression, and stress start in residency (and likely in medical school).
Suicide risks	Frank, 1995; Samkoff, 1995; Stack, 1990	Physicians have 2.3 times the risk of death by suicide compared to the general population. Female physicians have suicide rates that are four times higher than the general female population. Suicide was found to be the most common cause of death in young physicians, accounting for 26% of deaths.
Alcohol and drug abuse	Booth, 2002; O'Connor, 1997	Physicians have an increased risk of prescription drug abuse. 10%–14% of doctors may become addicted to drugs or alcohol over their careers. Fentanyl is the most common drug of abuse. In one study, 18% of healthcare providers died or almost died before substance abuse was even suspected.

Table 4-3. (Continued)

Focus of Study	Author	Outcomes
Divorce	Rollman, 1997; Sotile, 1996	Divorce rates among physicians are estimated to be 10%–20% higher than in the general population.
		22%–24% cumulative incidence of divorce in pediatricians after 30 years of marriage
		Female physicians have a higher risk of divorce (37%) than their male counterparts (28%).
		Long work hours, "displacement" of relationship issues onto outside factors, physicians with higher levels of anger—all contribute to increased divorce rates in physician relationships.

promotes the inability to set appropriate limits, rewarding long hours and "workaholic" tendencies. Revealing weakness and vulnerabilities to others is often felt to be unacceptable, and defense mechanisms are created that make it difficult to ask for help when needed (Miller, 2000). The set-up for stress, depression, and burnout can ultimately lead, if not addressed, to potential severe outcomes such as substance abuse, personal relationship issues, and even suicide.

Happiness in the Workplace

In physician workforce studies, pediatricians seem to be happier overall in their work-life balance than other primary care and subspecialty providers (family practice and internal medicine). In comparison with general internists, general pediatricians are more likely to spend the majority of time in the office versus the hospital, to have lower complexity patients in terms of medical and psychosocial problems, to be female, to work part time and to have a lower income. Not surprisingly, they were least likely to report stress or burnout symptoms (18% and 13% respectively).

Pediatric subspecialists, in contrast, had much higher stress and burnout symptoms (23% and 26% respectively). They worked more hours (average 56 hours/week), spent more time in the hospital versus the office, and had a higher number of complex patients (Shugarman, 2001). In a 2003 study of pediatric critical care, the majority of practitioners were happy or very happy with their work, but one-third of practitioners in the 40–49 years old age group were planning to leave critical care and change specialties, either for general pediatrics, another subspecialty, or medical administration. Critical care overwork and burnout is an issue, as increases in referral volumes and complexity continue to rise. The ratio of research time to direct patient care time is decreasing, and groups continue to struggle with cost and staffing issues (Anderson, 2003; Mackey, D. 2008, personal communication).

Creating balance by self-limiting the number of work hours seems to be a popular choice, especially for female physicians as the above study shows. However, providers may be reluctant to do this for a number of reasons, not just financial. One study assessed the attitudes and perceptions of pediatric faculty about part time faculty positions and policies at a large Midwestern medical center. Interestingly, although 59% (women and practitioners with dependant children in particular) believed that part-time faculty were perceived as being less committed to their careers, 69% thought they should be eligible for all academic tracks and 73% believed they should be allotted extra time to obtain tenure. Seventy-eight percent supported policy changes, believing that this would aid in improving diversity, retention, and recruitment, especially of female faculty (Kahn, 2005).

Institutions and group practices are paying attention to burnout and attrition because of the impact on the bottom line. Literal costs of primary care physician turnover range from $236,000 for family practice to $264,345 for pediatrics (Buchbinder, 1999). In one Southwest academic medical center, the annual turnover cost $17–29 million (up to ~6% of their annual operating budget).

More than a quarter of the total turnover cost was due to nurse turnover (260 recruitments). There was low turnover of physicians in 1 year (56 recruitments) but replacement costs were so high that it accounted for the second largest element of total turnover cost (Waldman, 2004).

Many studies have identified why physicians leave practice, although there are very few studies that look at provider happiness in the workplace. Reasons for physician turnover (Table 4-4) include "misalignment" between the organization and the individual practice philosophy of the provider. Lack of decision-making in the practice plays a large role in this element of "discontent." Other factors are more personal, such as family considerations, location of the practice, and financial concerns. Opportunities for career development are important as well—practitioners are more likely to stay if there are research or faculty appointment/teaching possibilities, for example. There has

Table 4-4. Contributing Factors to Provider Turnover and Discontent (Snider, 1997)

Lack of autonomy
Inability to impact work environment
High workload
Long hours
Lack of control over time/schedule at work
Difficulty balancing home/work life

been no association between turnover and gender, age, marital status, race, or previous practice experience (Misra-Hebert, 2004).

Provider Well-being: A Win-Win for Practitioners and Patients

No matter what the job, it seems intuitive that the happier a worker is, the higher quality of work he/she produces. In medicine, not only does this hold true, but it also impacts the patient's experience, quality of care, thoroughness of care, and how well the patient adheres to the plan of care. In pediatrics, when the provider models positive self-care, it affects the patient and the entire family (Table 4-5).

Studies show that when physicians are "professionally satisfied" in their work, they provide better quality of care and produce more patient satisfaction (Haas, 2001). A national physician survey of 2325 doctors showed an association between having greater control over the workplace with higher emphasis on quality of care (Williams, 2002).

Physicians' global job satisfaction was also related to their patients' overall compliance with their treatment plans. This study's intriguing conclusion demonstrated the power of the provider–patient relationship: "This study is one of the few to demonstrate that how clinicians feel about their work can influence something as clinically significant as whether their patients carry out instructions, and it is the only study of which we are aware to link physicians' job satisfaction with patient actions that are critical to the management of their chronic diseases" (DiMatteo, 1993).

Table 4-5. Provider Wellness and Impact on Patient Care

When physicians are "professionally satisfied" in their work, they provide better quality of care and produce more patient satisfaction (Haas, 2001).

Primary care physicians who had good personal health habits provided better preventative medicine counseling and screenings for their patients (Frank, 2000).

Practitioners' personal disclosure of their own healthy diet and exercise patterns are more motivating and more believable regarding diet and exercise (Frank, 2000).

High job satisfaction and greater control over the workplace correlate with increased emphasis on quality of care (Williams, 2002).

When physicians are satisfied with their work, their patients are more compliant with their treatment plans (DiMatteo, 1993).

Satisfied and less stressed physicians have less job turnover, less health complaints and less disability claims (Haas, 2001).

Patients receive better care when physicians are not feeling depressed or burned out (Shanafeldt, 2002; Snider, 1997).

Even the practitioners' own personal healthcare plays a role in providing the best care for their patients! One study showed that primary care physicians who had good personal health habits provided better preventative medicine counseling and screenings for their patients. This study reports:

> This is one of the first demonstrations that physicians' personal health habits are more strongly and consistently correlated with related prevention activities than are many other personal and professional variables... If we value disease prevention, and if physicians' personal health practices are consistent predictors of their likelihood to be more active preventionists, we ought to try to cultivate healthy physicians (in undergraduate, graduate education and in CME). (Frank, 2000)

Another study showed patients health education videotapes about diet and exercise with and without a physician's personal disclosure of her own healthy diet and exercise patterns. Patients in the personal disclosure video group thought the physician was more motivating and more believable regarding diet and exercise (Frank, 2000).

To effectively model healthy habits, lifestyles, and preventative health care, we need to practice what we preach! Pediatricians are more likely to have a primary care provider than pathologists, internists, and other specialists, but studies show that 35%–56% of physicians do not have their own personal doctor, 28% do not have regular medical care, and 7% self treat. This is not due to younger practitioner age—the mean age in one study was 61 years old! "Physician, heal thyself" is not adequate when it comes to routine healthcare maintenance for healthcare professionals. As would be expected, those physicians without a regular provider were less likely to have been screened for colon, breast, and prostate cancer (Gross, 2000).

Staying Ahead of the Darkness: Preventing Burnout

Burnout in healthcare providers has been widely studied, with rates among practicing physicians ranging from 25% to 60%. Physicians with burnout have increased self-reports of suboptimal patient care (Shanafeldt, 2002). Far from being issues when a practitioner is in the prime of his/her career, depression, stress and other burnout criteria start in residency (and likely in medical school, although studies are lacking in this area). Christina Maslach, who created the Maslach Burnout Inventory, defines burnout as having three interlinked components: emotional exhaustion, depersonalization, and decreased personal accomplishment (Maslach, 1986). Certain personality traits in physicians have been identified that may increase the risk of burnout, including low self-esteem, feelings of inadequacy, dysphoria, obsessive worry, social anxiety, passivity, and withdrawal from others (McCranie, 1988). The top six factors felt to be most contributory to burnout are the same factors highlighted in provider discontent: lack of autonomy/managed care, inability to impact work environment, long hours, high workload, no control over time, and difficulty in juggling personal and professional life (Snider, 1997).

Breaking the "Culture of Silence"

Sharing difficult professional experiences with another colleague may seem at first to be extremely difficult because of the medical culture in which we are immersed. Sharing a difficult situation and asking for help has long been seen as revealing personal and professional weakness. It is important to transcend this barrier, to realize that this is one of the biggest façades in medicine, and to realize that the culture will only change as much as individual providers are willing to risk connecting with each other. Thankfully,

Table 4-6. Resources for Personal Wellness/Healing Healthcare

Resource	Type of Resource	Contact information
Circle of Healers, Humanistic Medicine Resources	Retreats, website resources for medical students	www.amsa.org/humed/
Schwartz Center Rounds	Multi-disciplinary Rounds on relationship-centered care in various hospitals around the country	http://www.theschwartzcenter.org/programs/index.html
Gold Foundation	Foundation that supports programs in medical education for humanism in medicine	www.humanism-in-medicine.org
Doctoring to Heal	Healthcare provider group-narrative writing	See article Rabow, 2001 for instruction on creating a group
Balint Groups	Interactive provider-led group usually focusing on doctor–patient interactions	www.balint.co.uk
Institute for the Study of Health and Healing (ISHI)	Workshops/retreats	www.commonweal.org/ishi
Finding Meaning in Medicine	Support group with set topics, incorporating story-telling, sharing, and reflection	On-line group available Resources/ in person group information available at www.meaninginmedicine.org
The Association of Healing Healthcare Advocates	Organization that inspires and supports healthcare models that exemplify human caring and healing	www.healinghealthcareassoc.org
American Academy on Physician and Patient		www.physicianpatient.org

(continued)

Table 4-6. (Continued)

Resource	Type of Resource	Contact information
Harmony Hill	Retreats for healthcare providers (esp. nurses) who work with cancer patients	www.harmonyhill.org/retreats/healthprof.html
Explorations in Work/Practice Options	AMA-AAP joint website with tools to assess work/practice options	www.ama-assn.org/go/workpracticeoptions
Pediatric Physician Health/Wellness website of AAP with excellent articles by Hanna Sherman	AAP website	http://practice.aap.org under Practice Basics
Finding Balance in a Medical Life (Dr. Lee Lipsenthal)	Retreats/programs for physicians, nurses, therapists, office staff, family of healthcare providers	www.findingbalanceproductions.com

there are now many formal and informal programs supporting this connection (see Table 4-6). The "new model" of medicine is based on relationship-centered care—for our patients and for each other, with the intention that "dis-ease" on a professional or personal level be addressed early on.

Burnout and depression, if not addressed may lead to drastic acts such as suicide. Although it is difficult to compile suicide data for healthcare providers, rates for physicians have always been higher than those for the general population. One of the more recent estimates is from a 1990 study that showed that physicians have 2.3 times the risk of death by suicide compared to the general population (Stack, 2001). There does not seem to be a difference across specialties, although there is a striking gender difference: female physicians have suicide rates that are four times higher than the general female population. In a 1980–1988 study, suicide was found to be the most common cause of death in young physicians, accounting for 26% of deaths (Samkoff, 1995). More recently, attention has turned to early recognition and treatment of mood disorders in healthcare providers, with removing barriers to seeking care. Physicians have traditionally been reluctant to seek professional help because of the potential of future problems with medical licensing, hospital privileges, and professional advancement (Center, 2003).

Abuse of drugs and alcohol is another way in which stress, burnout, and depression may manifest. Physicians have an increased risk of prescription drug abuse in comparison to the rest of the population (O'Connor, 1997). The "culture of silence" in medicine is such that often colleagues are unaware that a provider is in difficulty until they overdose—in one study, 18% of individuals died or almost died before substance abuse was even suspected (Booth, 2002). The Federation of State Physician Health Programs

Table 4-7. Early signs of stress/burnout (Gautam, 2004)
Increased physical problems or illnesses
Increased problems with relationships
Iincreased negative thoughts or feelings about people or things that you used to enjoy
Increased unhealthy behaviors (either doing "bad" things or stopping good things)
The inability to continue to push oneself

(www.fsphp.org) has a list by state of the physician health programs that provide consultation and support to assist healthcare providers with a variety of mental health issues. Mandated reporting of impaired providers to the state medical board varies by state. Similar programs are in place for nurses as well, with similar issues around mandated reporting. In general, the focus is on returning the provider to active work after appropriate intervention and support is established.

Prevention of burnout requires self-knowledge and early intervention to identify and improve early signs of "dis-ease" well before signs and symptoms escalate. Dr. Mamta Gautam, in her book *IRONDOC*, highlights warning signs of stress (Table 4-7). These include increased physical problems or illnesses, increased problems with relationships, increased negative thoughts or feelings about people or things that you used to enjoy, increased unhealthy behaviors (either doing "bad" things or stopping good things!), and the inability to continue to push oneself (Gautam, 2004). It is important to recognize that the culture of medicine is changing and that the time for a "culture of silence" is past. When a provider identifies early warning signs like the above and actively takes steps to prevent burnout, everyone benefits. Taking action bolsters internal connection to self, re-establishing the possibility for healing. Rachael Naomi Remen describes it this way: "Part of our responsibility as professionals is to fight for our sense of meaning—against fatigue, numbness, overwork and unreasonable expectations—to find ways to strengthen it in ourselves and in each other…It has become vital to remember the essential nature of this work and renew our sense of calling to preserve the meaning of the work for ourselves and for those who will follow" (Remen, 2001).

Providers' Wellness Practices: What Makes a Difference?

Even though each practitioner may choose a different aspect of wellness to work on, it is still useful to look at what other providers have found helpful. Studies in providers' wellness practices are few but give us the opportunity to "not reinvent the wheel." It may also inspire one approach versus another or give new possibilities for daily "practice of well-being."

Table 4-8. Contributing Factors for Provider Wellness (Weiner, 1998, 2001)

Cultivating relationships (friends, family, spouse/significant other)

Spiritual/ religious activities (prayer, church activities)

Caring for self (vacations, exercise, counseling, hobbies, eating nutritious food, avoiding drugs/ alcohol)

Positive work practices

Autonomy

Able to control aspects of work environment (policies, schedule, work hours, etc.)

Creating meaning/satisfaction in work

Limiting work hours

Choosing particular type of medicine

Concentrating on success, having a positive attitude

One study, looking at predictors of psychological well-being among physicians, found that a high level of support from the practitioner's closest relationship, lower levels of practice stress, and the ability to maintain one's individual identity around family members were the most relevant factors (Weiner, 1998). This group of authors questioned why there is so much information about physician impairment but so little information on positive practices that physicians incorporate to improve their wellbeing. Their later study, which qualitatively assessed physicians' wellness promotion practices, found that responses clustered into five primary areas. The first was relationships, including involvement with community, family, friends, or colleagues. The second was religion or spirituality, participating in church activities, attending services, praying, or reading the Bible. The third was self-care, including various self-care actions such as taking vacation, exercising, meditating, having a hobby, being nutritionally mindful, avoiding drugs and alcohol, getting counseling and treatment for depression, and leaving unhealthy relationships. The fourth was work practices, including creating meaning and satisfaction from work, limiting, practice, or choosing a certain type of medical practice. The fifth was philosophical approaches, ranging from concentrating on success and being positive to creating and maintaining balance in one's life (Table 4-8) (Weiner, 2001).

The Power of Personal Narrative

Personal narrative (writing stories) was studied to see what experiences in physician's practices increased their sense of meaning and purpose of their work. Researchers identified common themes in narrative analyses of physicians' stories written during "Meaningful Experiences in Medicine" workshops. Three major themes emerged when stories were analyzed for commonalities in providers' professional experiences: a difference the provider made in someone's life, a connection made with a patient, and a change in the provider's perspective (Horowitz, 2003). This correlates nicely with the California Medical Association study, in which practitioners identified their relationships with their patients as the greatest source of their satisfaction (CMA, 2001).

One simple way of "doing" narrative is to "journal"—taking time (5–10 minutes or longer if desired) to write about something concerning your work—a good day, a bad event, a connection. The possibilities are endless. Since this writing is only for you, it can take any form you like…structured sentences or free form, prose or poetry. Often writing can tap into our emotions, and can be a wonderful outlet for stress. It may be surprising or humorous, sad or joyful.

A daily practice that healthcare providers might use as a way to connect with their own meaningful work experiences is highlighted by Rachael Remen in one story from her book, *My Grandfather's Blessings*. Three questions may be used as a journaling tool, as in the story, or simply as a personal ritual for daily meditation or reflection: "What surprised me today? What moved or touched me today? What inspired me today?" (Remen, 2000).

Writing has been used in groups of physicians and medical students as well. Its power lies in breaking the medical "culture of silence" as common experiences are identified and shared. "Doctoring to Heal," started by Michael Rabow and Stephen McPhee in 1996, is an easily established personal reflection program where providers' written narratives about clinical experiences around a set topic are shared and discussed. Practitioners who have participated in the "Doctoring to Heal" program report a strengthening of their personal and professional identity, improved connectedness with their colleagues, gleaning useful techniques for their practice from others' experiences, and improved balance and wellbeing (Rabow, 2001). The referenced article gives examples and instructions on how to start a "Doctoring to Heal" group, and could easily be adapted for other healthcare providers as well.

THE BENEFITS OF SPIRITUALITY

Spirituality and religion have traditionally been tricky topics in medicine. Physicians feel ill-prepared to talk about spiritual issues, and in pediatrics there is the added concern about age-appropriate spiritual beliefs and family culture. Although physicians struggle with how and when (and even if it is appropriate) to include a discussion of spirituality in medical care, a *Newsweek* poll showed that 72%of Americans say they would welcome a conversation with their physician about faith (Kalb, 2004). Other studies have corroborated this as well. Although end-of-life care in adults routinely addresses spiritual beliefs and care, pediatric critical and end-of-life care have not incorporated spirituality as fully as might be useful. This is now being addressed in the pediatric literature.

There are distinct differences between spirituality and religion; one definition of spirituality that highlights the difference between the two is:

> Religion organizes the collective spiritual experiences of a group of people into a system of beliefs and practices...Spirituality is a broader concept than religion and is primarily a dynamic, personal, and experiential process. Features of spirituality include quest for meaning and purpose, transcendence (the sense that being human is more than simple material existence), connectedness (eg, with others, nature, or the divine), and values (eg, love, compassion, and justice)." (Mueller, 2001)

Religion is thus a formal practice of spirituality. Rachael Naomi Remen describes the essence of the spiritual realm in the following way:

> The spiritual is inclusive. It is the deepest sense of belonging and participation. We all participate in the spiritual at all times, whether we know it or not...The most important thing in defining spirit is the recognition that the spirit is an essential need of human nature. There is something in all of us that seeks the spiritual. This yearning varies in strength from person to person but it is always there in everyone. And so, healing becomes possible. (Remen, 1998)

Spirituality and religion may be very good medicine personally for the healthcare provider. Studies have shown that people who are involved in religious activities live longer; have less cardiovascular disease and hypertension; have less risk of depression, anxiety, substance abuse, and suicide; and have better coping skills with illness (Mueller, 2001).

SPIRITUALITY IN PEDIATRICS

When a pediatric practitioner has religious or spiritual beliefs and/or practices, they are more likely to talk with patients and families about spirituality and to have their beliefs influence their treatment plans (especially in one study of neonatal intensivists). In one study of pediatric oncologists, 85% of them described themselves as spiritual, incorporating such activities as prayer, the reading of sacred texts, and attending religious services. Over half believed that their spiritual and/or religious beliefs influenced their interactions with their pediatric oncology patients and their colleagues (Ecklund, 2007). However, another study has shown a "spiritual paradox," in that while 76% of pediatricians thought their patients'/families' spirituality and/or religion were relevant to their practice, over half never or rarely talked with their patients/families about their spiritual/religious beliefs. Those who received formal training in addressing religious/spiritual issues with patients in residency were more likely to talk with their patients, but only 13% reported such training. Increase of formal training in residency programs may not be the solution, as it seems that the main criteria for whether a practitioner incorporates spiritual assessment into the clinical setting depends on the personal spiritual/religious life of the pediatrician! (Grossoehme, 2007). Other barriers to providing "psychosocial spiritual care" (PSS) particularly in end-of-life care, were identified by groups of primary care providers, including pediatricians. These included a culture of medicine that did not support empathic processing (for the provider) of end-of life experiences with their patients, time for adequate discussion of spirituality/religion with patients/ families, and a training system that sees PSS as a "soft" subject in medical school. After training, the medical practice environment was seen as equally challenging, with its lack of time to engage in emotionally challenging conversations, lack of reimbursement, provider dissatisfaction, and risk of emotional investment (Chibnall, 2004).

SPIRITUALITY AND HEALING VERSUS CURING

When a clinician is able to hold the larger viewpoint and context that spirituality provides, the concept of healing versus curing emerges. There may be many rich opportunities to be present and to be of service to a "noncurable" patient and their family in ways that facilitate healing, such as coming to terms with illness (in age appropriate ways), supporting constructive and positive family dynamics, helping siblings, and providing comfort care during the dying process for physical symptoms. This can be healing to practitioner, patient, and family alike.

These concepts were the foundation for the creation of Aggressive Comfort Care (ACT) in pediatric palliative care. It was created in response to the many children with chronic life-threatening disorders or cancer who were continuing to undergo curative medical treatments, tests and procedures, despite their end-stage disease process. Realizing that parents would never want to "withdraw" medical care or treatments for their child, ACT is a full-scale, patient-centered approach to palliative care. It is an aggressive approach to symptom management in the most non-invasive way possible that provides integrative mind-body-spirit care to the child and family. Psychosocial and spiritual needs are acknowledged in a variety of age-appropriate ways and play a large role in encouraging the individual to "discuss their fears, concerns and distress about the dying process while also enabling them to find meaning and purpose in the experience" (Calabrese, 2007). The ACT approach could be taught and incorporated into pediatric residency and fellowship programs, allowing for mentoring and skills development in palliative care as well as emphasis on the importance of spirituality and attention to psychosocial spiritual care for pediatric patients.

SPIRITUAL WELLNESS: THE BIG PICTURE

The practitioner's spiritual wellness can play a particular supportive role in self-care. Spirituality can increase our sense of connectedness, meaning, and purpose and create opportunities for transcendent experiences (ones that extend beyond the usual limits of ordinary experience). For pediatric practitioners who work with critically ill or chronically ill children, the spiritual element may help with the stressors inherent in their practice: communicating bad news, being witness to suffering, coping with patients' and families' emotional reactions, and working with terminally ill and dying patients. Many physicians feel a sense of isolation, not helped by the "culture of silence" in medicine, as they cope with their own emotions of grief, loss, and pain daily. Having a "spiritual outlet," in addition to other wellness practices, may be a way to constructively cope and thrive in the midst of these intense life experiences. Taking time to reflect on transcendent experiences in medical practice, whether through journaling, prayer, personal reflection, groups such as "Doctoring to Heal," or art, can provide a different and vastly larger context and viewpoint for daily work and life. For some providers, this recognition and "self-honoring" of their work can prevent creation of less useful coping mechanisms, such as becoming hardened and callous, clinical, and brusque.

Cultivating spiritual wellness is intensely personal. One medical model for inquiring about patients' and families' spirituality, the HOPE Questions, can be used as a starting point for providers' self-inquiry as well. The first step (**H**) is to assess basic spiritual resources, and identify sources of **h**ope, meaning, comfort, strength, peace, love and connection. The second and third steps (**O** and **P**) identify any use of **o**rganized religion and/or **p**ersonal spirituality and **p**ractices. The fourth step (**E**), in patients is used to assess the **e**ffects of personal spirituality and practices on their medical care and end-of-life issues (Anandarajah, 2001). In spiritual self-care for the provider, the fourth step could be used in a variety of ways, from inquiry into how spirituality might be an asset in their clinical care to how it could be used personally as a source of connection and renewal.

Creating Healthcare from "Sickcare": An Invitation

The need for transformation in medicine is not new. In 1978, Dale Garell posed a question: "Can we learn a way of life that not only minimizes the "risk" of being a physician, but also maximizes the opportunity to provide the highest quality of medical care while at the same time encouraging our own satisfaction and professional and personal development?" (Garell, 1978). It is clear that if healthcare practitioners take their own wellbeing out of the practice of medicine, everyone suffers. As Zeev Neuwirth, an internist, states so succinctly: "If we are physically, emotionally and spiritually exhausted, it is unlikely that we will be able to provide the type of medical care and healing that our patients want and need" (Neuwirth, 2002). But this challenge may seem like an impossible task. How do we teach and incorporate body/mind/spirit wellness into our practices and medical school or residency curricula when we are stuck between a rock (time, finances) and a hard place (patient care)? In addition, how do we teach that which we struggle with in our own lives to our patients and students? We need the best parts of ourselves—the creative, compassionate, flexible, caring, determined parts—to create ways to circumvent the impossibility of the medical system. Compassion for ourselves is the first step, recognizing that it takes a different sort of discipline and focus to create a healthy lifestyle as a healthcare provider today (Table 4-9). Introspection via self-assessment is the second step to determine where to start, since many areas of wellness may lack attention: "What would nurture me the most? What would allow me

Table 4-9. Questions for Self-assessment and Reflection (Neuwirth, 2002; Remen, 2000)

What would nurture me the most?

What would allow me to personally and professionally grow?

What would help me to sustain the day-to-day challenges and to connect with my work's meaning?

How do I define health and healing?

What is my personal philosophy toward health and healing?

How do my behaviors and relationships reflect and represent those values?

What values would I want my patients and colleagues to recognize in my behaviors?

What might I do to increase the likelihood of those values being expressed?

to personally and professionally grow? What would help me to sustain the day-to-day challenges and to connect with my work's meaning?" (Remen, 2000). Zeev Neuwirth uses these and other questions as a way to further this introspection, emphasizing the need to re-evaluate our personal philosophies toward medicine and healing: "How do I define health and healing? How do my behaviors and relationships reflect and represent those values? What values would I want my patients and colleagues to recognize in my behaviors? What might I do to increase the likelihood of those values being expressed?" (Neuwirth, 2002).

It may well be, as the Association for Healing Healthcare Advocates' motto states, that as we heal ourselves, we in turn heal our relationships and our communities (AHHCA, 2008). When each provider commits to their own healing and wellness in mind, body, spirit, and relationship, the choices and changes created extend beyond the individual into the larger domain of their medical practice and community circles. The provider becomes a role model and inspiration for positive change for colleagues, family, patients, the practice, and the larger medical community.

Healing Healthcare: Guiding Principles

Because of limited time and resources, it is useful to not "reinvent the wheel" when taking on transformation, whether on a personal, professional, or institutional level. There are many groups that are actively working on wellness issues from the perspective of transforming the healthcare environment. One working group, in addressing these issues, created a list of guidelines entitled, "Principles to Transform Healthcare." (Principles, 2004) These principles are described as being "a distillation of the wisdom of the many members of the Association of Healing Health Care Projects and the Relationship-Centered Care Network [Fetzer Institute]" (Table 4-10).

Table 4-10. Principles to Transform Healthcare: Healing Healthcare
and Relationship-Centered Care (2004)

Create caring relationships. Acknowledge the importance of self-awareness, self-care, and self-growth. Beginning with self, establish an ethic of love, forgiveness, unconditional positive regard, and service; then extend this ethic as the core of all relationships in health care. Develop these relationships to sustain health of self, patients, heath care team, organization, community, and environment.

Respect each person's experience as valid. Respect the practice of relationship-centered care and healing health care in all its unique representations, without bias toward or against any religion, race, sex, position or rank, community, or culture. All change toward creating health and healing is valued, great or small.

Respect the person's own power and self-healing processes. Place control with the person receiving the care. Appreciate the patient's meaning of the health-illness condition, and base care on his or her needs and values.

Value and practice personal responsibility for health, intentions, and actions. Individual lifestyle choices, actions, and practices largely determine the outcome of health. Provide information to support the person/patient in being an informed decision-maker.

Honor the sacred. Pay attention to and respect the most precious aspects of each person and place. Respect the person's dignity, uniqueness, and integrity (mind-body-spirit unity). Create sanctuary—space and time to reconnect with wholeness and something greater than oneself. Honor the ancient as well as the visionary.

Hold economic models responsible and accountable to the outcome of health. Acknowledge and attend to the relationship between wise use of economic resources and health.

Adopt an attitude and practice of continuous learning and improvement. Challenge ideas; remain open-minded and receptive to innovation and experimentation; respond to the changing environment with unchanging commitment to these principles.

Connect with others. Build and sustain conscious connections/partnerships with other individuals and groups who share this intention for transforming health care.

Create a compelling vision that is inclusive of all providers and citizens. Respect the integrity of the community, and participate actively in community development and dialogue. A sustained intention with action for the wellbeing of others endures all obstacles.

Start now, act locally, keep going, and support each other. Many local actions are global action—the transformation of health care.

Create caring relationships. Acknowledge the importance of self-awareness, self-care, and self-growth. Beginning with self, establish an ethic of love, forgiveness, unconditional positive regard, and service; then extend this ethic as the core of all relationships in health care. Develop these relationships to sustain health of self, patients, heath care team, organization, community, and environment.

Respect each person's experience as valid. Respect the practice of relationship-centered care and healing health care in all its unique representations, without bias toward or against any religion, race, sex, position or rank, community, or culture. All change toward creating health and healing is valued, great or small.

Respect the person's own power and self-healing processes. Place control with the person receiving the care. Appreciate the patient's meaning of the health-illness condition, and base care on his or her needs and values.

Value and practice personal responsibility for health, intentions, and actions. Individual lifestyle choices, actions, and practices largely determine the outcome of health. Provide information to support the person/patient in being an informed decision-maker.

Honor the sacred. Pay attention to and respect the most precious aspects of each person and place. Respect the person's dignity, uniqueness, and integrity (mind-body-spirit unity). Create sanctuary—space and time to reconnect with wholeness and something greater than oneself. Honor the ancient as well as the visionary.

Hold economic models responsible and accountable to the outcome of health. Acknowledge and attend to the relationship between wise use of economic resources and health.

Adopt an attitude and practice of continuous learning and improvement. Challenge ideas; remain open-minded and receptive to innovation and experimentation; respond to the changing environment with unchanging commitment to these principles.

Connect with others. Build and sustain conscious connections/partnerships with other individuals and groups who share this intention for transforming health care.

Create a compelling vision that is inclusive of all providers and citizens. Respect the integrity of the community, and participate actively in community development and dialogue. A sustained intention with action for the wellbeing of others endures all obstacles.

Start now, act locally, keep going, and support each other. Many local actions are global action—the transformation of health care.

These principles are the basis of a new model of healthcare, one based in relationships. They promote ethical service given with the highest professional and personal regard for others in a way that creates and supports conscious connections with other transformers of healthcare. Economic responsibility for the wise use and allocation of healthcare finances is championed, and care is given based on respect for the individual and their personal experience and needs. Healthcare is provided with emphasis on lifestyle-based personal responsibility for health, and honors the sacred in the body/mind/spirit interface. Being committed to holding a vision of healing healthcare in constantly changing healthcare environments is paramount, with continuous learning, improvement, innovation and experimentation as core expressions for healing healthcare throughout the institution.

Holding the Vision of Wellness: Doing the Work

We are the ones we have been waiting for.

—*Hopi Elder*

Once a provider is committed to honoring personal wellness as a way to further his/her professional work, there are many avenues to explore. Table 4-6 is a list of resources that can be tailored to an individual's choice on where to start. Many practitioners are already incorporating healing healthcare into their practices; others often ask "How do I know if I am 'doing' the work?" Healthcare providers who are holding the vision of a "new model" of healing healthcare may have work "discontent" and see where the gaps are in patient care, professional satisfaction or personal life. They may be the "rabble-rousers" or "ruckus-creators" in the practice, or may be the "go-to" person in the group. Anyone with *any* job description in healthcare, can hold the vision and do this work—secretaries, janitorial staff, dietary aides, nursing assistants, medical and nursing students, lab techs, and on and on. Anywhere there is human interaction, there is potential for creating a relationship to further healing. When providers work together to create interprofessional and institutional support for wellbeing, the possibility emerges for the entire medical system to change.

Not only is transformation of medical culture and practice possible, it is inevitable. Care must be taken so that further changes in the way heath care is practiced and delivered support the wellbeing of all practitioners, which in turn will reinforce excellent patient and family care. In his poem "Two Tramps in Mud Time," Robert Frost writes "Only where love and need are one, and the work is play for mortal stakes, is the deed ever really done for Heaven and the future's sakes."

Learning how to sustain and nurture ourselves in today's escalating demands of medical practice is a requirement for sustainable medical care, not a privilege or selfish act. In the world today, the "mortal stakes" have never been higher—for patients or providers.

Bullet Points/ "Take-home" Points

- Know what your personal stressors are and look for early signs of stress. Intervene before burnout occurs.
- Choose one area of wellness to focus on first.
- What are the qualities of your medical practice that support your happiness and well-being?
- Wellness is a fluctuating integrative concept that spans physical, emotional, spiritual, institutional, and collegial realms. Expect that when you personally affect one of these areas, that the others will start to shift in positive ways too.

- Model respectful and caring interactions with peers—help break the "culture of silence" in medicine.
- Take care of your physical well-being with regular medical and dental care. Establish care with a primary care provider if you do not have one currently.
- Consider sharing the article "When the Patient is a Doctor: Becoming an Effective Physician's Physician" with your personal healthcare providers (Kaufman, 1998).
- Consider a daily journaling practice or starting a narrative group, such as "Doctoring to Heal."

REFERENCES

Anandarajah, G., & Hight, E. (2001). Spirituality and medical practice: Using the HOPE questions as a practical tool for spiritual assessment. *American Family Physician, 63*(1), 86.

Anderson, M. R., Jewett, E. A., Cull, W. L., Jardine, D. S., Outwater, K. M., & Mulvey, H. J. (2003). Practice of pediatric critical care medicine: Results of the Future of Pediatric Education II Survey of Sections Project. *Pediatric Critical Care Medicine, 4*(4), 412–417.

Ardell, D. B., & Langdon, J. G. (1989). *Wellness: The body, mind and spirit.* Dubuque, Iowa: Kendall/Hunt Publishing Company.

Arizona State University, Wellness Definition. ©Arizona Board of Regents, 2000.

The Association of Healing Healthcare Advocates. Retrieved May 10, 2008, from www.healinghealthcareassoc.org

Booth, J. V., Grossman, D., Moore, J., Lineberger, C., Reynolds, J. D., Reves, J. G., et al. (2002). Substance abuse among physicians: A survey of academic anesthesiology programs. *Anesthesia and Analgesia, 95*(4), 1024–1030.

Buchbinder, S. B., Wilson, M., & Melick, C. F., & Powe, N. R. (1999). Estimates of costs of primary care physician turnover. *The American Journal of Managed Care, 5*, 1431–1438.

Calabrese, C. L. (2007). ACT—for pediatric palliative care. *Pediatric Nursing, 33*(6), 532–534.

California Medical Association. And then there were none: The coming physician supply problem. ©2001 CMA. Retrieved April 24, 2008, from www.cmanet.org/upload/Physician_Supply_(Acrobat).pdf

Center, C., Davis, M., Detre, T., Hansbrough, W., Hendin, H., Laszlo, J., et al. (2003). Confronting depression and suicide in physicians: A consensus statement. *Journal of the American Medical Association, 289*(23), 3161–3166.

Chibnall, J., Bennett, M. L., Videen, S., Duckro, P. N., & Miller, D. K. (2004). Identifying barriers to psychosocial spiritual care at the end of life: A physician study group. *American Journal of Hospice & Palliative Medicine, 21*(6), 419–426.

Dawson, D., & Reid, K. (1997). Fatigue, alcohol and performance impairment. *Nature, 388*, 235.

DiMatteo, M. R., Shelbourne, R. D., Hays, L., Ordway, L., Kravitz, R. L., & McGlynn, E. A. (1993). Physicians' characteristics influence patients' adherence to medical treatment: Results from the Medical Outcomes Study. *Health Psychology, 12*(2), 100.

Ecklund, E. H., Cadge, W., Gage, E., & Catlin, E. A. (2007). The religious and spiritual beliefs and practices of academic pediatric oncologists in the United States. *Journal of pediatric hematology/oncology, 29*(11), 736–742.

Fetzer Institute: Definition of relationship-centered care. Retrieved from July 1, 2004 from www.fetzer.org/rcc

Frank, E. (1995). The women physicians' health study: Background, objectives and methods. *Journal of the American Medical Women's Association, 50*, 64–66.

Frank, E., Breyan, J., & Elon, L. (2000). Physician disclosure of healthy personal behaviors improves credibility and ability to motivate. *Archives of Family Medicine, 9*, 287–290.

Frank, E., Rothenberg, R., Lewis, C., & Belodoff, B. (2000). Correlates of physicians' prevention-related practices. *Archives of Family Medicine, 9*, 359–367.

Garell, D. C. (1978). Some reflections on physicians' well-being. *New Physician 27*(4), 32–33.

Gautam, M. (2004). *IRONDOC: Practical Stress Management Tools for Physicians.* Book Coach Press, Ottawa, ON, Canada, 2004.

Gross, C. P., Mead, L. A., Ford, D. E., & Klag M. J. (2000). Physician, heal thyself? Regular source of care and use of preventive health services among physicians. *Archives of Internal Medicine, 160,* 3212.

Grossoehme, D. H., Ragsdale, J. R., McHenry, C. L., Thurston, C., DeWitt, T., & VandeCreek, L. (2007). Pediatrician characteristics associated with attention to spirituality and religion in clinical practice. *Pediatrics, 119*(1), e117–e123.

Haas, J. S. (2001). Physician discontent: A barometer of change and need for intervention. *Journal of General Internal Medicine, 16*(7), 496–497.

Hendrie, H. P., Claire, D. K., Brittain, H. M., & Fadul, P. E. (1990). A study of anxiety/depressive symptoms of medical students, housestaff and their spouses/partners. *Journal of Nervous and Mental Disease, 178,* 204–207.

Horowitz, C. R., Suchman, A. L., Branch, Jr., W. T., & Frankel, R. M. (2003). What do doctors find meaningful about their work? *Annals of Internal Medicine, 138*(9), 772–775.

Kahn, J., Degen, S., Mansour, M., Goodman, E., Zeller, M. H., Laor, T., et al. (2005). Pediatric faculty members' attitudes about part-time faculty positions and policies to support part-time faculty: A study at one medical center. *Academic Medicine, 80,* 931–939.

Kalb, C. (2003). "Faith and Healing" *Newsweek.* Retrieved September 27, 2004, from http://msnbc.msn.com/id/3339654/site/newsweek/

Kaufman, M. (1998). When the patient is a doctor: Becoming an effective physician's physician. *Ontario Medical Review, 65,* 50–51.

Landrigan, C. P., Rothschild, J. M., Cronin, J. W., Kaushal, R., Burdick, E., Katz, J. T., et al. (2004). Effect of reducing interns' work hours on serious medical errors in intensive care units. *New England Journal of Medicine, 351*(18), 1838–1848.

Lipsenthal, L. (2007). *Finding balance in a medical life,* From http://www.findingbalanceproductions.com/product_detail.asp?ProductID=74356&SessionID={32DF80CB-BEDB-4C2F-A3B5-8618ED4A1B65

Marvel, M. K., Epstein, R. M., Flowers, K., & Beckman, H. B. (1999). Soliciting the patient's agenda: Have we improved? *Journal of the American Medical Associatio, 281*(3), 283–287.

Maslach, C., & Jackson, S. E. (1986). *Maslach burnout inventory—manual* (2nd ed.). Palo Alto, CA: CPP/Consulting Psychologists Press.

McCranie, E. W., & Brandsma, J. M. (Spring 1988). Personality antecedents of burnout among middle-aged physicians. *Behavioral Medicine, 67*(4), 30–36.

Miller, M. N., McGowen, K. R., & Quillen, J. H. (2000) The painful truth: Physicians are not invincible. *Southern Medical Journal, 93*(10), 966–973.

Misra-Hebert, A., Kay, R., & Stoller, J. K. (2004). A review of physician turnover: Rates, causes, and consequences. *American Journal of Medical Quality, 19*(2), 56–66.

Mueller, P. S., Plevak, D. J., & Rummans, T. A. (2001). Religious involvement, spirituality, and medicine: Implications for clinical practice. *Mayo Clinic Proceedings, 76*, 1225.

Neuwirth, Z. E. (January 2002). Reclaiming the lost meanings of medicine. *Medical Journal of Australia, 176*(2), 78.

O'Conner, P. G., & Spickard, A. (1997). Physician impairment by substance abuse. *Medical Clinics of North America, 81*, 1037–1052.

Ostbye, T., Yarnall, K. S., Krause, K. M., Pollak, K. I., Gradison, M., & Michener, J. L. (2005). Is there time for management of patients with chronic diseases in primary care? *Annals of Family Medicine, 3*, 209–214.

"Principles to Transform Health Care: Healing Health Care and Relationship-Centered Care" From Impasse to Breakthrough: A National Summit. Retrieved August 13, 2004, from http://www.breakthroughsummit.org/principles.cfm

Rabow, M. W., & McPhee, S. J. (2001). Doctoring to heal: Fostering wellbeing among physicians through personal reflection. *Western Journal of Medicine, 174*, 68–69.

Remen, R. N. (2001). Recapturing the soul of medicine. *Wesernt Journal Medicine, 174*, 4–5.

Remen, R. N. (2000). *My grandfather's blessings: Stories of strength, refuge and belonging* (pp. 116–119). New York: Riverhead Books.

Remen, R. N. (Winter 1998). On defining spirit. *Noetic Sciences Review, 47*, 64. Retrieved September 28, 2004, from http://www.noetic.org/publications/review/issue47/r47_Remen%20.html

Rollman, B. L., Mead, L. A., Wang, N., & Klag, M. J. (1997). Medical specialty and the incidence of divorce. *New England Journal of Medicine, 336*(11), 800–803.

Samkoff, J. S., Hockenberry, S., Simon, L. J., & Jones R. L. (1995). Mortality of young physicians in the United States, 1980–1988. *Academic Medcine, 70*, 242–244.

Schwartz, A. J., Black, E. R., Goldstein, M. G., Jozefowicz, R. F., & Emmings, F. G. (1987). Levels and causes of stress among residents. *Journal of Medical Education, 62*, 744–753.

Shanafelt, T. D., Bradley, K. A., Wipf, J. E., & Back, A. L. (2002). Burnout and self-reported patient care in an internalm residency program. *Annals of Internal Medicine, 136*(5), 358.

Shugarman, R., Linzer, M., Nelson, K., Douglas, J., Williams, R., Konrad, R.; Career Satisfaction Study Group. (2001). Pediatric generalists and subspecialists: determinants of career satisfaction. *Pediatrics. 108*(3), E40. Retrieved April 19, 2008, from www.peds.org/cgi/content/full/108/3/e40

Snider, M., & Svenko, D. (January 1997). *The physician burnout project*. Sacramento, CA: El Dorado-Sacramento Medical Society.

Sotile, W. M., & Sotile, M. O. (1996). *The medical marriage: A couple's survival guide*. New York: Carol Publishing.

Stack, S. (June 2001). Occupation and suicide. *Social Science Quarterly, 82*(2), 392.

University of Arizona PIM Definition of Integrative Medicine. ©Program in Integrative Medicine, University of Arizona, 2003.

Waldman, J. D., Kelly, F., Aurora, S., & Smith, H. L. (2004). The shocking cost of turnover in health care. *Health Care Management Review, 29*(1), 2–7.

Weiner, E. L., Swain, G. R., & Gottlieb, M. (1998). Predictors of psychological wellbeing among physicians. *Families, Systems & Health, 16*, 419–430.

Weiner, E. L., Swain, G. R., & Gottlieb, M. (2001). A qualitative study of physicians' own wellness-promotion practices. *Westernal Journal of Medicine, 174*, 19–23.

Williams, E. S., Konrad, T. R., Linzer, M., McMurry, J., Pathman, D.E., Gerrity, M., et al. (2002). SGIM career satisfaction study group. *Health Services Research, 37*(1), 121–143.

World Health Organization: Preamble to the Constitution of the World Health Organization as adopted by the International Health Conference, New York, June 19–22, 1946; signed on July 22, 1946 by the representatives of 61 States (Official Records of the World Health Organization, no. 2, p. 100) and entered into force on April 7, 1948.

5

Research and Education in Integrative Pediatrics

SUNITA VOHRA AND TRISH DRYDEN

KEY CONCEPTS

- Research and education opportunities in pediatric integrative medicine abound. Collaboration between complementary and alternative medicine (CAM) and conventional providers, researchers, and educators may yield the greatest potential to ensure public safety, improve health, and increase the availability of qualified and knowledgeable CAM and conventional health care practitioners in pediatric integrative medicine.
- Research needs to expand beyond studies of utilization or efficacy, and assess safety and cost-effectiveness. Existing research networks can be utilized to address clinical questions, including identification of "best cases."
- Excellence should determine research funding, and phased step-wise approaches to clinical research are necessary. Understanding potential mechanism of action should not be a necessary prerequisite to conducting clinical research, as translational research in CAM may be "bedside to bench," rather than bench to bedside.
- Education in pediatric integrative medicine needs to foster and promote an evaluation culture across and within disciplines that is inclusive of research literacy and research capacity building skills, teacher education, and instructional methods and delivery models that enhance collaborative, child and family-centered practice, and evidence-informed approaches to ethical clinical decision-making.
- Building partnerships and sharing resources between and among CAM and conventional health care educators and researchers to

create opportunities for interprofessional education, networking and collaboration in-person and through innovative web-based programs, and simulation are key components of an effective education strategy.

■

Introduction

Integrative pediatrics is a new field, and there is a tremendous need for research and educational initiatives to help it grow. In this chapter, we identify gaps in knowledge and suggest topics and strategies to help address them. Multiple challenges and opportunities exist; some can be approached with methods that are tried and true, while others require innovation and collaboration between conventional and complementary providers, working together to achieve optimal health and healing for children. Since we are "looking ahead," our goal is to challenge researchers and educators with topics that have been relatively neglected, rather than recap successes to date.

In this chapter, we will use several related terms. For our purposes, complementary and alternative medicine (CAM) describes those practices and products currently outside mainstream conventional medicine; "integrative" refers to the coming together of conventional and complementary in a collaborative, mutually respectful fashion (Boon, Verhoef, O'Hara, & Findlay, 2004; National Center for Complementary and Alternative Medicine, 2007) and "interprofessional education" is when two or more professions learn with, from and about each other to improve collaboration and the quality of care (UK Centre for the Advancement of Interprofessional Education, 2007).

Research

Evidence of the safety and efficacy of individual CAM treatments is essential, but it represents just one facet of the research that is needed. For example, there is a paucity of clinical research that compares CAM therapies with each other or with conventional interventions. Very little research has been done on the cost-effectiveness of CAM. And although there is great opportunity for scientific discovery in the study of CAM treatments, it is an opportunity largely missed. Such investigations are hindered by shortages of established scientists engaged in CAM research, which tends to involve subject matter beyond the conventional scientist's knowledge base. CAM also needs a cadre of new junior researchers

—Committee on the Use of Complementary and Alternative
Medicine by the American Public, 2005.

To date, the most common form of research into pediatric CAM has been a pleth-ora of utilization studies. Dozens exist; more are underway. While the epidemiology of CAM use is helpful, the questions that are asked most often by patients and clinicians about any therapy are: Does it work? Is it safe? Apart from safety and efficacy, CAM researchers should consider evaluation of cost-effectiveness, as this is relevant to individuals as well as governments, insurance companies, and other payers. The long-term benefit of cost-effectiveness research may be that more CAM therapies are covered, reducing the financial burden on families who seek integrative care. Policy-makers are challenged to create evidence-based policy and clinical practice guidelines rely on best evidence—in both instances, CAM would benefit from rigorous safety, efficacy, and cost-effectiveness data.

In this section of the chapter, we review novel approaches to gathering evidence about the safety, efficacy, and cost-effectiveness of CAM. We also review the unique challenges faced by CAM researchers with regards to methodology, ethics, and funding.

SAFETY

Safety research involving conventional pharmaceuticals has revealed some important lessons that may be relevant to CAM researchers. Unlike efficacy, safety research demands a population-based approach. Since serious adverse events tend to be rare, clinical trials are usually not large enough to detect them (Barnes, 2003; Boudville et al., 2006; Shekelle, Adams, Chassin, Hurwitz, & Brook, 1992). Moreover, clinical trials are notorious for under-reporting harms (Papanikolaou, Christidi, & Ioannidis, 2006; Papanikolaou & Ioannidis, 2004). At present, serious adverse events are usually identified from passive post-marketing surveillance (i.e., relying on volunteers to identify and report potential harms) (Health Canada, 2007; US Food and Drug Administration, 2007). Passive surveillance to determine safety is impeded by vast under-reporting of potential adverse events (e.g., it is believed that only one in 10 serious drug-related adverse events is reported) (Alvarez-Requejo et al., 1998; Goldman, 1998; Hartmann, Doser, & Kuhn, 1999). Under-reporting of potential harms seems to be exaggerated for CAM products. For example, only one in 50 community pharmacists reported adverse events related to potential interactions between natural health products and prescription drugs (Charrois et al., 2007).

At present, safety data for CAM practices consist almost exclusively of case reports. Retrospective in nature, these reports have been of varying quality, and do not form the necessary foundation to determine causation. For example, when considering the most common pediatric CAM practice in North America, spinal manipulation, systematic review of adverse events identified only 14 reports, despite examining 8 major electronic databases from inception to 2004 (Vohra, Johnston, Cramer, & Humphreys, 2007). The review found that adverse events associated with pediatric spinal manipulation are either rare or they are under-reported. Inconclusive at best, this study points to an important gap in CAM research. Specifically, if this is the state of knowledge of safety for the most common of CAM therapies, there is considerable room for improvement.

Safety of popular CAM therapies is often assumed. Passive surveillance, relying primarily on voluntary case reports, grossly under-estimates harms. Given the widespread use of CAM, documenting safety is important and feasible.

Safety of CAM product use in children has also received little specific attention. A recent review of herb-drug interactions found an absence of pediatric pharmacokinetic trials even though natural health products and prescription medications are regularly used in children. In the absence of such studies, potential NHP-drug interactions are inferred on theoretical grounds from laboratory reports or (usually adult) case reports (Johnston & Vohra, 2005, 2006; Roth, Johnston, & Vohra, 2006).

Better ways to document safety exist. In particular, active surveillance "seeks to ascertain completely the number of adverse events via a continuous pre-organized process." This can be done with sentinel sites, drug event monitoring, or registries. In contrast to passive surveillance, active surveillance provides better quality data through both improved quantity and quality of adverse event reporting (Health Canada—ICH Steering Committee, 2003). The opportunities for CAM safety research are numerous, as pediatric data are lacking for most products and practices. As informed consent demands awareness of potential risks, there is an urgent need to accumulate this data.

Since CAM use is widespread, there is a tremendous opportunity to conduct community-based active surveillance to assess safety. When such research has been done, notably to assess the safety of acupuncture in adults, the results have been reassuring (MacPherson & Thomas, 2005; White, Hayhoe, Hart, & Ernst, 2001). It is particularly important that CAM professions not view safety research as a threat, but embrace it as an opportunity to document what they presume to be true. It is preferable to measure safety, not assume it (the absence of reported harms is not equivalent to data confirming safety). Prospective rigorous population-based safety data are more compelling than any amount of reassurances. Since CAM use is so common, it should not be unduly difficult for safety research to take place. With such data, it may be easier for integrative medicine programs to flourish, and for hospitals to consider including CAM within their suite of services.

A unique opportunity for translational research arises from CAM safety studies. In conventional medicine, "translational research" usually refers from bench to bedside, whereby basic science discoveries are applied for clinical use. Since clinical CAM use has far out-stripped basic science understanding, it is possible that CAM safety research could promote translational research in the opposite direction (i.e., bedside to bench). When potential CAM-related adverse events are identified, it is important they be examined by a multidisciplinary team with relevant content expertise to assess the likelihood of causation. If causal harms are identified, safety researchers should then focus on identifying potential mechanisms of action and strategies to mitigate risk. Adverse events could therefore inform potential mechanism of action, shedding new light on our understanding of how CAM "works."

> --
> Safety research affords new opportunities to understand the mechanism of action of some CAM therapies.
> --

It seems reasonable that therapies that have been examined for potential harms, and therefore have accurate risk assessments, should be promoted over those for which harms remain unknown, or poorly documented. Safety is relative, not absolute, and must always be considered in light of potential benefit for potential risks. There is no single right answer about healthcare decisions, but one that must be made in light of a given child's health state, as well as their family's health-related beliefs, priorities, and values.

EFFICACY

The challenge for CAM researchers to assess efficacy is that there are thousands of products and hundreds of practices, each potentially used for multiple conditions. Given the immense resources, time, and effort it would require, the current gold standard for assessing clinical efficacy, the randomized controlled trial (RCT), is simply not a practical approach to assess each potential intervention-condition pair. In this section, we will consider case-based research such as best case series and N-of-1 trials, as well as the advantages offered by collaborative research networks and mixed methods approaches.

Conventional pharmaceutical research is predicated on understanding mechanisms of action, and moving from Phase I to Phase III clinical trials in an orderly fashion before proceeding to routine clinical use. Since CAM use is already widespread amongst the general population, including children, it can capitalize on this through innovative approaches to identify efficacious therapies, such as best case series and N-of-1 trials.

Best case series describes an approach adopted by the National Cancer Institute (NCI) in 1991 to identify CAM therapies associated with tumor regression (NCI, 2006). Most often, CAM providers identify potential cases to NCI, which conducts a detailed investigation to identify the likelihood of a causal relationship. Best cases by definition are a biased sample, but if various providers independently report remarkable outcomes with the same intervention, it seems worthy of further consideration. Hypothesis-generating in nature, the best-case series has fulfilled this objective by identifying some promising therapies for more rigorous evaluation, such as the effect of a macrobiotic diet. NCI's primary goal is to determine if sufficient case report evidence is available to justify NCI-initiated prospective research for specific CAM practices as anti-cancer therapies (personal communication). To date, NCI does not have any pediatric "best cases" in their series, which seems surprising given the use of CAM in pediatric oncology (Kelly et al., 2000; McCurdy, Spangler, Wofford, Chauvenet, & McLean, 2003; Sawyer, Gannoni, Toogood, Antoniou, & Rice, 1994; Yeh, Lee, Chen, & Li, 2000).

There is a tremendous opportunity for CAM providers to use this approach to show-case their most successful therapeutic approaches in children. Dedicated journals now exist for CAM research and pediatric CAM research networks abound (Integrative Pediatrics Council; *BMC Complementary and Alternative Medicine; Canadian Pediatric Complementary and Alternative Medicine Network; Explore: The Journal of Science & Healing; Freshwinds Children's Complementary Therapy Network; Journal of Alternative and Complementary Medicine.*) Case reports are not a means to prove efficacy, but they can be a useful way to highlight successful approaches, to stimulate further research interest (Anwar, Kabir, Botchu, Khan, & Gogi, 2004; Burge, n.d.). When different prac-titioners independently report successful results for the same intervention-condition pair, thereby creating a "best-case series," their approach seems worth investigating further. Since case reports are particularly prone to bias, it is necessary to follow up with more rigorous approaches, such as N-of-1 trials.

CAM therapies are often highly individualized, and research methods need to take this heterogeneity into account, or they will systematically under-estimate treatment effect.

The highly individualized approach of CAM therapies makes designing appropriate RCTs challenging, if not impossible. N-of-1 refers to a form of single subject design, a randomized multiple crossover trial performed in a single subject (see Table 5-1). It has a long tradition in psychological research (Kazdin, 1982; Guyatt et al., 1990) and has been used in medicine to generate treatment information when evidence from RCTs is not available or applicable (Guyatt et al., 1988). N-of-1 allows for individualized approaches to therapy, while utilizing randomization and blinding to assess treatment effect. N-of-1 is also a potentially useful way to determine which CAM therapies warrant further

Table 5-1. Inclusion and Exclusion Criteria for N-of-1 Trials

Inclusion Criteria	Exclusion Criteria
Chronic, stable condition	Acute illness with rapid or spontaneous improvement
Treatment effectiveness in doubt	Treatment leads to cure or permanent change in condition
Treatment has quick onset and offset	
Patient/caregiver eager to take part	

Table 5-2. Recommended Resources about N-of-1 Trials

- Guyatt, G., Sackett,D., Adachi, J., Roberts, R., Chong, J., Rosenbloom, D., et al. (1988). A clinician's guide for conducting randomized trials in individual patients. *Canadian Medical Association, 139*(6), 497–503.

- Guyatt, G. H., Jaeschke, R., & Roberts, R. N-of-1 randomized clinical trials in pharmacoepidemiology. *Pharmacoepidemiology* (3rd ed.). Strom, B. Toronto, ON: John Wiley & Sons Inc., 2000: 615–632.

- Guyatt, G., Jaeschke, R., & McGinn, T. *Therapy and validity: N-of-1 randomized controlled trials. Users' guides to the medical literature: A manual for evidence-based clinical practice.* Chicago, IL: American Medical Association, 2002: 275–90.

- Keller, J. L., Guyatt, G. H., Roberts, R. S., Adachi, J. D., & Rosenbloom, D. (1988). An N-of-1 service: applying the scientific method in clinical practice. *Scandinavian Journal of Epidemiology, 147*, 22–29.

evaluation. Like CAM itself, N-of-1 is not one size fits all—this approach cannot answer every clinical question, but is especially helpful to assess the efficacy of natural health products (which happen to be the most common form of CAM used) in chronic stable conditions (see Table 5-2).

CAM research can learn important lessons from conventional medicine, pairing innovative design with methods that are tried and true. In particular, there is a critical need for a stepwise approach to clinical trials, else researchers risk spectacularly negative results in large Phase III trials that have been inadequately planned. The importance of Phase I/II research shouldn't be overlooked, even if mechanisms of action data are not fully understood. Experienced trialists need to partner with CAM providers to determine the most appropriate dose, duration, indication, and what outcomes to assess. The need for collaboration across disciplines is paramount.

Research collaboration can help advance pediatric integrative medicine in a rapid fashion. Other successful pediatric research networks should be emulated, such as Children's Oncology Group, which is currently conducting 150 concurrent studies with 40,000 patients being treated according to Children's Oncology group protocols

(Children's Oncology Group, n.d.) Academic pediatric integrative medicine programs should develop a set of common outcome measures for all to use in a systematic fashion. Such outcomes-based research is an efficient form of generating hypotheses, allowing promising therapies to be identified rapidly. Moreover, such collaboration allows for multicenter trials to be developed and implemented.

CAM research networks now exist within academic centers (Consortium of Academic Health Centers for Integrative Medicine, n.d.) as well as those between academics and community-based providers for example, PedCAM (*Canadian* Pediatric Complementary and Alternative Medicine Network, n.d.). There is also a need for strong collaborative partnerships between content experts, and methodological experts. There is also a need to promote cross-training, so that CAM providers can develop research expertise, and researchers can learn in-depth about specific CAM therapies. Some funders are promoting such cross-training, such as the National Center for CAM (National Center for Complementary And Medicine, 2007) and Sick Kids' Foundation (SickKids Foundation, 2007). Such collaboration has identified that CAM research may benefit from broader approaches, combining quantitative and qualitative methods in a single study.

Mixed-methods research, combining quantitative and qualitative approaches, has benefited CAM research. Rather than focusing only on "specific" effects, CAM researchers have found it useful to consider "non-specific" effects, and intended as well as unintended effects. In particular, patients have described that CAM approaches have helped them with personal transformation and becoming "unstuck," phenomena that would have been poorly captured had open-ended qualitative research not been conducted simultaneously with quantitative approaches. It seems that researchers do not always fully anticipate some of the effects that are seen, and should therefore, in quantitative fashion, assess what changes took place, and qualitatively, to assess how they affected people's lives.

COST-EFFECTIVENESS

CAM may offer important approaches to help empower patients, to let them achieve healing even if there isn't a cure, and be more functional in their lives. CAM researchers need to be creative in how such outcomes are measured, including return to school/work and improved quality of life (Verhoef et al., 2007). In this fashion, the economic impact of CAM therapies can be captured, as well as the direct health effects. Governments, insurance companies, and other payers need data to be convinced. Does using CAM cost society less money in the long-run? If it isn't cheaper, they will need to be convinced what added value CAM offers. Expense is not the only measure, as improved quality of life also "counts." Researchers also need to carefully examine the health promotion aspects of integrative approaches, which may result in less money spent on chronic disease management.

UNIQUE ISSUES IN CAM RESEARCH DESIGN, ETHICS, AND FUNDING

CAM researchers must be pragmatic in their approaches. Clinical evidence cannot wait until we fully understand the mechanism of action underlying specific therapeutic approaches. Nonetheless, the quality of the research does not have to be compromised. Indeed, despite our current imperfect understanding of how many CAM therapies work, the quality of CAM RCTs and systematic reviews meet or exceed those of conventional medicine (Klassen, Pham, Lawson, & Moher, 2005; Lawson, Pham, Klassen, & Moher, 2005).

A unique challenge faced by CAM researchers is the role of patient preference. In drug trials, research subjects can only access novel agents through participation in research. Access to CAM is not prescription-controlled, and patients may strongly prefer to try the therapy, rather than tolerate being randomized to placebo. This difficulty in recruiting patients into CAM trials is a barrier that some have overcome through use of waiting list controls (i.e., eventually all subjects will receive the CAM therapy, making them more tolerant of participating in research). The role of patient preference and its impact on randomized clinical trials has been explored in conventional medicine for some time (Brewin & Bradley, 1989) and is being explored in CAM research (Melchart et al., 2002). More work is needed to fully appreciate the impact of patient preference on outcomes, particularly for children.

CAM researchers require diverse approaches to assess complex therapies. Fortunately, sophisticated approaches to study complex interventions have been developed, such as the Medical Research Council framework for the development and evaluation of RCTs for complex interventions to improve health (Campbell et al., 2000). Specific consideration has been given to whole systems research, and how to improve sham controls and blinding for complex interventions such as acupuncture (Verhoef et al., 2005; White, Filshie, & Cummings, 2001). Some may benefit from reviewing recommended approaches to clinical trials when blinding is not possible (CONSORT, 2007).

ETHICS

The ethics of pediatric CAM are founded on core principles of beneficence, nonmaleficence, and a fundamental respect for autonomy in conjunction with the best interests of the child. There is a pressing need for good quality data with regards to safety and efficacy to guide decisions, making pediatric CAM research an emerging priority. Although CAM use is common in children (Jean & Cyr, 2007; Hanson et al., 2007; Sibinga, Shindell, Casella, Duggan, & Wilson, 2006), institutional review boards (IRB) may not receive the reassuring safety data they are accustomed to in applications to conduct pediatric research. Conventional medicine has studied children last, and animal and adult data have always been available prior to pediatric research. Since children often already receive CAM, there is no reason they should be asked to wait to benefit from CAM research. A fundamental challenge is potential IRB discomfort with pediatric CAM research, creating an opportunity to educate IRBs so that pediatric CAM studies receive appropriate reviews. If a researcher can demonstrate that children are already exposed to a particular therapy, then it seems reasonable that formal evaluation of that therapy through participation in research affords children greater protection, not less.

FUNDING

As any researcher knows, good quality research requires appropriate funding. Although CAM use is common, and clearly relevant to the taxpayers who support publicly funded research, many granting agencies remain reluctant to fund CAM studies. Debates exist in academic circles about the relative value of CAM research (Colquhoun, 2007). Impairing CAM research further, even dedicated agencies that were created to support CAM research, such as NCCAM or NCI OCCAM, describe challenges in obtaining appropriate peer review, a problem that is exacerbated in the relatively small community of pediatric CAM researchers. Some of the dedicated pediatric CAM networks, centers, and other initiatives described previously could offer a source of potential reviewers who are expert in content and/or methodology to ensure fair, appropriate peer review.

Excellence should determine which studies are funded, but it seems unreasonable for grant reviewers to demand data that do not exist as a necessary prerequisite. Not infrequently in CAM research, clinical use far exceeds basic science understanding of mechanisms of action. Neither IRBs nor granting agencies should limit CAM research to therapies with well-defined mechanisms of action. Clinical studies to assess safety or efficacy can shed new light on potential mechanisms of action, as "translational" research in CAM is backwards (bedside to bench). This approach does not negate a phased approach to clinical research. Phase I and II trials should precede Phase III trials, so as to avoid expensive, large negative clinical trials that are criticized for inappropriate interventions or outcome assessment and therefore offer limited new knowledge. Funders can insist that researchers justify their methodological choices, without creating barriers due to lack of current understanding about potential mechanisms of action. The two issues are not equivalent, and funders should be encouraged to distinguish between them.

Pediatric CAM research needs appropriate funding and qualified peer review. Widespread clinical use of CAM suggests that translational research in this field may be "bedside to bench," whereby therapies that have clinical effect (beneficial or deleterious) can be further explored in the lab to assess their potential mechanism of action.

Education

Since the public utilizes both conventional healthcare and complementary and alternative medicine (CAM), the Commission believes that this reality should be reflected in the education and training of all health practitioners. Thus, the education and training of conventional health professions should include CAM, and the education and training of CAM practitioners should include conventional healthcare. The result will be conventional providers who can discuss CAM with their patients and clients, provide guidance on CAM use, collaborate with CAM practitioners, and make referrals to them, as well as CAM practitioners who can communicate and collaborate with conventional providers and make referrals to them.

—*White House Commission (2002)*

In 2002, the White House Commission's Complementary and Alternative Health Care Policy Final Report recommended a number of key strategies in the education and training of both CAM and conventional healthcare practitioners for the purpose of ensuring public safety, improving health, increasing the availability of qualified and knowledgeable CAM and conventional healthcare practitioners, and to enhance collaboration among healthcare professions (Table 5-3). Data indicate that pediatric use of CAM products and practices is increasing with the highest rates of use in children with a variety of chronic conditions such as arthritis, cystic fibrosis, cancer, and autism (Braganza, Ozuah, & Sharif, 2003; Cohen & Kemper, 2005; Feldman et al., 2004; Jean & Cyr, 2007; National Center for Complementary and Alternative Medicine, 2007). Concerns continue to be raised about the clinically and legally appropriate use of CAM in pediatrics. For example, families who choose CAM for their children may substitute conventional medical treatment for CAM products and practices or delay getting conventional medical treatment (Cohen & Kemper, 2005). In addition, 18% of children in a recent study used herbal medicines and prescription medicine in combination and 75% of their families believed that CAM had no potential for adverse effect (Jean & Cyr, 2007). Consistent with previous studies (Crawford, Cincotta, Lim, & Powell, 2006; Prussing, Sobo, Walker, Dennis, & Kurtin, 2004), 53% of the CAM users did not inform their pediatrician that they were using CAM. Finally, increased interest in and changing attitudes about CAM by pediatricians (Sawni & Thomas, 2007) and increased interest by both pediatricians and CAM professionals in the development and utilization of various pediatric CAM and related networks (Weeks, 2007) suggests that CAM and pediatric education continues to be an important topic among healthcare professionals, researchers, policy makers, and the public.

In this section of the chapter, we will explore educational strategies to increase safety, develop research literacy and capacity, improve health, and enhance collaboration. We conclude with a discussion of future directions in integrative pediatric education.

Table 5-3. White House Commission on Complementary and Alternative Health Care Policy

The education and training of CAM and conventional practitioners should be designed to ensure public safety, improve health, and increase the availability of qualified and knowledgeable CAM and conventional practitioners, and enhance the collaboration among them.

Conventional health professional schools, postgraduate training programs, and continuing education programs should develop core curricula of knowledge about CAM that will prepare conventional health professionals to discuss CAM with their patients and clients and help them make informed choices about the use of CAM.

CAM education and training programs should develop curricula that reflect the fundamental elements of biomedical science and conventional health care relevant to and consistent with the practitioners' scope of practice.

CAM and conventional education and training programs should develop curricula and other methods to facilitate communication and foster collaboration between CAM and conventional students, practitioners, researchers, educators, institutions, and organizations.

Increased Federal, state, and private sector support should be made available to expand and evaluate CAM faculty, curricula, and program development at accredited CAM and conventional institutions.

Expansion of eligibility of CAM students at accredited institutions for existing Federal loan programs should be explored.

The Department of Health and Human Services should conduct a feasibility study to determine whether appropriately educated and trained CAM practitioners enhance and/or expand health care provided by primary care teams.* This feasibility study could lead to demonstration projects to identify: 1) the type of practitioners, 2) their necessary education and training, 3) the appropriate practice settings, and 4) the health outcomes attributable to the addition of these practitioners and services to comprehensive care.

The Department of Health and Human Services and other Federal Departments and Agencies should convene conferences of the leaders of CAM, conventional health, public health, evolving health professions, and the public; of educational institutions; and of appropriate organizations to facilitate establishment of CAM education and training guidelines. Subsequently, the guidelines should be made available to the states and professions for their consideration.

Feasibility studies of postgraduate training for appropriately educated and trained CAM practitioners should be conducted to determine the type of practitioners, practice setting, and their impact on clinical competency, quality of health care, and collaboration with conventional providers.

Practitioners who provide CAM services and products should complete appropriate CAM continuing education programs that include critical evaluation of CAM to enhance and protect the public's health and safety.

White House Commission on Complemenatary and Alternative Health Care Policy [Online] March 2002 Chapter 4, 51. Accessed July 16, 2007, from http://whccamp.hhs.gov/fr4.html

ENSURING SAFETY, BUILDING CAPACITY

Increasingly, as CAM for children becomes more widely accepted (Loman, 2003; Sanders et al., 2003) consumers, health care practitioners, government agencies, professional associations, and researchers are asking important questions about the safety and effectiveness of CAM as a healthcare intervention for children (Cohen & Kemper,

2005; Moher, Soeken, Sampson, Ben-Porat, & Berman, 2002). Furthermore, increased use of and reimbursement for CAM interventions brings an increased requirement for accountability. Consequently, healthcare practitioners and the public need to know which CAM products and therapies work best, for which children, and under what conditions. Clear and accurate information on the relative safety and risk of harm of CAM practices and products for children, either directly or indirectly through unwarranted emotional or financial burden (Cohen & Kemper, 2005), needs to be generated through sound research as discussed earlier in the chapter, with resulting best evidence widely disseminated across healthcare professions and translated to practice. Education for all healthcare practitioners in pediatric CAM needs to address fundamental issues of safety and efficacy and responsible professional judgment.

Cohen and Kemper (2005) provide an important framework to guide pediatricians in making responsible, ethical, appropriate and legally defensible clinical decisions in regards to pediatric CAM.

1. Do parents elect to abandon effective care when the child's condition is serious or life threatening?
2. Will use of the CAM therapy otherwise divert the child from imminently necessary conventional treatment?
3. Are the CAM therapies selected known to be unsafe and/or ineffective?
4. Have the proper parties consented to the use of the CAM therapy?
5. Is the risk-benefit ratio of the proposed CAM therapy acceptable to a reasonable, similarly situated clinician, and does the therapy have at least minority acceptance or support in the medical literature?

Underlying the clinical decision-making process implicit in Cohen and Kemper's questions are key assumptions about the educational preparation of health professionals in subjects such as informed consent, ethical and legal responsibilities, and requirements in relation to clinical practice with children and families, research literacy—the ability to find, understand, critically assess, and apply research evidence to practice (Dryden & Achilles, 2005)—including the capacity to assess relative risks and benefits of CAM treatment from a western biomedical perspective, and attitudes towards evidence-based practice.

Data on profession-specific competencies and curriculum in research literacy, evidence-based practice, ethics and clinical decision-making is complex to identify and assess across and within CAM professions. Results of a 2004 descriptive study on the degree of inclusion of research literacy and evidence-based approaches to practice within CAM educational programs (naturopathic medicine, chiropractic, massage therapy, homeopathic medicine, traditional Chinese medicine and acupuncture, and western herbal medicine) in Canada (Dryden et al., 2004) indicate that the length of educational programs vary greatly both within and across disciplines. Two-thirds of participants stated that their school offered research curricula within the academic program, although no common definition emerged for "research course," "research literacy," and "research capacity." In addition, the diversity of teacher experience and training in research in CAM educational programs tended to extend to curriculum development in general, influencing a school's ability to address the overall development of research literacy and evidence-based practice education (Table 5-4).

The concept of "readiness" emerged as a means of predicting the existence of research curriculum and/or a research program within a particular school and in some cases, across a whole discipline and provided a useful framework. The three major themes that emerged were *institutional readiness* in CAM schools to develop and deliver research curricula and support a program of applied research and evidence based practice, *societal readiness* by province/territory in Canada to recognize and regulate CAM professions

Table 5-4. Readiness for Delivering and Developing Research Literacy Curricula in CAM Schools

Institutional Readiness

Perceived differences in fiscal resources for public vs. private educational institutions

Evaluation and research values embedded in the culture of the school

Financial stability

Salaried teachers and the provision of teacher training

Research literacy/capacity resources (libraries, designated research librarians, computers, publication subscriptions, Internet and database access)

Societal Readiness

Legislative certification, regulation, or recognition

Accreditation of schools and availability of student bursaries

Primacy of the Western, evidence-based approach to health practice

Market driven trends—graduate employment rates, profitability, and competitiveness between schools

Student preferences—shorter and more affordable programs, closer to home

Professional Readiness

Codes of ethics, standards of practice

Competency-based guidelines

Pre-requisite educational level for entry to programs

Diversity of instructional design and delivery

Existence of innovative learning models

Research requirement: Literacy amongst complementary and alternative health care practitioners—phase I and phase II. Natural Health Products Directorate, Health Canada. 2004. Accessed online August 25, 2007, from http://www.hc-sc.gc.ca/sr-sr/pubs/nhp/research_literacy_e.html

and academic institutions, and the degree of *professional readiness* within each of the disciplines studied. Challenges and opportunities in developing research curricula and an evidence-based approach to practice in CAM professionals' educations were seen as highly interdependent and best addressed synergistically and collaboratively on several fronts: (1) fostering and promoting a culture of professionalism and inquiry in CAM education and practice; (2) increasing knowledge of research language/ terminology and developing national standards and competencies in research literacy; (3) increasing teacher education; (4) developing instructional methods and delivery models to enhance reflective practice, critical thinking, and evidence-based approaches to clinical decision- making; (5) building partnerships and sharing resources between and among CAM and conventional healthcare educational institutions and professions, and creating opportunities for interprofessional education and collaboration.

Implementing Cohen and Kemper's model on clinical decision-making in integrative pediatrics requires all healthcare practitioners to have ready access to safety and efficacy data and the skills to critically evaluate and translate research evidence to practice. Basic access to the best evidence for healthcare professionals and healthcare students varies widely depending on such diverse variables as profession-specific and individual values in regards to evidence-based practice and life-long learning, computer literacy, access to the Internet and access to peer-reviewed journals. In addition to accessing infor-mation, although research evidence in pediatric CAM is growing rapidly, not enough is known about many CAM practices and products in pediatric populations, making evidence-based decision-making, regardless of level of research literacy skills, challeng-ing for all. Both classroom and web-based (Centennial College, n.d.) courses in research literacy for those healthcare professionals, both conventional and CAM, who do not have training in finding, critically appraising, and applying best evidence to practice is a fundamental starting point.

Currently, not enough is known about the kinds and types of pediatric-specific curricula undertaken in the professional training of CAM practitioners at either the undergraduate (pre-diploma, pre-licensure) or continuing education level. From the American Academy of Pediatrics (AAP) policy statement on CAM first published in 2003 and reaffirmed in 2006, only chiropractic is sited as having specific curricula in pediatrics (American Academy of Pediatrics, 2006). Lee and Kemper (2000) in their study on pediatric practice characteristics in homeopathy and naturopathy stated that although nearly all the study cohort reported treating children, fewer than half of the practitioners reported any formal pediatric training. Numerous open-access websites advertise continuing education in pediatric CAM profession-specific educa-tion in homeopathy, massage, naturopathy, chiropractic, herbal medicine, traditional Chinese medicine, and acupuncture. Little is known about the content and quality of these educational programs. The same can be said about the lack of published research comparing and evaluating continuing medical, nursing and allied health curricula in pediatric CAM.

SAFETY AND EFFICACY

As discussed earlier in this chapter, the need for more research on the safety and efficacy of CAM use in children and the importance of utilizing research methods such as active surveillance, case reporting, best case series, and N-of-1 studies, suggest important directions in the development of curricula in both conventional and CAM healthcare education. Ensuring that all healthcare practitioners develop basic competency in maintaining accurate health records and reporting adverse events is fundamental to the development of a safety research agenda in integrative pediatrics. Given the diversity of educational preparation across and within CAM and conventional healthcare professions and profession-specific differences in expectations, values and requirements for public accountability, this is no small task. Developing customized reporting practices for adverse events in CAM modalities, in coordination with best-practice guidelines inclusive of "duty to report" competencies and professional values, will help to address this issue. As a model, existing standardized documentation of adverse events such as the NHP reporting requirements developed by the Natural Health Products Directorate, Health Canada for clinical trials of NHPs (Health Canada, n.d.) and manufactured NHPs (Health Canada, 2001) could be adapted for individual CAM modalities.

Funded educational and networking opportunities that prepare CAM practitioners, educators and leaders to actively participate with conventional practitioners, educators and researchers in the development of integrative pediatric research agendas will help to stimulate growth in this area. Similarly, providing all healthcare practitioners with opportunities to learn how to participate in, design and write clear case reports and case series, and N-of-1 studies will build research capacity and lead to better understanding of the use and safety of CAM products and practices for children. In addition, as clinical CAM use far outweighs basic science understanding, it is possible that CAM safety research could support translational research by promoting educational opportunities that enhance the iterative relationship between "bench and bedside." The National Institutes of Health (NIH) and Canadian Institutes of Health Research (CIHR) co-sponsored a conference on the Biology of Manual Therapies (Conference on the Biology of Manual Therapies, 2005) that provided an important example of a strategic and collaborative educational and networking forum for building integrative research agendas. By bringing together basic science and clinical researchers, conventional and CAM practitioners, educators and practice leaders, the conference opened an important and inclusive interprofessional dialogue. The outcomes from the conference guided the development of NCCAM's strategic agenda for CAM research in manual therapies. Similar international and interprofessional educational and research capacity building opportunities need to be developed to coordinate and drive a safety and efficacy research agenda for integrative pediatrics.

INNOVATIVE STRATEGIES

Although it is beyond the scope of this chapter to comprehensively assess what is being taught in integrative pediatrics to conventional healthcare practitioners, policy papers, and studies from the American Academy of Pediatrics (2006), in Nursing and Allied Health (Fenton & Morris, 2003; Laurenson, MacDonald, McCready, & Stimpson, 2006) suggest that there is strong interest and activity. In integrative medicine education, NCCAM's funding of fifteen complementary and alternative medicine (CAM) education project grants (National Centre for Complementary & Alternative Medicine, 2002) to encourage and support the incorporation of CAM information into medical, dental, nursing, and allied health professional school curricula, into residency training programs, and into continuing education courses is a significant capacity-building initiative. Outcomes of this educational initiative and the ongoing work from policy/advocacy groups such as the 36 medical school members of the Consortium of Academic Health Centres (CAHCIM—Consortium of Academic Health Centers for Integrative Medicine, n.d.), and the parallel CAM members of the Academic Consortium for Complementary and Alternative Health Care (ACCAHC) developed by the Integrated Health Care Policy Consortium (IHPC—Integrated Health Care Policy Consortium, n.d.), the CAM in Undergraduate Medical Education (CAM in UME—Complementary and Alternative Medicine Issues in Undergraduate Medical Education, 2007) initiative, and the Canadian Interdisciplinary Network for Complementary and Alternative Medicine Research (IN-CAM) Network (Canadian Interdisciplinary Network for Complementary & Alternative Medicine Research, n.d.) continue to advance the development of integrative medicine education. IHPC has also developed a focused education-specific initiative, the National Education Dialogue (NED—Integrated Health Care Policy Consortium, n.d.) to promote and support inter-institutional collaboration among CAM and conventional educators.

The growing numbers of integrative pediatric medicine-specific networks and interest groups such as PedCAM (Canadian Pediatric Complementary and Alternative Medicine Network, n.d.), Provisional Section on Contemporary, Holistic, and Integrative Medicine of the American Academy of Pediatrics (AAP SCHIM—Provisional Section on Complementary, Holistic, and Integrative Medicine, n.d.), International Pediatric Integrative Medicine Network (I-PIM—Provisional Section on Complementary, Holistic, and Integrative Medicine) and IPC (Integrative Pediatrics Council) and Pangea (*Pangea—A conference for the future of pediatrics*) indicates the centrality and growing importance of developing integrative pediatric education as a specialty or clinical focus of integrative medicine. In addition, the increasing numbers of web-based networks for both conventional and CAM practitioners and researchers (Canadian Interdisciplinary Network for Complementary & Alternative Medicine Research n.d.; Canadian Pediatric Complementary and Alternative Medicine Network, n.d.; Freshwinds

Children's Complementary Therapy Network, n.d.) to share information, education and resources, in conjunction with increased interest in interprofessional education for collaborative, patient-centred care (European InterProfessional Education Network, n.d.), suggests a number of key directions for ensuring safety, building capacity and enhancing communication and collaboration between and among both conventional and CAM practitioner groups. In addition, the provision of clinical fellowships and cross-training opportunities such those provided by the National Grants Program (SickKids Foundation, n.d.) until recently, are further examples of innovative educational strategies in integrative pediatric medicine. Along with its research grants in complementary and alternative healthcare (CAHC) and pediatrics, the Sick Kids Foundation developed scholarships for students enrolled in a masters program in any discipline related to the study of pediatrics and complementary and alternative healthcare practices, including natural health products, and funded an innovative cross-training program open to both conventional and complementary researchers and practitioners. The cross-training program provided complementary care practitioners with opportunities to further develop their research knowledge by working with conventional researcher, or conventional researchers with the opportunity to job-shadow, or train with a complementary care practitioner, or complementary care researchers who conducted research in the adult population but who wanted to deepen their knowledge of a particular child health issue, and organizations which wanted to develop a curriculum to support research capacity building in the area of complementary and alternative healthcare for children and youth. The National Centre for Complementary and Alternative Medicine (NCCAM) CAM Practitioner Research Career Development Award (National Centre for Complementary & Alternative Medicine, n.d.) to provide training for CAM practitioners who have an interest in pursuing a research career. This initiative provides up to 5 years of support for a CAM practitioner with a clinical doctorate who has never been a principal investigator on an NIH research, career, or fellowship grant. The award provides the CAM practitioner with protected time to focus on broad research training under the guidance of a mentor.

Another important example of a capacity-building educational initiative is the creation of searchable digital learning repositories such as the one created by the Complementary and Alternative Medicine in Undergraduate Medical Education (CAM in UME) Project. Collaboratively developed by representatives from all medical schools in Canada, CAM researchers and CAM practitioners, the CAM in UME searchable digital repository of teaching/learning resources and peer-reviewed curriculum guidelines, also provides an overarching framework and set of competencies (Table 5-5) to guide and assist medical school educators in implementing CAM teaching in their individual schools. Lessons learned from work currently underway at the CAM in UME project suggest that "effective curriculum change requires clear, open, two-way communication." This is probably all the more important when the change is controversial, unfamiliar, or misunderstood, as may be the case with education about CAM (*Complementary and Alternative Medicine Issues in Undergraduate Medical Education,* 2007). The CAM in UME project

Knowledge-based Competencies

- K1. Describe CAM and how CAM can be classified. List and describe commonly used CAM therapies in Canada.

- K2. Describe and discuss the potential challenges and benefits of Integrative Medicine (IM).

- K3. List CAM therapies that are commonly used by patients for specific diseases or health concerns (list to be determined locally by the instructor). Identify how CAM use is related to socio-demographic characteristics, values and beliefs.

- K4. Describe the potential impact of selected CAM therapies (list to be determined locally by the instructor) on stress reduction, illness prevention, health promotion.

- K5. Identify potential safety issues associated with selected CAM therapies (list to be determined locally by the instructor). This may include: interactions with other CAM therapies, interactions with conventional medicine, side effects, and/or contraindications.

- K6. Identify reliable sources to establish the current state of evidence for the following CAM therapies (list to be determined locally by the instructor).

- K7. Know where to find information on:

  - Natural Health Product Regulations (federally regulated);

  - Regulation and credentialing of common CAM practices in the student's province, medical licensing;

  - Medical licensing and regulation of physicians practicing CAM in the student's province; and

  - Medical licensing and regulation of physicians referring patients to CAM practitioners in the student's province.

- K8. Compare the conventional/biomedical paradigm with various complementary paradigms with respect to concepts such as reductionism, holism, experimental efficacy, clinical effectiveness, standards of evidence, clinical trials, wellness, healing, and placebo response.

- K9. Identify barriers to professional and ethical issues that arise in the establishment of collaborative relationships between physicians and CAM practitioners and discuss potential strategies for addressing these issues.

Skills-based Competencies

- S1. Critically appraise the evidence pertaining to selected CAM therapies for the prevention and treatment of specific conditions (list to be determined locally by the instructor)

- S2. Discuss the subject of CAM with patients in a respectful, non-judgmental, and professional manner, including:

  - Taking a patient history of CAM use;

  - Responding to patients in a manner which reflects some minimal knowledge of CAM, as well as cultural sensitivity, and appreciation for the values and beliefs of the patient;

  - Informing and advising patients regarding CAM; and

  - Acknowledging the limitations of one's own knowledge regarding CAM

(continued)

91

Table 5-5. (Continued)

- S3. Communicate respectfully and effectively, with permission of the patient, with CAM practitioners about assessment, treatment, decision-making, referrals, and patient safety.

Attitude-based Competencies

- A1. Reflect on your own culturally based values and belief systems, attitudes, and CAM related knowledge, and describe how these may affect your approach to self-care, health, wellness, healing, and the practice of conventional medicine and CAM.

- A2. Demonstrate respect for the beliefs and choices of patients who use CAM.

The CAM in UME Project, Accessed online August 25, 2007, from http://www.caminume.ca/documents/competencies.pdf

cites increasing opportunities for interprofessional education (IPE) as a key strategy for building communication and research capacity. Many learning objects and modules in integrative pediatrics currently exist at various conventional and CAM educational institutions and on websites. An internationally funded collaborative project that comprehensively develops core competencies and resources in integrative pediatrics, similar to the CAM in UME model, would serve to bring together and make more accessible existing educational resources, identify gaps, and create opportunities for interprofessional dialogue, curriculum development and could become accessible to all.

Other examples of capacity building educational initiatives include the work being done by the Education Working Group (EWG) of the Consortium of Academic Health Centres for Integrative Medicine (CAHCIM—Consortium of Academic Health Centers for Integrative Medicine, n.d.) to facilitate the incorporation of teaching of Integrative Medicine (IM) into all levels of medical education and to increase the application of IM principles and practices to all healthcare disciplines. To advance this mission, the EWG develops and implements a variety of plans for faculty training and collaborative resource-sharing in member institutions. The EWG is currently working on two major educational initiatives: developing faculty capacity for implementing curricular change in integrative medicine education, and developing integrative medicine training opportunities and longitudinal tracks in residency education. In addition, the work of the National Education Dialogue (NED) of the Integrated Health Care Policy Consortium (IHPC—Integrated Health Care Policy Consortium, n.d.) outlines a multi-year strategy through IHPC's Education Task Force. Through its working groups and larger meetings, NED promotes cross-disciplinary collaboration among educators from conventional and complementary and alternative healthcare institutions. The National Education Dialogue's priorities include:

- promoting and supporting inter-institutional collaboration among educators, including the development of regional models;
- developing CAM and conventional educational resources and materials to foster understanding of the value each discipline offers for quality care;

- exploring shared values, skills and attitudes among disciplines; and
- creating a website of resources which can assist educators in advancing their local initiatives.

The centerpiece of NED's work is facilitating model programs to foster inter-institutional partnerships in health professions education. Creating integrative pediatric medicine working groups in these organizations would help to focus and create synergy between and among these groups and help to move the integrative pediatric medicine agenda forward.

ENHANCING COLLABORATION

Interprofessional education (IPE) as defined by the UK Centre for the Advancement of Interprofessional Education (CAIPE) occurs "when two or more professions learn with, from and about each other to improve collaboration and the quality of care" (UK Centre for the Advancement of Interprofessional Education, 2007). IPE includes all such learning in academic and work-based settings before and after qualification, and adopts an inclusive view of "professional". Best practices in implementing interprofessional education, remains an open question. Outcomes from several IPE studies currently underway will help direct the kinds and types of education in the future that will enhance team performance and will help to provide models for integrated pediatric medicine education. Information from existing integrated medicine programs indicate that professionals from both CAM and conventional medicine need ample opportunity to learn with, from and about each other in order to build trust and enhance collaboration. Prior to opening the integrative medicine clinic at Harvard Medical School's, Osher Institute, David Eisenberg (Eisenberg, 2006)brought the conventional and CAM practitioners together who were to work at the newly created clinic, one day per week for six months prior to the opening of the clinic, to build trust and integrate treatment plans. Other organizations, such as Friends of Complementary and Alternative Therapies Society (FACTS—Friends of Complementary and Alternative Therapies Society, n.d.) have successfully used an integrated grand rounds model in the education of interprofessional teams to stimulate collaboration, explore synergies, and resolve potential conflicts. Significantly, FACTS is inclusive of patients/clients and their families as key stakeholders in their organization and educational programs. Key to the development of effective, coordinated and sustainable strategies for integrative pediatric medicine education will be the valuable contributions of families, advocacy groups, labour, community, industry and government to developing, evaluating and ultimately utilizing the benefits of collaborative educational initiatives, and knowledge translation.

FUTURE DIRECTIONS

Continuing to create a culture of inquiry and collaboration in integrative pediatrics requires the ongoing development of core competencies for all healthcare practitioners, inclusive of research literacy and research capacity, evidence-based approaches to clinical decision-making and interprofessional, child- and family-centred, collaborative practice skills. Developing core competencies in interprofessional collaborative practice requires that CAM and conventional health practitioners be given adequate opportunity to learn from, with and about each other in an atmosphere of mutual respect. It is not yet known at what point (or at which points) in a health care professional's education that interprofessional team and integrative medicine skills are best introduced; nor is it known which educational strategies are the most effective for knowledge retention and enhanced interprofessional and integrative behaviors. Face-to-face learning opportunities are highly valued and can be very effective. Increasing use and evaluation of web-based education and hybrid educational strategies (combined in-person and online learning) will continue to shed light on better, more cost-effective educational interventions. The use of high fidelity (in-person) simulation and web-based simulation including the use of online educational gaming strategies, holds interesting potential, as a means of enhancing interprofessional education (Wideman et al., 2007). Educational gaming strategies using simulated integrated pediatric medicine case-based scenarios could be used to train interprofessional teams in a simulated, web-based environment. A shared model of funding for such a collaboration would provide overall ongoing course and technical support management to ensure sustainability of such a project.

Evaluating the effectiveness of educational interventions intended to build interprofessional and integrative skills and attitudes for healthcare professionals continues to be a rich field for research exploration. The use of team-based objectively structured clinical examinations (TOSCEs) (Singleton, Smith, Harris, Ross-Harper, & Hilton, 1999) is one example of an innovative strategy to assess interprofessional competencies. Clinical practicums and educational settings which are intended to increase the opportunities for health professionals from all disciplines to interact and work together in teams are useful but need careful planning and implementation to ensure that roles, responsibilities, and clinical decision-making processes are clear and appropriately shared by the team and not dominated by one profession or another that may be perceived to have, or may actually have, more power than another. Healthcare professionals that work in geographical proximity can find ways to interact and build on the potential for collaborative practice but may need easily accessible and so-called "just-in-time" educational opportunities, and mentoring in each other's clinical roles and responsibilities in order to build trust and enhance integrative approaches to practice.

What we can be sure of in the future of integrative pediatric education, is that increased utilization of the Internet through interprofessional networks, web-based learning including educational simulation and gaming, and the use of collaborative authoring and communication cyber spaces such as Wikis, blogs, and Facebook, will alter the ways and the speed at which we can communicate and build collaborative communities of practice. The future of CAM pediatric education is both simple—effective educational strategies currently exist—and complex. The systemic barriers that currently maintain CAM and conventional health education in silos and as parallel systems of healthcare delivery, are remarkably resilient to change. The high utilization of both CAM and conventional practices and products by children and their families, will continue to put pressure on educators and educational systems to rethink, and for many to include for the first time, innovative curricula and delivery models at all levels of healthcare professional preparation. Education that enhances team performance, interprofessionalism, and collaborative patient-centred practice are the fundamental building blocks of a truly integrative pediatric medicine.

Acknowledgments

The authors gratefully acknowledge the contributions of Cecilia Bukutu and Connie Winther for help with editing and referencing and Amy Moen for proofreading and citation help with this chapter. Sunita Vohra receives salary support from the Canadian Institutes of Health Research and the Alberta Heritage Foundation for Medical Research.

REFERENCES

Alvarez-Requejo, A., Carvajal, A., Begaud, B., Moride, Y., Vega, T., & Arias, L.H. (1998). Under-reporting of adverse drug reactions. Estimate based on a spontaneous reporting scheme and a sentinel system. *European Journal of Clinical Pharmacology, 54*, 483–488.

American Academy of Pediatrics. (2006). *Scope of practice issues in the delivery of pediatric health care policy in complementary and alternative health care. Healthcare policy statement, 2003 reaffirmed in 2006.* Retrieved October 15, 2007, from http://aappolicy.aappublications.org/cgi/content/full/pediatrics;111/2/426#T2

Anwar, R., Kabir, H., Botchu, R., Khan, S.A., & Gogi, N. (2004) How to write a case report. *Student BMJ, 12*, 60–61.

Barnes, J. (2003). Quality, efficacy and safety of complementary medicines: Fashions, facts and the future. part II: Efficacy and safety. *British Journal of Clinical Pharmacology, 55*, 331–340.

BMC Complementary and Alternative Medicine. (2007). Retrieved October 15, 2007, from http://www.biomedcentral.com/bmccomplementalternmed/

Boon, H., Verhoef, M., O'Hara, D., & Findlay, B. (2004). From parallel practice to integrative healthcare: A conceptual framework. *BMC Health Services Research, 4*(1), 15.

Boudville, I. C., Phua, K. B., Quak, S. H., Lee, B. W., Han, H. H., Verstraeten, T., et al. (2006). The epidemiology of paediatric intussusception in Singapore: 1997 to 2004. *Annals of the Academy of Medicine, Singapore, 35*(10), 674–649.

Braganza, S., Ozuah, P. O., & Sharif, I. (2003). The use of complementary therapies in inner-city asthmatic children. *The Journal of Asthma: Official Journal of the Association for the Care of Asthma, 40*(7), 823–827.

Burge, S. K. (n.d.) *Writing a clinical case report. Family & community medicine.* Retrieved October, 22, 2007, from http://familymed.uthscsa.edu/facultydevelopment/elearning/caseReportIntro.htm

CAMline (n.d.). *The evidence based complementary and alternative website for healthcare professionals.* Retrieved August, 13, 2007, from www.camline.ca

Campbell, M., Fitzpatrick, R., Haines, A., Kinmonth, A. L., Sandercock, P., Spiegelhalter, D. & Tyrer, P. (2001). Framework for design and evaluation of complex interventions to improve health. *BMJ,* 321, 694–696.

Canadian Interdisciplinary Network for Complementary & Alternative Medicine Research (IN-CAM*)* (n.d.). Retrieved August, 13, 2007, from http://www.incamresearch.ca/

Canadian Pediatric Complementary and Alternative Medicine Network (PedCAM). (n.d.). Retrieved August, 13, 2007, from www.pedcam.ca

Centennial College. (n.d.). *Research literacy for complementary and alternative health care practitioners: An online course.,* Retrieved October 15, 2007, from http://www.centennialcollege.ca/future/schs_ce_cac_research.jsp

Charrois, T. L., Hill, R. L., Vu, D., Foster, B. C., Boon, H. S., Cramer, K., et al. (2007). Community identification of natural health product-drug interactions. *Annals of Pharmacotherapy, 41*(7), 1124–1129.

Children's Oncology Group. (n.d.). *Cure search COG pioneering research.* Retrieved November 5, 2007, from http://www.curesearch.org/our_research/index_sub.aspx?id=1523

Cohen, M. H., & Kemper, K. J. (2005). Complementary therapies in pediatrics: A legal perspective. *Pediatrics, 115*(3), 774–780.

Colquhoun, D. (2007). Should NICE evaluate complementary and alternative medicines? *BMJ, 334*(7592), 507.

Committee on the Use of Complementary and Alternative Medicine by the American Public. (2005). *Complementary and alternative medicine in the United States* Washington: National Academy of Sciences.

Complementary and Alternative Medicine Issues in Undergraduate Medical Education (CAM in UME). (2007). Retrieved October 15, 2007, 2007, from http://www.caminume.ca/

Conference on the Biology of Manual Therapies, Bethesda Maryland, June 9–10, 2005. (2005). Retrieved October 15, 2007, from http://nccam.nih.gov/news/upcomingmeetings/manual-conference.htm

CONSORT. (2007). *CONSORT extension for non-pharmacological treatment (NPT) interventions.* Retrieved November, 6, 2007, from http://www.consort-statement.org/index.aspx?o=1287

Consortium of Academic Health Centers for Integrative Medicine. (n.d). *Consortium of academic health centers for integrative medicine.* Retrieved August 13, 2007, from http://www.imconsortium.org/cahcim/home.html

Consortium of Academic Health Centers for Integrative Medicine. *Education working group.* Retrieved October, 23, 2007, from http://www.imconsortium.org/cahcim/committees/education/home.html

Crawford, N. W., Cincotta, D. R., Lim, A., & Powell, C. V. (2006). A cross-sectional survey of complementary and alternative medicine use by children and adolescents attending the university hospital of Wales. *BMC Complementary and Alternative Medicine, 6*, 16.

Dryden, T., & Achilles, R. (2005). CAM health services and policy research in Canada—new directions: Abstracts from the first annual IN-CAM symposium, December 4–5, 2004, Toronto, Canada. *Journal of Complementary and Integrative Medicine, 2*(1), Article 3.

Dryden, T., Findlay, B., Boon, H., Mior, S., Verhoef, M., & Baskwill, A. (2004). *Research requirement: Literacy amongst complementary and alternative health care practitioners—phase I & phase II.* Ottawa, ON: Natural Health Products Directorate, Health Canada.

Eisenberg, D. M. (2004). *Keynote address. 2nd International Symposium on the Science of Touch.* Toward an Integrative Medicine, Montreal, Quebec. Montreal, Quebec.

Eisenberg, D. M. (2006). *Keynote address. North American Research Conference on Complementary and Integrative Medicine*, Edmonton, Alberta, May 24–27.

European InterProfessional Education Network (Eipen). (n.d.). Retrieved October 15, 2007, from http://www.eipen.org/

Explore: The Journal of Science & Healing. (2007). Retrieved October 15, 2007 from http://www.elsevier.com/wps/find/journaldescription.cws_home/703862/description?navopenmenu=-2

Feldman, D. E., Duffy, C., De Civita, M., Malleson, P., Philibert, L., Gibbon, M., et al. (2004). Factors associated with the use of complementary and alternative medicine in juvenile idiopathic arthritis. *Arthritis and Rheumatism, 51*(4), 527–532.

Fenton, M. V., & Morris, D. L. (2003). The integration of holistic nursing practices and complementary and alternative modalities into curricula of schools of nursing. *Alternative Therapies in Health and Medicine, 9*(4), 62–67.

Freshwinds Children's Complementary Therapy Network. (n.d.). Retrieved October 15, 2007, from http://www.freshwinds.org.uk/education/cctn/

Friends of Complementary and Alternative Therapies Society (FACTS). (n.d.). Retrieved October, 23, 2007, from http://www.thefacts.org/

Goldman, S. A. (1998). Limitations and strengths of spontaneous reports data. *Clinical Therapeutics, 20* (Suppl c), c40–c44.

Guyatt, G., Sackett, D., Adachi, J., Roberts, R., Chong, J., Rosenbloom, D., et al. (1988). A clinician's guide for conducting randomized trials in individual patients. *Canadian Medical Association Journal, 139*(6), 497–503.

Guyatt, G. H., Keller, J. L., Jaeschke, R., Rosenbloom, D., Adachi, J. D., & Newhouse, M. T. (1990). The n-of-1 randomized controlled trial: Clinical usefulness. Our three-year experience. *Annals of Internal Medicine, 112*(4), 293–299.

Hanson, E., Kalish, L. A., Bunce, E., Curtis, C., McDaniel, S., Ware, J., et al. (2007). Use of complementary and alternative medicine among children diagnosed with autism spectrum disorder. *Journal of Autism and Developmental Disorders, 37*(4), 628–636.

Hartmann, K., Doser, A. K., & Kuhn, M. (1999). Postmarketing safety information: How useful are spontaneous reports. *Pharmacoepidemiology and Drug Safety, 8* (Suppl 1), S65–S71.

Health Canada. (2001). *Guidelines for the Canadian pharmaceutical industry on reporting adverse reactions to marketed drugs (vaccines excluded)*. Retrieved October 15, 2007, from http://www.hc-sc.gc.ca/dhp-mps/medeff/report-declaration/guide/guide-ldir_indust_e.html

Health Canada. (2007). *Canadian adverse drug reaction monitoring program CADRMP adverse reaction database*. Retrieved October, 5, 2007, from http://www.hc-sc.gc.ca/dhp-mps/medeff/databasdon/agreement_accord_e.html

Health Canada (ICH Steering Committee). (2003). *Draft consensus guidelines, pharmacovigilance planning (PVP) E2E*. Retrieved October, 5, 2007, from http://www.hc-sc.gc.ca/dhp-mps/prodpharma/applic-demande/guide-ld/ich/consultation/e2e_step2_etape2_e.html

Integrated Health Care Policy Consortium. (n.d) (a). *Academic consortium for complementary and alternative health care (ACCAHC)*. Retrieved October 15, 2007, from http://ihpc.info/accahc/accahc.shtml

Integrated Health Care Policy Consortium. (n.d.) (b). *Integrated healthcare policy consortium*. Retrieved October 15, 2007, from www.ihpc.info

Integrated Health Care Policy Consortium. (n.d.). *National education dialogue to advance integrated healthcare: Creating common ground (NED)*. Retrieved October 15, 2007, from http://ihpc.info/ned/ned.shtml

Integrative Pediatrics Council. (n.d.). *Integrative pediatrics council*. Retrieved October 15, 2007, from http://www.integrativepeds.org/

Jean, D., & Cyr, C. (2007). Use of complementary and alternative medicine in a general pediatric clinic. *Pediatrics, 120*(1), e138–e141.

Johnston, B. C., & Vohra, S. (2006). Which medications used in paediatric practice have demonstrated natural health product-drug interactions? Part A: Evidence-based answer and summary. *Paediatrics & Child Health, 11*(10), 671–672.

Johnston, B. C., & Vohra, S. (2005) Treating C. difficile. *Canadian Medical Association Journal, 172*(4), 447–448.

Journal of Alternative and Complementary Medicine.(n.d.). Retrieved October 15, 2007, from http://www.liebertpub.com/publication.aspx?pub_id=26

Kazdin, A. E. (1982). *Single-case research designs: Methods for clinical and applied settings.* New York: Oxford University Press.

Kelly, K. M., Jacobson, J. S., Kennedy, D. D., Braudt, S. M., Mallick, M., & Weiner, M. A. (2000). Use of unconventional therapies by children with cancer at an urban medical center [see comment]. *Journal of Pediatric Hematology/Oncology, 22*(5), 412–416.

Klassen, T., Pham, B., Lawson, M., & Moher, D. (2005). For randomized controlled trials, the quality of reports of complementary and alternative medicine was as good as reports of conventional medicine. *Journal of Clinical Epidemiology, 58*(8), 763–768.

Laurenson, M., MacDonald, J., McCready, T., & Stimpson, A. (2006). Student nurses' knowledge and attitudes toward CAM therapies. *British Journal of Nursing, 15*(11), 612–615.

Lawson, M., Pham, B., Klassen, T., & Moher, D. (2005). Systematic reviews involving complementary and alternative medicine interventions had higher quality of reporting than conventional medicine reviews. *Journal of Clinical Epidemiology, 58*(8), 777–784.

Lee, A. C., & Kemper, K. J. (2000). Homeopathy and naturopathy: Practice characteristics and pediatric care. *Archives of Pediatrics & Adolescent Medicine, 154*(1), 75–80.

Loman, D. G. (2003). The use of complementary and alternative health care practices among children. *Journal of Pediatric Health Care, 17*(2), 58–63.

MacPherson, H., & Thomas, K. (2005). Short term reactions to acupuncture—a cross-sectional survey of patient reports. *Acupuncture in Medicine: Journal of the British Medical Acupuncture Society, 23*(3), 112–120.

McCurdy, E. A., Spangler, J. G., Wofford, M. M., Chauvenet, A. R., & McLean, T. W. (2003). Religiosity is associated with the use of complementary medical therapies by pediatric oncology patients. *Journal of Pediatric Hematology/Oncology, 25*(2), 125–129.

Melchart, D., Steger, H. G., Linde, K., Makarian, K., Hatahet, Z., Brenke, R., et al. (2002). Integrating patient preferences in clinical trials: A pilot study of acupuncture versus midazolam for gastoscopy. *Journal of alternative and Complementary Medicine, 8*(3), 256–274.

Moher, D., Soeken, K., Sampson, M., Ben-Porat, L., & Berman, B. (2002). Assessing the quality of reports of randomized trials in pediatric complementary and alternative medicine. *BMC Pediatrics, 2*, 2.

National Cancer Institute. (n.d.). *NCI best case series program.* Retrieved October 15, 2007, from http://www.cancer.gov/cam/bestcase_intro.html

National Center for Complementary and Alternative Medicine. (2007). *CAM use in children. Patterns of CAM use in children.* Retrieved August 25, 2007, from http://nccam.nih.gov/health/children/#3

National Center for Complementary And Medicine (NCCAM). (2007). *What Is CAM.* Retrieved October 5, 2007, from http://nccam.nih.gov/health/whatiscam/#3

National Centre for Complementary & Alternative Medicine. (2002). *Complementary and alternative medicine (CAM) education project grant (R25s).* Retrieved October 15, 2007, from http://nccam.nih.gov/research/r25/

National Centre for Complementary & Alternative Medicine (NCCAM). *CAM practitioner research career development award (K01).* Retrieved October, 23, 2007, from http://nccam.nih.gov/research/concepts/consider/camprac-k01.htm

Natural Health Products Directorate. Health Canada. *Adverse reaction report form for clinical trials natural health products.* Retrieved October 15, 2007, from http://www.hc-sc.gc.ca/dhp-mps/alt_formats/hpfb-dgpsa/pdf/prodnatur/adv_reac_rep_form_e.pdf

Pangea—A Conference for the Future of Pediatrics. (n.d.). Retrieved October, 23, 2007, from http://www.pangeaconference.com/

Papanikolaou, P. N., Christidi, G. D., & Ioannidis, J. P. (2006). Comparison of evidence on harms of medical interventions in randomized and nonrandomized studies. *Canadian Medical Association Journal, 174*(5), 635–641.

Papanikolaou, P. N., & Ioannidis, J. P. (2004). Availability of large-scale evidence on specific harms from systematic reviews of randomized trials. *The American Journal of Medicine, 117*(8), 582–589.

Provisional Section on Complementary, Holistic, and Integrative Medicine.(n.d.). Retrieved October, 23, 2007, from http://www.aap.org/sections/chim/education.htm

Prussing, E., Sobo, E. J., Walker, E., Dennis, K., & Kurtin, P. S. (2004). Communicating with pediatricians about complementary/alternative medicine: Perspectives from parents of children with down syndrome. *Ambulatory Pediatrics: The Official Journal of the Ambulatory Pediatric Association, 4*(6), 488–494.

Roth, D., Johnston, B. C., & Vohra, S. (2006). Which medications used in paediatric practice have demonstrated natural health product-drug interactions? Part B: Clinical commentary. *Paediatrics & Child Health, 11*(10), 673–674.

Sanders, H., Davis, M. F., Duncan, B., Meaney, F. J., Haynes, J., & Barton, L. L. (2003). Use of complementary and alternative medical therapies among children with special health care needs in southern Arizona. *Pediatrics, 111*(3), 584–587.

Sawni, A., & Thomas, R. (2007). Pediatricians' attitudes, experience and referral patterns regarding Complementary/Alternative medicine: A national survey. *BMC Complementary and Alternative Medicine, 7*, 18.

Sawyer, M. G., Gannoni, A. F., Toogood, I. R., Antoniou, G., & Rice, M. (1994). The use of alternative therapies by children with cancer. *The Medical Journal of Australia, 160*(6), 320–322.

Shekelle, P. G., Adams, A. H., Chassin, M. R., Hurwitz, E. L., & Brook, R. H. (1992). Spinal manipulation for low-back pain. *Annals of Interal Medicine, 117*(7), 590–598.

Sibinga, E. M., Shindell, D. L., Casella, J. F., Duggan, A. K., & Wilson, M. H. (2006). Pediatric patients with sickle cell disease: Use of complementary and alternative therapies. *Journal of Alternative and Complementary Medicine (New York, NY), 12*(3), 291–298.

SickKids Foundation. (n.d.). *National grants program.* Retrieved October 15, 2007, from http://www.sickkidsfoundation.com/grants/howtoapply.asp

SickKids Foundation. (2007). Retrieved October 15, 2007, from http://www.sickkidsfoundation.com/

Singleton, A., Smith, F., Harris, T., Ross-Harper, R., & Hilton, S. (1999). An evaluation of the team objective structured clinical examination (TOSCE) *Medical Education, 33*(1), 34–41.

UK Centre for the Advancement of Interprofessional Education (CAIPE). (2007). *About CAIPE.* Retrieved October, 5, 2007, from http://www.caipe.org.uk/index.php?sid=dc8d922129b6b758e09d1efeb6b25e50&page=mission

US Food and Drug Administration (FDA). (2007). *Managing the risks from medical product use: Part 3: How does the FDA conduct postmarketing surveillance and risk assessment?* Retrieved October, 5, 2007, from http://www.fda.gov/oc/tfrm/Part3.html

Verhoef, M. J., WAre, M. A., Dryden, T., Gignac, P., Weeks, L., Kania, A., et al. (2007). *Focus on Alternative and Complementary Therapies, 12*(3), 170–171.

Vohra, S., Johnston, B. C., Cramer, K., & Humphreys, K. (2007). Adverse events associated with pediatric spinal manipulation: A systematic review. *Pediatrics, 119*(1), e275–e283.

Weeks, J. (2007) *The integrator blog.* Retrieved October 15, 2007, from http://theintegratorblog.com/site/

White, A., Hayhoe, S., Hart, A., & Ernst, E. (2001). Adverse events following acupuncture: Prospective survey of 32 000 consultations with doctors and physiotherapists *BMJ, 323*(7311), 485–486.

White House Commission. (2002). *White house commission on complementary and alternative medicine policy. Final Report –March 2002.* Retrieved October, 22, 2007, from http://whccamp.hhs.gov/pdfs/fr2002_document.pdf

Wideman, H., Owston, R., Brown, C., Kushniruk, A., Ho, F., & Pitts, K. (2007). Unpacking the potential of educational gaming: A new tool for gaming research. *Simulation and Gaming and Interdisciplinary Journal, 38*(1), 9–29.

Yeh, C. H., Lee, T. T., Chen, M. L., & Li, W. (2000). Adaptational process of parents of pediatric oncology patients. *Pediatric Hematology and Oncology, 17*(2), 119–131.

II

Pediatric Perspectives on Specific Therapeutic Approaches

6

A Pediatric Perspective on Acupuncture

YUAN-CHI LIN AND SHU-MING WANG

KEY CONCEPTS

- Acupuncture is a discipline of traditional Chinese medicine that has evolved over two millennia. It employs the technique of inserting and manipulating hair-thin needles into acupuncture points for therapeutic and preventive purposes.
- Acupuncture is widely practiced in the United States today and has become a visible component of the current healthcare system.
- Acupuncture is often practiced in conjunction with other modalities and related techniques of traditional Chinese medicine. Some of these modalities include moxibustion, cupping, gwa sha, acupressure, and tui na.
- According to traditional Chinese medicine, there are six pathological factors that cause disease. These factors include wind, cold, heat, dampness, dryness, and fire. Practitioners of traditional Chinese medicine (TCM) obtain detailed histories and perform physical examinations on patients with the goal of assessing the underlying causes of the patient's illness and to gain insight into other symptoms and organ function.
- There are eight principal classifications of symptoms. These classifications include Yin or Yang, external or internal, cold or hot, and deficient or excess. The aim of therapy is to restore deficiencies or address excesses of Qi, thereby refurbishing the patient's health.
- There have been a number of studies conducted, including randomized controlled trials, systemic reviews, and meta-analysis, to evaluate the efficacy of acupuncture.
- Although much of the scientific research into acupuncture focuses on its efficacy in pain management, there is documented evidence that acupuncture is efficacious for the treatment of a number of other pediatric conditions as well.

- Although in rare circumstances, acupuncture can produce complications, it is a very safe intervention in the hands of a competent practitioner.

■

History of Acupuncture

Acupuncture is a modality of traditional Chinese medicine (TCM), the use of which can be traced back more than 3,000 years ago. The word acupuncture is derived from Latin *acus* "with a needle" and *pungere* "puncture through the skin." It is commonly performed by inserting special hair-thin needles into the skin at specific sites known as acupuncture points. These points are connected to one another along meridians. TCM is not an ideological belief. It is a system of thoughts and practices that is based on the investigation of the natural phenomena, the understanding of the principles of realism, and their application to prevent and treat human ailments.

The ancient book of TCM is Huang Di Nei Jing (Yellow Emperor' Classic of Internal Medicine), which was compiled around 305–204 BCE. This text composed of two volumes "Shu Wen" and "Ling Shu." Each has 81 chapters in a question-and-answer format between dominion Huang Di and his divine Chi Po. The text describes the theoretical foundation of Chinese medicine, diagnosis and treatment methods, and acupuncture.

The Shang Han Lun is the treatise on cold disease damage by Zhang Zhong Jing. It mentions six divisions, which include Tai Yang (larger yang), Yang ming (yang brightness), Shao Yang (lesser yang), Tai Yin (larger yin), Shao yin (lesser yin), and Jue Yin (absolute yin). It also describes the prescriptions of ingredients for adult and pediatric diseases that occurred in the Han dynasty (25–220 AD). Chen Yi (1035–1117 AD) described the differential diagnosis of pediatric symptoms, and through his efforts, pediatric medicine became a discipline of Chinese medicine. Won Chen, during the Ming dynasty (1368–1644 AD), also addressed pediatric treatment in excess and deficiency states.

The first known European account of the use of acupuncture comes from a sixteenth-century Roman Catholic church in Canton, China, reported by Portuguese, Dutch, Danish, and French missionaries. "A Treatise on Acupunction" by a surgeon named James Morss Churchill, published in 1823, was the first English text known to describe the practice. The treatise attributes to acupuncture great success in the treatment of rheumatic conditions, sciatica, and back pain. Churchill's book generated increased interest in acupuncture as a treatment modality in the late nineteenth century.

In 1972, Mr. James Reston described the alleviation by acupuncture of his postoperative pain following an emergency appendectomy in a front-page article in *The New*

York Times. The article brought increased interest and awareness of acupuncture to the United States. Stories about the use of acupuncture for anesthesia during major surgery in China began appearing in the Western press. This popular interest led to scientific efforts to test the clinical effectiveness and determine the underlying mechanism of acupuncture for analgesia. In 1974, California became the first state in the United States to make acupuncture a legal experimental procedure. In 1996, the Food and Drug Administration changed the status of acupuncture needles from Class III to Class II medical devices, determining that acupuncture needles are regarded as safe and effective when used appropriately by licensed practitioners.

Acupuncture and Related Techniques

There is no universally accepted anatomical or histological configuration to acupuncture points or meridians. Acupuncture points are determined and described in functional rather than structural terms. Most of these points are located in minute grooves or in depressions in the skin's surface. On palpation, acupuncture points are frequently tender. After insertion of the needle, manual stimulation of the acupuncture needle produces a temporary sensation known as "De Qi," which means grasping or obtaining the energy. "De Qi" is described as a pressure, soreness, heaviness, or distension emanating from the point where the acupuncture needle is inserted.

Acupuncture is often practiced in conjunction with other modalities of traditional Chinese medicine. Some of these methods and techniques include moxibustion, cupping, gwa sha, acupressure, and tui na.

Moxibustion is a therapy that is complementary to acupuncture and is often used in conjunction with it. Moxibustion is the burning of moxa (*Artemisia vulgaris*) over the region of the desired acupuncture points, which can facilitate the energy flow in the body. This burning of the moxi can be used indirectly, with the acupuncture needles, or directly over the skin.

Cupping is the practice of creating a vacuum over the patient's skin. The vacuum is created inside specially designed glass "cups," which are placed over the skin at the desired locations. The cups are usually bell-shaped, and commonly, 2 to 12 cups can be placed on the subject's back or abdomen. The vacuum is achieved by drawing the air out of the space inside the cup, either using an air vacuum or by filling the cup with heated air, which produces the vacuum effect as it cools. Cupping is commonly used to treat respiratory disease and musculoskeletal pain.

Gwa sha is a technique in which the skin is scrapped in strokes by a round-edged instrument. The traditional tool used for gwa sha is a porcelain Chinese spoon. This scraping occurs across the upper back, shoulder, and posterior neck region. When gwa sha is employed to promote healing, the practitioner feels that he or she is scraping on the top of underlined sandy tissue. "Gwa" means scraping and "sha" means "sand."

Tui na is a form of Chinese manipulative therapy that employs finger pressure, friction, or massage. Tui na was mentioned in the Di Nei Jing (Yellow Emperor's Classic of

Internal Medicine). The practitioner may press or rub over the musculoskeletal tissue or joints. Tui na has been used for the treatment of musculoskeletal, digestive, respiratory, or chronic stress disorders. Acupressure is similar to Tui na in that it also employs hand and finger pressure over the acupuncture points.

Theories of Acupuncture

The theories of traditional Chinese medicine, including acupuncture, evolved from thoughtful observation and explanation of the nature phenomena, including the concepts of "Yin" and "Yang" and "the five phases."

The concept of Yin and Yang is apparent, but its implication is philosophical. Yin and Yang are co-dependent, existing in a constant state of dynamic balance. They are natural phenomena that exist within the body and can be transformed into each other. Yin is associated with rest, coldness, passivity, darkness, inwardness, and diminishment. Yang is associated with activity, hot, activity, brightness, outwardness, and augmentation. Health requires a balance of Yin and Yang in the body, while disease is characterized by a disharmony or imbalance between them.

The theory of five phases is based on the concept that all phenomena in the universe are the products of the evolution of five elements: fire, earth, metal, water, and wood. The concepts behind the five phases correspond with normal physiology and abnormal pathology, and they influence the management of ailments. There are two distinct cycles associated with the five phases—the "sheng" cycle, and the "ke" cycle. The "sheng" cycle is a creation cycle. In its initial stage, earth is created from fire, metal is originated from earth, metal engenders water, water promotes wood to grow, and wood fuels the fire. Each phase has a corresponding Yin and Yang channel, analogous with meridians in the body. The "ke" cycle is a controlling/limiting cycle. The root of wood/tree can split earth, earth can block water, water can extinguish the fire, fire can melt the metal, and metal can cut the wood. The controlling sequence ensures that balance is maintained in the five phases. The mutual generating and controlling relationship is the model for many of Yin and Yang's balancing processes.

The balance of Yin and Yang within the body promotes the flow of "Qi" (pronounced "chee"). Qi signifies power, movement, and a force similar to energy. Qi is a functional, active part of the body and is not easily definable. All Qi that resides in human beings and living creatures is the result of interaction between the Qi of Heaven and the Qi of Earth. Qi is an energy equivalent that can manifest at the physical and spiritual level. It flows through a complex system of meridians in the body, maintaining life and health. Diseases and illnesses are byproducts of obstruction or inadequate flow of Qi through the meridians. The flow of Qi may be restored by the insertion of the acupuncture needles into acupuncture points.

Practitioners of acupuncture routinely take detailed patient medical histories and details of present illnesses when pursuing the differential diagnosis. Attention is focused on the characteristic of the pulse and the manifestation of the tongue. According to TCM, six pathological factors that may cause disease include wind, cold, heat, dampness, dryness, and fire. The goal of history taking and physical examination of the patient is to assess the patient's balance of Yin and Yang, and to gain insight into other symptoms and organ function.

There are eight principal classifications of symptoms of disease or illness. They include Yin or Yang, external or internal, cold or hot, and deficient or excess. The aim of therapy is to restore deficiencies or to address the excesses of Qi, thereby restoring health.

Basic Scientific Evidence

Basic scientific research has focused on the understanding of acupuncture from a neurobiological perspective. The acupuncture-induced elevation of pain threshold is gradual at onset, with a peak effect at 20–40 minutes, followed by an exponential delay with a half-life of approximately 16 minutes (Figure 6-1) (Ulett, Han, & Han, 1998). A greater cumulative effect was observed when multiple acupuncture points were stimulated simultaneously and the injection of local anesthetics into the acupuncture point prior to the acupuncture stimulation abolished the expected analgesic effect.

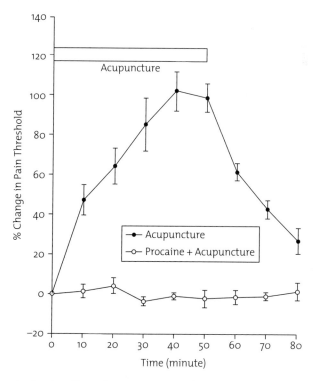

FIGURE 6-1. Analgesic effect of acupuncture in human volunteers. (Adapted from Electroacupuncture: mechanisms and clinical application. *Biological Psychiatry* 1998; 44:129–138.)

An intact sensory afferent system is essential for the transmission of acupuncture signals. Elevation of pain threshold was observed in an acupuncture-naïve rabbit infused with cerebral spinal fluid obtained from another rabbit post-acupuncture stimulation. Acupuncture stimulation releases a neuromodulatory substance into the cerebral spinal fluid. Administration of the opioid antagonist naxolone blocked the analgesic effect induced by acupuncture (Pomeranz, 1996; Pomeranz & Chiu, 1976).

Following the development of electroacupuncture, detailed information regarding the mechanism of acupuncture analgesia was revealed. The research studies revealed that low-frequency electroacupuncture induces the release of enkephalin and beta-endorphin and high- frequency electroacupuncture induces the release of dynorphin in an animal model (Figure 6-2) (Han et al., 1991; Han, 2003, 2004).

The analgesic effect of acupuncture had no correlation with the duration of acupuncture stimulation. That is, more than 40 minutes of acupuncture stimulation actually has no analgesic effect (Han, Li, & Tang, 1981; Han, Tang, Huang, Liang, & Zhang, 1979). This tolerance to acupuncture analgesia is the result of the release of anti-opioids, for example, cholecystokinin octapeptide (CCK-8). By administering CCK-8 antagonist, Han and colleagues were able to reverse this acupuncture tolerance phenomenon (Han, Ding, & Fan, 1986).The peripheral acupuncture stimulations activated various regions in the brain that are involved in the production of opioid precursors. Pan and colleagues

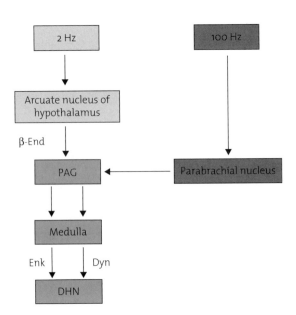

FIGURE 6-2. The release of opioid peptides after different frequencies of electrical acupuncture stimulation. (Adapted from Acupuncture: neuropeptide release produced by electrical stimulation of different frequencies. *Trends in Neurosciences* 2003; 26:17–22.)

(Pan, Castro-Lopes, Coimbra, & 1994, 1996, 1997) discovered an overlap of central path-ways between noxious stimulation and acupuncture stimulation. They demonstrated that acupuncture and pain both activated the hypothalamus-pituitary-adenocortical axis but at different nuclei of the hypothalamus. With the advancement of diagnostic imaging techniques, that is positron emission tomography (PET), single-proton emis-sion computer tomography (SPECT), and functional magnetic resonance imaging (fMRI), scientists have been able to study the central pathways of acupuncture nonin-vasively. With the use of PET, scientists have confirmed that the areas of the left anterior cingulum, superior frontal gyrus, bilateral cerebellum, and insular and right medial and inferior frontal gyri are activated by acupuncture stimulation. These areas of the brain are also activated in both acute and chronic pain conditions (Biella et al., 2001; Hsieh et al., 2001). Pariente and colleagues (Pariente, White, Frackowiak, & Lewith, 2005) dis-covered that the activation of right dorsolateral prefrontal cortex, anterior cingulated cor-tex, and midbrain may not be specific to acupuncture stimulation but that the activation of insula ipsilateral to the acupuncture stimulation is specific to acupuncture stimulation. With the use of SPECT, Newberg and colleagues (Newberg et al., 2005) found that patients with a history of chronic pain had asymmetrical uptake in the thalamic regions. However, after 20–25 minutes of acupuncture stimulation, they found a reversal of asymmetric uptake of thalamus that coincided with the reduction of pain in the patients.

The hypothalamus-limbic system is part of the acupuncture central pathway. Functional MRIs have been used to explore the central pathways of acupuncture. Acupuncture stimulation caused enhancement of blood-oxygenation-level-dependent (BOLD) signals at hypothalamus and nucleus accumbens but a reduction of BOLD signals at the rostral part of the anterior cingulate cortex, amygdale formation, and the hippocampal complex (Wu et al., 1999). Acupuncture stimulation caused a reduction of BOLD signals at the nucleus accumbens, hypothalamus, amygdale, hippocampus, para hippocampus, ventral tegmental area, anterior cingular gyrus, caudate, putamen, temporal lobe, and insula (Hui et al., 2000, 2005).

The nucleus accumbens, hypothalamus, amygdale, and anterior cingular gyrus are involved in transmitting acupuncture stimulation from peripheral to the higher cortex. When the images are captured, the duration of acupuncture manipulation from differ-ent studies and the sensation of "De Qi," which is experienced by the experimental sub-jects, may determine whether the BOLD signals should be enhanced or reduced in these areas. Other regions of the brain found to be associated with acupuncture stimulation are insula and periaquaductal grey regions (Liu et al., 2004; Wang et al., 2007). Langevin et al. (2001) described that the acupuncture needle is being grasped by connective tissue because of collagen and elastic fibers winding and tightening around the needle during needle rotation. A mechanical coupling is developed between needle and tissue. Using rat abdominal wall explants as an experimental model, they found that needle rotation was accompanied by marked thickening of the subcutaneous connective tissue layer in the area surrounding the needle during manipulation and that there was no structural

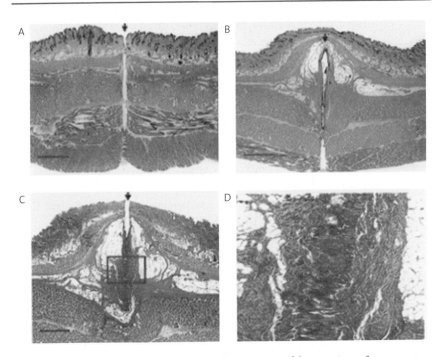

FIGURE 6-3. The local connective tissue changes caused by rotation of acupuncture needle and direct insertion of acupuncture needle without rotation. (Adapted from Mechanical signaling through connective tissue: mechanism for therapeutic effect of acupuncture *FASEB* 2001; 15:2275–2282.)

change in dermis, muscle, or abdominal wall muscles other than displacement by the thickened subcutaneous tissue layer. Masson trichrome staining showed collagen winding around the needle track with acupuncture needle rotation, clearly supporting the hypothesis that connective tissue winds around the needle during needle rotation (Figure 6-3a–d). Winding of connective tissue around the needle results in a marked amplification of the mechanical coupling between the needle and the local connective tissue (Langevin, Churchill, & Cipolla, 2001). Once the acupuncture needle becomes coupled to tissue, movements of the needle may send a signal through connective tissue via deformation of the extracellular matrix. The pulling of collagen fibers during needle manipulation may transmit a mechanical signal, through deformation of the extracellular matrix, to cells such as fibroblasts that are abundant in connective tissue. The subsequent signal transduction events may contribute to the effect of "De Qi."

Clinical Evidence of Pediatric Acupuncture

In order to validate the effectiveness of acupuncture in various clinical conditions, a rigorous scientific study design should be applied through randomization, double-blinded,

Table 6-1. Acupuncture Points in the Literature for Problems

Clinical Entity	Acupuncture Points
Asthma	LI-4, 11; UB-13; LU-7, 9,10; ST-36; Sp-6; KI-3
Migraine	GB-20, 40, 41, 42; GV-20; LI-3; TH-3, 5
Allergy rhinitis	EX-HN 3, 8; ST-36
Nocturnal enuresis	CV-3,4,6, UB-23, 28, 32, 33, 60; Sp-6,9; KI-3; ST-44
PONV[a]	PC-6, UB-10,11; GB 34; K-K9[b]
Postop abdominal pain	ST-36

[a]PONV: Postoperative nausea and vomiting.
[b]Korean hand acupuncture point.

or sham-controlled intervention. Although several specific problems related to acupuncture clinical research are frequently mentioned in the literature—most notably that acupuncture is an intervention that advocates individualized treatment—the number of high-quality adult acupuncture clinical studies is rapidly increasing. Only a few pediatric acupuncture clinical research studies have been conducted, and the majority of pediatric acupuncture clinical studies in literature are case reports and treatment outcomes.

Most pediatric acupuncture studies consist of case reports, case series, or intervention studies poorly designed for efficacy assessment. Only a few studies have followed the rigorous scientific guidelines, and the results derived from even these studies may be invalid owing to small sample size, active sham, placebo control, and limited duration of treatment, and follow-up period. These studies involve acupuncture for the treatment of asthma, chronic pain, smoking cessation, nocturnal enuresis, postoperative vomiting, postextubation strider, postoperative pain, chemotherapy-induced nausea and vomiting, and allergic rhinitis. The acupuncture points used in these studies are summarized in Table 6-1.

ASTHMA

In TCM, acute asthma attacks can be differentiated into cold, heat, or yang deficiency patterns on the basis of the presentation. Usually the cold pattern of an asthma attack is brought on by respiratory tract infection, stress, or allergy. In contrast, the heat pattern is brought on by the attack of wind-heat, in which patients tend to exhibit signs of heat. The deficiency pattern usually responds well to bronchodilator treatment. Based on the description in TCM, the patient simply gives up the struggle to fight for breath and has no strength left. Many acupuncture points used for asthma treatment, for example LI-4, are commonly used to expel wind in both cold and heat patterns. BL-13 and LU-9 are commonly used simultaneously to tonify the lung. Other acupuncture points such as LI-11, LU-7, LU-10, PC-6, ST-36, SP-6, and KI-3 are primarily used for ventilating the lungs, invigorating the spleen, and tonifying the kidneys.

The majority of publications available in the literature are case reports and series of treatments. Gruber and colleagues (2002) conducted the following clinical study to test the efficacy of laser acupuncture as a prophylactic treatment for children and adolescents with exercise-induced asthma. A total of 44 children and adolescents were randomized into single laser acupuncture treatment and a placebo-controlled group. The interventions were administered in random order on two consecutive days. Pulmonary functions were measured before intervention and after intervention using cold-air challenge. The investigators found there was no difference between laser acupuncture and the placebo-controlled groups in force expiratory volume in 1 second (FEV_1) and maximal expiratory airflow at 25% remaining vital capacity (Figure 6-4).

Stockert and colleagues (2007) enrolled 17 children between 6 and 12 years of age with intermittent or mild persistent medical asthma in a randomized, placebo-controlled, double-blinded pilot study. Eight children were randomly assigned to receive laser acupuncture for 10 weeks and probiotic treatment in the form of oral drops for 7 weeks. Nine children were randomly placed into the control group to receive a non-functional laser pen and were given placebo drops. Laser acupuncture and probiotics significantly decreased mean weekly bronchial hyper-reactivity. They did not find ten weeks of laser acupuncture and probiotic treatment to have a significant effect on FEV_1, quality of life criteria, and the use of additional medication. The laser acupuncture group had fewer days of acute febrile infections when compared to the control group. The laser acupuncture and probiotics had a beneficial clinical effect on bronchial hyper-reactivity in school-age children with intermittent or mild persistent asthma and, this effect may be helpful in the prevention of acute respiratory exacerbations.

HEADACHE

In traditional Chinese acupuncture theory, pain is the result of the obstruction of vital energy "Qi." The application of acupuncture and related interventions to the appropriate acupuncture points can restore the flow of vital energy and eliminate or reduce pain, for example, migraine. Acupuncture analgesia has a neurophysiological basis, that is, an intact nervous system is needed for the transmission of acupuncture signals from the peripheral to the central nervous system (Lim, Loh, Kranz, & Scott, 1977), thereby altering the central and peripheral secretion of neurotransmitters and the release of endogenous opioids. Several acupuncture points are recommended in the adult literature as treatment for migraine (Figure 6-5) (Allais et al., 2002).

Pintov and colleagues (Pintov et al., 1997) investigated the effectiveness of acupuncture in childhood migraines. Twenty-two children with migraines were randomly divided into true acupuncture groups and placebo acupuncture groups. Ten healthy children were included as controls. Opioid activity in blood plasma was assayed by the total (panopioid) activity with an opiate radioreceptor assay and the β-endorphin-like

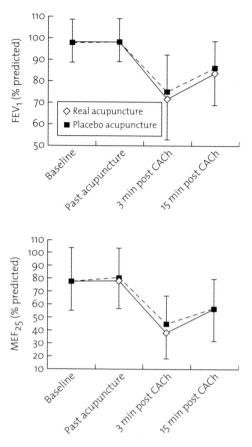

FIGURE 6-4. The changes of EFV$_1$ and MEF$_{25}$ before and after laser acupuncture. (Adapted from Laser acupuncture in children and adolescents with exercise induced asthma. *Thorax* 2002; 57:222–225.)

immunoactivity by radioimmunoassay. The true acupuncture led to a significant clinical reduction of migraine frequency and intensity. The total panopioid activity in plasma showed a gradual increase in the true acupuncture group that correlated with the clinical improvement. After the tenth treatment, the values of opioid activity in the true acupuncture group were similar to those of the control group, whereas the plasma of the placebo acupuncture group showed insignificant changes in plasma opioid activity. Similarly, a significant increase in the β-endorphin level was observed in the children of the true acupuncture group as compared to pretreatment or the placebo acupuncture groups. This suggests that acupuncture may be an effective treatment in children with migraine headaches by enhancing the release of endogenous opioids. A prospective, randomized, double-blind, placebo-controlled trial of low-level laser acupuncture was performed in 43 children with chronic headache. Patients were randomized to receive a

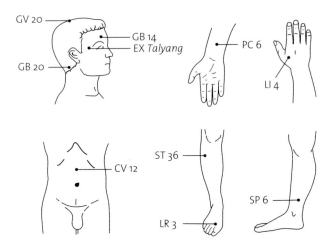

FIGURE 6-5. The acupuncture points used for migraine prophylaxis. (Adapted from Acupuncture in the Prophylactic Treatment of Migraine Without Aura: A Comparison with Flunarizine. *Headache* 2002; 42(9):855–861.)

course of four treatments over four weeks with either active or placebo laser. The mean number of headaches and the severity of headache per month decreased significantly in the laser acupuncture treatment group (Gottschling et al., 2007).

SMOKING CESSATION

A double-blinded, randomized, placebo-controlled clinical study was conducted (Yiming et al., 2000) to evaluate the efficacy of laser acupuncture treatment and sham acupuncture in a group of 330 adolescent smokers. At 4 weeks' and 3 months' follow-up, there was no significant difference in the rates of smoking cessation in the true and sham acupuncture groups.

NOCTURNAL ENURESIS

Nightly bedwetting affects about 10% of 7-year-old children, with a wide range of frequencies between populations (Monda & Husmann, 1995). The affliction is often linked to major social maladjustments and occupies considerable time in general practice. From the age of seven there is a spontaneous cure rate of 15% per year, such that few remain affected after the age of 16 years. There are two types of nocturnal enuresis: type I, primary, with at least three nightly episodes in children over 7 years of age, where the child has always had the disorder; and type II, secondary, where the child has been dry for at least six months, but enuresis has recurred. Acupuncture and its related techniques can be used for nocturnal enuresis. Capozza and colleagues (Capozza et al., 1991) randomized 40 children with primary nocturnal enuresis into desmopressin, acupuncture, desmopressin plus acupuncture, and placebo-controlled groups. They found that children in both the desmopressin and acupuncture group had a high percentage of dry nights and that the combination of desmopressin and acupuncture together appeared to be most effective.

Radmayr, Schlager, Studen, and Bartsch (2001) randomized 40 children who suffer from monosymptomatic nocturnal enuresis to receive desmopressin treatment or laser acupuncture treatment. The investigators found that the children of both groups had an initial mean frequency of 5.5 wet nights per week. At a 6-month follow-up, a completed success rate of 75% in the desmopressin group and 65% of laser acupuncture group was found. The investigators did not find statistical significance between these two interventions. A systemic review and meta-analysis by Bower et al. provides tentative evidence for the efficacy of acupuncture for the treatment of childhood nocturnal enuresis (Bower, Diao, Tang, & Yeung, 2005).

POSTOPERATIVE NAUSEA AND VOMITING

Postoperative vomiting is a significant problem that can cause wound dehiscence, electrolyte imbalance, and other complications. Multiple problems were identified in studies investigating the use of acupuncture to manage pediatric postoperative vomiting conducted before 1997. Some of these problems included small sample size, the timing of acupuncture stimulation, perioperative anesthetic techniques, and appropriate control groups (Wang & Kain, 2002). Schlager, Offer, and Baldissera (1998), using laser stimulation of the P6 point in children undergoing strabismus surgery, found that the intervention significantly decreased postoperative vomiting.

Chu and colleagues (1998) applied acupressure with acuplaster to BL-10, BL-11, and GB-34 acupuncture points as prophylactic treatment for postoperative vomiting in children undergoing strabismus surgery. The investigators randomized a total of 65 children between ages of 3 and 14 years into a placebo or an acuplaster group. The interventions were administered the night before surgery, and anesthetic techniques were standardized using halothane, nitrous oxide, and oxygen. They found that significantly fewer patients developed postoperative vomiting in the acuplaster group as compared to the placebo group during the first 24 hours following surgery.

Shenkman and colleagues (1999) used acupressure-acupuncture at the P-6 point on the wrist. A total of 100 children were enrolled into this study, and were randomized into the study and sham groups. The study group of children received acubands bilaterally and the sham group received no pressure beads at two sham points prior to induction. After induction, acupuncture needles were substituted for the beads and were left in place until the next day. Standardized anesthetic management was administered to all participants. The investigators did not find significant differences in the episodes of emesis between the two groups.

Schlager, Boehler, and Puhringer (2000) applied acupressure at the K-K9 acupuncture points 30 minutes before induction and kept the acupressure in place for 24 hours in a group of children undergoing strabismus surgery (Figure 6-6a,b). They found that children in the acupressure group had a significantly lower incidence of vomiting as compared to the placebo group.

Somri and colleagues (2001) compared the anti-emetic effect of P6 acupuncture with ondansetron and a placebo in a group of children receiving dental surgery. They found a significant decrease in the number of patients who vomited and also in the total number of vomiting episodes in two treatment groups as compared with the placebo group. There was no difference between the acupuncture and ondansetron groups.

Rusy, Hoffman, and Weisman (2002) used electrical stimulation of acupuncture point P6 as a prophylactic postoperative nausea and vomiting treatment for children undergoing tonsillectomy with or without adenoidectomy. The investigators also found that children who received true electrical stimulation at acupuncture points PC6 had significantly less postoperative nausea and vomiting.

Wang and Kain (2002) applied 0.2 cc of D50 glucose solution into bilateral acupuncture point PC6 as a prophylactic anti-emetic treatment for children after surgery. They found that bilateral acupuncture points PC6 injections are as effective as intravenous droperidol in preventing early postoperative nausea and vomiting in children. A systematic review supports the use of acupuncture point PC6 stimulation in patients without anti-emetic prophylaxis. Acupuncture point PC6 stimulation seems to reduce the risk of nausea but not vomiting (Lee & Done, 2004).

Butkovic and colleagues (2005) compared the use of laser acupuncture and metoclopramide in preventing the development of postoperative nausea and vomiting. The investigators found that bilateral laser acupuncture PC6 stimulations are as effective as metoclopramide in preventing the development of postoperative nausea and vomiting in children.

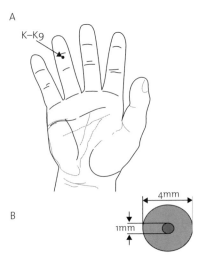

FIGURE 6-6. (a) The Korean hand acupuncture point K-K9. (b) The acupressure bead. (Adapted from Korean hand acupressure reduces postoperative vomiting in children after strabismus surgery. *British Journal of Anaesthesia*, 2000; 85:267–270.)

Kabalak, Akcay, Akcay, and Gogus (2005) found that transcutaneous electrical acupuncture point stimulation is as effective as ondansetron in preventing postoperative vomiting following pediatric tonsillectomy. A meta-analysis of the acupunture points stimulation effect on postoperative nausea and vomiting in children indicates that acupressure and acupuncture are effective treatment modalities for reducing postoperative vomiting in children. Acupuncture treatment is as effective as medication in reducing vomiting in children (Dune & Shiao, 2006). Acupuncture is also found to be effective as a treatment for chemotherapy-induced nausea and vomiting in adults. A crossover study was conducted in a group of children who received emetogenic chemotherapy (Reindl et al., 2006). Eleven children were enrolled into the study. The patients were randomized to receive acupuncture plus anti-emetics or anti-emetics alone. Twenty-two courses with or without acupuncture were compared. The benefits of acupuncture in adolescents with respect to the reduction of additional anti-emetic medication were observed. Acupuncture therapy enabled patients to experience higher levels of alertness during chemotherapy and reduced chemotherapy-induced nausea and vomiting. Acupuncture may reduce anti-emetic medication and episodes of vomiting in pediatric oncology.

POSTEXTUBATION STRIDOR

Laryngospasm sometimes occurs after tracheal extubation. Bloodletting acupuncture has been used for treatment for various upper respiratory tract problems, particularly those of laryngeal origin. A randomized controlled trial of 76 pediatric patients revealed that acupuncture with bloodletting at the LU-11 acupuncture point at the end of the operation may prevent laryngospasm. If laryngospasm developed, patients were immediately treated with acupuncture at either the LU-11 or LI-1 acupuncture points. The laryngospasm was relieved within one minute of acupuncture in all patients (Lee et al., 1998). However, Saghaei and Razavi (2001) conducted a randomized control study to determine whether bloodletting acupuncture can reduce the presence and severity of postextubation stridor. They found that acupuncture bloodletting was ineffective in reducing the severity of postextubation stridor.

Pain Management

Kim, Kim, and Yu (2006) applied capsicum plaster on to acupuncture points ST-36 to reduce the postoperative pain in children undergoing hernia repair (Figure 6-7a). One hundred and eight children were enrolled in the randomized controlled trial. Children in capsicum plaster at acupuncture points ST-36 had significantly decreased postoperative pain (Figure 6-7b) and reduced opioid analgesic consumption during the first 24 hours after surgery. Zeltzer and colleagues (2002) reported a study on the feasibility and acceptability of an acupuncture and hypnosis intervention for chronic pediatric pain. They found that children who received acupuncture and hypnosis treatment reported that it relaxed them and improved their pain.

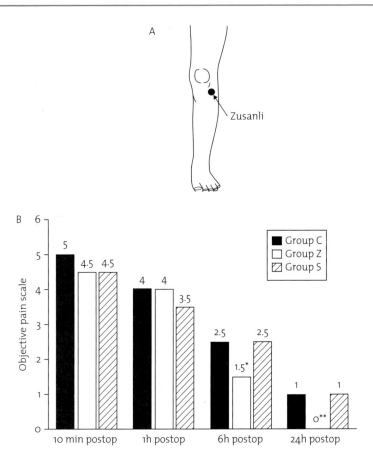

FIGURE 6-7. (a) The location of stomach 36 (ST-36). (b) The differences of pain after surgery. (Adapted from The effect of capsicum plaster in pain after inguinal hernia repair in children. *Paediatric anaesthesia* 2006; 16:1036–1041.)

Allergy Rhinitis

Ng and colleagues (2004) compared the therapeutic effect of acupuncture for children with persistent allergic rhinitis. Sixty-two children were randomized into true and sham acupuncture groups, and the outcome measures included daily rhinitis scores, symptom-free days, and visual analog scales before and after intervention. All participants received an intervention twice a week for a total of eight weeks. There were significantly lower daily rhinitis scores and more symptom-free days for the group receiving active acupuncture, during both the treatment and follow-up periods. The visual analog scale scores for immediate improvement after acupuncture were also significantly better for the active acupuncture group. There was no significant difference in daily relief medication scores and blood eosinophil counts between the active and sham acupuncture groups. Acupuncture treatment was effective in decreasing the symptom scores for persistent allergic rhinitis and increasing the symptom-free days.

Acupuncture Points

A unit of measurement called a "cun" is used to locate the acupuncture points. We use patients' body habitus for the measurements. One cun is equal to the space between the distal interphalangeal joint and the proximal interphalangeal joint on the middle finger or the width of the thumb.

LI-4 (he gu): "Union Valley" is located between the first and second metacarpal bones in the deep depression of the web space.

PC-6 (nei guan): "Inner Gate" is located 2–3 cun above the transverse crease of the wrist, between the tendons of m. palmaris longus and m. flexor carpi radialis.

SP-6 (san yin jiao): "Three Yin Intersection" is located 3 cun above the tip of medical malleolus on the posterior border of the tibia.

ST-36 (zu san li): "Leg Three Miles" is located 3 cun below the patella and 1 cun lateral to the crest of the tibia.

BL-23 (shen shu): "Kidney shu" is located 1.5 cun lateral to the lower border of the spinous process of second lumbar vertebra.

LR-3 (tai chong): "Supreme torrent" is located in the junction of first and second metatarsal bones.

Conclusion

Multiple series case treatments for pediatric patients were reported. There are limited clinical trials being published in the peer review literature. More clinical research should be conducted in the future with larger sample sizes, and valid sham intervention to confirm whether acupuncture and related interventions are effective as treatments for various medical problems in the pediatric population. With the development of translation medicine, problems that are more clinical in nature are being investigated under image techniques, and various markers have been identified as predictors for the therapeutic effect of treatments.

A desired medical therapy should address the pediatric patient as a whole and emphasize wellbeing. Wellbeing is more than absence of diseases; it calls attention to optimal functioning and considers a patient's background, family, belief, and culture. Scientific research supports the value of acupuncture for the prevention and treatment of nausea and vomiting and in pain management. When referring pediatric patients for acupuncture treatment, it is beneficial to ask patients to maintain a symptom diary, to discuss with the patients what their treatment preferences and expectations are, to review issues of safety and efficacy with them, to identify and refer patients to qualified pediatric providers, and to set up a follow-up visit to review the treatment results.

We anticipate more scientific evidence will soon become available that will help consumers to determine the efficacy of acupuncture and its related interventions for many clinical problems in pediatric population.

REFERENCES

Allais, G., De Lorenzo, C., Quirico, P. E., Airola, G., Tolardo, G., Mana, O., et al. (2002). Acupuncture in the prophylactic treatment of migraine without aura: A comparison with flunarizine. *Headache, 42*(9), 855–861.

Biella, G., Sotgiu, M. L., Pellegata, G., Paulesu, E., Castiglioni, I., & Fazio, F. (2001). Acupuncture produces central activations in pain regions. *Neuroimage, 14*(1 Pt 1), 60–66.

Bower, W. F., Diao, M., Tang, J. L., & Yeung, C. K. (2005). Acupuncture for nocturnal enuresis in children: A systematic review and exploration of rationale. *Neurourology and Urodynamics, 4*(3), 267–272.

Butkovic, D., Toljan, S., Matolic, M., Kralik, S., & Radesic, L. (2005). Comparison of laser acupuncture and metoclopramide in PONV prevention in children. *Paediatric Anaesthesia, 15*(1), 37–40.

Capozza, N., Creti, G., De Gennaro, M., Minni, B., & Caione, P. (1991). The treatment of nocturnal enuresis. A comparative study between desmopressin and acupuncture used alone or in combination. *Minerva Pediatrica, 43*(9), 577–582.

Chu, Y. C., Lin, S. M., Hsieh, Y. C., Peng, G. C., Lin, Y. H., Tsai, S. K., et al. (1998). Effect of BL-10 (tianzhu), BL-11 (dazhu) and GB-34 (yanglinquan) acuplaster for prevention of vomiting after strabismus surgery in children. *Acta Anaesthesiologica Sinica, 36*(1), 11–16.

Dune, L. S., & Shiao, S. Y. (2006). Metaanalysis of acustimulation effects on postoperative nausea and vomiting in children. *Explore (NY), 2*(4), 314–320.

Gottschling, S., Meyer, S., Gribova, I., Distler, L., Berrang, J., Gortner, L., et al. (2007). Laser acupuncture in children with headache: A double-blind, randomized, bicenter, placebo-controlled trial. *Pain.*

Gruber, W., Eber, E., Malle-Scheid, D., Pfleger, A., Weinhandl, E., Dorfer, L., et al. (2002). Laser acupuncture in children and adolescents with exercise induced asthma. *Thorax, 57*(3), 222–225.

Han, J. S. (2003). Acupuncture: Neuropeptide release produced by electrical stimulation of different frequencies. *Trends in Neuroscience, 26*(1), 17–22.

Han, J. S. (2004). Acupuncture and endorphins. *Neuroscience Letters, 361*(1–3), 258–261.

Han, J. S., Chen, X. H., Sun, S. L., Xu, X. J., Yuan, Y., Yan, S. C. et al. (1991). Effect of low- and high-frequency TENS on Met-enkephalin-Arg-Phe and dynorphin A immunoreactivity in human lumbar CSF. *Pain, 47*(3), 295–298.

Han, J. S., Ding, X. Z., & Fan, S. G. (1986). Cholecystokinin octapeptide (CCK-8): Antagonism to electroacupuncture analgesia and a possible role in electroacupuncture tolerance. *Pain, 27*(1), 101–115.

Han, J. S., Li, S. J., & Tang, J. (1981). Tolerance to electroacupuncture and its cross tolerance to morphine. *Neuropharmacology, 20*(6), 593–596.

Han, J., Tang, J., Huang, B., Liang, X., & Zhang, N. (1979). Acupuncture tolerance in rats: Anti-opiate substrates implicated. *Chinese Medical Journal, 92*(9), 625–627.

Hsieh, J. C., Tu, C. H., Chen, F. P., Chen, M., Yeh, T., & Cheng, H. (2001). Activation of the hypothalamus characterizes the acupuncture stimulation at the analgesic point in human: A positron emission tomography study. *Neuroscience Letters, 307*(2), 105–108.

Hui, K., Liu, J., Makris, N., Gollub R. L., Chen, A. J., Moore, C. I., et al. (2000). Acupuncture modulates the limbic system and subcortical gray structures of the human brain: evidence from fMRI studies in normal subjects. *Human Brain Mapping, 9*, 13–25.

Hui, K. K., Liu, J,. Marina, O., Napadow, V., Haselgrove, C., Kwong, K. K., et al. (2005). The integrated response of the human cerebro-cerebellar and limbic systems to acupuncture stimulation at ST 36 as evidenced by fMRI. *Neuroimage, 27*(3), 479–496.

Kabalak, A. A., Akcay, M., Akcay, F., & Gogus, N. (2005). Transcutaneous electrical acupoint stimulation versus ondansetron in the prevention of postoperative vomiting following pediatric tonsillectomy. *Journal of Alternative and Complementary Medicine, 11*(3), 407–413.

Kim, K. S., Kim, D. W., & Yu, Y. K. (2006). The effect of capsicum plaster in pain after inguinal hernia repair in children. *Paediatric Anaesthesia, 16*(10), 1036–1041.

Langevin, H. M., Churchill, D. L., & Cipolla, M. J. (2001). Mechanical signaling through connective tissue: A mechanism for the therapeutic effect of acupuncture. *FASEB Journal, 15*(12), 2275–2282.

Langevin, H. M., Churchill, D. L., Fox, J. R., Badger, G. J., Garra, B. S., & Krag, M. H. (2001). Biomechanical response to acupuncture needling in humans. *Journal of Applied Physiology, 91*(6), 2471–2478.

Lee, A., & Done, M. L. (2004). Stimulation of the wrist acupuncture point P6 for preventing postoperative nausea and vomiting. *Cochrane Database of Systematic Reviews, 3*, CD003281.

Lee, C. K., Chien, T. J., Hsu, J. C., Yang, C. Y., Hsiao, J. M., Huang, Y. R., et al. (1998). The effect of acupuncture on the incidence of postextubation laryngospasm in children. *Anaesthesia, 53*(9), 917–920.

Lim, T. W., Loh, T., Kranz, H., & Scott, D. (1977). Acupuncture—effect on normal subjects. *Medical journal of Australia, 1*(13), 440–442.

Liu, W. C., Feldman, S. C., Cook, D. B., Hung, D. L., Xu, T., Kalnin, A. J., et al. (2004). fMRI study of acupuncture-induced periaqueductal gray activity in humans. *Neuroreport, 15*(12), 1937–1940.

Monda, J. M., & Husmann, D. A. (1995). Primary nocturnal enuresis: A comparison among observation, imipramine, desmopressin acetate and bed-wetting alarm systems. *Journal of Urology, 154*(2 Pt 2), 745–748.

Newberg, A. B., Lariccia, P. J., Lee, B. Y., Farrar, J. T., Lee, L., & Alavi, A. (2005). Cerebral blood flow effects of pain and acupuncture: A preliminary single-photon emission computed tomography imaging study. *Journal of Neuroimaging, 15*(1), 43–49.

Ng, D. K., Chow, P. Y., Ming, S. P., Hong, S. H., Lau, S., Tse, D., et al. (2004). A double-blind, randomized, placebo-controlled trial of acupuncture for the treatment of childhood persistent allergic rhinitis. *Pediatrics, 114*(5), 1242–1247.

Pan, B,. Castro-Lopes, J. M., & Coimbra, A. (1994). C-fos expression in the hypothalamo-pituitary system induced by electroacupuncture or noxious stimulation. *Neuroreport, 5*(13), 1649–1652.

Pan, B., Castro-Lopes, J. M., & Coimbra, A. (1996). Activation of anterior lobe corticotrophs by electroacupuncture or noxious stimulation in the anaesthetized rat, as shown by colocalization of Fos protein with ACTH and beta-endorphin and increased hormone release. *Brain Research Bulletin, 40*(3), 175–182.

Pan, B., Castro-Lopes, J. M., & Coimbra, A. (1997). Chemical sensory deafferentation abolishes hypothalamic pituitary activation induced by noxious stimulation or electroacupuncture but only decreases that caused by immobilization stress. A c-fos study. *Neuroscience, 78*(4), 1059–1068.

Pariente, J., White, P., Frackowiak, R.S., & Lewith, G. (2005). Expectancy and belief modulate the neuronal substrates of pain treated by acupuncture. *Neuroimage, 25*(4), 1161–1167.

Pintov, S., Lahat, E., Alstein, M., Vogel, Z., & Barg, J. (1997). Acupuncture and the opioid system: implications in management of migraine. *Pediatric Neurology, 17*(2), 129–133.

Pomeranz, B. (1996). Scientific research into acupuncture for the relief of pain. *Journal of Alternative and Complementary Medicine, 2*(1), 53–60; discussion 73–55.

Pomeranz, B., & Chiu, D. (1976). Naloxone blockade of acupuncture analgesia: Endorphin implicated. *Life Sciences, 19*(11), 1757–1762.

Radmayr, C., Schlager, A., Studen, M., & Bartsch, G. (2001). Prospective randomized trial using laser acupuncture versus desmopressin in the treatment of nocturnal enuresis. *European Urology, 40*(2), 201–205.

Reindl, T. K., Geilen, W., Hartmann, R., Wiebelitz, K. R., Kan, G., Wilhelm, I., et al. (2006). Acupuncture against chemotherapy-induced nausea and vomiting in pediatric oncology. Interim results of a multicenter crossover study. *Support Care Cancer, 14*(2), 172–176.

Rusy, L. M., Hoffman, G. M., & Weisman, S. J. (2002). Electroacupuncture prophylaxis of postoperative nausea and vomiting following pediatric tonsillectomy with or without adenoidectomy. *Anesthesiology, 96*(2), 300–305.

Saghaei, M., & Razavi, S. (2001). Bloodletting acupuncture for the prevention of stridor in children after tracheal extubation: a randomised, controlled study. *Anaesthesia, 56*(10), 961–964.

Schlager, A., Boehler, M., & Puhringer, F. (2000). Korean hand acupressure reduces postoperative vomiting in children after strabismus surgery. *British Journal of Anaesthesia, 85*(2), 267–270.

Schlager, A., Offer, T., & Baldissera, I. (1998). Laser stimulation of acupuncture point P6 reduces postoperative vomiting in children undergoing strabismus surgery. *British Journal of Anaesthesia, 81*(4), 529–532.

Shenkman, Z., Holzman, R.S., Kim, C., Ferrari, L. R., DiCanzio, J., Highfield, E. S., et al. (1999). Acupressure-acupuncture antiemetic prophylaxis in children undergoing tonsillectomy. *Anesthesiology, 90*(5), 1311–1316.

Somri, M., Vaida, S. J., Sabo, E., Yassain, G., Gankin, I., & Gaitini, L. A. (2001). Acupuncture versus ondansetron in the prevention of postoperative vomiting. A study of children undergoing dental surgery. *Anaesthesia, 56*(10), 927–932.

Stockert, K., Schneider, B., Porenta, G., Rath, R., Nissel, H., & Eichler, I. (2007). Laser acupuncture and probiotics in school age children with asthma: A randomized, placebo-controlled pilot study of therapy guided by principles of Traditional Chinese Medicine. *Pediatric Allergy and Immunology, 18*(2), 160–166.

Ulett, G. A., Han, S., & Han, J. S. (1998). Electroacupuncture: mechanisms and clinical application. *Biological Psychiatry, 44*(2), 129–138.

Wang, S. M., & Kain, Z. N. (2002). P6 acupoint injections are as effective as droperidol in controlling early postoperative nausea and vomiting in children. *Anesthesiology, 97*(2), 359–366.

Wang, S. M., Constable, R. T., Tokoglu, F. S., Weiss, D. A., Freyle, D., & Kain, Z. N. (2007). Acupuncture-induced blood oxygenation level-dependent signals in awake and anesthetized volunteers: A pilot study. *Anesthesia and Analgesia, 105*(2), 499–506.

Wu, M. T., Hsieh, J. C., Xiong, J., Yang, C. F., Pan, H. B., Chen, Y. C., et al. (1999). Central nervous pathway for acupuncture stimulation: Localization of processing with functional MR imaging of the brain—preliminary experience. *Radiology, 212*(1), 133–141.

Yiming, C., Changxin, Z., Ung, W. S., Lei, Z., & Kean, L. S. (2000). Laser acupuncture for adolescent smokers—a randomized double-blind controlled trial. *American Journal of Chinese Medicine, 28*(3–4), 443–449.

Zeltzer, L. K., Tsao, J. C., Stelling, C., Powers, M., Levy, S., & Waterhouse, M. (2002). A phase I study on the feasibility and acceptability of an acupuncture/hypnosis intervention for chronic pediatric pain. *Journal of Pain and Symptom Management, 24*(4), 437–446.

7

A Pediatric Perspective on Aromatherapy

MAURA FITZGERALD AND LINDA L. HALCÓN

KEY CONCEPTS

- Essential oils have been used therapeutically and, for the most part, safely for millennia.
- Essential oils are widely available to the general public and are currently used by many adults and children.
- Clinicians need basic understanding of clinical aromatherapy in order to credibly and safely advise their patients.
- Generalizing about essential oils is inappropriate because each has unique properties.
- Children and teens have different oil preferences relative to adults and also show some variation for scent preference based on ethnicity and gender.

■

Introduction

DEFINITION OF CLINICAL AROMATHERAPY

The word "aromatherapie" was first coined by the French chemist Gattefossé in the early 1900s. After suffering a severe burn in a laboratory accident, Gattefosse healed the wounds by applying topical lavender oil. He then spent the rest of his career investigating the healing properties of essential oils or "aromatherapie." Today aromatherapy often refers to nearly anything with a pleasant odor, including scented candles or potpourris. Although all essential oils are volatile and thus odorous, this common understanding of aromatherapy is misleading for several reasons: (a) many pleasant smelling substances have nothing to do with essential oils; (b) some essential oils have an unpleasant odor; (c) inhalation is not the only way that aromatic oils can be used therapeutically; and (d) the word does not suggest that knowledge or caution are needed. In healthcare, it is preferable to use the term "clinical aromatherapy," defined as the intentional use of plant essential oils by qualified providers to promote and improve health or to treat disease.

SCOPE OF CHAPTER

This chapter will provide an overview of clinical aromatherapy, with examples focusing on the use of essential oils in children and adolescents. The reader will gain knowledge of the sources and processing of essential oils, as well as some of their properties and mechanisms of action. A brief history of the therapeutic use of essential oils provides the context for a discussion of current uses and common application methods are described. The chapter concludes with a review of key recent essential oils research on common health conditions among adults and children and a discussion of safety concerns.

History of Essential Oils

Most essential oil historians trace the first use of distilled essential oils to at least 5000 years ago. The earliest discoveries of distillation apparatus can be traced to that period. Evidence of early essential oil production has been found in Asia, the Middle East, North Africa, and Europe. Aromatic plant oils were used in embalming and for a variety of known health and cosmetic purposes in the ancient world. During the Middle Ages and, increasingly during the Renaissance, essential oils and hydrosols were used in perfumes, cosmetics and in health and specific industries (e.g., glove making).

Modern aromatherapy appeared in Europe in the early part of the twentieth century. Besides Gattefossé, other early modern pioneers in aromatherapy included Marguerite Maury, who set up the first aromatherapy clinics in Europe and Jean Valnet, a French medical doctor who treated many medical and psychiatric conditions successfully using essential oils. The practice of aromatherapy is part of the larger field of botanical medicines and is increasingly recognized as a specialty field within herbalism (Battaglia, 2003; Lavabre, 1990; Lawless, 1995).

Description

Essential oils are complex mixtures of organic compounds that are produced by and stored in certain plants. Each essential oil is a unique chemical combination that may include hydrocarbons (terpenes), oxygenated compounds (alcohols, aldehydes, ketones, esters phenols, ethers and oxides, peroxides, furans, lactones and acids), and sulfur or nitrogen compounds (Tisserand & Balacs, 1995). Essential oils may be obtained from the roots, leaves, bark, resin, fruit, or flower petals of a plant. Some plants yield more than one type of essential oil; for example, neroli (*Citrus aurantium* var. *amara*) is produced from the flower of the bitter orange tree, whereas petitgrain oil (*Citrus aurantium* subsp, *amara*) is obtained from the leaves (Battaglia, 2003). Some essential oils may be grown in different parts of the world under varying climatic conditions, resulting in a degree of natural variability in their chemical profiles (Tisserand & Balacs, 1995). Some plants have developed essential oils with distinctly different chemical compositions or chemotype. For example, thyme has six major therapeutic chemotypes and rosemary has three (Battaglia, 2003).

Once the plant or plant part is harvested, the essential oil is commonly extracted by *distillation*. Essential oils found in the fruit of citrus plants, however, are extracted by *expression*. A quality control chemical analysis such as gas chromatography can be performed to verify that the percentage of each constituent in the essential oil meets the standard set for that specific essential oil (Battaglia, 2003; Tisserand & Balacs, 1995). In order to reduce the risk of contamination with pesticides or fertilizers, organic cultivation and processing methods are recommended and becoming more common.

Essential oils used clinically should be labeled with the common and botanical name of the plant, part of the plant used, chemotype or variety if applicable, the country of origin, volume of oil, and the supplier. Batch numbers and expiration dates are desirable, but often not supplied. If the essential oil is diluted, the carrier oil or dilutant should be listed along with the percent of pure essential oil in the mixture. If the essential oil purchased is a blend (more than one essential oil) all oils included should be listed. Ideally, the proportion of each oil in a blend should be listed; however, most suppliers consider this proprietary information. Additional information on the label may indicate whether the product was organically grown or has been certified. When purchasing or using essential oils it is important to note the botanical as well as common name, as there are essential oils that have similar common names, such as true lavender (*Lavandula offinialis* or *Lavandula angustifolia*) and spike lavender (*Lavandula spica* or *Lavandula latifolia*) or Roman chamomile (*Chamaemelum nobilis*) and German chamomile (*Matricaria recutita*). There are many species of plants that are commonly called eucalyptus or tea tree, illustrating the importance of knowing the Latin name as an identifier.

Methods of Administration

The method and route of essential oil administration depend on the desired dosage, condition being treated, characteristics of the patient, including age and medical condition, properties of the essential oil, professional practice parameters, safety data, and patient preference (Halcón, 2002). Essential oils are commonly applied topically, by inhalation, by oral ingestion, or occasionally by rectal and vaginal routes. In the United States, inhalation and topical application are most common; however, a few oral enteric-coated essential oils, such as peppermint and oregano, are available as over-the-counter supplements (Table 7-1).

The topical route is recommended when local, external action is desired, such as when treating a skin condition, wound, or muscular pain. Essential oils are lipid-soluble and are absorbed when applied to the skin; therefore, the topical route is also an option to achieve systemic effects such as relaxation. With few exceptions, essential oils are never applied topically at full-strength but rather, are diluted with carrier oils. Carrier oils are vegetable oils derived from seeds or nuts and include: sweet almond, avocado, canola, evening primrose, jojoba, olive, rosehip, safflower, sesame, and sunflower (Battaglia, 2003). Essential oils used topically generally should be diluted to concentrations of 1%–10% (Table 7-2). Dilution reduces the risk of skin irritation and increases the potential area of distribution. It is recommended that concentrations of 0.5%–2% be used with children because their skin is more permeable and more susceptible to irritation (Buckle, 2003).

Inhalation is often the best route for respiratory and sinus conditions (colds, sore throats, sinus congestion, cough) and for affecting mood and cognition (anxiety, tension, relaxation, stress, alertness, insomnia). There are a number of ways in which an essential oil can be presented for inhalation. The simplest is to place a small amount (1–4 drops) of the essential oil on a tissue or cotton ball and inhale. Devices that diffuse or vaporize the essential oil either heat the essential oil or have an air pump that disperses the essential oil into the air. Steam inhalation is beneficial for treatment of colds and sinus or upper respiratory tract infections.

Ingestion of essential oils is controversial. It is much more common in France where physicians may prescribe oral or rectal doses of essential oils (Battaglia, 2003). Most aromatherapy organizations do not endorse the use of oral essential oils except by licensed providers with prescribing authority (Battaglia 2003; Buckle, 2003). Although not generally available in the United States, rectal suppositories containing essential oils are commonly used by medical aromatherapists in France. Given the high absorption potential of this route, it should be considered equivalent to oral administration and restricted to authorized prescribers. The vaginal route (douche, pessary, or tampon soaked in diluted essential oil) is occasionally used to treat vaginal infections.

Proposed Mechanisms of Biologic Effect

The roles of essential oils in plants are not fully understood but include preventing and treating infections, healing wounds, and repelling animal, and insect predators (Halcón, 2002). Likewise, there is still much to be learned about the mechanisms and actions of essential oils in humans. A wide range of physiological and psychological actions are attributed to essential oils, including analgesic, anti-inflammatory, antimicrobial, antiseptic, decongestant, digestive, insecticide, relaxant, and sedative properties (Battaglia, 2003; Buckle 2003). This is largely based on observation and analysis of the chemical components. More recent laboratory testing, particularly on antimicrobial properties, has enlarged the body of scientific knowledge (D'Auria, 2005; Halcón & Milkus, 2004; Hammer, Carson & Riley, 2004; Hammer, Carson, Riley, & Nielsen, 2006; Nelson, 1997; Papadopoulos, Carson, Hammer, & Riley, 2006; Tisserand & Balacs, 1998). Each essential oil has a different profile of actions but there is overlap as many oils share similar chemical compounds. Essential oils that are high in monoterpene alcohols (true

Table 7-1. Methods of Administration of Essential Oils

Inhalation

Place 2–5 drops of essential oil(s) on a tissue or cotton ball.

Diffusion device: Follow the manufacturer's directions for application of essential oil. (Do not use flame- based devices around children.)

Spray bottle: Mix 2–10 drops essential oil(s) in 1 ounce (30 ml) of water in a spray bottle. Shake immediately before spraying.

Steaming: Add 3–6 drops of essential oil(s) into steaming water (not boiling). Place a towel over the head to direct the steam to the face. Close eyes. Steam for 5 minutes. Children must be attended at all times.

Topical

Compress: Add 5–10 drops of essential oil(s) to 200 ml of water (warm or cold). Dip in compress material, wring out and cover area. Wrap in plastic wrap and cover with a towel to maintain temperature.

Massage: Dilute essential oil(s) in a carrier oil or lotion and apply to the skin with gentle rubbing or therapeutic massage. Use low concentrations 1%–5%. The younger the child, the more dilute the solution should be. Common recommendations are infants and young children 0.5%–1%, school age children 1%–3%, adolescents and adults 2%–5%. Start with lower dilutions and increase if needed (Refer to dilution table).

Bath

Foot bath: Add 2–5 drops to bowl of warm water.

Full bath: Add 4–8 drops to 5 cc of dispersal solution (unscented bath oil, whole milk, milk power).

Protect eyes from splashing.

---

lavender, clary sage) or in phenols (thyme, oregano) are strongly antibacterial. Those high in esters (Roman chamomile, geranium) tend to be antispasmodic and calming (Battaglia 2003; Buckle 2003). The activity profile of each oil is based on its unique combination of chemical compounds. True lavender (*L. angustifolia*), composed of 30%–40% monoterpene alcohols (linalool, geraniol), 46%–53% esters (linalyl acetate, lavandulyl acetate) and many other compounds, has analgesic, antibacterial, antiseptic, sedative, and other effects (Battaglia 2003).

Essential oils are absorbed either through the skin or the mucous membranes, for example of the nasopharynx, trachea, or lungs. The rate of absorption depends on location (skin, mucous membranes), patient characteristics (skin condition, circulation), size of the area of application, essential oil concentration of the mixture, and viscosity of the carrier oil. The more volatile components of an essential oil both evaporate and absorb more quickly. Covering the area of application will reduce evaporation and increase absorption (Tisserand & Balacs, 1995). The rate and amount of absorption is increased with larger areas of application, good circulation and the use of massage

Table 7-2. Dilution Chart for Essential Oils

Drops of Essential Oil Placed in Carrier Oil or Lotion	Amount of Carrier Oil or Lotion (ml)	Solution (%)
1	5	1
2	5	2
3	5	3
4	5	4
5	5	5
1	10	0.05
1	20	0.25

or heat. Rate of absorption is also higher if skin break down is present (Buck, 2004; Buckle, 2003).

Measuring the level of systemic absorption of the essential oil is complicated by the heterogenous chemical structure of each essential oil. Often analysis is done by measuring two or three of the constituents that comprise the bulk of the essential oil. In an analysis of true lavender (*Lavandula angustifolia*) plasma concentrations of linalool and linalyl were measured. Lavender was applied to the skin in a 2% solution, and blood samples were drawn at intervals up to 90 minutes. A peak level of 120 ng/ml for linalool and 90 ng/ml for linalyl acetate was reached at 20 minutes. Neither component was detected at 90 minutes (Tisserand & Balacs 1995). Although this provides evidence for systemic absorption, there is little known about essential oil dosing, effects of pathophysiological processes on therapeutic actions, or interactions with medications, herbal preparations or homeopathic remedies.

Although the exact mechanisms of action are unknown, several possibilities are likely. In topical applications essential oils are absorbed locally, resulting in direct effects (including anti-inflammatory, anti-spasmodic, or antiseptic effects) on the tissue. With inhalation, there seem to be a central nervous system (CNS) response that forms the primary basis for the use of essential oils for mental calming or stimulation. It is postulated that inhalation of essential oils either triggers the olfactory nerve or that the volatile molecules are absorbed into the circulation through the mucous membranes of the nasal sinus. In either case, the primary site of CNS action is believed to be the limbic system, generating an effect on arousal and emotional response (Battaglia, 2003; Tisserand & Balacs 1995). Because of the volatile nature of the essential oils, there is always some inhalation, even in topical application.

Emotional and cognitive reactions to an essential oil may also be due to an individual's response to the odor or smell memory. Odors or scents evoke memories that, in turn, engender a variety of feelings and thoughts that may arouse, relax, or induce stress (Buckle, 2003). A number of studies have been carried out in animal models and in humans to better delineate effects of specific essential oils on cognition, memory, and emotional response. Results of these studies demonstrate complex interactions between the effects of essential oils, types of mental processes, and subject factors, such as preference for a given essential oil (Buchbauer, Jirovetz, Jager, Dietrich, & Plank, 1991; Buchbauer, Jirovetz, Jager, Plank, & Dietrich, 1993; Moss, Cook, Wesnes, & Duckett, 2003; Sakomota, Minoura, Usui, Ishizuka, & Kanba, 2005).

Review of Clinical Applications

Aromatherapy texts and articles describe the use of essential oils in a variety of clinical situations for children and adults (Battaglia, 2003; Buckle, 2003; Maddocks-Jennings & Wilkinson, 2004; Price & Parr, 1996). However, most recommendations are based on observational and experiential data, there is little human research on adults and even less involving children. Existing studies are often pilot work with small sample size and inadequate power to detect statistical differences. Many studies couple aromatherapy with another therapy such as massage or deep breathing, making it difficult to measure the effect of each separately. Some published studies also use a number of essential oils in a blend, making it difficult to evaluate the effects of individual oils, or if there was no effect, to determine if there might have been an effect for one of the essential oils that was masked by antagonistic or synergistic interactions. Even when the study includes randomization and a placebo control it is difficult to blind the subject and evaluator because of the distinctive odors of essential oils. Many studies do not have adequate information about the procedures and methodology, and often the essential oil(s) used are listed only by common rather than botanical name. Chemical analyses of essential oils are often not included in published reports. Early studies tended not to note the presence or absence of adverse effects although more recent studies are more likely to include this valuable information. Clinical conditions for which there is some research regarding efficacy of aromatherapy include pain, insomnia, dermatologic conditions, anxiety, and nausea.

The majority of research and experiential data is based on experience with adults and then applied to children; however, children may have scent preferences that are quite different from the preferences of adults. Generally children are more likely to react positively to sensory experiences with which they have some familiarity. Children become familiar with smells in the home where they are exposed to cooking odors, perfumes, and plants. When the scent preferences of 87 school age boys and girls of Latino and non-Latino Caucasian ethnicity were compared, it was noted that subjects preferred lemon (*Citrus limon*), sweet orange (*Citrus sinensis*), spearmint (*Mentha spicata*), and peppermint (*Mentha piperita*) over ginger (*Zingiber officinalis*) and lavender (*Lavandula angustifolia*). Girls were more likely to report feeling happy when smelling sweet orange than boys, and male Latino boys were more likely to describe peppermint as energetic than non-Latino Caucasian boys. Children usually identified the smell with a common substance such as spearmint with gum; however, some children described much more evocative scent triggered memory associations stating it reminded them of "a flower in Ecuador" or "my grandmother's house." Nearly all children in the study were willing to try aromatherapy, with only one subject dropping out. Children also were willing to continue to smell all six of the study essential oils even if they reported not liking one of the smells (Fitzgerald et al., 2007).

PAIN MANAGEMENT

Many essential oils are purported to be useful for pain management through analgesic and anxiolytic effects, including true lavender (*Lavandula angustifolia*), peppermint (*Mentha piperita*), rosemary (*Rosmarinus officinalis*), lemongrass (*Cymbopogon, citratus*) and Roman chamomile (*Chamaemelum nobile*). The mechanism of analgesia is uncertain but it is postulated that it is related to modulation of pain perception by inhibiting nociceptive impulses or by activating the endogenous opioid system, which suppresses the pain impulses (Gobel, Schmidt, & Soyka, 1994). The aromatherapy may also change pain perception by setting a more pleasant environment or distracting from the pain experience (Gedney & Glover, 2004; Kerr, Casey, & Fillingim, 2004).

Essential oils or strong smells present at the time of a painful procedure may change the subject's immediate response or later memory of the event. Goubet and colleagues conducted two studies on the effect of an odorous substance (vanillin, not an essential oil) on the pain response of neonates undergoing heel stick procedures or venipuncture. In the first study, neonates were randomly assigned to exposure to vanillin scent in advance and during the blood draw (familiar scent), exposure to scent only during the blood draw (unfamiliar scent), and to have no scent. Infants in the familiar-scent category displayed a faster decrease in pain behaviors (crying, grimacing, movement) than the non-familiar and no-scent groups (Goubet, Rattaz, Pierrat, Bullinger, & Lequien, 2003). A second study confirmed the previous findings and established that exposure to the odor in the crib versus exposure with mother did not affect pain response (Goubet, Strasbaugh, & Chesney, 2007). Adults exposed to essential oils of lavender or rosemary or a distilled water control indicated no change in pain rating between groups at the time the painful stimulus was administered. However, in retrospective evaluation subjects reported less pain intensity and pain unpleasantness after lavender treatment (and a trend in that direction with rosemary) as compared to the control group. The researchers postulated that the use of essential oils might have provided a pleasant olfactory stimulus that led to more positive post-procedure appraisal (Gedney, Glover, & Fillingim, 2004).

Essential oils are often suggested for the treatment of headache. A series of experiments that mimicked the possible mechanisms of headache and then tested the effect of peppermint and eucalyptus essential oils were conducted on 32 healthy adult male subjects. The situations were (a) increasing pressure applied to the scalp and the middle finger of the right hand, (b) thermal pain induced by an electrical voltage, and (c) ischemic pain produced by applying a collar around the head and inflating it while the subject rhythmically bit on an object. Different strengths and combinations of peppermint (*Mentha piperita*) and eucalyptus (*Eucalyptus* unknown sp.) diluted in ethanol and a placebo control of ethanol were applied to the subjects' forehead and temples and left on for 3 minutes. Measurements included EMG activity of the temporal muscle, EEG, self-report of pain, and current mood state. Peppermint and eucalyptus oil mixture in ethanol had a stronger impact on muscle-relaxation and on performance-related activity and concentration. Sensitivity to pressure was not reduced by any preparation, but peppermint in ethanol was the strongest in reducing ischemic pain. Eucalyptus in ethanol and the placebo resulted in no significant reductions (Gobel, Schmidt, & Soyka, 1994).

Essential oils have traditionally been used for abdominal conditions such as irritable bowel, constipation, and functional abdominal pain. Essential oils classified as antispasmodics or carminatives (the property of relaxing abdominal muscles and improving peristalsis) such as Roman chamomile (*Chamaemelum nobile*), sweet fennel (*Foeniculum vulgaris*), peppermint (*Mentha piperita*), and ginger (*Zingiber officinalis*) are frequently recommended (Battaglia, 2003); however, most clinical research has focused on the use of peppermint.

Research on the effectiveness of therapies for treatment of abdominal pain or irritable bowel syndrome (IBS) is challenging, due to lack of understanding of the pathophysiology of many gastrointestinal conditions, overlap and multiplicity of symptoms, and variation in expression of symptoms. Systematic reviews and meta-analysis of enteric-coated peppermint and traditional therapies (including peppermint) for IBS in both children and adults have reported mixed results. A review of clinical trials reported that eight out of 12 placebo-controlled studies found significant results in favor of peppermint (Grigoleit & Grigoleit, 2004), while another review of eight randomized control trials reported three with evidence favoring peppermint, two showing no effect and three with inadequate methodological information (Pittler & Ernst, 1998). Research problems commonly cited included lack of common diagnostic criteria, brief evaluation periods, and not including a washout period between cross-overs. A review of clinical research on a number of conventional and CAM therapies for IBS found similar issues on most studies of treatment for IBS; the authors concluded that there is no strong evidence based research for many common IBS treatments (Fennerty, 2003).

The pain reduction efficacy of peppermint essential oil in children with IBS was evaluated in a randomized, double-blind, controlled trial that included 42 subjects 8 years of age or older, who met the Manning or Rome criteria for IBS. Subjects received either peppermint oil as Colpermin (an enteric capsule containing 187 mg of peppermint oil) or a placebo three times daily. The study lasted 2 weeks, which may be an inadequate amount of time for full evaluation. The children receiving the peppermint showed significant improvement in severity of pain and no significant difference in other GI symptoms such as abdominal rumbling, distention, belching, or gas. There were no adverse drug reactions reported. The investigators concluded that peppermint oil is useful for the treatment of pain related to IBS in children (Kline, Kline, Di Palma, & Barbero, 2001).

Although not a study of children, a randomized, placebo-controlled, double-blind study of 96 adults diagnosed with functional dyspepsia tested enteric capsules of peppermint oil and caraway oil to alleviate symptoms. There was a statistically significant reduction in pain, pressure, heaviness, and fullness, and an increase in ratings of clinical improvement (May, Kohler, & Schneider, 2000).

Massage with aromatherapy was studied for the treatment of dysmenorrhoea in Korean college students. Sixty-seven female college students were randomized to treatment, placebo and control groups. The treatment group received 15 minute abdominal massage with a 4% solution of lavender (*L. officinalis*), clary sage (Salvia *sclarea*), and rose (*Rosa centifolia*) in almond oil carrier, while the placebo group received 15-minute abdominal massages with almond oil only and the control group received no therapy. To attempt to blind the participants, both placebo and treatment groups were told they were receiving aromatherapy. Intensity of menstrual cramps was measured using a visual analog scale, along with impact on daily life. The aromatherapy group demonstrated a decrease in severity of cramps over both the placebo (massage only) and the no treatment groups. No side effects were reported in any group (Han, Hur, Buckle, Choi, & Lee, 2006).

Further study of the aromatherapy for pain management is needed, particularly in pediatrics. However the relative safety of aromatherapy and the difficulty of managing chronic pain have led many researchers to suggest the use of aromatherapy alone or coupled with massage therapy as an adjunctive therapy, along with other pain management strategies (Buckle, 1999; Howarth, 2004; Snyder & Wieland, 2003).

DERMATOLOGY AND SKIN INFECTIONS

Aromatherapy has traditionally been used for the treatment of skin conditions ranging from dry or irritated skin to burns and wounds. There is little systematic research on any one condition and most citations are of observational clinical data without controls, or are single-case reports. For example, Forbes and Schmid (2006) report a case in which lavender essential oil was successfully used to treat plantar warts in an immunosuppressed adult cancer patient. These types of reports are encouraging and suggest value in further research; but they do not constitute strong evidence.

Essential oils commonly recommended for acne include bergamot (*Citrus bergamia*), geranium (*Pelargonium graveolens*), juniper (*Juniperus communis*), palma rosa (*Cymbopogon martinii*), German chamomile (*Matricaria recutita*), and tea tree (*Melaleuca alternifolia*) (Battaglia, 2003; Bensouilah, 2002). Topical tea tree (*M. alternifolia*) was compared to benzoyl peroxide in a randomized single-blind study of 124 subjects. Subjects applied either a 5% solution of tea tree oil solution (*M. alternifolia*) in a water-based gel or a 5% solution of benzoyl peroxide in water-based lotion applied to their faces (daily) for the 3-month study period. Although subjects were not told which preparation they were using, it was possible to identify the tea tree oil by smell; thus they were not considered blinded. Change in total number of lesions and skin tolerance was assessed monthly by an investigator who was blinded. Both preparations reduced mild to moderate acne. The benzoyl peroxide group improved faster and to a greater degree, but side effects of scaling, pruritus, and dryness were also greater (Basset, Pannowitz, & Arnetson, 1990). The authors also noted that a 5% solution of tea tree oil is fairly dilute and that stronger solutions might result in stronger effects.

The treatment of head lice (*Pediculus humanus capitis*) is a common concern in children and interest in essential oils has increased as lice have become resistant to commonly used chemical insecticides and concern has increased about the toxicity of these chemicals. An in vitro study was conducted to evaluate the reaction of head lice to hair treated with multiple experimental preparations, including single essential oils of tea tree (*Melaleuca alternifolia*), true lavender (*Lavandula angustifolia*), and peppermint (*Mentha piperita*), essential oil blends, coconut oil, a DEET (*N,N*-Diethyl-3-methylbenzamide) preparation and an inert water-based gel (control). Transmission inhibition, irritancy, and avoidance activity of the lice was observed. Investigators determined that none of the preparations (including DEET) demonstrated enough benefit to be recommended. However a number of the essential oil preparations were as effective as DEET with tea tree shown to have superior repellent and antifeedant properties (Canyon & Speare, 2007). In another in vitro study, peppermint (*M. piperita*), eucalyptus (species not identified), lavender (*L. angustifolia*), and orange (*Citrus sinensis*) essential oils singly and in combination were compared to a control ethanol and isopropanol-based mixture. All of the preparations were evaluated for their knock-down effect on head lice. All essential oils showed significant knock-down effect with peppermint in a 10% concentration having the greatest effect, while a 10% concentration of peppermint and eucalyptus in lotion was similar to a commercial pedicidal lotion (Audino, Vassena, Zerba, & Picollo, 2007). Commercial head lice products containing tea tree oil are widely available.

Although essential oils are sometimes recommended for eczema, they should be used with caution. In pilot study, eight children (ages 3–7) with atopic eczema were randomly assigned to either scalp massage alone or scalp massage with aromatherapy. The children received massage one time per week by a massage therapist and mothers provided daily massage after consultation with the therapist. Mothers in the aromatherapy group selected three essential oils, which were then mixed in equal parts and diluted to a 2% solution in almond oil; a total of eight different essential oils were used and each child had a unique blend. Mothers rated change in daytime irritation and nighttime disturbance and mothers and medical practitioners rated general improvement. The study was conducted for 8 weeks. Nighttime and daytime disturbance scores dropped equally for both groups and general improvement scores were the same, indicating no benefit

from the addition of the essential oil. In a follow-up evaluation, night-time disturbance scores increased for the aromatherapy group and the authors expressed concern
that contact dermatitis was provoked by the essential oil (Anderson, Lis-Balchin, &
Kirk-Smith, 2000).

There is considerable and growing international literature on the use of plant essential
oils against pathogenic microorganisms (Hayashi, Kamiya, & Hayashi, 1995; Maudsley &
Kerr, 1999). In vitro studies suggest that some essential oils and their chemical components have strong bactericidal action (Gustafson et al., 1998; Carson, Hammer, &
Riley, 1996). Over the past 30 years, there have been many reports of the efficacy of
tea tree oil (*Melaleuca alternifolia*) against bacterial pathogens. Many *Staphylococcus
aureus* isolates (both antibiotic-susceptible and antibiotic-resistant) have been found
to be susceptible to tea tree oil (Carson, Cookson, Farrelly, & Riley, 1995; Christoph,
Stahl-Biskup, & Kaulfers, 2001; May, Chan, King, Williams, & French, 2000), suggesting that it may be an effective adjunctive wound-care treatment. Initial case studies and
pilot studies in humans appear encouraging. Tea tree oil was an active ingredient in a
wound-care protocol used successfully to treat two cases of chronic MRSA-infected
osteomylitis (Sherry, Boeck, & Warnke, 2001). Many essential oils have been recommended to treat wounds in aromatherapy textbooks, including myrrh (*Commiphora
myrrha*), German chamomile (*Matricaria recutita*), everlasting (*Helichrysum italicum*),
and lavender (*Lavandula angustifolia*) (Battaglia, 2003).

NAUSEA

Aromatherapy is often recommended for nausea of any type, including motion sickness and post-operative or chemotherapy-related nausea. Research on postoperative
nausea has had mixed results. A randomized, placebo control trial of 33 adult postoperative ambulatory surgery patients were exposed to 2 × 2 gauze pads prepared with
2 ml of peppermint essential oil (*Mentha piperita*), 1 ml of isopropyl alcohol 70%, or 2 ml
isotonic saline and told to inhale with deep breathing. Nausea scores reduced in all
three groups with no significant difference between groups. The authors postulated that
the deep breathing, which is frequently recommended to relieve nausea, might have
been a confounding factor (Anderson & Gross, 2004). Alternatively, in a three-group
randomized, placebo-controlled study of 18 women postoperative for gynecological
surgery, there was a statistically significant reduction in nausea in the group receiving
peppermint essential oil as compared to the control (no treatment) and the placebo
group (peppermint essence) (Tate, 1997).

INSOMNIA

Many essential oils are believed to have properties that will improve sleep; however
specific studies or evidence are lacking. Wheatley (2005) noted that there is some evidence to support the use of true lavender (*Lavandula angutifolia*), [Roman] chamomile

(*Chamaemelum nobilis*), and ylang ylang (*Cananga odorata*) for sleep, but that the evidence is incomplete and difficult to fully evaluate. The effect of lavender (*L. angustifolia*) on sleep was measured in a sample of 31 young adults who were monitored in a sleep lab for three nights. During the second and third nights, subjects held and inhaled a vial of lavender essential oil or distilled water (control) for 2 minutes out of each of four 10-minute periods before going to sleep. The order of exposure to lavender or water varied. Lavender was shown to increase the percentage of deep or slow-wave sleep (measured by polysomnogram) and also increased subjects' reported vigor in the morning. In female subjects, lavender increased stage-2 light sleep and decreased rapid eye movement and wake after sleep onset latency, but it in males, it had an opposite effect (Goel, Kim, & Lao, 2005).

Lavender (*Lavandula angustifolia*) was also tested for sleep in a singleblind, randomized pilot study of ten adults with mild insomnia. After baseline assessment, subjects were randomized into two groups, with group one receiving lavender (*L. angustifolia*) essential oil first and almond oil second, and group two receiving the reverse. Subjects were not informed of the identity of the products. Treatments were administered by the subjects at home using a home diffusion device and there was a washout period of 1 week between treatments. A clinically significant improvement in sleep was seen with the lavender group, with a tendency toward stronger effect in women and younger participants (<39 years of age) (Lewth, Godfrey, & Prescott, 2005).

Lavender administered with a foot and leg massage was delivered to 12 children in a residential home for children with autism. The aromatherapy massage was provided on three nights (1 week apart), within 2 hours before going to bed (massage had been included as an daytime activity previous to the study so that the children were familiar with it). Subjects' sleep was monitored every half-hour through the night. Analysis compared aromatherapy massage nights to non-massage nights and there was no statistically significant difference between groups; however, the authors noted that their sample size was too small to detect clinically meaningful changes (Williams, 2006).

CHILDHOOD CANCER

The use of complementary and alternative therapies in the treatment of children with cancer has been described in a number of studies over the past decade (Bold & Leis, 2001; Fernandez, Stutzer, Maewilliam, & Fryer, 1998; Friedman et al., 1997; Kelly et al., 2000; Martel et al., 2005; Molasiotis & Cubbin, 2004). Patients and their parents described their use of a variety of therapies largely to improve health, reduce symptoms, and to feel more involved in care. The use of aromatherapy, either alone or with massage, in hospitals and in palliative care of children is considered to be safe and possibly useful for reduction of symptoms of pain, anxiety, and improvement of sleep (Styles, 1997). However, there are no large studies of individual essential oils' efficacy in children with cancer.

Although there is little published aromatherapy research in children, there is a growing body of research in adult cancer patients, usually for symptom management (Ernst, 2001; Kite et al., 1998; Zappa & Cassileth, 2003). Many of these studies are also hampered by small sample size, and often aromatherapy treatment is coupled with massage. In an analysis of eight randomized controlled trials, the use of aromatherapy resulted in a short-term reduction of anxiety in four studies, although the effects on other symptoms such as depression, pain, and nausea were mixed. The researchers concluded that replication, longer follow-up and larger studies are needed to determine benefit (Fellowes, Barnes, & Wilkinson, 2004).

In a randomized, controlled study of 46 adults with cancer in a day-treatment unit, subjects were divided into standard care or standard care plus aromatherapy massage. Groups were compared on measures of mood, quality of life, and intensity of symptoms. No differences were noted, but all of the patients in the aromatherapy massage group wished to continue the therapy (Wilcock et al., 2004). In a randomized, control trial, 42 adult patients with advanced cancer were assigned to massage, aromatherapy massage, or no treatment to evaluate the effects on sleep. Sleep improved in both the aromatherapy massage and massage groups, and depression decreased in the massage group; there was no change on pain intensity, anxiety, or quality of life indicators in any group (Soden, Vincent, Craske, Lucas, & Ashley, 2004). In a randomized study of 103 adult cancer palliative care patients, subjects were assigned to massage or aromatherapy massage groups. There was reduced anxiety after each treatment and overall improvement in psychological, quality of life, and physical indicators for both groups, with the aromatherapy massage group improving to a greater degree (Wilkinson, Aldridge, Salmon, Cain, & Wilson, 1999). Imanishi et al. (2007) noted short-term reduction of anxiety in adults receiving twice-weekly aromatherapy massage. Wilkinson et al. (2007) compared 288 adult cancer patients randomly assigned to aromatherapy massage or usual care finding clinically significant reduction in anxiety in the treatment group but no long-term difference between groups. Finally, Grahman, Browne, Cox, and Graham (2003) studied aromatherapy by itself in cancer patients undergoing radiation therapy. A blend of essential oils of [true] lavender (*L. angustifolia*), bergamot (*C. bergamia*) and cedar wood (*Cedrus atlantica*) were administered by inhalation to 313 subjects. Anxiety and depression were measured, with a reduction in anxiety seen only in the control group.

Infant Apnea

Olfactory stimulation as a therapy to prevent apnea was studied in 14 preterm newborns with recurrent apnea despite use of caffeine and doxapram. Although the intervention, vanillin, was not an essential oil, there may be a relationship to essential oils as olfactory stimulants. Each infant served as his own control. The protocol was carried out over 3 days, day 1 to establish baseline, day 2 vanillin was introduced and infants were observed, and day 3 all vanillin was removed and infants were observed without scent.

Nursing staff was aware of the scent, but not the purpose of the study. A decrease of 44% in apnea without bradycardia and 45% in apnea with severe bradycardia was noted on day of scent exposure. There was no significant difference in apnea with moderate bradycardia (Marlier, Gaugler, & Messer, 2005).

ANXIETY

Aromatherapy is often recommended to reduce stress and anxiety. The difference between state and trait anxiety and stress is often not well defined or differentiated in the recommendations. It is difficult to find tools to measure state anxiety in young children. In a systematic review of aromatherapy studies, Cooke and Ernst (2000) did not find strong evidence for the long-term treatment of anxiety with essential oils, but they did note a transient anxiolytic effect in many studies. Muzzarelli, Force, and Sebold (2006) randomized 118 adults about to undergo colonoscopy or esophagogastroduodenos-copy to treatment (lavender essential oil) or placebo control (unscented grapeseed oil). Pre- and post-state anxiety was measured, and there was no identified difference between groups. The authors noted that the pre-procedure anxiety level of both groups was high and that the fast-paced environment and short period of time for exposure to the essential oil may have overwhelmed any effect aromatherapy could have had. Both experimental and control groups reported that they found the scent pleasant.

Safety Concerns and Risks of Aromatherapy

Aromatherapy, especially when used topically or by inhalation, is a relatively safe therapy. However, there are safety issues to address. Common problems are toxicity from accidental ingestion and poisoning, skin irritation, allergic reactions, and pho-totoxicity. Drug interactions are not well-delineated but should be considered, particu-larly if the essential oil is taken orally.

Toxicity may be acute or chronic (Tisserand & Balacs, 1995). Acute toxicity often occurs with a single, large dose whereas chronic toxicity is associated with the use of smaller amounts over a longer time. Acute toxicity levels have been estimated using the Lethal Dose 50 (LD50) or the point at which 50% of subjects die from either oral or dermal exposure. Testing is conducted on animals (rodents and rabbits), and then extrapolated to humans. LD50 results should be interpreted cautiously since human physiology and skin characteristics differ from animal models. Tisserand and Balacs (1995) categorized essential oils into four levels of toxicity, from most toxic (LD50 up to 1 g/kg) to least toxic (LD50 over 5 g/kg). The most toxic essential oils, such as penny-royal, wormwood, and tansy, are never to be used in aromatherapy practice. However, some oils in the LD50 1–2 g/kg range, such as tea tree and basil, are in common use.

Acute toxicity is also evaluated by studying case reports of poisoning in humans. Based on these data, most essential oils have been found to be safe in the small quantities

(1–5 drops) in which they are usually recommended. However, aromatherapists sometimes use novel essential oils or essential oils of new chemotypes with no readily available safety analysis (Lis-Balchin, 1999). Although the LD50 for most essential oils exceeds the quantity in a standard bottle, severe reactions for some oils have been reported in both children and adults when quantities of 5–15 ml. were ingested (Tisserand & Balacs, 1995). There are many recorded cases of accidental poisoning in children, usually between 1 and 3 years of age. In some cases outcomes were severe, including death (Battaglia, 2003; Buckle, 2003; Tisserand & Balacs, 1995; Wilkinson 1991). It is important to discuss these issues with parents, as often they see complementary therapies as risk-free, as has been noted in case reports of accidental ingestions (Wilkinson, 1991). An accidental ingestion of an essential oil should be considered dangerous and poison control should be contacted. In order to reduce the chance of accidental ingestions:

1. Treat essential oils as medications and keep them out of the reach of young children;
2. Buy essential oils only in bottles with an integral drop dispenser to minimize the potential for ingesting large amounts; and
3. Buy essential oils that are clearly labeled, with labeling that includes all essential oils in a blended product and the carrier oil that was used for dilution.

Chronic toxicity is more difficult to assess as there are few published studies on the cumulative effects of specific essential oils. Symptoms are likely to be minor, such as nausea or headaches, and easily attributed to other causes. If children using an essential oil on an ongoing basis have vague or unexplained symptoms, it may be best to stop use for a period of time and evaluate. Henly, Lipson, Korach, and Bloch (2007) reported three case reports of prepubertal boys with unexplained gynecomastia. All three were using a topical product (shampoo, hair gel, lotion, or ointment) containing essential oil of lavender (*L. angustifolia*) and in one case lavender and tea tree (*M. alternifolia*). In all three cases the gynecomastia resolved when the product was discontinued. The authors noted estrogenic and antiandrogenic activity in in vitro testing of the essential oils and attributed the boys' condition to topical exposure to essential oils. Critiques of this report noted that there may be other unknown environmental factors, the possible role of other product ingredients was not investigated, the dose or amount of essential oil exposure was not well-delineated, and there is a notable lack of reports of estrogenic effects among workers in the essential oil industry who would likely have much higher exposure (Kalvan, 2007; Kemper, Romm, & Gardiner, 2007). Again, however, effects specifically in children have not been well studied.

Additionally, there are minimal data available on potential drug interactions. Although systemic levels of essential oils are quite low when used by inhalation or topically, children using a number of medications should be introduced to essential oils slowly to adequately evaluate potential interactions.

When essential oils are applied to the skin there is risk of irritation, sensitization or allergic reaction, and phototoxicity (Tisserand & Balacs, 1995). Data on skin irritation are inconsistent because (a) they often are derived from animal studies; (b) sensitivity is idiosyncratic; (c) damaged skin reacts differently than intact skin; and (d) children often have more sensitive skin than adults. Skin irritation, usually manifested as contact dermatitis, occurs most often with essential oils that are high in aromatic aldehydes, oxidized hydrocarbons or phenols (Buckle, 2003; Guba, 1999 part I). Only a few essential oils are classified as severely or strongly irritant, and none of those are commonly used in aromatherapy practice. Moderately irritant oils include cinnamon (*Cinnamomum zeylanicum*), oregano (*Origanum vulgare*), clove (*Eugenia caryophyllata*), and thyme (*Thymus vulgaris*); however, irritation can occur with any essential oil (Tisserand & Balacs, 1995).

To reduce the likelihood of irritation, essential oils for topical use should always be diluted in a carrier oil or lotion. Patch testing may be used to help determine if an essential oil will cause irritation in an individual. In order to conduct a patch test, dilute the essential oil in a carrier oil to at least double the intended strength. Apply the resulting solution to a small area of skin and cover with a small bandage for 24–48 hours. Observe for redness or other reactions. Any essential oil is likely to cause irritation if it comes in contact with the eyes or mucous membranes. For emergency treatment in these types of exposures, rinse the area with a bland vegetable oil (Guba, 1999, part I). If vegetable oil is not readily available, wash the skin with soap and rinse with water. If redness persists, a mild hydrocortisone ointment may be used on the skin.

Allergic sensitization also may occur with essential oil applications. Maddocke-Jennings (2004) reported two cases of allergic sensitivities that developed after multiple exposures. In the first case, a student who was learning aromatherapy massage experienced swollen, tingling and reddened hands which progressed to tracheal edema and shortness of breath. She was treated with antihistamines and recovered. The second case involved a student who experienced lightheadedness, tachycardia, and nausea after inhaling an essential oil. This student was removed from the source and monitored; no other treatment was necessary. The author noted that these are the only two cases of sensitivity to develop in this aromatherapy training program over a 10-year period. Essential oils with severe or strong risk of inducing sensitization are not commonly used (Tisserand & Balacs, 1995). There is a slight increase in risk for sensitivity associated with the use of lemongrass (*Cymbopogon citratus*), lavender (*Lavandula angustifolia or latifolia*), may chang (*Litsea cubeba*), and ylang ylang (*Cananga odorata*) essential oils. Additionally, there may be cross-reactivity between essential oils and similar plants, for example Roman chamomile (*Chamaemelum nobile*) should not be used if there is a known allergy to plants from the *Compositae* family (Battaglia, 2003).

Phototoxicity or increased sensitivity to ultraviolet light may occur with essential oils that contain furanocoumarins. Phototoxicity is a concern with topical application on exposed skin and is most likely to occur with bergamot (*Citrus bergamia*), lime (*Citrus medica*), cumin (*Cuminum cyminum*), and angelica (*Angelica archangelica*). It may also occur with lemon (*Citrus limonum*), bitter orange (*Citrus aurantium var. amara*), and grapefruit (*Citrus paradisi*) (Guba, 1999, part I). Some preparations containing bergamot have had the furanocoumarins removed and will be labeled bergaptene-free or furanocoumarin-free (FCF) (Tisserand & Balacs, 1995). Children with light skin tones are at higher risk for phototoxicity and subsequent sunburn.

There is a body of largely anecdotal and sometimes contradictory information in the aromatherapy literature suggesting that some essential oils may be contraindicated in specific medical conditions. For example, it is often suggested that essential oils of rosemary (*Rosmarinus officinalis*), thyme (*Thymus vulgaris*), or sage (*Salvia sclarea*) are contraindicated when patients have high blood pressure, or that fennel (*Foeniculum vulgaris*), hyssop (*Hyssopus officinalis*), or sage (*Salvia sclarea*) should not be used in patients with epilepsy. Guba (1999 part II) makes the case that these prohibitions may not be supported by science in that they are sometimes based on reports following toxic ingestions, and that documentation on the original observations sometimes cannot be found. In most cases, aromatherapy used by inhalation or topical application is unlikely to produce untoward systemic effects. However in a recent case study, Stafstrom (2007) documents seizures in a 7-month-old who was given an oral homeopathic remedy with thuja (*Thuja accidentialis*) and was receiving a herbal chest rub of sage (*Salvia officinalis*), eucalyptus, wintergreen (*Artemisia absinthium*), peppermint (*Mentha peperita*), and camphor (*Cinnamomun camphora*) several times a day. Wintergreen, thuja, and camphor are described as hazardous essential oils not recommended for general use (Battaglia, 2003; Tisserand & Balacs, 1995). The relative safety of aromatherapy was highlighted in an 8-year, observational study. In this study, 8,058 women on a childbirth unit received aromatherapy by topical application or inhalation. Only 1% of this sample reported side effects to the aromatherapy: nausea and vomiting was reported in 0.8% of cases, rash/itching in 0.2%, hay fever/watery eyes in 0.03%, and precipitous labor in 0.1% (Burns, 2000).

Essentials oils are generally a safe and gentle therapy; however, as noted above, there are a number of cautions. To increase the level of safety, incorporate the following guidelines when using essential oils in pediatric practice:

1. Educate parents in principles of safe application.
2. Store essential oils in airtight dark glass containers in a cool place in order to slow oxidation.
3. Limit oral applications unless prescribed as medications by healthcare providers who have had extensive training in essential oils.
4. Use only two to three drops of essential oils at a time for inhalation applications.
5. Use only diluted essential oils for topical applications (generally 1%–3%).

6. Consider the size and condition of the child when determining dose, use smaller and more dilute doses for children who are very young, medically fragile, seriously ill, or taking a number of medications.

7. Conduct a patch test when there is a history of sensitivity or multiple allergies.

Licensure

There is no national certification for aromatherapists in the United States. Individuals who have completed a qualifying program of study may sit for the registration exam offered through the Aromatherapy Registration Council (www.aromatherapycouncil. org). Upon passing this multiple choice examination covering basic therapeutic essential oils and safety principles, persons may use the title "Registered Aromatherapist." There are many aromatherapy education programs of varying lengths and foci. A few of these programs aim specifically to teach health professionals, and some offer their own certifications. Some of these programs are recognized through the National Associations for Holistic Aromatherapy (www.naha.org) (Lee, 2003). For more information about essential oils and other complementary therapies, web-based modules for the public, and for health professionals may be accessed free at www.csh.umn.edu under the headings, "Taking Charge of Your Health" and "Education."

Conclusion

Although the role of aromatherapy in specific health conditions needs to be better researched, it has been demonstrated to be a safe option for a variety of health concerns in children. Specific applications depend on the child's condition, size, and preferences, and the comfort and knowledge level of parents and providers.

REFERENCES

Anderson, C., Lis-Balchin, M., & Kirk-Smith, M. (2000). Evaluation of massage with essential oils on childhood atopic eczema. *Phytotherapy Research, 14*(6), 452–456.

Anderson, L. A., & Gross, J. G. (2004). Aromatherapy with peppermint, isopropyl alcohol or placebo is equally effective in relieving postoperative nausea. *Journal of PeriAnesthesia Nursing, 19*, 29–35.

Audino, P. G., Vassena, C., Zerba, E., & Picollo, M. (2007). Effectiveness of lotions based on essential oils from aromatic plants against permethrin resistant *Pediculus humanus capitis. Archives of Dermatological Research, 299*, 389–392.

Bassett, I. B., Pannowitz, D. L., & Barnetson, R. S. (1990). A comparative study of tea tree oil versus benzoyl peroxide in the treatment of acne. *Medical Journal of Australia, 153*(8), 455–458.

Battaglia, S. (2003). *The complete guide to aromatherapy* (2nd ed.). Brisbane, Australia: The International Centre of Holistic Aromatherapy.

Bensouilah, J. (2002). Aetiology and management of acne vulgais. *International Journal of Aromatherapy, 12*(2), 99–104.

Bold, J., & Leis, A. (2001). Unconventional therapy use among children with cancer in Saskatchewan. *Journal of Pediatric Oncology Nursing, 18*, 16–25.

Buck, P. (2004). Skin barrier function: Effect of age, race and inflammatory disease. *International Journal of Aromatherapy, 14*, 70–76.

Buckle, J. (1999). Use of aromatherapy as a complementary treatment for chronic pain. *Alternative Therapies, 5*(5), 42–51.

Buckle, J. (2001). The role of aromatherapy in nursing care. *Nursing Clinics of North America, 36*(1), 57–73.

Buckle, J. (2003). *Clinical aromatherapy: Essential oils in practice* (2nd ed). Edinburgh: Churchill Livingstone.

Buchbauer, G., Jirovetz, L., Jager, W., Dietrich, H., & Plank, C. (1991) Aromatherapy: Evidence for sedative effects of the essential oil of lavender after inhalation. *Z Naturforsch (Journal of Biosciences), 46*, 1067–1072.

Buchbauer, G., Jirovetz, L., Jager, W., Plank, C., & Dietrich, H. (1993). Fragrance compounds and essential oils with sedative effects upon inhalation. *Journal of Pharmaceutical Sciences, 82*, 660–664.

Burns, E., Blamey, C., Lloyd, A. J., & Barnetson, L. (2000). The use of aromatherapy in intrapartum midwifery practice: An observational study. *Complementary Therapy in Nurse Midwifery, 6*, 33.

Canyon, D., & Speare, R. (2007). A comparison of botanical and synthetic substances commonly used to prevent head lice (*Pediculus humanus* var. *capitits*). *International Journal of Dermatology, 46*, 422–426.

Carson, C., Cookson, B., Farrelly, H., & Riley, T. (1995). Susceptibility of methicillin-resistant Staphylococcus aureus to the essential oil of Melaleuca alternifolia. *Journal of Antimicrobial Chemotherapy, 35*(3), 421–424.

Carson, C., Hammer, K., & Riley, T. (1996). In-vitro activity of the essential oil of Melaleuca alternifolia against Streptococcus spp. *Journal of Antimicrobial Chemotherapy, 37*(6), 1177–1178.

Christoph, F., Stahl-Biskup, E., & Kaulfers, P.-M. (2001). Death kinetics of *Staphylococcus aureus* exposed to commercial tea tree oils s.l. *Journal of Essential Oils Research, 13*(Mar/Apr), 98–102.

Cooke B., & Ernst, E. (2000). Aromatherapy: A systematic review. *British Journal of General Practice, 50*, 493–496.

D'Auria, F. D., Tecca, M., Strippoli, V., Salvatore, G., Battinelli, L., & Mazzanti, G. (2005). Antifungal activity of *Lavandula angustifolia* essential oil against *Candida albicans* yeast and mycelial form. *Medical Mycology, 43*, 391–396.

Ernst, E. (2001). A primer of complementary and alternative medicine commonly used by cancer patients. *Medical Journal of Australia, 174*, 88–92.

Fellowes, D., Barnes, K., & Wilkinson, S. (2004). Aromatherapy and massage for symptom relief in patients with cancer. *Cochrane Database of Systematic Reviews.* Issue 3, Art. No.: CD002287. DOI:10.1002/14651858.CD002287.pub2.

Fennerty, B. (2003). Traditional therapies for irritable bowel syndrome: An evidence-based approach. *Reviews in Gastroenterological Disorders, 3*(suppl.2), S18–S24.

Fernandez, C. V., Stutzer, C. A., Macwilliam, L., & Fryer, C. (1998). Alternative and complementary therapy use in pediatric oncology patients in British Columbia: prevalence and reasons for use. *Journal of Clinical Oncology, 16*, 1279–1286.

Fitzgerald, M., Culbert, T., Finkelstein, M., Green, M., Johnson, A., & Chen, S. (2007). The effect of gender and ethnicity on children's attitudes and preferences for essential oils: A pilot study. *Explore: Journal of Science and Healing, 3*(4), 378–385.

Forbes, M. A., & Schmid, M. M. (2006). Use of OTC essential oils to clear plantar warts. *The Nurse Practitioner, 31*(3), 53–57.

Friedman, T., Slayton, W. B., Allen, L. S., Pollock, B. H., Dumont-Driscoll, M., Mehta, P., et al. (1997). Use of alternative therapies for children with cancer. *Pediatrics, 110*(6), e1.

Gedney, J. J., Glover, T. L., & Fillingim, R. B. (2004). Sensory and affective pain discrimination after inhalation of essential oils. *Psychosomatic Medicine, 66,* 599–606.

Gobel, H., Schmidt, G., & Soyka, D. (1994). Effect of peppermint and eucalyptus oil preparations on neurophysiological and experimental algesimetric headache parameters. *Cephalalgia, 14,* 228–234.

Goel, N., Kim, H., & Lao, R. P. (2005). An olfactory stimulus modifies nighttime sleep in young men and women. *Chronobiology International, 22*(5), 889–904.

Goubet, N., Rattaz, C., Pierrat, V., Bullinger, A., & Lequien, P. (2003). Olfactory experience mediates response to pain in preterm newborns. *Developmental Psychobiology, 42,* 171–180.

Goubet, N., Strasbaugh, K., & Chesney, J. (2007). Familiarity breeds content? Soothing effect of a familiar odor on full-term newborns. *Journal of Developmental and Behavioral Pediatrics, 28*(3), 189–194.

Graham, P. H., Browne, L., Cox, H., & Graham, J. (2003). Inhalation aromatherapy during radiotherapy: Results of a placebo-controlled double-blind randomized trial. *Journal of Clinical Oncology, 21*(12), 2372–2376.

Grigoleit, H. G., & Grigoleit, P. (2004). Peppermint oil in irritable bowel syndrome. *Phytomedicine, 12,* 601–606.

Guba, R. (1999). Toxicity myths…the actual risks of essential oil use. Part I. *Aromatherapy Today, 11,* 28–35.

Guba, R. (1999). Toxicity myths…the actual risks of essential oil use. Part II. *Aromatherapy Today, 12,* 16–22.

Gustafson, J. E., Liew, Y. C., Chew, S., Markham, J., Bell, H., & Wyllie, S. G. (1998). Effects of tea tree oil on *Escherichia coli. Letters in Applied Microbiology, 26*(3), 194–198.

Halcón, L. (2002). Aromatherapy: Therapeutic applications of plant essential oils. *Minnesota Medicine, 85*(11), 42–46.

Halcón, L., & Milkus, K. (2004). Staphylococcus aureus and wounds: A review of tea tree oil as a promising antimicrobial. *American Journal of Infection Control, 32,* 402–408.

Hammer, K., Carson, C., & Riley, T. (2004). Antifungal effects of *Melaleuca alternifolia* (tea tree) oil and its components on *Candida albicans, Candida glabata* and *Saccharomyces cerevisiae. Journal of Antimicrobial Chemotherapy, 53*(6), 1081–1085.

Hammer, K., Carson, C., Riley, T., & Nielsen, J. (2006). A review of the toxicity of *Melaleuca alternifolia* (tea tree) oil. *Food and Chemical Toxicology, 44*(5), 616–625.

Han, S., Hur, M., Buckle, J., Choi, J., & Lee, M. S. (2006). Effect of aromatherapy on symptoms of dysmenorrhea in college students: a randomized placebo-controlled clinical trial. *Journal of Alternative and Complementary Medicine, 12*(6), 535–541.

Hayashi, K., Kamiya, M., & Hayashi, T. (1995). Virucidal effects of the steam distillate from Houttuynia cordata and its components on HSV-1, influenza virus, and HIV. *Planta Medica, 61*(3):237-41.

Henley, D. V., Lipson, N., Korach, K., & Bloch, C. A. (2007). Prepubertal gynecomastia linked to lavender and tea tree oils. *New England Journal of Medicine, 356*(5), 479–485.

Howarth, A. (2004). The use of aromatherapy for the management of chronic pain. *International Journal of Clinical Aromatherapy, 1*(1), 29–32.

Hunt, V., Randle, J., & Freshwater, D. (2004). Paediatric nurses attitudes to massage and aromatherapy massage. *Complementary Therapies in Nursing and Midwifery, 10,* 194–201.

Imanishi, J., Kuriyama, H., Shigemori, I., Watanabe, S., Aihara, Y., Kita, M., et al. (2007). Anxiolytic effect of aromatherapy massage in patients with breast cancer. *Evidence-based Complementary and Alternative Medicine*. eCAM doi:10.1093/ecam/nem073

Kalyan, S. (2007). Prepubertal gynescomastia linked to lavender and tea tree oils(letter to the editor) *New England Journal of Medicine, 356*(24), 2542.

Kelly, K. M., Jacobson, J. S., Kennedy, D. D., Braudt, S. M., Malick, M., & Weiner, M. (2000). Use of unconventional therapies by children with cancer at an urban medical center. *Journal of Pediatric Hematology and Oncology, 22*, 412–416.

Kemper, K. J., Romm, A. J., & Gardiner, P. (2007). Prepubertal gynescomastia linked to lavender and tea tree oils (letter to the editor) *New England Journal of Medicine, 356*(24), 2541–2542.

Kerr, J., & Casey, M. (2004). Aromatherapy and the perception of pain. *International Journal of Clinical Aromatherapy, 1*(1), 24–28.

Kite, S. M., Maher, E. J., Anderson, K., Young, T., Young, J., Wood, J., et al. (1998). Development of an aromatherapy service at a cancer centre. *Palliative Medicine, 12*, 171–180.

Kline, R. M., Kline, J. J., Di Palma, J., & Barbero, G. J. (2001). Enteric-coated, pH-dependent peppermint oil capsules for the treatment of irritable bowel syndrome in children. *Journal of Pediatrics, 138*, 125–128.

Lavabre, M. (1990). *Aromatherapy workbook* (pp. 3–9). Rochester, Vermont: Healing Arts Press.

Lawless, J. (1995). *The illustrated encyclopedia of essential oils: The complete guide to the use of oils in aromatherapy and herbalism* (pp. 14–21). London: Element Books Ltd.

Lee, C. O. (2003). Clinical aromatherapy part II: Safe guidelines for integration into clinical practice. *Clinical Journal of Oncology Nursing, 7*(5), 597–598.

Lewith. G. T., Godfrey, A. D., & Prescott, P. (2005). A single-blinded, randomized pilot study evaluating the aroma of *Lavandula augustifolia* as a treatment for mild insomnia. *Journal of Alternative and Complementary Medicine,* 11(4), 631–637.

Lis-Balchin, M. (1999). Possible health and safety problems in the use of novel plant essential oils and extracts in aromatherapy. *Journal of the Royal Society for the Promotion of Health, 119*(4), 240–243.

Maddocke-Jennings, W. (2004). Critical incident: Idiosyncratic allergic reactions to essential oils. *Complementary Therapies in Nursing and Midwifery, 10*(1), 58–60.

Maddocks-Jennings, W., & Wilkinson, J. (2004). Aromatherapy practice in nursing: Literature review. *Journal of Advanced Nursing, 48*(1), 93–103.

Marlier, L., Gaugler, C., & Messer, J. (2005). Olfactory stimulation prevents apnea in premature newborns. *Pediatrics, 115*(1), 83–88.

Martel, D., Bussieres, J. F., Theoret, Y., Lebel, D., Kish, S., Moghrabi, A., et al. (2005). Use of alternative and complementary therapies in children with cancer *Pediatric Blood Cancer, 44*, 660–668.

Maudsley, F., & Kerr, K. G. (1999). Microbiological safety of essential oils used in complementary therapies and the activity of these compounds against bacterial and fungal pathogens. *Support Care Cancer, 7*(2),100–102.

May, J., Chan, C. H., King, A., Williams, L., & French, G. L. (2000). Time-kill studies of tea tree oils on clinical isolates. *Journal of Antimicrobial Chemotherapy, 45*(5), 639–643.

May, B., Kohler, S., & Schneider, B. (2000). Efficacy and tolerability of a fixed combination of peppermint oil and caraway oil in patients suffering from functional dyspepsia. *Alimentary Pharmacology and Therapeutics, 14*, 1671–1677.

Molassiotis, A., & Cubbin, D. (2004). Thinking outside the box: Complementary and alternative therapies use in paediatric oncology patients. *European Journal of Oncology Nursing, 8*, 50–60.

Moss, M., Cook, J., Wesnes, K., & Duckett, P. (2003). Aromas of rosemary and lavender essential oils differentially affect cognition and mood in healthy adults. *International Journal of Neuroscience, 113*, 15–38.

Muzzarelli, L., Force, M., & Sebold, M. (2006). Aromatherapy and reducing preprocedural anxiety: A controlled prospective study. *Gastroenterology Nursing, 29*(6), 467–471.

Nelson, R. R. (1997). In-vitro activities of five plant essential oils against methicillin-resistant Staphylococcus aureus and vancomycin-resistant Enterococcus faecium. *Journal of Antimicrobial Chemotherapy, 40*(2), 305–306.

Papadopoulos, C., Carson, C., Hammer, K., & Riley, T. (2006). Susceptibility of pseudomonads to *Melaleuca alternifolia* (tea tree) oil and components. *Journal of Antimicrobial Chemotherapy, 58*(2), 449–451.

Pittler, M. H., & Ernst, E. (1998). Peppermint oil for irritable bowel syndrome: a critical review and meta-analysis. *The American Journal of Gastroenterology, 3*(7), 1131–1135.

Price, S., & Parr, P. P. (1996). *Aromatherapy for babies and children.* San Francisco: Thorsons.

Sakamoto, R., Minoura, K., Usui, A., Ishizuka, Y., & Kanba, S. (2005). Effectiveness of aroma on work efficiency: Lavender aroma during recesses prevents deterioration of work performance. *Chemical Senses, 30*, 683–691.

Sherry, E., Boeck, H., & Warnke, P. (2001). Topical application of a new formulation of eucalyptus oil phytochemical clears methicillin-resistant Staphylococcus aureus infection. *American Journal of Infection Control, 29*(5), 346.

Stafstrom, C. E. (2007). Seizures in a 7-month-old child after exposure to the essential plant oil thuja. *Pediatric Neurology, 37*(6), 446–448.

Snyder, M., & Wieland, J. (2003). Complementary and alternative therapies: What is their place in the management of chronic pain? *Nursing Clinics of North America, 38*, 495–508.

Soden, K., Vincent, K., Craske, S., Lucas, C., & Ashley, S. (2004). A randomized controlled trial of aromatherapy massage in a hospice setting. *Palliative Medicine, 18*(2), 87–92.

Styles, J. (1997). The use of aromatherapy in hospitalized children with HIV disease. *Complementary Therapies in Nursing, 3*, 16–20.

Tate, S. (1997). Peppermint oil: A treatment for postoperative nausea. *Journal of Advanced Nursing, 26*, 543–549.

Tisserand, R., & Balacs, T. (1995). *Essential oil safety.* Edinburgh: Churchill Livinstone.

Wheatley, D. (2005) Medicinal plants for insomnia: A review of their pharmacology, efficacy, and tolerability. *Journal of Psychopharmacolgy, 19*(4), 414–421.

Wilcock, A., Manderson, C., Weller,R., Walker, G., Carr, D., Carey, A. M., et al. (2004). Does aromatherapy benefit patients with cancer attending a specialist palliative care day centre? *Palliative Medicine, 18*(4), 287–290.

Wilkinson, H. F. (1991). Childhood ingestion of volatile oils. *Medical Journal of Australia, 154*, 430–431.

Wilkinson, S., Aldridge, J., Salmon, I., Cain, E., & Wilson, B. (1999). An evaluations of aromatherapy massage in palliative care. *Palliative Medicine, 13*, 409–417.

Wilkinson, S. M., Love, S. B., Westcombe, A. M., Gambles, M. A., Burgess, C. C., Cargill, A., et al. (2007). Effectiveness of aromatherapy massage in the management of anxiety and depression in patients with cancer: A mulricenter randomized controlled trial. *Journal of Clinical Oncology, 25*(5), 532–539.

Williams, T. I. (2006). Evaluating effects of aromatherapy massage on sleep in children with autism: A pilot study. *Evidence-Based Complementary and Alternative Medicine, 3*(3), 73–77.

Zappa, S. B., & Cassileth, B. (2003). Complementary approaches to palliative oncology care. *Journal of Nursing Care Quarterly, 18*(1), 22–26.

8

A Pediatric Perspective on Chiropractic

KAREN ERICKSON, ELISE G. HEWITT, AMY LYNNE WATSON,
ANTHONY L. ROSNER, AND RANDY L. HEWITT

KEY CONCEPTS

- Chiropractic is the third largest heath care profession in the United States after medicine and dentistry, and the most utilized type of holistic health care.
- All chiropractors are trained to treat infants and children. Chiropractors have the option of furthering their specialization through post-doctorate training certification in pediatric chiropractic.
- There is a growing body of evidence in the literature as well as growing clinical experience that shows chiropractic to be a gentle, safe, and effective treatment for many conditions experienced by the pediatric population.
- Chiropractic care is safe and effective during pregnancy for back pain, when diagnostic imaging and medication may be contraindicated.
- Chiropractic care during pregnancy may have beneficial effects on the fetus, and may reduce labor time and certain complications during delivery.
- Chiropractic care for newborns includes gentle palpation and adjustment of the spine and cranium to eliminate any structural stress experienced by the infant during pregnancy or delivery.
- Birth trauma, nursing dysfunction, torticollis, colic, and reflux are some of the conditions in infants that can be successfully treated with chiropractic manipulation.
- Research shows that back pain in childhood is a strong predictor of back pain in adulthood. Chiropractic is appropriate for treating the growing incidence of back pain and headaches in children from the use of backpacks, computers, and hand-held devices.

- Chiropractors may be a part of a multidisciplinary healthcare team that treats various developmental and neurological disorders including ADHD and autism.
- Chiropractors have an increasing role in treating pediatric sports and other injuries to facilitate rapid and complete healing, and prevent chronic conditions.
- Research shows that chiropractic has a modulating effect on the nervous system and may reduce stress hormones like cortisol.

■

Introduction

A growing body of research is emerging that supports what chiropractors and parents have observed for years: pediatric chiropractic is a gentle, safe, and effective treatment for many common pediatric conditions. Chiropractic is a uniquely American healing art that was founded in 1895 in Davenport, Iowa, and today has licensed practitioners in all 50 states, and countless countries around the world. Chiropractic is the third largest health care profession in the United States, and is the most commonly utilized of all the holistic healing arts. Most major insurance carriers cover chiropractic.

All chiropractors are trained in specific examination and adjusting techniques appropriate for infants and children. Additionally, there are many post-graduate courses in pediatric chiropractic offering continuing education credit, as well as diplomate certification in pediatric chiropractic. As the clinical field of pediatric chiropractic research expands every year, there is a need for research with larger cohorts and better methodology to provide "best practices" for this growing subspecialty.

Chiropractic Rationale and Therapeutic Interventions

Chiropractors employ a variety of techniques to restore normal biomechanics to the articulations of the spine, cranium, and extremities and modulate neurological and physiological function (Haldeman, 2004). Joint aberration is variously termed a joint restriction, joint dysfunction, or a subluxation. The procedures used to address this condition are interchangeably called adjustments, manipulations, chiropractic manipulative therapy, or spinal manipulative therapy. An adjustment may be performed with the hands or with the aid of a mechanical instrument.

LOCAL AND SYSTEMIC EFFECTS OF SUBLUXATION

A subluxation affects function on both local and systemic levels. On a local level, a subluxation disrupts normal joint kinematics, causes irritation to related neurological

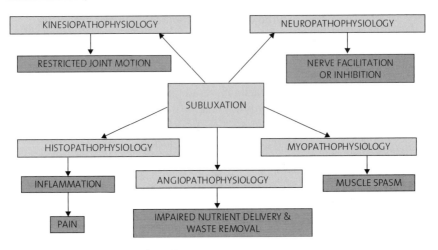

FIGURE 8-1. Local effects of a subluxation.

structures, affects resting muscle tone, disrupts blood flow to affected structures and alters normal cell histology, leading to inflammation and pain (Figure 8-1). Clinically, a subluxation presents as restricted segmental range of motion at the affected joint, muscle spasm in local paraspinal musculature, and pain to palpation in the area of the subluxation. A subluxation can disrupt normal physiological function far from the site of articular derangement. These changes are mediated through altered afferent input to the brainstem, cerebellum, thalamus, and cerebrum (Haldeman, 2004). For example, Edwards found that neck muscle spindle afferent activation, such as can occur secondary to a cervical subluxation, may influence central cardio-respiratory control via the intermedius nucleus of the medulla and the nucleus tractus solitarii (Edwards 2007).

CHIROPRACTIC ADJUSTMENTS

Chiropractors employ a variety of adjustment techniques to address a number of variables, including therapeutic intent, and characteristics of both the patient and presenting condition. Adjustments can be categorized based upon the velocity and amplitude of the procedure. Some techniques (such as diversified and Gonstead methods) use a high-velocity, low-amplitude thrust (HVLA), while others (such as craniosacral therapy, sacro-occipital technique, Network and muscle energy technique) use a low-velocity, low-amplitude manoeuvre (LVLA).

Most HVLA adjusting techniques create an audible click, termed a cavitation, as the joint is brought from the physiological space into the para-physiological space (Figure 8-2). This sound occurs as a result of a change in gas pressure within the enclosed joint capsule of the affected segment and indicates that a physiological alteration has occurred in the cellular structures of the affected joint (Leach, 1994). LVLA adjusting techniques bring a joint to the end of its passive range of motion using low-force or non-force procedures. Craniosacral therapy and other LVLA cranial techniques focus on gently

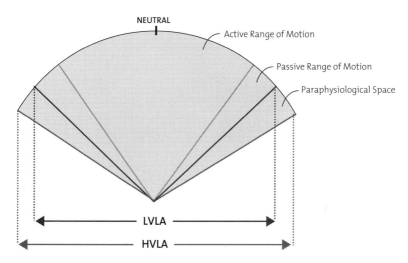

FIGURE 8-2. Range of movement in diarthrodial joints: In a LVLA (low velocity low amplitude) manoeuvre or adjustment, a joint is brought through the passive range of motion to the elastic barrier of resistance. A HVLA (high velocity low amplitude) differs in that a precise adjustment moves the joint beyond this initial barrier of resistance into the paraphysiological space, creating a cavitation. or "popping sound," causing the joint range of motion to be restored. (Based on Sandoz's chart in Leach 1994, and Bartol's chapter in Gatterman 1995.)

restoring normal motion to the cranial bones with the aim of relieving tension on and restoring function to underlying soft tissues, including the dura matter and cortical tissue (Upledger, 1983). No cavitation occurs with LVLA maneuvers, since the procedure stops before the joint enters the paraphysiological space.

SAFETY OF CHIROPRACTIC ADJUSTING

Delivering a chiropractic adjustment to a child is a relatively safe procedure. A systematic review of adverse events by Vohra in 2007 examining the literature of the past 110 years revealed 11 cases of moderate or severe adverse events following spinal manipulation in children, 7 of which involved a chiropractor (Vohra et al., 2007). Balanced against an estimated 30 million pediatric visits to the chiropractor in the US in 1997 (Lee et al., 2000), the estimated relative risk of adverse events in the pediatric population appears to be exceedingly small.

To increase safety, the chiropractor modifies the adjustive procedure to account for the hyperflexible pediatric spine. This hyperflexibility results from the combination of immature cartilaginous bone and hyper-elastic ligaments, especially the zygapophyseal joints of the spine (Fysh, 2002). Procedural modifications to adapt the adjustive procedure to the hyperflexibility of the pediatric spine include modified contact and patient positioning, decreased force, and decreased amplitude of thrust (Fysh, 2002) (Figure 8-3).

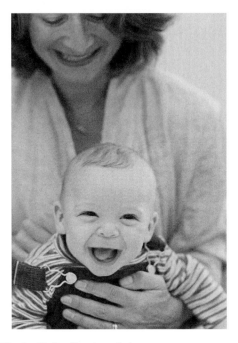

FIGURE 8-3. Elise Hewitt, D.C. adjusting a baby.

Physiological Therapies, Nutritional Supplementation, Exercise, and Lifestyle Advice

Chiropractors may employ a variety of physiotherapeutic techniques to support and enhance the adjustive procedure and the child's overall health including gentle soft tissue massage, cryotherapy, heat, electrical stimulation, lymphatic drainage, and visceral manipulation. A basic tenet of chiropractic is that, in addition to full joint mobility, true health requires good nutrition to increase function and decrease inflammation, proper rest, and an active lifestyle in an environment free of toxins and stress.

Frequency and Duration: Curative versus Preventative Care

CURATIVE CARE

During the initial visit, the chiropractor takes a complete history and performs an examination to evaluate both the child's chief complaint and overall health status, paying special attention to the joints of the spine, cranium, and extremities. Duration and frequency of care for this curative segment depend upon many elements including: (a) the overall health status and age of the child, (b) the severity of the initial event that caused the subluxation, and (c) the duration of the subluxation at the time of initial visit (Fallon, 2005). Healing time is inversely proportional to age; the younger the child, the shorter the duration and frequency of care needed to reach articular stabilization. Conversely, event severity is directly proportional to treatment duration and frequency (Fysh, 2002). Once curative care is completed, and stabilization and full function have been restored, the child is released from care.

PREVENTATIVE CARE

Subluxations don't always cause pain or inflammation as they do in adults, because of the elasticity of the child's ligamentous and articular structures. Just as a cavity in a child's tooth, the subluxation can go undetected without regular chiropractic check-ups. Chiropractors recommend periodic spinal checkups for children, the frequency of which depend upon the child's age, but vary from monthly in the first 12 months of life, to once every 3 to 4 months in the older child (Fysh, 2002).

The body has an inherent ability to self-regulate and chiropractors postulate that subluxations in the spine may interfere with these self-regulatory abilities, resulting in non-symptomatic physiological dysfunction and eventual symptomatic disease. Research is beginning to elucidate how chiropractic adjustments produce beneficial systemic physiological changes. In a 2007 double-blind, placebo-controlled study, Bakris found chiropractic adjustments to the cervical spine are "associated with marked and sustained reductions in blood pressure similar to the use of two-drug combination therapy" (Bakris, 2007). By measuring changes in somatosensory-evoked potentials in the frontal and parietal regions of the brain, Haavik-Taylor and Murphy demonstrated that cervical spinal adjusting,when compared to a passive head movement control group, alters cortical somatosensory processing and sensorimotor integration, thus leading to cortical plastic changes (Haavik-Taylor, 2006). These changes in blood pressure and cortical brain activity following an adjustment illustrate both the subluxation's ability to interfere with host systemic health and the adjustment's capability to restore and enhance health.

Etiology of the Subluxation in Children

INTRAUTERINE CONSTRAINT

A newborn infant may be engaged in their mother's pelvis with their neck in a biomechanically stressed position, causing joint and muscle imbalances. Once outside the womb, the infant may display a preference for certain positions of the neck, with or without signs of discomfort. This can lead to nursing difficulty, torticollis, and/or plagiocephaly. Abnormal posture may go unnoticed, dismissed as within normal variance, or lead to clinical diagnosis and treatment. Chiropractic offers a valuable resolution of conditions caused by intrauterine constraint.

BIRTH TRAUMA

Many factors influence the force on the infant's spine during delivery, including the method of delivery (vaginal or caesarean), the presentation (vertex or breech), and use of interventions (vacuum extraction or forceps). Even with optimal position and a minimum amount of added force applied during delivery, the delicate spine may still be subject to assorted forms of injury. Various examples of severe neonatal morbidity and mortality attributed to birth trauma have been documented in the medical literature (Brand, 2006; Gottleib, 1993; Hughes, 1999; Tobwin, 1969). Serious sequelae of birth trauma may require surgical intervention and/or extended intensive care best managed in a hospital setting. Less severe birth trauma may present with more subtle signs and symptoms displayed by comparatively healthy newborns that may respond favorably to chiropractic manual therapy, namely KISS Syndrome and Blocked Atlantal Nerve Syndrome.

KISS Syndrome

Heiner Biedermann, MD, has proposed a concept known as the KISS (Kinematic Imbalances due to Sub-occipital Strain) syndrome. The strain exerted on suboccipital structures at birth may lead to symptomology that goes unnoticed, considered benign and self-limiting, but that may have an underestimated long-term effect on infant health. He describes two main forms of this syndrome he has observed in his pediatric practice: KISS I and II (Figures 8-4 and 8-5).

> KISS I is characterized by fixed lateroflexion: torticollis, unilateral microsomia, asymmetry of the skull, C-scoliosis of the neck and trunk, asymmetry of the gluteal area, asymmetry of motion of the limbs, and retardation of motor development of one side.

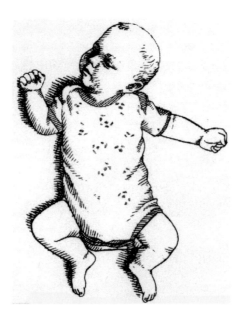

Figure 8-4. KISS I.

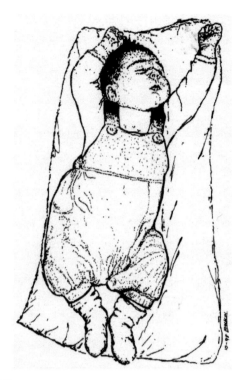

Figure 8-5. KISS II.

KISS II involves fixed retro-flexion: hyperextension (during sleep), (asymmetric)
occipital flattening, shoulders pulled up, fixed supination of the arms, inability to lift trunk from ventral position, orofacial muscular hypotonia, difficulty
breast-feeding on one side. Biedermann reports using spinal manipulation to
successfully treat over 20,000 infants with both forms of KISS syndrome, with
no serious complications (Biedermann, 2005)

Blocked Atlantal Nerve Syndrome

Blocked Atlantal Nerve Syndrome has "three characteristic groups of symptoms: (a)
Disturbance of motor responses, both in postural-tonic and kinesiological-phasic portion; (b) A brain-stem component net central disturbance of negative regulatory systems; (c) Inclination to infections in the throat, nose and ear" (Gutman, 1990). Perinatal
trauma can have lasting effects on the atlanto-occipital joints, and this can lead to a variety of structural, postural, functional, and kinesological disturbances including torticollis, cranial asymmetry, delayed motor response, increased infections, and impairment
of the hip, and sacroiliac joints. The infants studied showed improved symptomology
following manual adjusting of the atlas (Gutman, 1990).

DEVELOPMENT OF SPINAL CURVATURES AND STAGES OF LOCOMOTION

A child's entire spine is kyphotic at birth (Figure 8-6). The cervical lordosis forms by the third month as the child develops head control, especially in the prone "tummy time." Proper spinal curvature formation is essential for shock absorption and spinal health in adulthood (Corrigan, 1998). The presence of chronic subluxations in the spine, cranium, or extremity articulations can interfere with proper curvature formation and early motor development (Viholainen, 2002) Subluxations in the cervical or upper thoracic regions of the spine inhibit lifting and turning of the head in the prone position. The presence of cervical or thoracic subluxation may contribute to SIDS by preventing the baby from being able to lift and turn the head while prone (Koch, 1998, 2002). The lumbar lordosis develops towards the end of the first year of life, as the child becomes weight-bearing during the acts of standing and walking. The sagital spinal curves contribute to balance, movement facilitation and shock absorption, protecting the vertebrae, intervertebral discs, ligaments, joint capsules, muscles and tendons from the gravitational forces involved in locomotion and an upright posture.

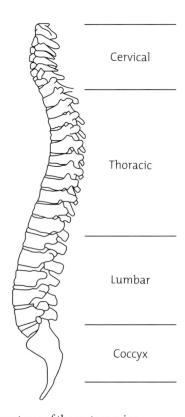

Cervical

Thoracic

Lumbar

Coccyx

FIGURE 8-6. Normal curvatures of the mature spine.

Subluxation can impede the formation of these curvatures (often called a military or straight spine), create discomfort and premature spinal degeneration (Wiegand, 2003), as well as interfere with early motor development affecting brain patterning and coordination. See Table 8-1 for symptoms of subluxation. The connection between improper development of the stages of locomotion and the appearance of the learning disability, dyslexia, is still poorly understood. Viholainen found significant motor development differences in the first 2 years of life between children with familial risk of dyslexia and those without such a family risk (Viholainen, 2002). Nicolson found that 80% of children with dyslexia had cerebellar impairment as demonstrated on behavioural and neuro-imaging tests (Nicolson, 2001). By modulating neurological function through correction of joint restriction, chiropractic may have a role in alleviating developmental delay in children (Figure 8-7).

Table 8-1. Symptoms of an Infant/Toddler that May Indicate the Presence of a Subluxation Impairing Proper Development of Spinal Curvatures and/or Locomotion

Dislikes lying in prone position

Poor head control

Persistent head tilt

Asymmetrical crawl

Abnormal gait

Delayed walking

Frequent tripping and falling

Poor balance

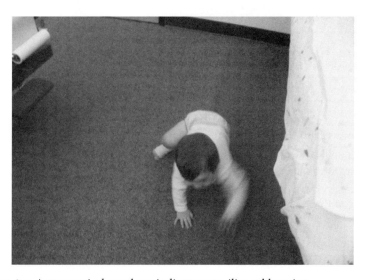

FIGURE 8-7. Asymmetrical crawl can indicate sacro-iliac subluxation.

Recognizing the Child Who Needs a Chiropractic Evaluation

Subluxation can originate in a seemingly benign fall while the child learns to stand and walk, or in a more obvious trauma, such as a fall from a bicycle, motor vehicle accident, playground fall, or sports injury. Table 8-2 lists conditions that respond to chiropractic care. Table 8-3 lists behavioral changes often seen when a subluxation occurs following a fall or other trauma. An alert pediatrician may detect the presence of subluxations by history and examination as outlined in Table 8-4.

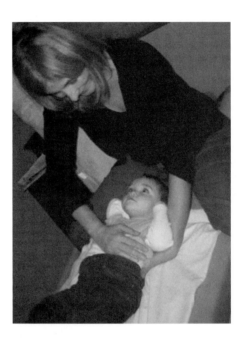

Chiropractic Care for Conditions of the Neonate and Infant

Infants can safely be adjusted within minutes of birth. Whether the birth is "normal" and uncomplicated, or "difficult" with medical intervention, the birth process exerts significant forces on the infant's delicate spinal column (Geutjens, 1996; Tobwin, 1969). There is a growing body of literature showing that chiropractic is effective at treating many conditions such as *torticollis* (Colin, 1998; Fallon, 1997; McCoy Moore, 1997; Smith-Nguyen, 2004; Toto, 1993), *colic* (Klorgart, 1989; Leach, 2002; Mercer, 1999; Olfsdottir, 2001; Pluharet, 1991; VanLoon, 1998; Wiberg, 1999), *nursing dysfunction* (Cuhel & Powell, 1997; Hewitt, 1999; Holtrop, 2000; Sheader, 1999; Vallone, 2004, 2007), *constipation* (Eriksen, 1994; Falk, 1990; Hewitt, 1993; Marko, 1994; Quist, 2007),

Table 8-2. Pediatric Conditions that Respond to Chiropractic Care

Neonate—Infant

    Colic/irritability

    Plagiocephaly

    Sutural ridging

    Torticollis/Head tilt

    Brachioplexus irritation

    Poor sleep

    Nursing dysfunction

    Gastroesophageal reflux disease (GERD)

    Chronic constipation

    Sleep apnea or snoring

    Asymmetrical crawl or gait

Toddler

    Chronic ear infections

    Chronic upper respiratory infections

    Asthma

    Growing pains/foot or leg cramping

    Primary nocturnal enuresis

    Incontinence (bowel or bladder)

    Pervasive developmental disease*

    Seizures

School-Age Child and Adolescent

    Back pain

    Neck pain

    Headaches

    Scoliosis

    Spondylolisthesis

    Extremity injuries (chronic ankle sprains, shoulder pain, knee pain, etc.)

    Chronic abdominal pain

*Including autism, sensory integration disorder, ADD, ADHD, learning disabilities.

Table 8-3. Changes Following a Fall that Indicate the Presence of a Subluxation

Characteristic	Change
Attitude	Increased grumpiness, clinginess, frustration
Appetite	Decreased appetite, increased abdominal discomfort
Sleep	Sudden change in sleep habits—frequent waking, nightmares, difficulty falling asleep
Bowel habits	Sudden onset of constipation or diarrhea

Table 8-4. Clues Indicating the Presence of a Spinal Subluxation

Clues in the History

In utero constraint

Prolonged or precipitous labor

Abnormal presentation or position during birth

Assisted delivery (forceps, vacuum extraction, Caesarean section)

Multiples (twins, etc.)

Nursing difficulties

Poor latch

Irritated/painful maternal nipples

Plugged ducts/mastitis

Refusal to nurse on one side

Irritability

Sleep issues

Easily awakens

Wakes often

Difficulty falling asleep

Constipation/abdominal discomfort

Unsteady gait/frequent tripping

Delayed developmental skills (gross motor, fine motor, verbalization)

History of chronic infection (upper respiratory, otitis media, etc.)

History of trauma

Clues in the Examination

Head tilt with or without rotation

Plagiocephaly

Sutural overlap/ridging

Hyperactive startle reflex

Hyperactive gag reflex

Weak or shallow latch

Decreased TMJ excursion

Inadequate weight gain

Discomfort in prone position

Postural asymmetry

Positive Adams test for scoliosis

Decreased range of motion (spine or extremities)

Abnormal gait

Pronation syndrome

Pain (back, neck, extremity)

Muscular hypertonicity and/or weakness

and *reflux or GERD* (Alcantara, 2005; Haldeman, 1974; Hipperson, 2004; Kiyomi, 1978). The rationale for treating visceral conditions with chiropractic is its modulating effect on the autonomic nervous system, allowing end organs to function normally (Whelan, 2002).

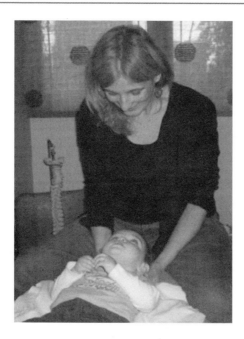

CONGENITAL AND POSITIONAL PLAGIOCEPHALY

Tension in the dural lining of the cranial bones secondary to intrauterine constraint or birth trauma can prevent the skull from expanding in response to brain growth. This results in a flattening of the cranium adjacent to the area of dural tension. Congenital and positional plagiocephaly respond well to spinal and cranial adjustment (Philips, 1996; Quezeda, 2004). Cranial adjusting reduces dural tension, allowing the cranial bones to expand as the brain enlarges. While the supine sleeping position prevents SIDS, it can increase pressure on the occiput, resulting in asymmetric cranial growth. Positional plagiocephaly can result when an infant has torticollis or a persistent preference for rotation to one side, leading to the development of a unilateral flattening of the parieto-occipital region of the cranium. Mild cases respond to stretching exercises and regular prone positioning. Severe cases are treated with molding helmets (Morrison & Chariker, 2006). Chiropractic restores normal range of motion to the cervical spine, eliminating persistent rotation, allowing the skull shape to normalize over time. Chiropractic can be used in lieu of or concurrently with a molding helmet.

Chiropractic for the Toddler and Preschool-Aged Patient

OTITIS MEDIA

Chiropractic evaluation for children at the onset of otitis media is recommended to reduce antibiotics usage. Children who have already experienced a case of otitis media

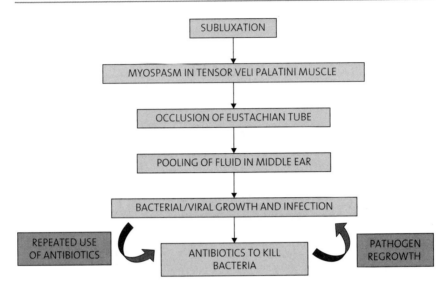

FIGURE 8-8. How a subluxation can create otitis media.

should be referred for chiropractic care to prevent a cycle of recurrence. There is strong evidence for the chiropractic management of otitis media. Subluxation of the C1 vertebra and/or cranium may lead to constriction or closure of the Eustachian tube, which creates a pooling of fluid in the middle ear cavity (Figure 8-8).

Chiropractors use gentle upper cervical adjustment, cranial adjusting of the temporal, parietal and occipital bones, and lymphatic drainage to assist Eustachian tubes drainage (Philips, 1992). The majority of otitis media cases treated with spinal manipulation resolve within 10 days, most responding to fewer than 5 adjustments (Fallon, 1997; Fysh, 1996) and many requiring only one or two treatments (Froehle, 1996; Peet, 1996; Phillips, 1992). Acute cases showed faster improvement with chiropractic, and much lower incidence or recurrence or surgical intervention (Fallon, 1998). Patients undergoing manipulation encountered fewer surgeries or subsequent episodes of acute otitis media (Mills, 2003).

CHRONIC UPPER RESPIRATORY INFECTION

Chiropractic has a valuable role in the integrative approach to upper respiratory infection. These conditions may begin with bacterial or viral etiology, but can progress to become a low-level chronic condition consisting of sinus congestion, post-nasal drip, coughing, lung congestion, and reactive airway disease. Vertebral subluxations may increase the work of breathing, decreasing oxygenation and forcing the overuse and spasm of the secondary muscles of respiration including trapezius, anterior scalenes, sternocleidmastoid and pectoral muscles. In addition to spinal and rib adjustments to ease respiratory effort and improve tissue oxygenation, chiropractors integrate myofascial release or massage, shiatsu reflex points for the lungs and sinuses, lymphatic drainage techniques, and craniosacral and visceral manipulation to the respiratory diaphragm and thoracic outlet. Two studies show chiropractic manipulation and endo- nasal and nasal-specific techniques were effective at resolving sinusitis in adults (Folweiler, 1995; Oliver, 1998).

ASTHMA

Spinal manipulation has been proposed as part of an integrative approach to asthma for two reasons. First, vertebral subluxations appear to produce reflex irritations of the somatic and autonomic nervous system, which could affect respiratory control mechanisms; second, from neurological and biomechanical points of view, chest wall function or bronchial airway tone can be adversely affected by subluxation (Dhami, 1992).

Four randomized clinical trials plus a pilot, three cohort studies, one crossover investigation, and four case studies involving over 550 patients offer support for chiropractic in the management of asthma (Ali, 2002; Balon, 1998; Bockenhauer, 2002; Bronfort, 2002; Garde, 1994; Guiney, 2005; Hunt, 2000; Jamison, 1986; Killinger, 1995; Lines, 1993; Nilsson, 1995, 1998; Peet, 1995, 1997). Case reports present a positive clinical effect of spinal manipulation for asthma (Beyeler, 1965; Nilsson, 1988). In some studies, lung function improvements per se may not have been detectable (Balon, 1998; Bronfort, 2002), but quality of life scores improved by 10%–28% (Bronfort, 2002). Several reports and case studies show a reduction in medication use for asthma after manipulation (Garde, 1994; Jamison, 1986; Lines, 1993; Peet, 1995, 1997). The largest randomized clinical trial to date, comparing different manipulative techniques in the management of asthma, is currently underway by Ali et al. in Australia. Preliminary results show manipulation may decrease cortisol and increase immunoglobulin A levels (Ali 2002).

ENURESIS

Studies involving over 200 patients suggest that chiropractic may play a role in managing primary nocturnal enuresis (Blomerth, 1994; Gmmell, 1989; Lebouef, 1991; Reed, 1994). Secondary diurnal enuresis caused by sacral joint trauma (common after falls) can alter bladder innervation by the sacral plexus located on the anterior surface of the sacrum. Chiropractic sacral adjustment restores normal neuro-modulation to the bladder, increasing the sensation of fullness and sphincter control.

Chiropractic Care for Conditions of the School-Aged Child and Adolescent Back Pain in the Pediatric Population

Chiropractic has an important role in the integrative approach to treating pediatric back pain (Lee, 2001). In school children, the lifetime prevalence of low back pain has been estimated to be 20% to 51% (Balague, 1999; Olsen, 1992; Timela, 1997; Viry, 1999). Thirty-five percent of children with low back pain at 15 reported continuous or recurrent pain at 18 and 23 years of age, and had three times the incidence of disc herniation on MRI (Hestbaek, 2004). Children's physical and psychological response to pain increases their risk of chronic pain in adulthood (Finley, 2005; Harreby, 1995, 1997). It is imperative that the most efficacious, cost-effective, minimally invasive, and evidence-based interventions like chiropractic be put into practice to reduce the incidence of pediatric pain.

Ergonomic factors play a major role in the etiology of pediatric back pain. Improper use of backpacks is the major cause of neck and back pain affecting 97% of school children, with female student showing double the incidence (Ancaster, 2006; Chow, 2005; Sheir-Neiss, 2003; Skaggs, 2006; Wall, 2003). The average backpack weight is 17% of the student's body weight (Ancaster, 2006), in excess of the 10% proposed by pediatric chiropractors. One-third of Italian schoolchildren carried more than 30% of their body weight. Students without back pain were more likely to attend a school that banned the use of backpacks between classes (Sheir-Neiss, 2003). The increased contact pressure and asymmetric shoulder loading apparent with average backpack loads of 22% of body weight were associated with significant pain and injury (Macias, 2005). The use of backpacks has been linked to reduced lung capacity, especially in children with adolescent idiopathic scoliosis (Chow, 2005).

One cohort (Hayden, 2003) and three case studies (Hession, 1993; Kazemi, 1999; King, 1996) involving chiropractic spinal manipulation for low back pain in the pediatric and adolescent population have been reported. A recent prospective study showed that a majority of pediatric patients with low back pain [especially acute] respond positively to chiropractic treatment (Hayden, 2003). Spondylolysis is caused by hyperextension with rotation, causing injury to the posterior elements of the spine, most commonly at L-5, L-4, and L-3. Sports that commonly cause spondylolysis are gymnastics, wrestling, and weightlifting (Moeller, 2001).

Studies of adolescent lumbar disc herniation, demonstrate the most prudent course of healthcare: begin with conservative chiropractic care and progress until a positive outcome is attained (Hession, 1993; Kazemi, 1999; King, 1996). Hession describes a progression from chiropractic flexion-distraction to side-posture manipulation, with full recovery experienced by 8 weeks with no recurrence of complaints 16 months after treatment (Hession, 1993). Kazemi depicts a 120-week course of chiropractic treatment, yielding a Tae Kwon Do martial artist subjected to extreme physical challenge, pain-free at 1 year of follow-up (Kazemi, 1999). King reports an adolescent who begins chiropractic care, but ultimately undergoes surgery for disc removal after just 3 weeks of visits to both chiropractic and neurosurgeon (King, 1996).

NECK AND SHOULDER PAIN IN THE PEDIATRIC POPULATION

The prevalence of neck, shoulder, and back pain is increasing in the pediatric and adolescent population, suggesting "a new disease burden of degenerative musculoskeletal disorders in future adults" (Grimer, 2006; Hakala, 2002). Chiropractic is ideally suited to alleviate neck and shoulder pain, which increases with computer usage exceeding 2 to 3 hours per day (Ehrmannet, 2002). A major review found chiropractic manipulation reduced pain and enhanced range of motion for chronic and sub-acute neck pain in adults (Coulter, 1995). A randomized trial showed 85% of the manipulated group and 69% of the mobilized group reported improvement, but the decrease in pain was 1.5 times higher in the chiropractic group (Cassidy, 1992). Manual manipulation is superior to physical therapy for persistent neck pain (Koes, 1993). More studies on chiropractic for pediatric neck pain are needed. Chiropractic is a safe and effective treatment option in the integrative approach to pediatric neck pain.

PEDIATRIC HEADACHE

Up to 90% of all school age children experience headache. It is a common reason for pediatric office visits and the third most common reason for school absenteeism (Brna, 2005; Collin, 1985). Most patients continued to have headaches into adulthood, although the headache classification often changes over time. The severity of headache when first diagnosed is a predictor for headache chronicity (Brna, 2005). Cervicogenic headaches in children can come from cervical and/or occipital injury or subluxation. Chiropractors see pediatric headaches associated with repetitive stress, trauma to the head, neck, shoulder, and thoracic spine caused by computers and backpacks, poor posture, irregular meals or dehydration, bruxism, braces, and stress.

There is strong evidence that chiropractic is effective for migraine, cervicogenic, and tension-type headaches in adults (Bronfort, 2001; Nelson, 1998; Parker, 1978; Stodolny, 1989; Vernon, 1995; Wight, 1978). Nilsson's randomized controlled trial on cervicogenic headaches found chiropractic decreased headache intensity, frequency and analgesic use (Nilsson, 1995). While clinical trials on pediatric patients have yet to be performed, case series and case reports on chiropractic care for pediatric headache patients show positive results (Anderson-Peacock, 1996; Hassel, 2004; Hewitt, 1994; Luellen, 2004), suggesting that children with headaches respond to chiropractic care. The most common type of secondary headache that chiropractors treat is sinus headache associated with upper respiratory infection. Gentle chiropractic adjustments and cranial adjusting, as well as lymphatic massage, help drain lymph nodes, sinuses and Eustachian tubes.

TEMPOROMANDIBULAR DYSFUNCTION AND PEDIATRIC HEADACHES

Temporomandibular dysfunction (TMD) from dental malocclusion, braces, clenching, and grinding (bruxism) is a commonly overlooked pediatric syndrome that can be concomitant with headaches. TMD is often associated with upper cervical subluxation and cranial restrictions. Chiropractors evaluate patients for TMD and alleviate the symptoms of jaw pain and headache with adjustments, massage and other therapeutic modalities. Chiropractors often collaborate with dentists or TMD specialists when treating this condition.

SCOLIOSIS

Several animal model studies show idiopathic scoliosis associated with aberrant vertebral growth, actually producing scoliosis by surgically placing *external ring fixers* and *spinal staples* to mechanically alter vertebral growth and create a 35–40 degree scoliosis in 8 weeks. Histological analysis revealed disorganized chondrocyte development and paraphyseal density in the region of the staple blades (Aronsson, 1999; Bylski-Austrow, 1999) and elevated synthetic activity on the convex side of the scoliosis (Antoniou, 2001). Chiropractors hypothesize that mechanical forces associated with spinal subluxations act like the "staples" and contribute to the development of scoliosis. Because the spine is rapidly growing in adolescents, abnormalities of chondrocyte development caused by subluxations may contribute to scoliosis. Periodic chiropractic evaluation and treatment to restore normal biomechanics to the spine may reduce the development of scoliosis in at-risk individuals.

Morningstar and Woggon did a retrospective study on 19 patients whose Cobb angles ranged from 15 to 52 degrees. After 4 to 6 weeks of chiropractic care, including other rehabilitative therapies, there was an average reduction of the scoliosis Cobb angle of 62% or 17 degrees. Nine of the 19 patients were no longer classified as scoliotic (Morningstar, Woggon, & Lawrence, 2004) Morningstar and Woggon point out that scoliosis patients tend to have "Librarian posture" with a forward head tilt, caused by an extension malposition of the occiput and atlas. The loss of cervical lordosis often precedes the onset of scoliosis. Subluxation at the atlanto-occipital junction affects the proprioceptive spinocerebellar loop resulting in idiopathic scoliosis. Clinically, reestablishing the cervical lordosis with chiropractic manipulation before addressing the thoraco/lumbar curvatures produced the best results. In addition to chiropractic, specific spinal isometric exercises, proprioceptive neuromuscular re-education, cervical and lumbar lordosis restoration, muscle and ligament rehabilitation, and vibration therapy where utilized (Morningstar et al., 2004). There have been many case reports of chiropractic causing cessation of back pain in older scoliosis patients (Tarola, 1994). A study by Lantz did not report significant changes in curvature pre- and post-chiropractic treatment (Lantz, 2001), but Menke re-evaluated Lantz's data and found that subsets of patients with greater amounts of curvature within five vertebral joints were responsive to chiropractic manipulation (Menke, 2006).

Chiropractors are trained to evaluate children for scoliosis, and often conduct in-school scoliosis screenings. The medical approach to scoliosis is to x-ray and "wait and see" for the rate and extent of progression, utilizing bracing or surgical rod insertion to limit progression. Chiropractors also conduct x-ray evaluation and monitor patients, but offer a pro-active approach to restoring musculoskeletal and biomechanical function and alignment, possibly preventing the onset or limiting the progression of scoliosis. The ideal integrative approach to pediatric scoliosis includes a regime of chiropractic care with monitoring of scoliotic progression or regression.

CHIROPRACTIC AND DEVELOPMENTAL, BEHAVIORAL, AND NEUROLOGICAL DISORDERS

Research by chiropractic neurologists demonstrate that brain de-synchronization seen in the Pervasive Developmental Disorder (PDD) spectrum, including autism, Asperger's and ADHD can be corrected by stimulating contra lateral spinal mechanicoreceptors (Melillo, 2004; Pedro, 2005). Integrative treatment for autism includes structured education, supportive family counselling, behavior modification training, diet modification, including heavy metal testing and detoxification, casein and gluten-free diet, and medication (Barnes, 1997). A number of case studies involving autistic children treated with chiropractic show encouraging outcomes (Aguilar, 2000). The fact that autism appears to be grounded in a broad spectrum of metabolic disorders (Neimark, 2007) suggests that an integrative approach including chiropractic deserves more research.

Chiropractic's ability to modulate the nervous system is the rationale for the chiropractic management of ADHD (Giesen et al., 1989). The correction of cervical kyphosis may improve symptoms of ADHD, according to one author (Bastecki, 2004). A handful of case studies and single-subject design studies show good results with manipulation, but there is not enough evidence to make a broad hypothesis (Bastecki, 2004; Elster, 2003; Giesen, 1989; Lovett, 2006; Phillips, 1991). Given the wide use of medications that are expensive and have side effects (Sandefur, 1987), further research on the chiropractic treatment of ADHD is warranted. Although no outcome studies on chiropractic's effect on learning disabilities and sensory integration disorder have been done, chiropractic has been shown to improve central nervous system processing which is thought to be key in these disorders (Haavik-Taylor, 2007).

CHIROPRACTIC FOR INJURIES AND SPORTS-RELATED CONDITIONS

Chiropractic is an effective and safe treatment for pediatric sports and other injuries. A child doesn't have to be involved in a sport to develop a condition that requires care. Sports-related conditions encompass many of the everyday dents and dings that affect children. Toddlers fall, siblings wrestle, young children and teens play individual and team sports, carry heavy backpacks, and use computers and hand-held devices. Chiropractors can acquire post-graduate specializations in sports care. A doctor of chiropractic can become recognized as a Certified Chiropractic Sports Physician (100 hours) or Diplomate of the American Chiropractic Board of Sports Physicians (300 hours).

Sports injuries, whether from trauma, misuse, or disuse, frequently result in joint restrictions and mechanoreceptor alterations causing pain, tissue damage, muscle tension, dys-coordination, and limited mobility. Therapeutic exercises alone applied to a dysfunctional joint will result in impaired reflexive training. Chiropractic manipulation restores full mobility to affected articulations, restoring normal mechanoreceptor function (Figure 8-2) and stimulating organized, rather than random, deposition of reparative structural and neurological tissue. For the athlete who has noticed the first, often subtle signs of incomplete joint function (such as tension, soreness, "cracking," or limitation of movement), chiropractic care is the first line of defense against a more serious injury.

Head Injuries

Chiropractic care for concussion or other less severe forms of head trauma focuses on the cranial sutures as well as the relationship between the head and neck. Addressing the atlanto-occipital articulation is of key importance in relieving the common occurrence of persistent headache and neck pain associated with cervical sprain/strain following trauma (Evans, 1992). Many chiropractors utilize cranial adjusting techniques to restore normal function of the cranial sutures. Chiropractic is contra-indicated for acute head injury involving fracture, unconsciousness, or subdural hematoma, but may be appropriate for patients who have had previous head injury and are medically stable.

Upper Extremity Conditions

Upper extremity musculo-tendonous strains take the form of rotator cuff, deltoid, medial/lateral elbow conditions, and wrist injuries fall into three categories: joint subluxations, musculo-tendonous strains, and joint sprains. Common references to "tennis elbow" and "pitcher's shoulder" indicate that overuse is the cause of the condition. Chiropractic manipulation and adjunctive therapies are judiciously used throughout the kinematic chain for sprain injuries. Manipulation often yields significant, immediate relief. Intermittent treatment promotes resolution within a few days to a couple of weeks, with toddlers having the quickest response.

Lower Extremity Conditions

A hamstring strain can be the downstream sequelae of lumbar peripheral nerve irritation. Falls causing spinal hyperextension or hyperflexion are commonly caused by trampolines, contact, or speed-related sports. Musculo-tendonous conditions such as snapping hip syndrome (iliotibial band tendonitis), trochanteric bursitis, hamstring and groin strains, infrapatellar tendonitis ("Jumper's knee"), lateral knee pain (iliotibial band syndrome), and patellofemoral pain syndromes (PFPS) are common in the proximal lower extremity due to the biomechanics of running/walking/kicking activities and sports. Foot and ankle conditions such as pronation syndrome and Achilles tendonitis not only cause pain, but adversely affect lower extremity biomechanics. The lumbar, sacroiliac, hip and knee, and ankle joints, and their related musculature serve as a foundation for the biomechanical function of the lower extremity; they are addressed in lower extremity conditions utilizing manipulation, massage, physiotherapy, exercise, and foot orthotics to diminish pronation. Our society pays substantial costs associated with injury chronicity and the resultant sedentary lifestyles.

A combination of regular care (several times per year), acute injury treatment, and a heightened awareness of subclinical problems (a subtle limp or stiffness) keeps children active.

COMMUNICATING CHIROPRACTIC CARE TO PATIENTS AND THEIR FAMILIES

a. **Safe** Chiropractic adjustments are safe, with adverse events being exceedingly rare. The "cracking" or "popping" sound elicited by gentle spinal and extremity manipulation is merely the result of a rapid change in joint fluid pressure – harmless, brief, and nearly painless. The pediatrician's discussion of the safety of manipulation should encourage patients and their parents to seek chiropractic care before trying riskier interventions.

b. **Effective and Practical** A visit to the chiropractor helps educate the child about how the body works in a very tangible way. Chiropractic's hands-on care teaches the child to sense the difference between proper and improper function, full or limited range of motion, and painful or non-painful movements. Once the pediatrician explains the relationship between joint mobility and neuromuscular control to the child and parent, consenting to a treatment plan of chiropractic becomes a pragmatic step.

c. **Affordable** Much like physical therapy or exercise, chiropractic care often requires repeat visits to the chiropractor. Although this may be perceived as costly in the short run, chiropractic is a relative healthcare bargain (Legorreta, 2004). Eliminating joint restriction, muscle imbalance, and promoting mechanoreceptor control is cost-effective, saving money and time, and minimizing re-injuries.

Pediatric Chiropractic Care: Summary and Conclusions

Chiropractors fill a unique niche in integrative pediatrics by giving parents and pediatricians an effective, safe, gentle, and natural way to address many common childhood conditions. Manual adjusting, physiotherapy techniques, exercise, nutritional analysis, and lifestyle advice are some of the therapeutic tools used by the chiropractor to restore normal kinematics to the joints of the spine, cranium, and extremities and support physiological homeostasis. By using these chiropractic tools, improvements have been seen in pediatric conditions ranging from colic and nursing dysfunction in the neonate, to otitis media and asthma in the toddler, to back pain, headache, and sports injury in the school-age child, adolescent, and teen.

You can find a qualified chiropractor experienced in Pediatrics in your area by contacting the American Chiropractic Association or ACA at: http://www.amerchiro.org or call: 703 276 8800. You can also contact a directory of pediatric chiropractors at: www.acapedscouncil.org.

REFERENCES

Aguilar, A. L., Grostic, J. D., & Pfleger, B.(2000). Chiropractic care and the behavior in autistic children. *Journal of Clinical Chiropractic Pediatrics, 5*(1), 293–304.

Aker, P. S., & Cassidy, D. (1990). Torticollis in infants and children: A report of three cases. *Journal of the Canadian Chiropractic Association, 34*(1), 13–19.

Alcantara, J., & Anderson, R. (2005). Chiropractic care of a pediatric patient with symptoms associated with gastroesophageal reflux disease. *Journal of Chiropractic Education, 19*(1), 43.

Alexander, J. M., Leveno, K. J., Hauth, J., Landon, M. B., Thom, E., Spong, C. Y., et al. (2007). Atlas vertebra realignment and the achievement of arterial pressure goal in hypertensive patients: A pilot study. *Journal of Human Hypertension, 21*, 347–352.

Amulu, W. C. (1998). Autism, asthma, irritable bowel syndrome, strabismus and illness susceptibility: A case study in chiropractic management. *Today's Chiropractic, 27*(5), 32–47.

Ancaster News, September 1, 2006. Retreived September 08, 2006 from www.ancasternews.com/an/news_65044.html

Anderson-Peacock, E. S. (1996). Chiropractic care of children with headaches: Five case reports. *Journal of Clinical Chiropractic Pediatrics, 1*(1), 18–27.

Anderson, C. D., & Partridge, J. E. (1993). Seizures plus attention deficit hyperactivity: A case report. *ICA International Review of Chiropractic, 49*, 35–37.

Antoniou, J., Arlet, V., Goswami, T., Aebi, M., & Alini, M. (2001). Elevated synthetic activity in the convex side of scoliotic intervertebral discs and endplates compared with normal tissues. *Spine, 26*(10), E198–E206.

Aronsson, D. D., Stokes, I. A., Rosovsky, J., & Spence, H. (1999). Mechanical modulation of calf tail vertebral growth: Implications for scoliosis progression. *Journal of Spinal Disorders, 12*(2), 141–6.

Asher, M. A., & Burton, D. C. (1999). A concept of idiopathic scoliosis deformities as imperfect torsion(s). *Clinical Orthopaedics and Related Research, July* (364), 11–21.

Bagnell, K. (2004). The Bagnell System for breech presentation. *Today's Chiropractic, Jan/Feb*, 36–42.

Balague, F., Dutoit, G., & Waldburger, M. (1988). Low back pain in schoolchildren: An epidemiological study. *Scandinavian Journal of Rehabilitative Medicine, 20*(4), 175–179.

Balague, F., Troussier, B., & Salminen, J. J. (1999). Non-specific low back pain in children and adolescents: Risk factors. *European Spine Journal, 8*(6), 429–438.

Bartol, K. M. (1995). Osseous manual thrust techniques. In M. I.Gatterman, (Ed.), *Foundations of chiropractic: Subluxation.* Chicago: Mosby.

Bastecki, A. V., Harrison, D. E., & Haas, J. W. (2004). Cervical kyphosis is a possible link to attention-deficit/hyperactivity disorder. *Journal of Manipulative and Physiological Therapeutics, 27*(8), 525e1–525e5.

Beyeler, W. (1965). Experiences in the management of asthma. *Annals of the Swiss Chiropractic Association, 3*, 111–117.

Berg, G., Hammar, M., Moller-Neilsen, J., Linden, U., & Thorbald, J. (1988). Low back pain during pregnancy. *Obstetrics and Gynecology, 71*(1), 71–75.

Bergmann, T. F. (2004). High-velocity low-amplitude manipulative techniques. In S. Haldeman (Ed.), *Principles and practice of chiropractic* (p. 755). New York: McGraw-Hill Professional.

Biedermann, H. (1992). Kinematic imbalances due to sub-occipital strain in newborn infants. *Journal Manual Medicine, 6*, 151–156.

Biedermann, H. (2005). Manual therapy in children: Proposals for an etiologic model. *Journal of Manipulative and Physiological Therapeutics, 28*, 211.e1–211.e15.

Blomerth, P. R.(1994). Functional nocturnal enuresis. *Journal of Manipulative and Physiological Therapeutics,17*(5), 335–338.

Bluestone, C. D., & Klein, J. O. (1988). *Otitis media in infants and children* (p.175). Philadelphia, PA: WB Saunders Company.

Bockenhauer, S. E., Julliard, K. N., Lo, K. S., Huang, K. E., & Sheth, A. M. (2002). Quantifiable effects of osteopathic manipulative techniques on patients with chronic asthma. *Journal of the American Osteopathic Association, 102*(7), 371–375.

Bolton, P. S. (1985). Torticollis: A review of etiology, pathology, diagnosis, and treatment. *Journal of Manipulative and Physiological Therapeutics, 8*(1), 29–32.

Boog, G. (2004). Alternative methods for external cephalic version in the event of breech presentation. *J Gynecol Obstet Biol Reprod, 33*, 94–98.

Borowiz, S. M., Cox, D. J., Tam, A., Ritterband, L. M., Sutphen, J. L., & Penberthy, J. K. (2003). Precipitants of constipation during early childhood. *Journal of the American Board of Family Practitioners, 16*, 213–218.

Brand, C., Furdon, S., & Clark, D. (2006) Recognizing neonatal spinal cord injury. *Advances in Neonatal Care, 6*(1), 15–24.

Brna, P., Dooley, J., Gordon, K., & Dewan, T. (2005). *Archives of Pediatrics & Adolescent Medicine, 159*(12), 1157–1160.

Bronfort, G., Assendelft, W. J. J., Evans, R., Haas, & M., Bouter, L. (2001). Effects of spinal manipulation for chronic headache: A systemic review. *Journal of Manipulative and Physiological Therapeutics, 24*(7), 457–466.

Bronfort, G., Evans, R. L., Kubic, P., & Filkin, P. (2002). Chronic pediatric asthma and chiropractic spinal maniulation: A prospective clinical series and randomized clinical pilot study. *Journal of Manipulative and Physiological Therapeutics, 24*(6), 369–377.

Burton, A. K., Clarke, R. D., McClune, T. D., & Tellotson, K. M. (1996). The natural history of low-back pain in adolescents. *Spine, 21*, 2323–2328.

Bylski-Austrow, D., Wall, E., & Kolata, R. (2000). Endoscopic mechanical spinal hemiepiphysiodesis modifies spine growth. Presented at The Orthopaedic Research Society 46th Annual Meeting; Orlando, FL.

Cantekin, E. I., McGuire, T. W., & Griffith, T. L. (1991). Antimicrobial therapy for otitis media with effusion ["secretory" otitis media]. *Journal of the American Medical Association, 266*(23), 3309–3317.

Cassidy, J. D., Lopes, A., & Young-Hing, K.(1992). The immediate effect of manipulation versus mobilization on pain and range of motion in the cervical spine: A randomized controlled trial. *Journal of Manipulative and Physiological Therapeutics, 15*(9), 570–575.

Chow, D. H., Ng, X. H., Holmes, A. D., Chang, J. C., Yao, R. Y., & Wong, M. S. (2005). Effect of backpack loading on the pulmonary capacities of normal schoolgirls and those with adolescent idiopathic scoliosis. *Spine, 30*(21), E649–E654.

Cohen, K. B. (1997). Chiropractic treatment of the musculoskeletal system during pregnancy. *Journal of the American Chiropractic Association, 34*(5), 33–34, 90.

Colin, N. (1998). Congenital muscular torticollis: A review, case study, and proposed protocol for chiropractic management. *Topics in Clinical Chiropractic, 5*(3), 27–33.

Collin, C., Hockaday, J. M., & Waters, W. E. (1985). Headache and school absence. *Archives of Disease in Childhood, 60*(3), 245–247.

Corrrigan, B., & Maitland, G. D. (1998). *Vertebral musculoskeletal disorders* (pp. 9–10). New York: Butterworth-Heinemann.

Coulter, I. Hurwitz, E., Coulter, I., Adams, A. H., Genovese, B., & Brook, R. H. (1995). The appropriateness of spinal manipulation and mobilizations of the cervical spine: Literature review, indications and ratings by a multidisciplinary expert panel. Santa Monica, CA: RAND Monograph No. DRU-982-1-CCR.

Croft, P. R., Macfarlane, G. J., Papageorgiou, A. C., Thomas, E., & Silman, A. J. (1998). Outcome of low back pain in general practice: A prospective study. *British Medical Journal, 316*, 1356–1359.

Cuhel, J. M., & Powell, M. (1997). Chiropractic management of an infant patient experiencing colic and difficulty breastfeeding: A case report. *Journal of Clinical Chiropractic Pediatrics, 2*(2), 150–154.

Dabbs, V., & Lauretti, W. (1995). A risk assessment of cervical manipulation vs NSAIDS for the treatment of neck pain. *Journal of Manipulative and Physiological Therapeutics, 18*(8), 530–536.

Delessio, D. J. (1986). Classification and treatment of headache during pregnancy. *Clinical Neuropharmacology, 9*(21), 121–131.

Dhami, M. S. I., & DeBoer, K. F. (1992). Systemic effects of spinal lesions. In S. Haldeman, (Ed.), *Principles and practice of chiropractic* (2nd ed., pp. 115–135). Norwalk, CT: Appleton & Lange.

Diakow, P. R., Gadsby, T. A., Gadsby, J. B., Gleddie, J. G., Leprich, D. J., & Scales, A. M. (1991). Back pain during pregnancy and labor. *Journal of Manipulative and Physiological Therapeutics, 14*(2), 116–118.

Diepenmaaat, A. C., van der Wal, M. F., de Vet, H. C., & Hirasing, R. A. (2006). Neck/shoulder, low back and arm pain in relation to computer use, physical activity, stress, and depression among Dutch adolescents. *Pediatrics, 117*(2), 412–416.

DiLorenzo, C.(2000). Childhood constipation: Finally some hard data about hard stools! *Journal of Pediatrics, 136*, 4–7.

Edward, I. J., Dallas, M. L., Poole, S. L., Milligan, C., Yanagawa, Y., Szabó, G., et al. (2007). The neurochemically diverse intermedius nucleus of the medulla as a source of excitatory and inhibitory synaptic input to the nucleus tractus solitarii. *Journal of Neuroscience, 27*(31), 8324–8333.

Ehrmann Feldman, D., Shrier, I., Rossignol, M., & Abenhaim, L. (2002). Risk factors for the development of neck and upper limb pain in adolescents. *Spine, 27*(5), 523–528.

El-Metwally, A., Salminen, J. J., Auvinen, A., Kautianen, H., & Mikkelsson, M. (2004). Prognosis of non-specific musculoskeletal pain in preadolescents: A prospective 4-year follow-up study till adolescence. *Pain, 110*, 550–559.

Elster, E. (2003). Upper cervical chiropractic care for a nine-year old male with Tourette's syndrome, attention deficit hyperactivity disorder, depression, asthma, insomnia, and headaches: A case report. *Journal of Vertebral Subluxation Research, 2003*(1), 1–11.

Eriksen, K. (1994). Effects of upper cervical correction on chronic constipation. *Chiropractic Research Journal, 3*, 19–22.

Evans, R. (1992). The postconcussion syndrome and the sequelae of mild head injury. *Clinical Neurology, 10*(4), 815–847 (Neurology Section, AMI Park Plaza Hospital , Houston , Texas).

Evans-Pritchard, A. (May 3, 1998). Science in the dock as the antibiotic miracle crumbles. *Sunday Times [London]*, p. 1.

Fallon J. (2005). The child patient: A matrix for chiropractic care. *Journal of Clinical Chiropractic Pediatrics, 6*(3), supplement.

Fallon, J. M., & Fysh, P. N. (1997). Chiropractic care of the newborn with congenital torticollis. Journal of *Clinical Chiropractic Pediatrics, 2*(1), 116–125.

Fallon, J. M. (1997). The role of the chiropractic adjustment in the care and treatment of 332 children with otitis media. *Journal of Clinical Chiropractic Pediatrics, 2*(2), 167–183.

Fallon, J., & Edelman, M. J. (1998). Chiropractic care of 401 children with otitis media: A pilot study. *Alternative Therapies in Health and Medicine, 4*(2), 93.

Fast, A., Shapiro, D., Ducommun, E. J., Friedmeann, L. W., Bouklas, T., & Floman, Y. (1987). Low-back pain in pregnancy. *Spine, 12*(4), 368–371.

Finley, G. A., Franck, L. S., Gronau, R. E., & von Baeyer, C. L. (2005). Why children's pain matters. *Pain Clinical Update, 13*(4), 1–6.

Folweiler, D. C. & Lynch, O. T. (1995). Nasal Specific technique as part of a chiropractic approach to chronic sinusitis and sinus headaches. *Journal of Manipulative and Physiological Therapeutics, 18*(1), 38–41.

Froom, J., Culpepper, L., Jacobs, M., DeMelker, R. A., Green, L. A., van Buchem, L., et al. (1997). Antimicrobials for acute otitis media? A review from the International Primary Care Network. *British Medical Journal, 315*(7100), 98–102.

Frodi, A. M. (1981). Contributions of infant characteristics to child abuse. *American Journal of Mental Deficiency, 85*, 341–349.

Froehle, R. M. (1996). Ear infection: A retrospective study examining improvement from chiropractic care and analyzing for influencing factors. *Journal of Manipulative and Physiological Therapeutics, 19*(3), 169–177.

Fysh, P. (2002). *Chiropractic care for the pediatric patient.* Arlington, VA: Int'l Chiropractors Assn. Council on Chiropractic Pediatrics.

Fysh, P. N. (1996). Chronic recurrent otitis media: Case series of five patients with recommendations for case management. *Journal of Clinical Chiropractic Pediatrics, 1*, 66–78.

Garde, R. (1994). Asthma and chiropractic. *Chiropractic Pediatrics, 1*, 9–16.

Gemmell, H. A., & Jacobson, B. H. (1989). Chiropractic management of enuresis: Time-series descriptive design. *Journal of Manipulative and Physiological Therapeutics, 12*(5), 386–389.

Gergen, P. J., & Weiss, K. B. (1990). Changing patterns of asthma hospitalization among children: 1979 to 1987. *Journal of the American Medical Association, 264*, 1688–1692.

Geutjens, G., Gilbert, A., & Helsen, K. (1996). Obstetric brachial plexus palsy associated with breech delivery. A different pattern of injury. *The Journal of Bone and Joint Surgery, 78*, 303.

Giesen, J. M., Center, D. B., & Leach, R. A. (1989). An evaluation of chiropractic manipulation as a treatment of hyperactivity in children. *Journal of Manipulative and Physiological Therapeutics, 12*(5), 353–363.

Goldberg, M. (2000). Oral and written testimony. Autism: Present challenges, future needs: Why the increased rates? Hearing before the Committee on Government Reform, House of Representatives, 106th Congress, April 6, 2000. Serial #106-180: 335–417.

Goodman, R. J., & Mosby, J. S. (1990). Cessation of a seizure disorder: Correction of the atlas subluxation complex. *Journal of Chiropractic Research Clinical Investigation, 6*(2), 43–46.

Gorman, R. F. (1995). Monocular visual loss after closed head trauma: Immediate resolution associated with spinal manipulation. *Journal of Manipulative and Physiological Therapeutics, 18*(5), 308–314.

Gottlieb, M. S. (1993). Neglected spinal cord, brain stem and musculoskeletal injuries stemming from birth trauma. *Journal of Manipulative and Physiological Therapeutics, 16*(8), 537–543.

Grantham, V. A. (1977). Backache in boys—a new problem. *Practitioner, 218*(1304), 226–229.

Grimmer, K., Nyland, L., & Milanese, S. (2006). Repeated measures of recent headache, neck and upper back pain in Australian adolescents. *Cephalalgia, 26*(7), 843–851.

Guiney, P. A., Chou, R., Vianna, A., & Lovenheim, J. (2005). Effects of osteopathic manipulative treatment on pediatric patients with asthma: A randomized controlled trial. *Journal of the American Osteopathic Association, 105*, 7–12.

Gutmann, G. (1990). Blocked Atlantal nerve syndrome in infants and small children. English translation in *International Review of Chiropractic, 46*(4), 37. Original German paper published in *Manuelle Medizin, 25*(5), 1987.

Guyton, A. C., & Hall, J. E. (2006). *Textbook of medical physiology* (pp. 771–779, 822). 11th ed., Philadelphia, PA: Elsevier Saunders.

Haavik-Taylor, H., & Murphy, B. (2007). Cervical spine manipulation alters sensorimotor integration: A somatosensory evoked potential study. *Clinical Neurophysiology, 118*(2), 391 402.

Haldeman, S. (1974). The influence of the autonomic nervous system on cerebral blood flow. *Journal of the American Chiropractic Association, 18,* 6–11.

Haldeman, S. (Ed.). (2004). *Principles and practice of chiropractic* (p.755). New York: McGraw-Hill Professional.

Hamm, R. N., Hicks, R. J., & Bemben, D. A. (1996). Antibiotics and respiratory infections: Are patients more satisfied when expectations are met? *Journal of Family Practice, 43*(1), 56–62.

Hakala, P. T., Rimpela, A. H., Saami, L. A., & Salminen, J. J. (2006). Frequent computer-related activities increase the risk of neck-shoulder and low back pain in adolescents. *European Journal of Public Health, 16*(5), 536–541.

Hakala, P., Rimpela, A., Salminen, J. J., Virtanen, S. M., & Rimpela, M. (2002). Back, neck, and shoulder pain in Finnish adolescents: National cross sectional surveys. *British Medical Journal, 325*(7367), 743.

Harreby, M. S., Neergaard, K., Hesselsoe, G., & Kjer, J. (1997). Are low back pain and radiological changes during puberty risk factors for low back pain in adult age? A 25-year prospective cohort study of 640 school children. *Ugeskr Langer, 159*(2), 171–174 [In Danish].

Harreby, M. S., Neergaard, K., Hesselsoe, G., & Kjer, J. (1995). Are radiological changes in the thoracic and lumbar spine risk factors for low-back pain in adults? A 25-year prospective study of 640 school children. *Spine, 20*(21), 2298–2302.

Hart, J. J. (1996). Pediatric gastroesophageal reflux. *American Family Physician, 54,* 2463–2472.

Hassel, T. N. (2004). Pediatric cephalgia. *Journal of Clinical Chiropractic Pediatrics, 6*(2), 383–386.

Hawk, C., Khorsan, R., Lisi, A. J., Ferrance, R. J., & Evans, M. W. (2007). Chiropractic care for nonmusculoskeletal conditions: A systematic review with implications for whole systems research. *Journal of Alternative and Complementary Medicines, 13*(5), 491–512.

Hayden, J. A., Mior, S. A., & Verhoef, M. J. (2003). Evaluation of chiropractic management of pediatric patients with low back pain: A prospective cohort study. *Journal of Manipulative and Physiological Therapeutics, 26*(1), 1–8.

Headache Classification Subcommittee of the International Headache Society. (2004). The International Classification of Headache Disorders. 2nd ed. *Cephalalgia, 24*(Suppl 1), 9–160.

Health Letter on the CDC, via Newsedge Corporation. May 11, 1998.

Hession, E. F., & Donald, G. D. (1993). Treatment of multiple lumbar disk herniations in an adolescent athlete utilizing flexion distraction and rotational manipulation. *Journal of Manipulative and Physiological Therapeutics, 16,* 185–192.

Hestbaek, L., Lebouef-Yde, C., Kyvik, O., Vach, W., Russell, M. B., Skadhauge, L., et al., (2004) Comorbidity with low back pain: A cross-sectional population-based survey of 12- to 22-year-olds. *Spine, 29*(13), 1483–1491.

Hewitt, E. G. (1994). Chiropractic care of a 13-year-old with headache and neck pain: A case report. *Journal of the Canadian Chiropractic Association, 38*(3), 160–162.

Hewitt, E. (1999). Chiropractic care for infants with dysfunctional nursing: A case series. *Journal of Clinical Chiropractic Pediatrics, 4*(1), 241–244.

Hewitt, E. G. (1993). Chiropractic treatment of a 7-month old with chronic constipation: A case report. *Chiropractic Technic, 5,* 101–103.

Hide, D. W., & Guyer, B. M. (1983). Prevalence of infantile colic. *Archives of Disease of Childhood, 57*(7), 559–560.

Himmel, W., Lippert-Urbanke, E., & Kochen M. M. (1997). Are patients more satisfied when they receive a prescription? The effect of patient expectations in general practice. *Scandinavian Journal of Primary Health Care, 15*, 118–122.

Hipperson, A. (2004). Chiropractic management of infantile colic. *Clinical Chiropractic, 7*(4), 180–186.

Hollbrook, B. (2005). Chiropractic treatment of childhood constipation: A review of the literature. *Journal of Clinical Chiropractic and Pediatrics, 6*, 427–431.

Holtrop, D. (2000). Resolution of suckling intolerance in a 6-month-old chiropractic patient. *Jour Manipulative Physiol Therapeutics, 23*, 615–618.

Holborow, C. (1975). Eustachian tube function: Changes throughout childhood and neuro-muscular control. *Journal of Laryngology and Otolaryngology, 89*, 47–55.

Hughes, C. A., Harley, E. H., Milmoe, G., Bala, R., & Martorella, A. (1999). Birth trauma in the head and neck. *Archives of Otolaryngology—Head & Neck Surgery, 125*, 193–199.

Hunt, J. (2000). Upper cervical chiropractic care of a pediatric patient with asthma: A case study. *Journal of Clinical Chiropractic Pediatrics, 1*, 3–9.

Jamison, J. R. (1986). Asthma in a chiropractic clinic: A pilot study. *Journal of the Australian Chiropractic Association, 16*, 138–144.

Kazemi M. (1999) Adolescent lumbar disc herniation in a tae kwon do martial artist: A case report. *Journal of the Canadian Chiropractic Association, 43*, 236–242.

Karma, P., Palva, T., Kouvalnainea, K., Karja, J., Makela, P. H., Prinssi, V. P., et al. (1987). Finnish approach to the treatment of acute otitis media: Report of the Finnish Consensus Conference. *Annals of Otolaryngology, Rhinology, and Laryngology Supplement, 129*, 1–19.

Keefe, Mr. (1988). Irritable infant syndrome: Theoretical perspectives and practice implications. *ANS Advances in Nursing Science, 10*(3), 70–78.

Khorshid, K. A., Sweat, R. W., Zemba, Jr., D. A., & Jemba, B. N. (2006). Clinical efficacy of upper cervical versus full spine chiropractic care on children with autism: A randomized clinical trial. *Journal of Vertebral Subluxation Research, 1*, 1–7.

Khorshid, K. A., Zemba, Jr., D. A., Zemba, B. N., & Sweat, R. W. (2003). Clinical efficacy of upper cervical versus full spine adjustment on children with autism. *Proceedings of the 7th Biennial Congress of the World Federation of Chiropractic*, Orlando, FL, May 1–3, 2003, pp. 328–329.

Killinger, L. Z. (1995). Chiropractic care in the treatment of asthma. *Palmer Journal of Research, 2*, 74–77.

King, L., Mior, S. A., & Devonshire-Zielonka, K. (1996). Adolescent lumbar disc herniation: A case report. *Journal of the Canadian Chiropractic Association, 40*, 15–18.

Kirkaldy-Willis, W. H., & Cassidy, J. D. (1985). Spinal manipulation in the treatment of low back pain. *Canadian Family Physician, 31*, 535–540.

Kiyomi, K. (1978). Autonomic system reactions caused by the excitation of somatic afferents: Study of cutaneo-intestinal reflex. In I. M. Korr (Ed.), *The neurobiologic mechanisms in manipulative therapy* (pp. 219–227). New York: Plenum.

Kleinman, L. C., Kosecott, J., Dubois, R. W., & Brook, R. H. (1994). The medical appropriateness of tympanostomy tubes proposed for children younger than 16 years in the United States. *Journal of the American Medical Association, 271*(16), 1250–1255.

Klougart, N., Nilsson, N., & Jacobsen, J. (1989). Infantile colic treated by chiropractors: A prospective study of 316 cases. *Journal of Manipulative and Physiological Therapeutics, 12*(4), 281–288.

Koch, L. E., Biedermann, H., & Saternus, K. (1998). High cervical stress and apnoea. *Forensic Science International, 97*(1), 1–9.

Koch, L. E., Koch, H., Graumann-Brunt, S., Stolle, D., Ramirez, J. M., & Saternus, K. S. (2002). Heart rate changes in response to mild mechanical irritation of the high cervical spinal cord region in infants. *Forensic Science International, 128*(3), 168–176.

Koes, B., Bouter, L., Van Mameren, H., Essers, A. H. M., Verstegen, G. M. J. R., Hofhuizen, D. M., et al. (1993). A randomized clinical trial of manual therapy and physiotherapy for persistent back and neck pain complaints: Subgroup analysis and the relationship between outcome measures. *Journal of Manipulative and Physiological Therapeutics, 16*(4), 211–219.

Korovessis, P., Koureas, G., Zacharatos, S., & Papazizis, S. (2005) Backpacks, back pain, sagittal spinal curves and trunk alignments in adolescents: A logistic and multinomial logistic analysis. *Spine, 30*(2), 247–255.

Lantz, C., & Chen, J. (2001). Effect of chiropractic intervention on small scoliotic curves in younger subject: A time series cohort design. *Journal of Manipulative and Physiological Therapeutics, 24*(6), 385–393.

Leach, R. A. (2002). Differential compliance instrument in the treatment of infantile colic: A report of two cases. *Journal of Manipulative and Physiological Therapeutics, 25*(1), 58–62.

Leach, R. (1994). *The chiropractic theories: Principles and clinical applications.* Philadelphia: Williams & Wilkins.

Lebouef, C., Brown, P., Herman, A., Leembruggen, K., Walton, D., & Crisp, T. C. (1991). Chiropractic care for children with nocturnal enuresis: A prospective outcome study. *Journal of Manipulative and Physiological Therapeutics, 14*(2), 110–115.

Le, C. T., Freeman, D. W., & Fireman, B. H. (1991). Evaluation of ventilating tubes and myringotomy in the treatment of recurrent or persistent otitis media. *Pediatric Infectious Disease Journal, 10*(1), 2–11.

LeDuc, J. W. (1996). World Health Organization strategy for emerging infectious diseases. *Journal of the American Medical Association, 275*(4), 318–320.

Lee, A. C., Li, D. H., & Kemper, K. J. (2000) Chiropractic care of children. *Archives of Pediatrics & Adolescent Medicine, 154*(4), 401–407.

Legorreta, A., Metz, D., Nelson, C., Ray, S., Chernicoff, H. O., & Dinubile, N. A. (2004). Comparative analysis of individuals with and without chiropractic coverage patient characteristics, utilization, and costs. *Archives of Internal Medicine, 164,* 1985–1992.

Lester, B. M., Boukydis, C. F. Z., Garcia-Coll, C. T., & Hole, W. T. (1990). Colic for developmentalists. *Symposium on infantile colic: Infant Mental Health Journal, 11,* 320–333.

Lines, D. (1993). A holistic approach to the treatment of bronchial asthma in a chiropractic practice. *Chiropractic Journal of Australia, 23,* 408.

Lovett, L. (2006). Behavioral and learning changes secondary to chiropractic care to reduce subluxations in a child with attention deficit hyperactivity disorder: A case study. *Journal of Vertebral Subluxation Research,* 1–6.

Luellen, J. (2004). Chiropractic care of adolescent migraine headache. *Journal of Clinical Chiropractic Pediatrics, 6*(2), 403–405.

Marko, S. K. (1994). Case study: The effect of chiropractic care on an infant with problems of constipation. *Chiropractic Pediatrics, 1,* 23–24.

Mayo Clinic. Retrieved October 1, 2007, from http://www.mayoclinic.org/pediatric-sleep-apnea/treatment.html

Mendez, F. J., & Gomez-Conesa, A. (2001). Postural hygiene program to prevent low back pain. *Spine, 26*(11), 1280–1286.

Moawad, A. H., Caritis, S. N., Harper, M., Wapner, R. J., Sorokin, Y., Miodovnik, M., et al. (2006) Fetal injury associated with cesarean delivery. *Obstetrics and Gynecology, 108*(4), 885–890.

Macias, B. R., Murthy, G., Chambers, H., & Hargens, A. R. (2005) High contact pressure beneath backpack straps of children contributes to pain. *Archive of Pediatric and Adolescent Medicine, 159*(12), 1186–1187.

Management of acute otitis media. Summary, evidence report/technology assessment No. 15, AHRQ Publication No. 01-E007, Rockville, MD: Agency for Health Research and Quality, Public Health Service, US Department of Health and Human Services, December 2000.

Macfarlane, J., Holmes, W., Macfarlane, R., & Britten, N. (1997). Influences of patients' expectations on antibiotic management of acute lower respiratory tract illness in general practice: Questionnaire study. *British Medical Journal, 315*(7117), 1211–1214.

Mangione-Smith, R., McGlynn, E. A., Elliott, M. N., Krogstad, P., & Brook, R. H. (1999). The relationship between perceived parental expectations and pediatrician antimicrobial prescribing behavior. *Pediatrics, 103*(4 Pt1), 711–771.

McCoy Moore, T., & Pfiffner, T. J. (1997) Pediatric traumatic torticollis: A case report. *Journal of Clinical Chiropractic Pediatrics, 2*(2):145-149.

McIntyre, I. N., & Broadhurst, N. A. (1996). Effective treatment of low back pain in pregnancy. *Australian Family Physician, 25*(9 suppl 2), S65-S67.

Melillo, R., & Leisman, G. (2004). *Neurobehavioral disorders of childhood* (p. 4). New York: Kluwer Academic/Plenum Publishers.

Menke, J., Plaugher, G., Carrari, C., Coleman, R., Vannetiello, L., & Bachman, T. (2006). Likelihood-evidential support and Bayesian re-analysis on a prospective cohort of children and adolescents with mild scoliosis chiropractic management. *Journal of the Arizona-Nevada Academy of Sciences*. Supplemental Issue; Accepted for publication 10/06.

Mercer, C., & Nook, B. C. (1999). The efficacy of chiropractic spinal adjustments as a treatment protocol in the management of infantile colic. *Proceedings of the 5th Biennial Congress*, Auckland, New Zealand, May 17–22, 1999, pp. 170–171.

Meyer, J. J., & Phillips, C. J. (1995). Chiropractic care, including craniosacral therapy, during pregnancy: A static-group comparison of obstetric interventions during labor and delivery. *Journal of Manipulative and Physiological Therapeutics, 18*(8), 525–529.

Mills, M. V., Henley, C. E., Barnes, L. L. B., Carreiro, J. E., & Degenhardt, B. F. (2003). The use of osteopathic manipulative treatment as adjuvant therapy in children with recurrent acute otitis media. *Archives of Pediatrics and Adolescent Medicine,157*(9), 861–866.

Moeller, J. L., & Rifat, S. F. (2001). Spondylolysis in active adolescents: Expediting return to play. *The Physician and Sportsmedicine, 29*(12). www.physsportsmed.com.

Morrison, C. S., & Chariker, M. (2006). Positional plagiocephaly: Pathogenesis, diagnosis, and management. *The Journal of the Kentucky Medical Association, 104*(4), 136–140.

Moss, A. I., Hamburger, S., Moore, R. M. Jr., Jeng, L. L., & Howie, L. G. (1988). *Use of selected medical device implants in the United States: Advance data* (p. 191). Hyattsville, MD: National Center for Health Statistics.

Morningstar, M., Woggon, D., & Lawrence, G. (2004). Scoliosis treatment using a combination of manipulative and rehabilitative therapy: A retrospective case series. *BMC Musculoskeletal Disorders, 5*, 32.

Nassar, N., Roberts, C. L., Barratt, A., Bell, J. C., Olive, E. C., & Peat, B. (2006). Systematic review of adverse outcomes of external cephalic version and persisting breech presentation at term. *Pediatric & Perinatal Epidemiology, 20*(2), 163–171.

National Center for Complementary and Alternative Medicine. A randomized controlled trial of the use of craniosacral osteopathic manipulative treatment and of botanical treatment in recurrent otitis media in children. Retreived September 11, 2002, from http://www.clinicaltrials.gov/ct…/NCT00010465?order=1&JServSessiionIdzone_ct=rdo2fm5sc

National Center for Health Statistics, Department of Health and Human Services, http://www.dhhs.gov.

Navuluri, N., & Navuluri, R. B. (2006). Study on the relationship between backpack use and back and neck pain among adolescents. *Nursing Health Science, 8*(4), 206–215.

Nelson, C. F., Bronfort, G., Evans, R., Boline, P., Goldsmith, C., & Anderson, A. V. (1998) The efficacy of spinal manipulation, amitriptyline and the combination of both therapies for the prophylaxis of migraine headache. *Journal of Manipulative and Physiological Therapeutics, 21,* 511–519.

Neurologic disorders, seizure disorders [epilepsy]. (1992). In *The Merck manual of diagnosis and therapy,* 17th ed. Rahway, NJ: Mercke, pp. 1436–1440.

Nicolson, R. I., Fawcett, A. J., & Dean, P. (2001). Developmental dyslexia: The cerebellar deficit hypothesis. *Trends in Neurosciences, 24*(9), 508–11.

Nilsson, N. H., Bronfort, G., Bendix, T., Madsen, F., & Weeke, B. (1995). Chronic asthma and chiropractic spinal manipulation: A randomized clinical trial. *Journal of Clinical and Experimental Allergy, 25*(1), 80–88.

Nilsson, N., & Christiansen, B. (1988). Prognostic factors in bronchial asthma in chiropractic practice. *Journal of the Australian Chiropractic Association, 18,* 85–87.

Nilsson, N. (1995). A randomized controlled trial of the effect of spinal manipulation in the treatment of cervicogenic headache. *Journal of Manipulative and Physiological Therapeutics, 18,* 435.

Nurko, S. (2000). Advances in the management of pediatric constipation. *Current Gastroenterology Reports, 2,* 234–240.

Olafsdottir, E., Forshei, S., Fluge, G., & Markestad, T. (2001). Randomised controlled trial of infantile colic treated with chiropractic spinal manipulation. *Archives of Diseases of the Child, 84*(2), 138–141.

Oliver, S. E., & LeFebvre, R. (1998). Sinusitis and sinus pain: Conservative chiropractic care. *Topics in Clinical Chiropractic, 5*(1), 39–47, 62–65,73–75.

Ostgaard, H. C., Andersson, G. B. J., & Karlsson, K. (1991). Prevalence of back pain in pregnancy. *Spine, 16*(5), 549–552.

Olsen, T. L., Anderson, R. L., Dearwater, S. R., Kriska, A. M., Cauley, J. A., Aaron, D. J., et al. (1992). The epidemiology of low back pain in an adolescent population. *American Journal of Public Health, 82*(4), 606–608.

Orenstein, S. R. (1997). Infantile reflux: Different from adult reflux. *American Journal of Medicine, 103,* S114–S119.

Orenstein, S. R. (1999). Gastroesophageal reflux. *Pediatrics in Review, 20,* 24–28.

Palmer College of Chiropractic Adjusting Manual. Davenport, IA: Palmer College of Chiropractic, 1983.

Palmer, D. D. (1910). *Science, art and philosophy of chiropractic.* Portland, OR: Portland Printing House Company.

Parker, G., Tupling, H. & Pryor, D. (1978). A controlled trial of the effect of spinal manipulation for migraine. *Australian and New Zealand Journal of Medicine, 8,* 589–593.

Pedro, V. M., & Leisman, G. (2005). Hemispheric integrative therapy in Landau-Kleffner syndrome: Applications for rehabilitation sciences. *International Journal of Neuroscience, 115*(8), 1227–1238.

Peet, J. B., Marko, S. K., & Piekarczyk, W. (1995). Chiropractic response in the pediatric patient with asthma: A pilot study. *Chiropractic Pediatrics, 1,* 9–13.

Peet, J. (1996). Case study: Chiropractic results with a child with recurrent otitis media accompanied by effusion. *Chiropractic Pediatrics, 2,* 8–10.

Peet, J. B. (1997). Case study: Eight year old female with chronic asthma. *Chiropractic Pediatrics, 3,* 9–12.

Phillips, C. J. (1991). Case study: The effect of utilizing spinal manipulation and craniosacral therapy as the treatment approach for attention deficit hyperactivity disorder. *Proceedings of the National Conference on Chiropractic and Pediatrics, 57–74.*

Phillips, C. J. (1992). Vertebral subluxation and otitis media: A case study. *Journal of Chiropractic Research and Clinical Investigation, 8*(2), 38–39.

Phillips, C. J. (1996). Craniosacral therapy. In C. Anrig & G. Plaugher (Eds.), *Pediatric chiropractic* (p. 55). Philadelphia: Williams & Wilkins.

Pluhar, G., & Schobert, P. D. (1991). Vertebral subluxation and colic: A case study. *Journal of Chiropractic Research and Clinical Investigation, 7,* 75–76.

Potisk, T. J. (2001). A case study of a five-year-old male with autism/pervasive development disorder who improved remarkably and quickly with chiropractic treatment. *Proceedings of the 6th Biennial Congress of the World Federation of Chiropractic,* Paris, France, May 21–26, 2001, p. 313.

Quezada, D. (2004). Chiropractic care of an infant with plagiocephaly. *Journal Clinical Chiro Pediatrics, 6,* 342–348.

Quist, D. M., & Duray, S. M. (2007). Resolution of symptoms of chronic constipation in an 8-year-old male after chiropractic treatment. *Journal of Manipulative and Physiological Therapeutics, 30*(1), 65–68.

Rapport, M. D., & Moffit, C. (2002). Attention deficit/hyperactivity disorder and methylphenidate: A review of height/weight, cardiovascular, and somatic complaint side effects. *Clinical and Psychological Review, 22,* 1107–1131.

Rautava, P., Lehonten, L., Helenius, H., & Sillanpaa, M. (1995). Infantile colic: Child and family three years later. *Pediatrics, 96*(1 Pt. 1), 43–47.

Reed, W. R., Beavers, S., Reddy, S. K., & Kern, G. (1994). Chiropractic management of primary nocturnal enuresis. *Journal of Manipulative and Physiological Therapeutics, 17*(9), 596–600.

Reis, S., Hermoni, D., Borkan, J. M., Bidermann, A., Tabenkin, C., & Orat, A. (1999). A new look at low back complaints in primary care: A RAMBAM Israeli family practice research network study. *The Journal of Family Practice, 48*(4), 299–303.

Rome, P. L. (1999). Perspective: An overview of comparative considerations of cerebrovascular accidents. *Chiropractic Journal of Australia, 29*(3), 87–102.

Rosner, A. (2003). CVA Risks in perspective. *Manuelle Medizin, 3,* 1–9.

Rubinstein, H. (1994). Case study: Autism. *Chiropractic Pediatrics, 1*(1), 22–23.

Sandefur, R., & Adams, E. (1987). The effect of chiropractic adjustments on the behavior of autistic children: A case review. *Journal of Chiropractic, 24*(12), 21–25.

Sando, I., Takahashi, H., & Matsune, S. (1991). Update on functional anatomy and pathology of human Eustachian tube related to otitis media with effusion [review]. *Otolaryngologic Clinics of North America, 24,* 795–811.

Schmidt, M. A. (1990). *Childhood ear infections* (p. 75). Berkeley, CA: North Atlantic Books.

Sergueef, N., Nelson, K. E., & Glonek, T. (2006). Palpatory diagnosis of plagiocephaly. *Complementary Therapies in Clinical Practice, 12*(2), 101–110. Epub 2006 Mar 29.

Sheader, W. (1999). Chiropractic management of an infant patient experiencing breastfeeding difficulties and colic: A case report. *Journal of Clinical Chiropractic Pediatrics, 4*(1), 245–247.

Sheir-Neiss, G. I., Kruse, R. W., Rahman, T., Jacobson, L. P., & Peli, J. A. (2003). The association of backpack use and back pain in adolescents. *Spine, 28*(9), 922–930.

Skaggs, D. L., Early, S. D., D'Ambra, G. P., Tolo, V. T., & Kay, R. M. (2006). Back pain and backpacks in school children. *Journal of Pediatrics and Orthopedics, 26*(3), 338–363.

Smith-Nguyen, E. J. (2004). Two approaches to muscular torticollis. *Journal of Clinical Chiropractic Pediatrics, 6*(2), 387–393.

Stodolny, J., & Chmielewski, H. (1989). Manual therapy in the treatment of patients with cervical migraine. *Journal of Manual Medicine, 4,* 49.

Strittmatter, M., Bianchi, O., Ostertag, D., Grauer, M., Paulus, C., Fischer, C., & Meyer, S. (2005) Altered function of the hypothalamic-pituitary-adrenal axis in patients with acute, chronic, and episodic pain. *Schmerz, 19*(2),109–116.

Taimela, S., Kujala, U. M., Salminen, J. J., & Viljanen, T. (1997). The prevalence of low back pain among children and adolescents: A nationwide, cohort-based questionnaire survey in Finland. *Spine, 22*(10), 1132–1136.

The Nation's Health [official newspaper of the American Public Health Association], November 2000, pp. 1, 12.

Tobwin, A. (1969). Latent spinal cord and brain stem injury in newborn infants. *Developmental Medicine and Child Neurology, 11,* 54–58.

Tomasz, A. (1994). Multiple-antibiotic-resistant pathogenic bacteria: A report on the Rockefeller University Workshop. *New England Journal of Medicine, 330*(17), 1247–1251.

Tarola, G. (1994). Manipulation for the control of back pain and curve progression in patients with skeletally mature idiopathic scoliosis: Two case studies. *Journal of Manipulative and Physiological Therapeutics, 17*(4), 253–257.

Toto, B. J. (1993). Chiropractic correction of congenital muscular torticollis. *Journal of Manipulative and Physiological Therapeutics, 16*(8), 556–559.

Travis, J. (1994). Reviving the antibiotic miracle? *Science, 264*(5157), 360–362.

Upledger, J. (1983). *Craniosacral therapy.* Seattle: Eastland Press.

Vallone, S. (2007). The role of subluxation and chiropractic care in hypolactation. *Journal of Clinical Chiropractic Pediatrics, 8*(1–2), 518–524.

Vallone, S. (2004). Chiropractic evaluation and treatment of musculoskeletal dysfunction in infants demonstrating difficulty breastfeeding. *Journal of Clinical Chiropractic Pediatrics, 6*(1), 349–368.

Van Ginkel, R., Reitsma, J. B., Buller, H. A., van Wijk, M. P., Tamimiau, J., & Benninga, M. A. (2003). Childhood constipation: Longitudinal follow-up beyond puberty. *Gastroenterology, 125,* 357–363.

Van Loon, M. (1998). Colic with projectile vomiting: A case study. *Journal of Chiropractic Pediatrics, 3,* 207–210.

Vandenplas, Y., Lifshitz, J. Z., Orenstein, S., Lifschitz, C. H., Shepherd, R. W., Casaubon, P. R., et al. (1998). Nutritional management of regurgitation in infants. *Journal of the American College of Nutrition, 17,* 308–316.

Vernon, H. T. (1995). The effectiveness of chiropractic manipulation in the treatment of headache: And exploration of the literature. *Journal of Manipulative and Physiological Therapeutics, 18,* 611.

Viholainen, H., Ahonen, T., Cantell, M., Lyytinen, P., & Lyytinen, H. (2002). Development of early motor skills and language in children at risk for familial dyslexia. *Developmental Medicine And Child Neurology, 44*(11), 761–769.

Vinson, D. C., & Lutz, L. J. (1993). The effect of parental expectations on treatment of children with a cough: A report from the ASPN. *Journal of Family Practice, 37*(1), 23–27.

Virji, A., & Britten, N. (1991). A study of the relationship between patients' attitudes and doctors' prescribing. *Family Practice, 8,* 314–319.

Viry, P., Creveuil, C., & Marcelli, C. (1999). Nonspecific back pain in children: A search for associated factors in 14-year old schoolchildren. *Review of Rheumatology* [English Edition] *66*(7–9), 381–388.

Vohra, S., Johnston, B. C., Cramer, K., & Humphreys, K. (2007). Adverse events associate with pediatric spinal manipulation: A systematic review. *Pediatrics, 119*, 275–283.

Wall, E. J., Foad, S. L., & Spears, J. (2003). Backpack and back pan: Where's the epidemic? *Journal of Pediatrics and Orthopedics, 23*(4), 437–439.

Watson, K. D., Papageorgiou, A. C., Jones, G. T., Taylor, S., Symmons, D. P. M., Silman, A. J., et al. (2002). Low back pain in schoolchildren: Occurrence and characteristics. *Pain, 97*(1–2), 87–92.

Webb, S., & Lloyd, M. (1994). Prescribing and referral in general practice: A study of patients' expectations and doctors' actions. *British Journal of General Practice, 44*(381), 165–169.

Wedderkopp, N., Lebouef-Yde, C., Andersen, L. B., Froberg, K., & Hansen, H. S. (2001). Back pain reporting pattern in a Danish population-based sample of children and adolescents. *Spine, 26*(17), 1879–1883.

Whalen, C. K., & Henker, B. (1988). Attention-deficit/hyperactivity disorder. In T. H. Olenduc,k., M. Hersen (Eds.), *Handbook of child psychopathy* (pp. 181–211). 3rd ed. New York: Plenum.

Whelan, T. L., Dishman, J. D., Burke, J., Levine, S., & Sciotti, V. (2002). The effect of chiropractic manipulation on salivary cortisol levels. *Journal of Manipulative and Physiological Therapeutics, 25*(3), 149–153.

Wiberg, J. M. M., Nordsteen, J., & Nilsson, N. (1999). The short-term effect of spinal manipulation in the treatment of infantile colic: A randomized controlled trial with a blinded observer. *Journal of Manipulative and Physiological Therapeutics, 22*(8), 517–522.

Wiegand, R., Kettner, N., Brahee, D., & Marquina, N. (2003). Cervical spine geometry correlated to cervical degenerative disease in a symptomatic group. *Journal of Manipulative and Physiological Therapeutics, 26*(6), 341–346.

Wickens, K., Pearce, N., Crane, J., & Beasley, R. (1999). Antibiotic use in early childhood and the development of asthma. *Clinical and Experimental Allergy, 29*(6), 766–771.

Wight, J. S. (1978). Migraine: A statistical analysis of chiropractic treatment. *Chiro J, 12*, 363.

Wu, W. H., Meijer, O. G., Uegaki, K., & Mens, J. M. A. (2004). Pregnancy-related pelvic girdle pain (PPP), I: Terminology, clinical presentation, and prevalence. *Eur Spine J, 13*, 575–589.

9

A Pediatric Perspective on Energy Therapies

MARY JANE OTT, LARRAINE BOSSI, AND JEANNE COLBATH

KEY CONCEPTS

- The National Center of Complementary and Alternative Medicine (NCCAM) lists energy healing as one of the five major "domains" (categories) of complementary and alternative therapies.
- The ability to learn and use energy healing is a natural human potential that can be actualized by anyone who has the desire and intent to learn and practice it.
- Therapeutic Touch, Reiki, and Healing Touch are taught and used in the care of patients in both hospital and ambulatory settings.
- Therapeutic Touch, Reiki, and Healing Touch are used by children and adults to support health and well-being and for first aide in the event of injury.
- Research indicates the effectiveness of these therapies to reduce anxiety and pain and to support relaxation and healing.

■

"...We will never understand the scientific basis of everything. We must be open to approaches that work even when we don't understand how or why they work."

—*Ralph Snyderman, MD, September 2000*

Introduction

This chapter will provide an overview of Therapeutic Touch, Reiki, and Healing Touch. These three different energy healing modalities are used across disciplines by health care providers in both hospital and ambulatory settings. Each modality will be described including definition, brief history, review of the literature (including common adult and pediatric applications), safety/risks, training, accreditation, and licensure issues. A list of professional organizations and additional suggested reading will be offered. Historically, these three energy healing modalities have been used primarily by nurses. However, there is an increasing interest in the clinical application of energy healing among physicians and other healthcare professionals as well as the lay public.

HEALING PRESENCE

Caring is the foundation of all healing arts as it is the force that transforms the recipient–provider relationship. Yet, in the current fast-paced healthcare environment, the ability to maintain a caring focus is becoming increasingly more difficult to achieve. Moving from a mechanistic task-oriented practice (of doing) to one that resonates with the human spirit (being) is key for establishing healing presence.

Moving from a mechanistic task-oriented practice (of doing) to one that resonates with the human spirit (being) is key for establishing healing presence.

The philosophies of touch or energy therapies are consistent with the healing paradigm, which understands the interconnectedness of the recipient and the practitioner. In fact, the influence of touch therapies as a means to connect with recipients has been recognized within the healing arts for years (Engebretson & Wardell, 2002). Since 1979, Jean Watson, nurse scholar, has written extensively on the science of caring. One of the basic tenets of her caring model, the Theory of Human Caring, is "transpersonal caring." Watson asserts that healthcare providers are the environment that brings in positive or negative healing potentials by virtue of setting mindful (consciousness) intentions (intentionality) to care prior to recipient interactions (Watson, 2005, p. 7). Healing presence creates an environment that facilitates physical, mental, emotional, and spiritual balance.

Use of energy therapies requires that the practitioner become a therapeutic agent through "presence."

Use of energy therapies requires that the practitioner becomes a therapeutic agent through "presence." The yogic greeting "namaste," which can be translated as, "the Light within me greets the Light within you," or "the God in me greets the God in you," best describes the feeling of presence. Such a feeling connotes an acknowledgment of being ready in the moment to listen empathetically without judgment, to open to one's own intuitive guidance, to release one's own ego attachments to the outcome, and to be an instrument of divine or universal love (Burhardt, 2002, p. 92).

Becoming present requires a shift in attention to the now (mindfulness). Even in a busy work environment, there are many ways to come into the present (Santorelli 1999, p. 33). For example, one could turn one's focus to the rhythm of a few focused breaths, or mindfully wash one's hands. One could also quietly say a calming word, phrase, or prayer such as "peace," "calm," "Thy will be done."

Without therapeutic presence, energy practitioners' work would be similar to the placebo effect in clinical trials. On many levels, presence transforms the practitioner into a therapeutic agent. As a multi-level continuing education model, each level of energy therapy training builds on the previously learned techniques and increases in complexity as the individual's development as a healer progresses in both the skill and art of being a compassionate practitioner.

Biological Mechanism

Currently, there is no consensus regarding the scientific mechanism of action involved in energy therapies. Eisenberg and his colleagues (1998) reported the use of energy healing tripled between 1990 and 1997. This steady increase in the practice of energy therapy has provided scientists and clinicians with the opportunity to study and build a better understanding of the mechanisms involved in energy therapies. A variety of theories and explanations have been explored: the balancing effect of subtle energies, a non-linear electromagnetic energy or biofield, theory of psychoimmunology, complex science concepts, including generalized entanglement, a vibrational field, and vital energy, or spirit (Becker, 1985; Cornelio & Warber, 2003; Engebretson & Wardell, 2007; Engebretson, 1998; Gerber, 2001; Hunt, 1996; Jonas & Crawford, 2003; Kiang, Marotta, Wirkus, Wirkus, & Jonas, 2002; Oschman, 2000; Rubik, 2002; Walach, 2005). In a recent article, Kerr and colleagues (2007) suggest that touch healing therapies such as Therapeutic Touch (TT) and Reiki induce cortical plasticity and sensory reorganization, which has a positive effect on pain remediation. The NIH National Center for Complementary and Alternative Medicine (NCCAM) classifies Therapeutic Touch, Reiki, and Healing Touch as an energy medicine therapy working in the biofield, the subtle energy field, to facilitate the body's own natural healing ability (www.nccam.nih.gov/health/backgrounds/energymed.htm, accessed July 28, 2007). While there are many similarities among these therapies, distinctions have been noted (Potter, 2003).

Therapeutic Touch: History, Definition, and Process

Therapeutic touch (TT) was developed in 1972 by Dr. Dolores Krieger, professor of nursing at New York University, and Dora Kunz, a fifth-generation healer. Developed initially for use by nurses, Krieger defined TT as a "method . . . of using the hands to direct human energies to help or heal someone who is ill" (Krieger, 1979, p. 1). Therapeutic

Touch International Association, Inc. (formerly Nurse Healers—Professional Associates International [NH-PAI]), the professional organization for TT defines it as, "a contemporary interpretation of several ancient healing practices, is an intentionally directed process of energy exchange during which the practitioner uses the hands as a focus for facilitating healing" (www.therapeutic-touch.org, accessed July 28, 2007). Therapeutic touch is done with the intention to help or heal and to enable the recipient to "re-pattern their energy in the direction of health," and to facilitate the "body's natural restorative processes" (www.therapeutic-touch.org, accessed July 28, 2007).

Initially taught in a master's level "Frontiers in Nursing" course at New York University (circa 1975), Therapeutic Touch is currently taught in more than 70 US nursing and medical schools as well as in 90 other countries. The study and practice of TT supports the cultivation of compassion, wellbeing, and job satisfaction among nursing and medical students (Cox & Hayes, 1998; Kemper, Larrimore, Dozier, & Woods, 2006; Krieger, 2002; McElliogott et al., 2003).

THERAPEUTIC TOUCH CLINICAL PROCESS

The TT provider must come from a clearly focused intention to support healing throughout the treatment, while at the same time not being attached to the outcome of the treatment. Intentionality, motivation in the best interests of the individual receiving the treatment, and the ability to know and consistently confront oneself, are essential components of being an effective practitioner (Krieger, 1979, p. 37). Krieger consistently teaches that:

> Therapeutic touch is not done with only the hands. It is an interiorization process called into being by compassion for someone who is in need and is coupled with a deep-seated, knowledgeable intentionality. The point of entry for this is a centering of consciousness that continues throughout the process; it is not a simple technique using the hands that can be mindlessly turned on and off (Krieger, 1998).

TT treatments are conducted with the recipient fully clothed, in a comfortable position, either sitting or lying down. Treatment frequently lasts 15 to 20 minutes. Those who are more sensitive to energy interventions, including neonates, young children, pregnant women, the elderly, the critically ill, and individuals with psychiatric disorders,

---

The TT provider must come from a clearly focused intention to support healing throughout the treatment, while at the same time not being attached to the outcome of the treatment.

---

respond more quickly. Their treatments may be only 5 or 10 minutes in duration. As with many healing modalities, TT can be administered in combination with other interventions.

The TT treatment is a dynamic, interactive process that moves through four phases that are distinct and may be repeated depending on the individual needs of the recipient (www.therapeutic-touch.org, accessed July 28, 2007). The four phases are (1) centering, (2) assessment, (3) intervention, and (4) evaluation and closure.

During centering, the practitioner brings their body, mind, and emotions to a state of quiet, focused consciousness. This is done "using the breath, imagery, meditation, and/or visualizations to open one's self to find an inner sense of equilibrium to connect with the inner core of wholeness and stillness" (www.therapeutic-touch. org, accessed July 28, 2007). During the second phase, the practitioner places his or her hands 2 to 6 inches away from the recipient's energy field and focuses on sensory cues while moving the hands from the individual's head to the feet in a rhythmic, symmetrical manner. The third phase has two parts: (1) clearing (also called unruffling) and (2) rebalancing the energy field. While clearing, the practitioner again moves his or her hands in a rhythmic, symmetrical manner from the head of the recipient to feet with the intention of "facilitating a symmetrical flow of energy through the field." (www.therapeutic-touch.org, accessed July 28, 2007). After clearing the energy field, the practitioner moves their hands to areas of the energy field that seem to need attention in order to re-establish order in the system. The fourth and final phase of evaluation and closure finishes the treatment and ends the session. Ongoing assessment

---

Intentionality, motivation in the best interests of the individual receiving the treatment, and the ability to know and consistently confront oneself, are essential components of being an effective Therapeutic Touch practitioner.

---

of the recipient's energy field is a continuous part of the treatment, which offers cues regarding the best time to end the session (www.therapeutic-touch.org, accessed July 28, 2007).

Therapeutic Touch: Selected Literature Review

THERAPEUTIC TOUCH: ADULT LITERATURE

The earliest reported research on Therapeutic Touch was done by Krieger in which she reported an increase of circulating hemoglobin levels as a result of TT treatments (Krieger, 1972, 1976). There were problems related to the study design; however, it provided the impetus for scientific study of an intervention that nurses found consistently helpful to patients. In 2006, Movaffaghi, Hasanpoor, Farsi, Hooshmand, and Abrishami reported significant changes in both hemoglobin and hematocrit among healthy student volunteers who received TT treatments. In 2008, Gronowicz and colleagues found that Therapeutic Touch treatments produced a significant increase (p = 0.04–0.01) in proliferation of fibroblasts, osteoblasts, and tenocytes in culture when compared to sham treatments.

There are numerous anecdotes and case reports as well as quantitative and qualitative research, which document the effectiveness of Therapeutic Touch to quiet the autonomic nervous system and elicit a sense of relaxation and peacefulness. TT has been used successfully in healthy adults to treat anxiety related to episodic stress (Olsen & Sneed, 1995) and to reduce tension, confusion, anxiety and increase in vigor (Lafreniere et al., 1999); Hurricane Hugo survivors (Olson, Sneed, Bonadonna, Ratliff, & Dias, 1992); institutionalized elderly recipients (Simington & Laing, 1993); students taking exams (Olson & Sneed, 1995); hospitalized adult psychiatric patients (Gagne & Toye, 1994); and pregnant patients with chemical dependency (Larden, Palmer, & Janssen, 2004).

Additionally, a variety of studies report positive outcomes using TT for pain relief in hospitalized adult cardiovascular patients (Heidt, 1981; Meehan, 1993; Quinn, 1984;); pre- and post-operative experiences of breast cancer surgery (Samarel, Fawcett, Davis, & Ryan 1998); tension headache (Keller & Bzdek, 1986); osteoarthritis (Gordon, Merenstein, D'Amico, & Hudgens, 1998); degenerative arthritis (Peck, 1997); sickle-cell anemia (Myers, Robinson, Guthrie, Lamp, & Lottenberg, 1999); musculoskeletal pain in the elderly; (Lin & Taylor, 1998); burn recipients (Clark, Turner, Gauthier, & Williams, 1998); phantom limb (Leskowitz, 1999, 2000a); and fibromyalgia (Denison, 2004). Smith, Arnstein, Rosa, and Wells-Federman (2002) described the effectiveness of integrating Therapeutic Touch into a cognitive behavorial pain treatment program. Patients who received TT and massage therapy during bone marrow transplant reported comfort benefits (Smith, Reeder, Daniel, Baramee, & Hagman 2003). An article published in 1998 by Rosa, Rosa, Sarner, and Barrnett concluded all TT claims were groundless; therefore, Therapeutic Touch was not appropriate as a therapeutic intervention. Critics of this study reported procedures involved in the study violated the essential practice requirement of Therapeutic Touch, resulting in inappropriate conclusions (Achterberg, 1998; Cox, 2003; Dossey, 2003; Leskowitz, 2000b).

There are three integrative reviews and two meta-analyses of the TT literature. One integrative review spans from 1985 to 1996 (Spence & Olson, 1997) and concluded that there was sufficient evidence at that time to support the use of TT to reduce anxiety and pain. The second review (Easter, 1997) included research done from 1981 to 1996 and concluded that there was a positive regard for Therapeutic Touch, that it should be taught as a part of basic clinical nursing education. Easter also acknowledged a need for more rigorous methodologies in its study.

Similarly, the meta-analytic reviews of five quantitative studies of psychological variables, and four quantitative studies of physiological variables conducted between 1986
and 1996, found that TT, "has a positive, medium effect on physiological and psychological variables" (Peters, 1999, p. 52). Winstead-Fry and Kijeck (1999) reported in their
meta-analysis of 13 controlled TT studies, that the effect of TT on reducing anxiety was
one of the most validated findings in the literature" (Winstead-Fry & Kijeck, 1999, p. 64).
They identified trends in the use of TT and made recommendations for future research.
Specifically, they proposed that practitioners must be granted sufficient time and space
to provide "real time" treatments rather than being limited to the five-minute treatments
that were performed in research protocols at the time. In contrast, a Cochrane integrated
review by O'Mathuna and Ashford (2004) reviewed four studies and concluded that there
was not sufficient evidence to support a benefit from TT in the healing of acute wounds.

Giasson and Bouchard (1998) reported that TT treatments significantly increased
terminal cancer recipients' sense of wellbeing. More recently, Kelly, Sullivan, Fawcett,
and Samarel (2004) found that women with breast cancer who received TT reported a
sense of calmness and relaxation. Therapeutic touch treatments have resulted in positive psychoimmunologic effects for both recipients and practitioners (Olson et al., 1997;
Quinn & Strelkauskas, 1993). Investigation of pandimensional field patterns showed parallel changes in both those giving and receiving TT treatments (Smith & Broida, 2007).
TT has been suggested as one way that nurses can support and nurture one another in
clinical practice (Ott & Mulloney, 1998). Recent studies have found that Therapeutic
Touch can have a positive effect on the practitioner providing the treatment (Barron,
Coakley, Fitzgerald & Mahoney, 2008; Moore, Ting & Rossiter-Thornton, 2008).

THERAPEUTIC TOUCH: PEDIATRIC LITERATURE

There have been four research studies, one integrative review, and one clinical review
published regarding the use of Therapeutic Touch in the pediatric population. In the
first published research article on the use of TT in children, Kramer (1990) examined the effectiveness of TT compared to casual touch in the stress response of 30
hospitalized children between the ages of 2 weeks and 2 years of age. The TT treatment
(Krieger/Kunz method) and the casual touch (stroking or patting the head, upper
torso, or arms) were done with the infants recumbent in a crib. The stress response
(pulse, peripheral skin temperature, and galvanic skin response) was measured at 3-
and 6-minute intervals. TT was found to significantly reduce the time needed to calm
children after stressful experiences.

Using a descriptive, phenomenological methodology, France (1993) studied the
TT experience of 11 healthy children ranging in age from 3 to 9 years old. Each child
received a series of 4 to 6 TT sessions, and participated in videotaped interviews and
were asked to draw about their experiences. The parents of the children in the study and
the investigators running the study kept diaries in which they described the children's
experiences during the TT sessions. The children described kinesthetic, visual, and

affective responses. Their body language reflected a relaxation response. Interestingly, the children reported that they could "feel" the energy.

Hughes, Meize-Grochowski, and Harris (1996) conducted a qualitative study in which they investigated the TT experience of 7 hospitalized psychiatric recipients, aged 12 to 16 years old. Thirty-one treatments were administered and the recipients were interviewed pre- and post-session. The participants described feeling relaxed and having an expanded awareness of body sensations both during and after the TT treatments. They also reported that the TT treatments improved their communication with the staff.

In a pilot study, Ireland (1998) randomly assigned 20 HIV-infected children ages 6 to 12 to TT or mimic TT groups in order to evaluate the effectiveness of TT in reducing state anxiety. While sitting in a chair, each child received a five-minute treatment. Data analysis indicated a statistically significant decrease in state anxiety in those children who received the TT treatment. Despite the limitations of the study, Ireland concluded that the findings provide preliminary support for the use of TT in reducing state anxiety of children with HIV infection and made recommendations for further study.

Ireland and Olson (2000) reviewed and analyzed the research on the effect of both massage therapy and TT on the pediatric population. They reviewed the four research studies previously mentioned and one unpublished dissertation testing the affect of TT on neonates. They concluded that like adults, "children seem to be comforted and calmed by TT" (p. 62). However, Ireland and Olson also stated that because there are too few controlled studies with children, and because placebo may have an effect, they cannot recommend TT.

Kemper and Kelly (2004) reported that the most frequent pediatric conditions treated by TT included anxiety and worry, anxiety and subjective dyspnea related to asthma, fatigue, insomnia, isolation (providing a sense of support and caring), and pain. The types of pain commonly treated include abdominal pain, arthritis, backache, burns, bruises, cancer pain, fibromyalgia, headache, and post-operative pain. They found that pediatric recipients consistently responded well to treatments and did not have adverse side effects. They indicated additional research is needed to determine: (1) the mechanism of action, (2) factors that predict treatment response, (3) the optimal duration and frequency of treatment, and (4) the costs and benefits of treatment. In addition, Kemper and Kelly (2004) described both Therapeutic Touch and Healing Touch as "extremely safe," (p. 252) stating that the major concern about the therapies is that in serious conditions they might be used by patients and families instead of effective medical therapies.

Critics often cite an unknown mechanism of action, research methodology (small sample size, randomization, statistical issues), treatment issues (practitioners needing to determine the length of treatment based on the recipient's needs), placebo effect, and the impact of interpersonal relationships as reasons to dismiss claims about the effectiveness of any energy healing. The success of future research on TT (as in all integrative therapies) relies heavily on addressing research methodology issues related to control, design, and statistical analysis.

Therapeutic Touch Training

Therapeutic Touch International Association, Inc. (formerly Nurse Healers—Professional Associates International [NH-PAI]), is the professional organization for TT. Its mission is, "to inspire and advance excellence in Krieger and Kunz TT as a healing practice and life way" (www.therapeutic-touch.org, accessed July 27, 2007). The organization provides a code of ethics and clearly delineated training and continuing education requirements. The Basic Level course involves a 12-contact-hour workshop covering both the cognitive and experiential aspects of TT. This is followed by one year of mentored practice during which time the practitioner in training provides at least two treatments per week. The layperson can provide treatments for family and friends. The healthcare professional, may, at the discretion of and with supervision from their mentor, provide treatments in a healthcare setting. Written documentation of the treatments and case reports are a component of the supervised mentorship.

The practitioner is then expected to complete an additional Intermediate Level course (14 contact hours) while maintaining contact with their mentor and peer colleagues. The Advanced Level course requires an additional 14 to 16 hours of training. A 1-year mentorship is required in order to become a Qualified Therapeutic Touch Practitioner. All training must be taught by a Qualified Therapeutic Touch Teacher who has met additional training requirements.

There is no licensure requirement for TT. It is expected that TT practitioners are committed to self-awareness, growth, and healing for themselves and others. Additionally, Therapeutic Touch practitioners are expected to maintain a relatively stable health pattern, demonstrate compassion or the desire to help others, and to continue ongoing knowledge (including research) and skill development. Additional training, experience, and mentorship are required for those who become qualified teachers of TT.

Reiki: History, Definition, and Process

During the early part of the twentieth century, Dr. Mikai Usui introduced Reiki in Kyoto, Japan. Dr. Usui was a Buddhist who meditated often, expanding his inner awareness (Petter, 1997, p. 25). During one of his meditations, Usui had a "satori," which is translated as a sudden understanding or a fleeting glimpse of a higher order (Petter, 1997, p. 25). Usui named the practice he learned from this experience Reiki. Rei, which means holy, spirit, mystery, gift, or invisible; combined with ki, translated as energy, talent, feeling, and nature. Reiki can also be understood as an offspring of Buddhist Qigong with a Shintoist influence (Petter, 1997, p. 18). Reiki is different from chi or prana, and more similar to their source states, yuanchi and mahaprana. These energies represent the primordial consciousness that gently encourages an individual's system toward its own unique balance (Miles, 2006, pp. 10–12).

By 1926, Usui had taught Reiki to a number of practitioners, and Reiki centers were established throughout Japan. Reiki came to the Western world when Hawayo Takata, born on the island of Kauai, Hawaii, in 1900 journeyed to Japan and was treated by Dr. Usui. Ms. Takata's granddaughter, Phyllis Furumoto, herself a Reiki Master, founded the Reiki Alliance in 1981, a year after Takata's death (Petter, 1997, p. 15).

REIKI CLINICAL PROCESS

A Reiki session, as practiced by Dr. Usui, begins with a brief meditation by the practitioner, referred to as Gassho, or "hands coming together" (Usui & Petter, 2003, p. 15). The recipient is fully clothed, reclining or sitting, and often soft ambient music is present (Miles, 2006, p. 10). With hands at the chest level, focusing on the breath and the middle fingers touching, the practitioner brings him or herself to a meditative state and connects with the Reiki energy. Next, the practitioner acknowledges the flow of Reiki energy through him or herself. He or she has the intention for the health and recovery of the recipient on all levels, allowing him or herself to become a tool for Reiki. With folded hands elevated to the third eye or brow chakra, the practitioner "asks" that his or her hands be guided to where the Reiki energy is needed. Most often the practitioner begins by placing her hands on the crown chakra, at the top of the head, then proceeding to a series of hand placements that correspond to each of the seven major charkas (crown, brow, throat, heart, solar plexus, sacral, root), ending with grounding at the recipient's feet.

Body scanning can often start and/or end a treatment. Alternatively, the practitioner may begin the session with a body scan and start hand placements in the body area that corresponds to signals picked up during the scan (Usui & Petter, 2003, p. 7). Although there are no rules for the length of treatment, each hand position is held for 2 to 5 minutes, depending on the practitioner's evaluation (Usui & Petter, 2003, p. 28).

Dr. Usui summarized a Reiki treatment in this way: So Chiryo (treatment) builds on Reiji-Ho (devotion/ intention) and Gassho (meditative posture/ attitude). Only when

---

Only when we can devote ourselves without being prejudiced by our thoughts and feelings, will we become an instrument for the universal life energy.

---

we can devote ourselves without being prejudiced by our thoughts and feelings, will we become an instrument for the universal life energy (Usui & Petter, 2003, p. 21). Miles (2006, p. 11) adds that Reiki very gently, quietly, and gradually opens an inner spiritual connection. This connection can help to transform negative attitudes while creating a sense of meaning and purpose.

Reiki: Selected Literature Review

REIKI: ADULT LITERATURE

Although Reiki was introduced in the US during the late 1930s, the professional literature did not report on Reiki until the 1990s. The predominant theme in the Reiki literature from 1990 to the present focuses on the feeling of peacefulness and calm produced by a Reiki session, and its application to self-care (Brathovde, 2006; Bullock, 1997; Burden, Herron-Marx, & Clifford, 2005; Engebretson & Wardell, 2002; Mansour, Laing, Leis, Nurse, & Denilkewich, 1998; Nield-Anderson & Ameling 2001; Swartz, 1995; Van Sell, 1996; Whalen, 2003; Witte & Dundes, 2001). As early as 1998, Sawyer discussed having a Reiki practitioner present during surgical procedures (Sawyer, 1998). Alandydy (1999) reported on ways to use Reiki to support surgical patients, both pre- and post-operatively. Since the integration of Reiki treatments into pre- and post-operative care at New Hampshire Hospital, more than 8000 Reiki treatments have been administered with consistent reports of positive effects (Miles, 2006). Edelbute (2003) reported that the Herbert Irving Child and Adolescent Oncology Center of Children's Hospital of New York-Presbyterian routinely offers Reiki. Schiller (2003) suggests Reiki as a way to introduce complementary therapies into clinical practice. Reiki as a clinical intervention in oncology nursing at Dana-Farber Cancer Institute and Children's Hospital Boston is described by Bossi, Ott, and DeCristofaro (2008).

A number of investigators conducted studies that attempted to measure the affects of Reiki sessions. Wetzel (1989) reported a positive change in haemoglobin and hematocrit levels in study participants who received Reiki. Wardell and Engebretson (2001) worked from the assumption that Reiki elicits the relaxation response, and used biological markers related to stress-reduction: state anxiety, salivary IgA and cortisol, blood pressure, galvanic skin response (GSR), muscle tension, and skin temperature. Significance was achieved in comparison of pre- and post-Reiki sessions for 23 participants who experienced anxiety reduction, salivary IgA increase, and systolic blood pressure decrease. Other results did not reach a level of significance, but suggested changes in the direction of relaxation (Wardell & Engebretson, 2001). Shiflett, Nayak, Miles, and Agostinelli (2002) describe the effect of Reiki treatments on the functional recovery of patients in rehabilitation after a stroke.

In 2004, Mackay, Hansen, and McFarlane reported on a study in which participants were randomly assigned into three groups: group 1 = no treatment, group 2 = Reiki treatment; and group 3 = placebo treatment. Heart rate, cardiac vagal tone, blood pressure, cardiac sensitivity to baro reflex, and breathing activity were measured. Significant results for decreased heart rate and diastolic blood pressure in the Reiki group were achieved when compared to both the placebo and control groups.

Rubrik, Brooks, and Schwartz (2006) recently reported on the role of experimental context and practitioner wellbeing when investigating the effect of a Reiki treatment on bacterial cultures.

Studies on the effect of Reiki sessions on individuals' perceptions of pain include a pilot study by Olson and Hanson (1997) in which pain was significantly relieved by Reiki. They treated 20 participants who reported pain from cancer, chronic back problems, and arthritis. In a subsequent phase II clinical trial, Olson, Hanson, and Michaud (2003) randomized 24 participants with advanced cancer to receive standard treatment plus rest, or standard treatment plus Reiki on Days 1 and 4. Patients receiving Reiki reported a significant decrease in their pain on Day 1 and 4.

Dressen and Singg (1998) found Reiki to be an effective modality for reducing pain, depression, and anxiety, as well as a shift to internal locus of control. Kenney (2001) found Reiki treatments to be effective in relieving some of the trauma experienced by Sarajevo torture survivors.

Miles (2003) reported decreases in pain and anxiety in HIV-positive individuals after Reiki treatments. Similarly, Schmehr (2003) provided a case study of an individual living with AIDS who used Reiki treatments (along with training received at a hospital clinic) to augment treatment of his depression, anxiety, substance abuse, adherence to medication regime, and ultimately his return to work. In 2006 Crawford, Leaver, and Mahoney reported the successful use of Reiki in decreasing memory and behavioral problems in people with mild cognitive and mild Alzheimer's disease. Tsang, Carlson, and Olson (2007) reported that Reiki treatments reduced cancer-related fatigue, pain, and anxiety, and improved recipients' quality of life. Lee (2008) conducted a systematic review of randomized clinical trials of Reiki that found most published trials suffered from methodological flaws, small sample sizes, lack of replication, and/or poor reporting.

REIKI: PEDIATRIC LITERATURE

Vitale (2007) conducted an integrative review of Reiki therapy research. Her summary of Reiki studies illustrates the scope of conditions considered for the use of Reiki: stress, relaxation, depression, pain, wound healing management, anxiety, and cancer fatigue. Although most of the Reiki literature involves adult subjects, the findings related to effects on pain, stress, anxiety, depression, and wound healing are applicable to the pediatric population.

Reiki Training

Reiki training began as an oral tradition by Dr. Usui, who later developed a Reiki handbook for his students. The handbook was subsequently translated into German by Frank Arjava Petter and published in 1997 (Petter, 1997). As Reiki training and practice became more prevalent in the US and Europe, three levels of training emerged: (1) First Degree Reiki, or Level I initiates the practitioner to hands-on treatment of self and others; (2) Second Degree or Level II confirms a practitioner's commitment to Reiki and adds the skill of distant, non-touch healing; and (3) Third Degree or Level III involves becoming a Reiki master, which includes the ability to initiate and train students in the practice of Reiki (Miles, 2006, p. 64). Licensing is not required by law for Reiki practice; however, there are Reiki organizations that offer licensing and/or certification for their students (Rand, 1998, pp. 26–27).

Healing Touch: History, Definition, and Process

Healing touch (HT) is one contemporary touch therapy that is gaining in popularity in clinical practice. It is estimated that over 50,000 individuals have been trained in HT (Personal communication Diane Wardell, 9/10/07). HT was developed in the 1980s by Janet Mentgen, RN BSN, who incorporated energy-based care into her holistic nursing practice in Colorado. Mentgen further developed and offered the program through the American Holistic Nurses Association. In 1996, Healing Touch International, Inc. was formed and the HT certification program was created.

In addition to being taught and practiced in the US, HT classes have been taught to international audiences in over 36 countries including Canada, Mexico, Australia, New Zealand, Europe, South Africa, South America, Cambodia, Korea, Tibet, Thailand, and India.

The basic supposition of HT is that energy permeates all matter (universal energy) and humans possess dynamic penetrating layers of energy (energy field). The practice of HT assumes that any disruption in the flow and/or balance in the energy system can cause physical, mental, emotional, or spiritual illness. HT is defined as a "relaxing, nurturing therapy" that uses gentle touch to assist in "balancing physical, mental, emotional, and spiritual well being" (www.healingtouchinternational.org, accessed July 28, 2007).

The basic supposition of HT is that energy permeates all matter (universal energy) and humans possess dynamic penetrating layers of energy (energy field).

HEALING TOUCH CLINICAL PROCESS

The HT practitioner begins a session by combining therapeutic presence, a sincere intention to help another person, with one or more techniques to facilitate healing. The focus is on the client's highest good and is not about curing. A typical session lasts 30 to 60 minutes, but may vary in length depending on the situation. Infants, the elderly, those seriously ill, or with certain psychiatric conditions are sensitive to energy therapy and require shorter treatment times. Recipients are fully clothed and may be either sitting or lying down.

After obtaining a history of the recipient's symptoms, the practitioner takes a few minutes to center and focus, and then conducts an assessment of the participant's subjective symptoms by performing a hand scan of the body to identify any energy imbalances. The practitioner then selects one or more local (specific site or problem area) or full body HT technique based on the assessment findings (Mentgen, 2001). A typical HT session concludes with the practitioner assisting the recipient in coming back to a fully awake state referred to as grounding. The practitioner will conduct a reassessment of the energy system and presenting symptoms, and will discuss with the recipient a mutually agreed upon plan to enhance self-care. Often, HT self-treatment is recommended as part of the treatment plan. Further, HT complements traditional medical care and may be used individually or in conjunction with other healing modalities such as imagery, music, or aromatherapy therapy.

HT can be integrated into clinical settings including intensive care units (Eschiti, 2007; Umbreit, 2000), hospitals (Loveland, Cook, Guerrerio, & Slater, 2004), and the community (Moss, 1998; Dubrey, 1999; Tovey, 2001). For example, HT has become a standard of care at Scripps Green Hospital in La Jolla, CA. All cardiac surgical and intensive care patients at Scripps Green are offered Healing Touch (King, 2005). Patient feedback indicates that HT has reduced pain and anxiety symptoms in many recipients.

Healing Touch: Selected Literature Review

HEALING TOUCH: ADULT LITERATURE

Research in the field of touch therapies presents the unique challenge of elucidating the biological mechanism supporting HT (Wardell & Weymouth, 2004). There are, however, a number of HT studies and anecdotes supporting its use for health promotion and for minimizing symptoms. Since 1993, HT International, the certifying body for HT, lists 92 abstracts of completed research studies and 24 research studies in progress (Healing Touch International Research Survey, 2006). The majority of studies relate to pain, psychological wellbeing, cancer, and focus on the adult population.

Wardell and Weymouth (2004) conducted an integrative review, covering the period from 1993 to 2003. Of the 30 quantitative HT studies, 7 were randomized trials. The findings were categorized by problem or study area, and included pain, cancer, immune system, cardiovascular, elderly, mental health, post-operative recovery, theoretical, and pediatrics. The authors concluded that although "many positive results of HT have been reported, none of the findings were conclusive."

Several studies have demonstrated effectiveness in reducing pain (Slater, 1996; Wardell, 2000; Wardell, Rintala, Duan, & Tan, 2006; Welcher & Kish, 2001; Weymouth & Sandberg-Lewis, 2000). For example, Cordes, Proffitt, and Roth (2002) conducted a study comparing an HT group with a mock HT group, and a control group. Forty-eight post-operative subjects with total knee replacements were recruited and randomly assigned to one of the three groups. While there was no effect on reported pain, a 30.6% increase in joint mobility as measured by goniometry reading was noted in the HT group. Interestingly, there was a 27% increase in joint mobility in the mock HT group.

Post-White and colleagues (2003) conducted a randomized controlled study involving 220 cancer patients, all of whom were randomly assigned to one of three groups: (1) HT, (2) massage therapy, and (3) presence of a caring practitioner (attention control). The results showed that both HT and massage therapy decreased perceived pain, but the HT group had lower fatigue levels over the 4-week intervention period.

A number of studies have also demonstrated positive mental health outcomes, such as: relief from depression (Bradway, 1998; Van Aken, 2004), alcoholism recovery (DuBrey, 2006), and stress reduction (Dowd, Kolcaba, Steiner, & Fashinpaur, 2007). Similarly, a number of studies have shown that recipients can expect HT to be useful in assisting with pain control, promoting relaxation, lessening stress, and enhancing spiritual and emotional wellbeing. (Brannon, 2002; Garret, 2006; Wilkinson, 2002). Feeling "cared for" is a common and important hospital quality metric. In one study, HT was shown to increase recipient satisfaction survey scores, as recipients who receive HT perceive the staff to be more sensitive to their needs (Garcia, 2004).

HEALING TOUCH: PEDIATRIC LITERATURE

Kemper and Kelly (2004) report that touch therapies are widely available in pediatric hospitals and have been useful as adjunctive therapy to decrease stress, anxiety, reduce pain, and promote an improved sense of wellbeing in both the recipient and the practitioner. For example, staff at the Cincinnati Children's Hospital Medical Center offers HT free of charge to hospitalized children.

Verret (2000) examined the effect of HT on a small sample of young children, ages 6 to 7, with disabilities who had mild to moderate chronic spasticity. Using a pre- and post-test design, the outcomes noted included weight gain, increased range of motion, decreased spasticity and improved motor skills. Speel (2002) also found that HT diminished spasticity and improved gait in a small sample of high school students with cerebral palsy.

Healing Touch Training

In 1990, The HT Certificate Program (HTCP) was created and endorsed by the American Holistic Nurses Association. HT is oriented towards nurses and other allied healthcare providers, but training is available to anyone interested in specialized energy-based healing training. Through out the HT classes, self-care is emphasized as a requisite foundation to being a HT practitioner. The curriculum consists of 124 hours of classroom education that includes didactic education on energy-based healing techniques and direct experience and supervision in performing HT. After completing the level 4 class, the HT student achieves HT apprentice status.

In preparation for the fifth-level class, the student spends 6 to 12 months as a HT apprentice by working closely with a certified HT practitioner (CHTP) and completes additional year of course work which focuses on client-practitioner relationships, establishment of a practice, and integration of activities within the health community. Additionally, the apprentice is required to write an in-depth written case study synthesizing their understanding and ability to demonstrate correct use of HT techniques.

After completion of level 5, practitioners can apply for certification as a Certified Healing Touch Practitioner. The Healing Touch International, Inc. Certification Board reviews each applicant and makes a determination as to whether the individual will be certified (www.healingtouchinternational.org, accessed September 18, 2007).

Certification is granted for 5 years, after which point the HT practitioner must complete 75 continuing education hours and submit a practice statement, a letter of support from and confirmation that the practitioner continues to abide by the HT International certification requirements.

Energy Therapies: Safety and Risks

Therapeutic Touch, Reiki, and Healing Touch are safe, gentle, non-invasive therapies that activate the autonomic nervous system, decreasing anxiety and pain, and eliciting a deep sense of peacefulness. These therapies are safe to use as part of self-care and as an adjunct to nursing or medical care. Energy therapies are indicated for those who desire it as a part of their treatment to support relaxation, and decrease anxiety and/or pain. Use of an energy therapy is clearly contraindicated if the recipient does not want it or if the practitioner feels they are not centered or otherwise in condition to offer

Table 9-1. Comparison between Healing Touch, Reiki, and Therapeutic Touch

Comparison Points	HT	Reiki	Therapeutic Touch
Techniques	Hands on or off the body	Hands on and off the body	Hands on or off the body
Practitioner Attunement needed before providing a session	No, any one can perform	Yes	No, any one can perform
Practitioner Intention	Directs the flow of energy	Allows the flow of energy	Directs the flow of energy
Pre-treatment assessment	Yes	No*	Yes
Pre-treatment centering or "Align with Higher Power"	Yes	Yes	Yes
Practitioner Certification	Yes	No	Yes**
Code of Ethics	Yes	Yes	Yes

*A subpopulation of Reiki practitioners use assessment.
**Therapeutic Touch practitioners and teachers are "qualified" to practice (not certified).
Adapted from Potter P. What are the distinctions between Reiki and TT? (2003) Clinical Journal of Oncology Nursing, pp. 89-91.

the treatment. As mentioned previously, those who are more sensitive to energy interventions (neonates, young children, pregnant women, the elderly, the critically ill, and people with psychiatric disorders), generally respond quickly and intensely to energy therapies. Individuals diagnosed with paranoia, thought disorders, or severe personality dissociation are not appropriate candidates for HT, as time-space orientation is altered during HT sessions (Hover & Kramer, 1997, p. 204).

There have been no reported cases of adverse effects in either the medical or the nursing literature. On rare occasions, those who are sensitive to this kind of therapy (neonates, sick infants, or the elderly) may experience transient dizziness, tingling, restlessness, or tearfulness. In some cases, recipients may experience feeling soothed or calmed, deep-muscle relaxation, dozing, joy, doubtful thoughts replaced by faith, and a feeling of being loved unconditionally.

Making a Referral

Referrals for all three types of energy therapies can be made by anyone. Nurses most often make the referrals; however, with increasing frequency, referrals are made by physician colleagues and other healthcare professionals. Patients and their families typically request energy therapy treatments based on their own experience or because energy therapies were recommended to them by another recipient. Current evidence supports the safety of Therapeutic Touch, Reiki, and Healing Touch and their usefulness in eliciting relaxation, and decreasing the subjective experience of anxiety and pain. Healthcare professionals can recommend these healing energy therapies and continue to monitor their effectiveness.

Acknowledgments

The authors gratefully acknowledge Angela Epshtein, MA, for her review and editing; Christine Fleuriel, MSLIS, Catherine Guarcello, MS, and Alison Clapp, MLIS, for assistance with the literature review; and their families for their ever-present support and encouragement.

REFERENCES

Achterberg, J. (1998). Clearing the air in the TT controversy. *Alternative Therapies, 4*(4), 100–101.

Alandydy, P. (1999). Using Reiki to support surgical patients. *Journal of Nursing Care Quality, 13*, 89–91.

Barron, A., Coakley, A., Fitzgerald, E., & Mahoney, E. (2008). Promoting the integration of Therapeutic Touch in nursing practice on an inpatient oncology and bone marrow transplant unit, *International Journal for Human Caring, 12*(2), 81–89.

Becker, R., & Selden, G. (1985). *The body electric: Electromagnetism and the foundation of life.* New York: Quill, William Morrow.

Bossi, L., Ott, M.J., & DeCristofaro, S. (2008). Reiki as a clinical intervention in oncology nursing practice. *Clinical Journal of Oncology Nursing, 12*(3), 489–494.

Bradway, C. (1998). The effects of healing touch on depression. *Healing Touch Newsletter: Research Edition, 8*(3), 2.

Brannon, J. (2002). A patient satisfaction survey for cancer patients experiencing healing touch at the cancer wellness center. *Healing Touch International Research Survey,* June, Lakewood, CO: Healing Touch International, Inc.

Brathovde, A. (2006) A pilot study: Reiki for self-care of nurses and healthcare providers. *Holistic Nursing Practice, 20,* 95–101.

Bullock, M. (1997). Reiki: A complementary therapy for life. *The American Journal of Hospice and Palliative Care, January/February,* 31–33.

Burden, B., Herron-Marx, S., & Clifford, C. (2005). The increasing use of Reiki as a complementary therapy in specialist palliative care. *International Journal of Palliative Nursing, 11,* 248–253.

Burhardt, M. (2002). *Spirituality: Living our connectedness,* Albany, NY: Delmar, a division of Thomson Learning.

Clark, A. J., Turner, J. G., Gauthier, D. K., & Williams, M. (1998). The effect of TT on pain and anxiety in burn patients. *Journal of Advanced Nursing, 28*(1), 10–20.

Cordes, P., Profitt, D., & Roth, J. (2002) *The effect of healing touch therapy on the pain and joint mobility experienced by patients with total knee replacements. In Healing Touch research survey.* Lakewood, CO: Healing Touch International.

Cornelio, D., & Warber, S. (2003). Social Construction of CAM. *Molecular Interventions, 3,* 182–185.

Cox, C., & Hayes, J. (1998). Experiences of administering and receiving TT in intensive care. *Complementary Therapies in Nursing and Midwifery, 4,* 128–132.

Cox, T. (2003). A nurse-statistician reanalyzes data from the Rosa TT study. *Alternative Therapies in Health and Medicine, 9*(1), 58–64

Crawford, S. E., Leaver, V. W., & Mahoney, S. D. (2006). Using Reiki to decrease memory and behavior problems in mild cognitive impairment and mild Alzheimer's disease. *Journal of Alternative & Complementary Medicine, 12,* 911–913.

Denison, B. (2004). Touch the pain away: New research on TT and persons with fibromyalgia syndrome. *Holistic Nursing Practice, 18,* 142–151.

Dossey, L. (2003). TT at the crossroads: observations on the Rosa study. *Alternative Therapies in Health and Medicine, 9*(1), 38–39.

Dowd, T., Kolcaba, K, Steiner, R, & Fashinpaur D. (2007). Comparison of a healing touch, coaching and a combined intervention on comfort and stress in younger college students. *Holistic Nursing Practice, 21*(4), 194–202.

Dressen, L. J., & Singg, S. (1998). Effects of Reiki on pain and selected affective and personality variables of chronically ill patients. *Subtle Energies and Energy Medicine, 9*(1), 51–83.

Dubrey, R. J. (1999) A quality assurance project on the effectiveness of healing touch treatments as perceived by patients at the wellness institute. In Healing Touch International research survey. 2006 Lakewood, CO: Healing Touch International.

Dubrey, R. (2006). The role of healing touch in the treatment of persons in recovery from alcoholism. *Counselor: The Magazine for Addiction Professionals, Dec,* 58–64.

Easter, A. (1997). The state of research on the effects of therapeutic touch. *Journal of Holistic Nursing, 15*(2), 158–175.

Edelblute, J. (2003). Pediatric oncology patients find help and hope in New York City. *Alternative Therapies, 9*(2), 106–107.

Eisenberg, D. M., Davis, R. B., Ettner, S. L., Appel, S., Wilkey, S., Van Rompay, M, et al. (1998). Trends in alternative medicine use in the United States 1990–1997: Results of a follow-up national survey. *Journal of the American Medical Association, 280*(18), 1569–1575.

Engebretson, J. (1998). A heterodox model of healing. *Alternative Therapies, 4*(2), 37–43.

Engebretson, J., & Wardell, D. W. (2002). Experience of a reiki session. *Alternative Therapies, 8*(2), 48–53.

Engbretson, J., & Wardell, D. (2007). Energy-based modalities. *Nursing Clinics of North America, 42*, 23–259.

Eschiti, V. (2007). Healing touch: A low tech intervention in high tech settings. *Dimensions in Critical Care Nursing, 26*(1), 9–14.

France, N. (1993). The child's perception of the human energy field using TT. *Journal of Holistic Nursing, 11*, 319–331.

Gagne, D., & Toye, R. (1994). The effects of TT and relaxation therapy in reducing anxiety. *Archives of Psychiatric Nursing, 7*(3), 184–189.

Garcia, K. (2004). Healing touch program survey at St. Joseph Hospital. In Healing Touch International research survey 2006. Lakewood, CO: Healing Touch International.

Garrett, N. (2006). A persuasive commentary and study: exploring perception of HT therapy as a positive treatment modality for wellness maintenance, physical and psychological concerns in adults. Unpublished Master's thesis in Social Work, New Mexico University. Healing Touch International research survey. 2006 Lakewood, CO: Healing Touch International.

Gerber, R. (2001). *Vibrational medicine.* 3rd ed. Rochester, VT: Bear & Company.

Giasson, M., & Bouchard. L. (1998). Effect of TT on the wellbeing of persons with terminal cancer. *Journal of Holistic Nursing, 16*(3), 383–389.

Gordon, A., Merenstein, J. H., D'Amico, F., & Hudgens, D. (1998). The effects of TT on patients with osteoarthritis of the knee. *Journal of Family Practice, 47*(4), 271–277.

Gronowicz, G., Jhaveri, A., Clarke, L., Aronow, M., & Smith, T. (2008). Therapeutic Touch stimulates the proliferation of human cells in culture, *The Journal of Alternative and Complementary Medicine, 14*(3), 233–239.

Healing Touch International research survey. 2006 Lakewood, CO: Healing Touch International.

Healing Touch International website. Retreived July 28, 2007, from www.healingtouchinternational.org

Heidt, P. (1981). Effect of TT on the anxiety level of hospitalized patients. *Nursing Research, 30*(1), 32–37.

Hover-Kramer, D., & Shames K. (1997). *Energetic approaches to emotional healing.* Albany, NY: Delmar Publishers.

Hughes, P. P., Meize-Grochowski, R., & Harris, C. (1996). TT with adolescent psychiatric patients. *Journal of Holistic Nursing, 14*(1), 6–23.

Hunt, V. (1996). *Infinite mind: Science of the human vibrations of consciousness.* 2nd ed. Malibu, CA: Malibu Publishing Co.

Ireland, M. (1998). TT with HIV-infected children: A pilot study. *Journal of the Association of Nurses in AIDS Care, 9*(4), 68–77.

Ireland, M., & Olson, M. (2000). Massage therapy and TT in children: state of the science. *Alternative Therapies, 6*(5), 54–63.

Jonas, W., & Crawford, C. (2003). *Healing, intention and energy medicine: Science, research methods and clinical implications.* New York: Churchill Livingstone.

Keller, E., & Bzdek, W. (1986). Effects of TT on tension headache pain. *Nursing Research, 35*(2), 101–105.

Kelly, A., Sullivan, P., Fawcett, J., & Samarel, N. (2004). Therapeutic touch, quiet time, and dialogue: Perceptions of women with breast cancer. *Oncology Nursing Forum, 31*(3), 625–631.

Kemper, K., & Kelly, E. (2004). Treating children with TT and HT. *Pediatric Annals, 33*(4), 249–252.

Kemper, K. J., Larrimore, D., Dozier, J., & Woods, C. (2006). Impact of a medical school elective in cultivating compassion through touch therapies. *Complementary Health Practice Review, 11*(1), 47–56.

Kennedy, P. (2001) Working with survivors of torture in Sarajevo with Reiki. *Complementary Therapies in Nursing & Midwifery, 7,* 4–7.

Kerr, C., Wasserman, R., & Moore, C. (2007). Cortical dynamics as a therapeutic mechanism for touch healing. *The Journal of Alternative and Complementary Medicine, 13*(1), 59–66.

Kiang, J. Marotta, D., Wirkus, M. Wirkus, M., & Jonas, W. (2002). External bioenergy increases intracellular free calcium concentration and reduces cellular response to heat stress. *Journal of Investigative Medicine, 50*(1), 38–45.

King, R. P. (2005). The integration of healing touch with conventional care at the Scripps center for integrative medicine. *Explore: The Journal of Science and Healing, 1*(2), 144–145.

Kramer, N. A. (1990). Comparison of TT and casual touch in stress reduction of hospitalized children. *Pediatric Nursing, 5*(16), 483–485.

Krieger, D. (1972). The response of in-vivo human hemoglobin to an active healing therapy by direct "laying on" of hands. *Human Dimensions, 1,* 12–15.

Krieger, D. (1976). Healing by the "laying on" of hands as a facilitator of bioenergetic change: The response of in-vivo human hemoglobin. *Psychoenergetic Systems, 1*(2), 121–129.

Krieger, D. (1979). *Therapeutic touch: How to use your hands to help or to heal.* Englewood Cliffs, NJ: Prentice-Hall, Inc.

Krieger, D. (1998). Therapeutic Touch, In Touch... *The Therapeutic Touch Networks of Canada Newsletter, 10*(2), Cover.

Kreiger, D. (2002). *TT as transpersonal healing.* New York: Lantern Books.

Lafreniere, D., Mutus, B., Cameron, S., Tannous, M., Giannotti, M., Abu-Zahra, H., & Laukkanen, E. (1999). Effects of TT on biochemical and mood indicators in women. *The Journal of Alternative and Complementary Medicine, 4*(5), 367–370.

Larden, C. N., Palmer, M. L., & Janssen, P. (2004). Efficacy of TT in treating pregnant inpatients who have a chemical dependency. *Journal of Holistic Nursing, 22*(4), 320–332.

Lee, M., Pittler, M., & Ernst, E. (2008). Effects of reiki in clinical practice: a systematic review of randomized clinical trials. *International Journal of Clinical Practice, 62*(6), 947–954.

Leskowitz, E. (1999). Phantom limb pain: Subtle energy perspectives. *Subtle Energies and Energy Medicine, 2*(8), 125–152.

Leskowitz, E. (2000a). Phantom limb pain treated with TT: A case report. *Archives of Physical Medicine and Rehabilitation, 81,* 522–524.

Leskowitz, E. (2000b). Un-debunking TT. *Alternative Therapies, 4*(4), 101–102.

Lin, Y., & Taylor, A. G. (1998). The effects of TT in reducing pain and anxiety in an elderly population. *Integrative Medicine, 1,* 155–162.

Lipinski, K. (2006). Finding Reiki: Applications for your nursing practice. *Beginnings, 26*(1), 6–7.

Loveland Cook, C. A., Guerrerio, J. F., & Slater, V. E., (2004). Healing touch and quality of life in women receiving radiation treatment for cancer: a randomized controlled trial. *Alternative Therapies, 10*(3), 34–40.

Mansour, A. A., Laing, G., Leis, A., Nurse, J., & Denilkewich, A. (1998). The experience of reiki. *Alternative and Complementary Therapies, 4*(3), 211–217.

Mackay, N., Hansen, S., & McFarlane, O., (2004). Autonomic nervous system changes during reiki treatment: A preliminary study. *The Journal of Alternative and Complementary Medicine, 10*(6), 1007–1081.

McElligott, D., Holz, M., Carollo, L., Sommerville, S., Baggett, M., Kuzniewski, S., et al. (2003). A pilot feasibility study of the effects of touch therapy on nurses. *Journal of the New York State Nurses Association, 34,* 16–24.

Meehan, M. T. C. (1993). TT and postoperative pain: A Rogerian research study. *Nursing Science Quarterly, 6*(2), 69–77.

Mentgen J. (2001). Healing touch. In J. D. Colbath, P. M., & Prawlucki (Eds.), *The nursing clinics of North America: Holistic nursing care*. Philadelphia, PA: WB Saunders Co.

Miles, P. (2003). Preliminary report on the use of Reiki for HIV-related pain and anxiety (Research Letter). *Alternative Therapies, 9*(2), 36.

Miles, P. (2006). *Reiki: A comprehensive guide*. New York: Penguin Group.

Moore, T., Ting, B., & Rossiter-Thornton, M. (2008). A pilot study of the experience of participating in a Therapeutic Touch practice group, *Journal of Holistic Nursing, 26*(1), 161–168.

Moss, N. (1998). Healing Touch offers an addition to traditional therapy in health care. *Rural Nurse Connection, 6*(5), 1, 3.

Movaffaghi, Z., Hasanpoor, M., Farsi, M., Hooshmand, P., & Abrishami, F. (2006). Effects of therapeutic touch on blood hemoglobin and hematocrit level. *Journal of Holistic Nursing, 24*(1), 41–48.

National Center for Complementary and Alternative Medicine. (2007). Reiki Clinical Trials. Retrieved July 24, 2007, from http://nccam.nih.gov/clinicaltrials/reiki.htm

The NIH National Center for Complementary and Alternative Medicine (NCAMM). Retrieved July 28, 2007, from www.nccam.nih.gov/health/backgrounds/energymed.htm

Nield-Anderson, L., & Ameling, A. (2001). Reiki: A complementary therapy for nursing practice. *Journal of Psychosocial Nursing and Mental Health Services, 39*, 42–49.

Nurse Healers—Professional Associates International (NH-PAI). Retrieved July 28, 2007, from www.therapuetic-touch.org

Olson, M., & Sneed, N. (1995). Anxiety and TT. *Issues in Mental Health Nursing, 16*, 97–108.

Olson, K., & Hanson, J. (1997). Using reiki to manage pain: A preliminary report. *Cancer Prevention & Control, 1*(2), 109–113.

Olson, M., Sneed, N., Bonadonna, R., Ratliff, J., & Dias, J. (1992). Therapeutic touch and post-hurricane Hugo stress. *Journal of Holistic Nursing, 10*(2), 120–136.

Olson, M., Sneed, N., LaVia, M., Virella, G., Bonadonna, R., & Young, M. (1997). Stress-induced immunosuppression and TT. *Alternative Therapies, 2*(3), 68–72.

Olson, K., Hanson, J., & Michaud, M. (2003). A phase II trial of reiki for management of pain in advanced cancer patients. *Journal of Pain and Symptom Management, 26*(5), 990–997.

O'Mathuna, D. P., & Ashford, R. L. (2004). TT for healing acute wounds. *The Cochrane Library*, Issue 4, 2004.

Oschman, J. L. (2000). *Energy medicine: The scientific basis*. New York: Livingstone.

Ott, M. J., & Mulloney, S. S. (1998). Therapeutic touch: Nurturing the nurse leader. *Nursing Management, 29*(6), 46–48.

Peck, S. (1997). The effectiveness of therapeutic touch for decreasing pain in elders with degenerative arthritis. *Journal of Holistic Nursing, 15*(2), 176–198.

Peters, R. (1999). The effectiveness of TT: A meta-analytic review. *Nursing Science Quarterly, 12*(1), 52–61.

Petter, F. A. (1997). *Reiki fire: New information about the origins of the Reiki power a complete manual*. Twin Lakes, WI: Lotus Press.

Post-White, J., Kinney, M. E. Savik, K., Gau, J. B., Wilcox, C., & Lerner, I. (2003). Therapeutic massage and healing touch improve symptoms in cancer. *Integrative Cancer Therapies, 2*(4), 332–344.

Potter, P. (2003). What are the distinctions between Reiki and Therapeutic Touch? *Clinical Journal of Oncology, 7*(1), 89–91.

Quinn, J. F. (1984). Therapeutic touch as energy exchange: Testing the theory. *Advances in Nursing Science, 2*(2) 42–49.

Quinn, J. F., & Strelkauskas, A. J. (1993). Psychoimmunologic effects of TT on practitioners and recently bereaved recipients: A pilot study. *Advances in Nursing Science, 4*(15), 13–26.

Rand, W. L. (1998). *The healing touch first and second degree manuel*. Southfield, MI: Vision Publications.

Rosa, L., Rosa, E., Sarner, L., & Barrett, S. (1998). A close look at therapeutic touch. *Journal of the American Medical Association, 279*(13), 1005–1010.

Rubik, B. (2002). The biofield hypothesis: Its biophysical basis and role in medicine. *Journal Alternative and Complementary Medicine, 8*(6), 703–717.

Rubrik, B., Brooks, A., & Schwartz, G. (2006). In vitro effect of Reiki treatment on bacterial cultures: Role of experimental context and practitioner wellbeing. *Journal of Alternative and Complementary Medicine, 12,* 7–13.

Samarel, N., Fawcett, J., Davis, M., & Ryan, R. (1998). Effects of dialogue and TT on preoperative and postoperative experiences of breast cancer surgery: An exploratory study. *Oncology Nursing Forum, 8*(25), 1369–1376.

Santorelli, S. (1999). *Heal thyself: Lessons on mindfulness in medicine.* New York: Bell Tower, a division of Crown Publishers.

Sawyer, J. (1998). The first Reiki practitioner in our OR. *Association of Operating Room Nurses Journal, 67,* 674–677.

Schiller, R. (2003). Reiki: A starting point for integrative medicine. *Alternative Therapies in Health & Medicine, 9,* 20–21.

Schmehr, R., (2003). Enhancing the treatment of HIV/AIDS with reiki training and treatment. *Alternative Therapies, 9*(2), 118, 120.

Shiflett, S., Nayak, S., Bid, C., Miles, P., & Agostinelli, S. (2002). Effect of reiki treatment on functional recovery in patients in poststroke rehabilitation: A pilot study. *Journal of Alternative and Complementary Medicine, 8*(6), 755–763.

Simington, J., & Laing, G. (1993). Effects of TT on anxiety in the institutionalized elderly. *Clinical Nursing Research, 2*(4):438–450.

Slater, V. (1996). Safety, elements and effects of healing touch on chronic non-malignant abdominal pain. Unpublished doctoral dissertation, University of Tennessee, College of Nursing, Knoxville, TN.

Smith, D., Arnstein, P., Rosa, K., & Wells-Federman, C. (2002). Effects of integrating TT into a cognitive behavioral pain treatment program. *Journal of Holistic Nursing, 20*(4), 367–387.

Smith, D., & Broida, J. (2007). Pandimensional field pattern changes in healers and healees: Experiencing therapeutic touch. *Journal of Holistic Nursing, 25*(4), 217–225.

Smith, M., Reeder, F., Daniel, L., Baramee, J., & Hagman, J. (2003). Outcomes of touch therapies during bone marrow transplant. *Alternative Therapies, 9*(1), 40–49.

Snyderman, R. (2000). CAM (complementary and alternative medicine) and the role of the academic health center. *Journal of Alternative Therapies, 6,* 96, 93.

Speel, L. (2002). A pilot study on the effect of healing touch-mind clearing and magnetic unruffling on high school students with mental and physical disabilities, In Healing Touch research survey. Lakewood, CO: Healing Touch International.

Spence, J., & Olson, M. (1997). Quantitative research on TT: An integrative review of the literature 1985–1995. *Scandinavian Journal of Caring Science, 11,* 183–190.

Swartz, L. (1995). First person experience. Reiki: how one patient became a practitioner. *Alternative and Complementary Therapies, 1,* 389–392.

Tovey, M. (2001). Healing Touch: An energy-based approach to student health. *School Nurse News,* March, pp. 29–31.

Tsang, K., Caralson, L., & Olson, K. (2007). Pilot crossover trial of Reiki versus rest for treating cancer-related fatigue. *Integrative Cancer Therapies, 6,* 25–35.

Umbreit, A. (2000). Healing touch: Applications in the acute care setting. *AACN Clinical Issues, 11*(1), 105–119.

Usui, M., & Petter, F. A. (2003). *the Original Reiki Handbook of Dr. Mikado Usual.* Twin Lakes, WI: Lotus Press.

Van Akin, R. (2004). The experiential process of healing touch for people with moderate depression, unpublished doctoral dissertation, Southern Cross University, Australia.

Van Sell, S. L. (1996). Reiki: an ancient touch therapy. *RN*, February, pp. 57–59.

Verret, P. (2000). Healing Touch as a relaxation intervention in children with spasticity. *Healing Touch Newsletter. 0*(3), 6–7.

Vitale, A. (2007). An integrative review of Reiki touch therapy research. *Holistic Nursing Practice, 21*, 167.

Walach, H. (2005). Generalized entanglement: A new theoretical model for understanding the effects of complementary and alternative medicine. *The Journal of Alternative and Complementary Medicine, 11*(3), 549–559.

Wardell, D. W. (2000). The trauma release technique: How it is taught and experienced in healing touch. *Alternative and Complementary Therapies, 6*(1), 20–27.

Wardell, D. W., & Engebretson, J. (2001). Biological correlates of Reiki Touch healing. *Journal of Advanced Nursing, 33*, 439–445.

Wardell, D., & Weymouth, K. (2004). Review of studies of Healing Touch. *Journal of Nursing Scholarship: Image, 36*(2), 147–154.

Wardell, D., Rintala, D., Duan, Z., & Tan, G. (2006). A pilot study of healing touch and progressive relaxation for chronic neuropathic pain in persons with spinal cord injury. *Journal of Holistic Nursing, 24*(4), 231–240.

Watson, J. (2005). *Caring Science as sacred science.* Philadelphia, PA: F. A. Davis.

Welcher, B., & Kish, J. (2001). Reducing pain and anxiety through Healing Touch. *Healing Touch Newsletter, 1*(3), 19.

Wetzel, W. S. (1989). Reiki healing: A physiologic perspective. *Journal of Holistic Nursing, 7*(1), 47–54.

Weymouth, K., & Sandberg-Lewis, S. (2000). Comparing the efficacy of Healing Touch and chiropractic adjustment in treating low back pain: A pilot study. *Healing Touch Newsletter, 00*(3), 7–8.

Whelan, K. M. (2003). Reiki therapy: The benefits to a nurse/Reiki practitioner. *Holistic Nursing Practice, 17*, 209–217.

Wilkinson, D., Knox, P., Chatman, J., Johnson, T., Barbour, N., Myles, Y., & Reel, A. (2002). The clinical effectiveness of Healing Touch. *Journal of Alternative and Complementary Medicine, 8*(1), 33–47.

Winstead-Fry, P., & Kijek, J. (1999). An integrative review and meta-analysis of TT research. *Alternative Therapies, 5*(6), 58–67.

Wirth, D., Brenlan, D., Levine, R., & Rodriguez, C. (1993). The effect of complementary healing therapy on post-operative pain after surgical removal of impacted third molar teeth. *Complementary Therapies in Medicine, 1*, 133–138.

Witte, D., & Dundes, L. (2001). Harnessing life energy or wishful thinking? Reiki, placebo reiki, meditation, and music. *Alternative and Complementary Therapies*, October, 304–309.

PROFESSIONAL ORGANIZATIONS AND RESOURCES

American Academy of Pediatrics Provisional Section on Complementary, Holistic, and Integrative Medicine
  Website: www.aap.org/sections/CHIM
American Holistic Medical Association
  Website: www.holisticmedicine.org
American Holistic Nurses' Association
  Website: www.ahna.org
Center for Frontier Medicine in Biofield Science
  Website: www.lach.web.arizona.edu/biofield.htm

Healing Touch International
  Website: www.healingtouchinternational.org
Healing Touch Program Classes
  Website: www.healingtouchprogram.com
International Association of Reiki Professionals (IARP)
  Website: www.IARP.org
International Center for Reiki Training
  Website: www.reiki.org
International Society for the Study of Subtle Energy and Energy Medicine
  Website: www.issseem.org
National Center for Complementary and Alternative Medicine
  Website: www.nccam.gov
Therapeutic Touch International Association, Inc. (Formerly Nurse Healers – Professional
Associates, International [NH-PAI])
  Website: www.therapeutic-touch.org
Reiki Alliance
  Website: www.reikialliance.com
Therapeutic Touch Network (Ontario)
  Website: www.therapeutictouchnetwk.com

ADDITIONAL SUGGESTED READINGS

Gerber, R. (2000). *Vibrational Medicine for the 21st Century: The Complete Guide to Energy Healing and Spiritual Transformation.* New York: HarperCollins.

Gray, J. and Gray, L. (2002). *Hand to Hand: The Longest-Practicing Reiki Master Tells His Story.* Reiki Xlibris Corporation, www.Xlibris.com.

Hover-Kramer, D. (2002). *HT— A Guidebook for Practitioners,* 2nd Edition. Albany, NY: Thomson Learning.

Hover-Kramer, D., Mentgen, J., Scandrett, Hibdon, S. (2002). *Healing Touch: A Resource for Health Professionals.* Albany, NY: Delmar Publishers.

Karagulla, S. and Kunz, D. (1989). *The Chakras and the Human Energy Fields,* Wheaton, IL: Theosophical Publishing House.

Krieger, D. (1993). *Accepting Your Power to Heal: The Personal Practice of TT.* Santa Fe, NM: Bear & Co.

Krieger, D. (1996). *TT Inner Workbook: Ventures in Transpersonal Healing.* New York: Lantern Books.

Kunz, D. (1995). *Spiritual Healing.* Wheaton, IL: Quest Books.

Lubeck, W., Petter, F., Rand, W.L. (2001). *The Spirit of Reiki: The Complete Handbook of the Reiki System.* Twin Lakes, WI: Lotus Press.

Macrae, J. (1988). *TT: A Practical Guide.* New York, N.Y: Knopf.

May, D. (2001). *The TT Handbook: Level One – Basic.* Ontario, Canada: Scribe Press.

May, D. (2003). *The TT Handbook: Levels Two and Three - Intermediate.* Ontario, Canada: Scribe Press.

Upczak, P. (1999). *Reiki: A Way of Life.* Nederland, CO: Synchronicity Publishing.

Wager, S. (1996). *A Doctor's Guide to TT: Enhancing the Body's Energy to Promote Healing.* New York: The Berkley Publishing Group.

10

A Pediatric Perspective on Exercise Medicine

AMANDA K. WEISS KELLY AND SUSANNAH M. BRISKIN

KEY CONCEPTS

- Exercise should be considered as an essential component of treatment for many chronic diseases including obesity, hypertension, diabetes, low bone mineral density, and depression.
- Athletes' performance may be improved by incorporating integrative techniques, such as imagery and biofeedback, into their preparatory routines.
- Forms of integrative medicine, such as massage, acupuncture, and yoga may be successfully used by athletes to treat and possibly prevent injury.

■

1. The skyrocketing rate of obesity in the United States will bring a dramatic increase in co-morbidities, such as hypertension and diabetes. Prescribing exercise as a form of treatment is a key component to successfully addressing these challenging problems.
2. Participating in weight-bearing exercise, such as running and jumping, during childhood and adolescence will help maximize bone density potential.
3. All family members should be encouraged to exercise. Don't underestimate the value of lifestyle activities, such as hiking, biking, or walking. They are simple ways to get all family members active and create an excellent opportunity for quality family time.

4. The use of complementary medicine by athletes is not only well accepted, but it is growing. As athletes try to gain any possible advantage over their competition they will expand their standard training and treatment techniques to include forms considered outside the realm of traditional medicine and exercise.

Basic Recommendations for Pediatric Exercise

1. Kids should be encouraged to participate in 60 to 90 minutes of physical activity every day.
2. This amount of exercise can be accumulated throughout the day and a bout of exercise can be considered beneficial as long as the session is a minimum of 10 minutes.
3. Physical activity may be achieved through organized sports participation with adult supervision. However, free play and lifestyle activities are equally beneficial if the above guidelines are followed.
4. If an individual is not currently active, it is best to start with 10 to 15 minutes a day of exercise and gradually increase it by 10% per week until the goal time is reached. Abrupt increases in training time and intensity may predispose an individual to injury or may discourage their participation due to a sudden lifestyle change.
5. Family participation should be strongly encouraged. This will allow for quality family time, demonstration of the parent as a role model, and facilitate the parent reaching their recommended exercise goal.

When evaluating the role of exercise in integrative medicine there are two distinct concepts to consider. The first is the use of exercise as a treatment option for disease. The second is the use of other forms of integrative medicine in the treatment of sport related pain and injury and performance enhancement.

Exercise as a form of Medicine

Exercise and sports participation may be useful in the prevention and treatment of many disease processes in children and adolescents including obesity, hypertension, insulin resistance, decreased bone mineral density, and depression.

OBESITY

Obesity is a growing epidemic in the United States with the prevalence of obesity rising from 5% in the 1960s to 17% in 2004 (Ogden, 2006). The increasing prevalence of obesity has been attributed to sedentary lifestyle, decreased physical activity and increased caloric consumption (Gungor, 2005; Ludwig, 2001). Unfortunately, most children who are obese become obese adults (Whitaker 1997). Obesity is related to a host of other chronic medical issues including hypertension, dyslipidemia, and type 2 diabetes, which are discussed separately, later in this section. Overall, childhood obesity is associated with a 1.5-fold increase in all causes of mortality and a 2-fold increase specifically in cardiovascular mortality during adulthood (Must, 1999).

Multiple randomized controlled trials have demonstrated the efficacy of increased physical activity in treating overweight and obesity in children (Balagopal, 2005; Epstein, 1984, 1985; Gutin, 2002; Owens, 1999; Ritchie, 2006). Encouraging "lifestyle exercise," such as biking and walking, may help in maintenance of weight loss as compared to calisthenics or aerobic exercise (Epstein, 1985). Including resistance training as part of an exercise regimen may also help improve subject retention in long-term weight loss programs (Sothern, 2000). Compared to diet change alone, exercise plus diet change has been found to improve fitness, and in some studies, to enhance weight loss (Epstein, 1985; Ritchie, 2006).

It is important to note that several studies have failed to note improvement in BMI or weight with exercise interventions in obese children (Woo, 2004). This is likely due to significant methodological variations in the type, frequency, and duration of exercise amongst studies. Also, variations in how quantity of exercise is assessed, such as questionnaires, heartrate monitors, or pedometers, make it difficult to compare studies. However, a recent comprehensive review notes that exercise programs performed 3 to 7 days each week, for 30 to 60 minutes each session, seem to be successful in reducing body fat in obese children (Strong, 2005). In addition to increasing physical activity, decreasing sedentary activities such as television watching, has been shown to improve weight loss in obese children (Epstein, 1995; Ritchie, 2006).

CARDIOVASCULAR DISEASE: HYPERTENSION, LIPID ABNORMALITIES, ATHEROSCLEROSIS

Hypertension in children is significantly more common in children now than it has been in the past (Flynn, 2005). Studies in the 1970s and 1980s found hypertension in 0.3% to 1.2% of adolescents, whereas more recent studies have found as many as 13% of adolescents with blood pressures persistently above the 95th percentile (Sorof, 2002).

The increasing prevalence of hypertension in children may be related to the increase in prevalence of obesity. Obese children have an increased risk for hypertension—as high as three times the risk (Freedman, 2001; Becque, 1988; Luma, 2006).

Luepker et al. evaluated BMI and blood pressure in 18,000 children in 1986 and 1996 and found that BMI had significantly increased during that time period and was associated with a corresponding rise in systolic blood pressures (Luepker, 1999).

Several investigators have demonstrated that exercise interventions can lower blood pressure in children (Becque, 1988; Hansen, 1991; Luma, 2006). One randomized, controlled trial demonstrated that aerobic exercise, over an 8-month time period, significantly reduced both systolic and diastolic blood pressure in a group of children aged 9 to 11 years old (Hansen, 1991). Other investigators demonstrated 6 to 12 mm Hg improvements in systolic and 3 to 5 mm Hg changes in diastolic blood pressure with a 3 to 6 month exercise regimen (Alpert, 2000). Another controlled trial found that improvements in blood pressure, triglycerides, and cholesterol with an exercise and diet change intervention were greater than with a behavioral counseling and diet change intervention (Becque, 1988). Lifestyle change, including exercise, is the recommended first step in treating primary hypertension in children (National High Blood Pressure Education Program, 2004).

Increased LDL, decreased HDL, and increased triglycerides are also linked with decreased physical activity, obesity, and type 2 diabetes in children (Becque, 1988; Cook, 2003; Freedman, 2001; Morrison, 1999). Atherosclerosis has been found at autopsy in young children, indicating that dyslipidemia in childhood can lead to coronary artery disease, which can persist into adulthood (Berenson, 1998; Strong, 1999). Exercise intervention seems to improve HDL and triglyceride levels, however it does not seem to have an effect on LDL or total cholesterol in children with abnormal lipid profiles (Strong, 2005).

Regular physical activity is a consistent recommendation from the American Heart Association for the treatment and prevention of hypertension, dyslipidemia, and atherosclerosis in children (Pratt, 2007).

INSULIN RESISTANCE

The rising rates of obesity have been connected to the increasing incidence of impaired glucose resistance and type 2 diabetes (Dietz, 2005; Gungor, 2005; Kaufman, 2005; Rosenbloom, 1999). Increased body fat and elevated BMI have both been directly associated to fasting insulin levels and inversely related to glucose clearance (Arslanian, 1998; Bacha, 2004; Caprio, 1999; Weiss, 2002).

The Diabetes Prevention Program trial demonstrated the effectiveness of physical activity in preventing type 2 diabetes and insulin resistance in adults. A lifestyle change in the Diabetes Prevention Program, which included 150 minutes of physical activity each week, a healthy diet and 7% weight loss, was even more effective than metformin in preventing the onset of type 2 diabetes in at-risk adults (DPPRG, 2002). Another study in adults performed in China found that exercise alone was more effective than diet alone and equivalent to diet plus exercise in reducing the risk for type 2 diabetes in at-risk individuals (Pan, 1997).

In children, one group found that level of fitness was a more significant predictor of fasting insulin level, than percent body fat (Allen, 2007), suggesting that increased physical activity may improve insulin sensitivity more in children than weight loss through caloric restriction. Other investigators have directly demonstrated that interventions that improve cardiovascular fitness in overweight children can lead to reduced fasting insulin levels (Carrel, 2005; Gutin, 2002; Janner, 2004). A large multi-center trial is now being performed to help determine the best methods for treating type 2 diabetes in children (Peterson, 2007).

BONE DENSITY

Regular weight-bearing exercise during childhood has been associated with increased bone mineral density in adulthood. When this exercise is continued into adulthood, the risk for osteoporosis and related fractures appears to be reduced (Marcus, 2001; Riddoch, 2000). The biggest improvements in bone mineral density with weight-bearing exercise seem to occur during Tanner stages II to IV (Bailey, 2000; Kohrt, 2004). High-intensity activities that include sprinting and jumping seem to be the most effective types of exercise in enhancing bone mineral accumulation (Heinonen, 2000).

DEPRESSION

Regular physical activity has been associated with improved self-esteem and self-concept, decreased anxiety, and decreased risk for depression in children (Calfas, 1994; Farmer, 1988). Sedentary children report higher levels of depression than active children (Allgower, 2001; Brown, 1982). In addition, introducing exercise programs to adolescents with depression may be effective in improving the depressive state (Nabkasorn, 2006). Finally, introducing exercise to obese adolescents has been successful in improving self-worth and self-esteem (Daley, 2006).

ENCOURAGING EXERCISE

Clearly, regular exercise can be useful in treating and preventing chronic disease in childhood. As a result, children should be encouraged to participate in regular physical activity. Children, whose parents exercise, especially if parents and children exercise together, are more likely to exercise and to report that they enjoy exercise. Children should enjoy physical activity and effort should be made to introduce several kinds of activity and then allow the children to select activities that they enjoy. In general, children should accumulate about 60 to 90 minutes of exercise each day. This can include organized sporting activities, free play and lifestyle exercise. Encouraging lifestyle activities, such as biking and walking, may improve maintenance of exercise in the future, as may the addition of strength training programs. Activities involving large muscle groups will enhance the amount of energy expended. Finally, early in an exercise program the intensity and duration of activity should be low, then gradually increased to prevent overuse injuries (Bar-Or, 2000).

Children tend to become less active during high school years. This is especially true for girls, so it is particularly important to encourage girls to remain physically active this time period (Sallis, 1993). In addition, sedentary activities, such as TV watching, should be limited as much as possible.

Integrative Medicine in Treating Injuries in Sport and Exercise

The use of complementary medicine by athletes is widespread. In one Danish study, 47% of women and 35% of men who attended a sports medicine clinic reported usage of complementary medicine. Some authors believe that athletes seek out alternative treatments due to their "disillusionment with conventional medicine" (Ernst, 1998); they will "do whatever it takes to get back on the field" (Anonymous, 2001); and they have an "urge to leave no option untried" (Ernst, 1995).

Adolescents, in general, seem to be very accepting of the use of complementary medicine. In a study at the University of Hawaii at Manoa use of complementary medicine was widespread among NCAA Division I athletes, with about 56% reporting the use of complementary medicine. There was a significant difference between genders, with women accounting for 67% and men 49% of the athletes using complementary medicine. Massage was the most commonly used form, at 38%. Other common treatments included acupuncture and Hawaiian-specific forms of alternative medicine. It is unclear if the use of complementary therapies was primarily for prevention or treatment of athletic injuries and illnesses. Of note, none of the subjects received referrals for alternative forms of treatment from their primary care physicians. However, the majority of athletes reported receiving treatment from both allopathic physicians and complementary medicine practitioners. This emphasizes the need for communication between practitioners, as well as disclosure by athletes of their use of complementary medicine to avoid adverse interactions (Nichols, 2006).

IMAGERY

Imagery is one of the most common forms of complementary medicine employed by athletes. Imagery is a mental process for guiding and managing sports performance. One proposed definition by Richardson states, "mental imagery refers to all of those quasi-sensory or quasi-perceptual experiences of which we are self-consciously aware and which exist for us in the absence of the stimulus conditions that are known to produce their genuine sensory or perceptual counterparts" (Richardson, 1969). In an unpublished report performed at the United States Olympic Training Center in 1989, over 90% of athletes reported using imagery. The vast majority, 97%, found imagery to be an effective technique (Jowdy, Murphy, Durschi in Murphy, unpublished).

Several forms of imagery interventions exist. The most common types used in sports are mental practice and pre-competition imagery rehearsal. Mental practice may or may not include imagery. It may involve only verbal rehearsal and may be performed covertly. The goal of mental practice is to improve skill acquisition. Pre-competition imagery involves rehearsing a sport-specific task or skill within ones' mind or performing a cognitive task in order to improve performance (Suinn, 1983).

The use of mental practice dates back to the 1890s (Jastrow, 1892). It is typically employed to aid in the acquisition of skills. Although controlled trials are difficult to perform, one large meta-analysis from the 1980s showed that individuals who use mental practice techniques perform about one-half of a standard deviation better on cognitive and motor tasks than individuals who do not perform mental practice. And the results were especially striking for cognitive tasks. The effects on motor and strength tasks were less impressive (Feltz & Landers, 1983). Mental practice techniques have been employed in a wide range of sports. Recent studies have demonstrated performance benefits in learning technically difficult skills in rhythmic gymnastics, as well as, in helping amateur golfers learn to putt successfully (Cagno, 2007; Kruisselbrink, 2006).

Athletes commonly term pre-competition imagery rehearsal "psyching up." Mental imagery is probably the most common form, but cognitive forms such as attentional focus or control, preparatory arousal, and self-confidence manipulations exist (Murphy, 1994).

One study to assess pre-competition imagery was done with 90 high school cross-country runners. The performance effect was measured after combining running technique instruction with motivational statements. The runners who received motivational and running technique statements significantly improved their performance on a 1 mile trial run when compared to controls (Miller & Donohue, 2003). Subsequent studies have revealed that individuals receiving motivational statements prior to long-distance running performed better than those who were taught attentional control (Donohue et al., 2005).

BIOFEEDBACK

Biofeedback is a commonly used technique to help reduce stress. Psychological stress has been consistently linked to athletic injury risk. Certainly stress can produce changes in level of attention, as well as physical changes in muscle tension and coordination, which may predispose an athlete to injury (Team Physician: Consensus Statement, 2006). However, psychological state can also affect performance. Biofeedback allows individuals to monitor their physiological responses through visual or auditory feedback. These responses are typically controlled automatically by the body, but are thought to be subject to volitional control once an individual is in a heightened state of awareness.

Biofeedback is just one method that elite runners use during activity to help monitor their physiologic state, and enhance performance by improving running economy (Morgan, 1985). Running economy, the steady-state oxygen consumption that occurs during a submaximal running velocity, is thought to be an important determinant of success in long distance runners (Conley, 1980). Biofeedback, when combined with relaxation, has been shown to improve running economy in trained long distance runners (Caird, 1999).

MASSAGE

Massage is another commonly used form of complementary medicine. Both can serve an important role when considering integrative medicine and sports. Although many forms of massage exist, sport massage is the most commonly studied. It is frequently used to promote muscle recovery after physical activity. The role of massage in the prevention and treatment of delayed-onset muscle soreness (DOMS) is frequently investigated. DOMS is characterized by muscle pain after eccentric exercise. The pain typically occurs with active movement, passive stretch, or palpation. The intensity of soreness tends to increase in the first 24 hours, peak by 48 hours, and subside within 7 days (Armstrong, 1984). It has been difficult to determine if massage improves muscle recovery. However, the perception of soreness associated with DOMS is clearly and consistently improved with the use of massage (Hilbert, 2001, 2003; Mancinelli, 2004; Moraska, 2005),

ACUPUNCTURE

Acupuncture is the penetration of the skin by stainless steel needles. This allows for stimulation of tissue either manually, electrically, or by heat. It has been used in Asian countries for centuries; however athletes throughout the world have begun to learn its value. It is thought to alleviate muscle tension, improve blood flow, and modulate the autonomic nervous system. Athletes have turned to acupuncture for treatment of injuries as well for improving recovery after exercise (Gustaven, 2003; Karvelas, 1996; Miyamoto, 1997). Acupuncture has also been found to improve immunologic function in elite athletes (Akimoto, 2003).

YOGA

Yoga is a commonly employed form of exercise for both recreational and elite athletes. It has become a mainstream form of conditioning. However, it can also be used as a form of treatment for athletic injury. Much like massage, yoga has been found to decrease peak muscle soreness in athletes (Boyle, 2003). Yoga has also been found to be as effective in improving lower extremity flexibility as a static stretching program (Casey, 2006).

Conclusion

Integrative medicine clearly plays an important role in pediatric sports medicine. Exercise is an effective form of disease treatment and prevention. It is becoming increasingly important with the growing epidemic of obesity and its concomitant chronic medical issues. Athletes at many levels of participation use a wide array of complementary medicine techniques to aid in performance, recovery, and injury treatment.

REFERENCES

Akimoto, T., Nakahori, C., Aizawa, K., Kimura, F., Fukubayashi, T., & Kono I. (2003). Acupuncture and responses of immunologic and endocrine markers during competition. *Medicine and Science in Sports and Exercise 35*, 1296–1302.

Allen, D. B., Nemeth, B. A., Clark, R., Peterson, S. E., Eickhoff, J., & Aaron, C. (2007). Fitness is a stronger predictor of fasting insulin levels than fatness in overweight male middle-school children. *The Journal of Pediatrics, 150*, 383–387.

Allgower, A., Wardle, J., & Steptoe A. (2001). Depressive symptoms, social support, and personal health behaviors in young men and women. *Health Psychology, 20*(3), 223–227.

Alpert, B. S. (2000). Exercise as a therapy to control hypertension in children. *International Journal of Adolescent Medicine and Health, 21*(suppl 2), S94–S96.

Anonymous. (2001). Warm up [Editorial]. *British Journal of Sports Medicine, 35*, 141.

Armstrong, R. B. (1984). Mechanisms of exercise-induced delayed onset muscular soreness: a brief review. *Medicine and Science in Sports and Exercise, 16*, 529–534.

Arslanian, S., & Danadian, K. (1998). Insulin secretion, insulin sensitivity and diabetes in black children. *Trends in Endocrinology and Metabolism, 9*, 194–199.

Bacha, F., Saad, R., & Gungot, N. (2004). Adiponectin in youth: Relationship to visceral adiposity, insulin sensitivity and beta-cell function. *Diabetes Care, 27*, 547–552.

Bailey, D. A., Martin, A. D., McKay, H. A., Whiting, S., & Mirwald, R. (2000). Calcium accretion in girls and boys during puberty: A longitudinal analysis. *Journal of Bone and Mineral Research, 15*, 2245–2250.

Barlow, S. E. (2007). Expert committee recommendations regarding prevention, assessment, and treatment of child and adolescent overweight and obesity: Summary report. *Pediatrics, 120*, S164–S192.

Brown R. S. (1982). Exercise and mental health in the pediatric population. *Clinics in Sports Medicine, 1*(3), 515–527.

Balagopal, P., George, D., Yarandi, H., Funanage, V., & Bayne E. (2005). Reversal of obesity-related hypoadiponectinemia by lifestyle intervention: A controlled, randomized study in obese adolescents. *The Journal of Clinical Endocrinology and Metabolism, 90*, 6192–6197.

Bar-Or, O. (2000). Juvenile obesity, physical activity and lifestyle changes. Cornerstones for prevention and management. *The Physician and Sportsmedicine, 28* (11), 51–58.

Becque, M. D., Katch, V. L., Rocchini, A. P., Marks, C. R., & Moorehead, C. (1988). Coronary risk incidence of obese adolescents: Reduction by exercise plus diet intervention. *Pediatrics, 81*, 605–612.

Berenson, G. S, Srinivasan, S. R., & Rao, W. (1998). Association between multiple cardiovascular risk factors and atherosclerosis in children and young adults. *The New England Journal of Medicine, 338*, 1650–1656.

Boyle, C. A., Sayers, S. P., Jensen, B. E., Headley, S. A., & Manos, T. M. (2003). Effect of chronic and acute yoga training on delayed onset muscle soreness. *Medicine and Science in Sports and Exercise, 35*, S240.

Cagno, A. D., Battaglia, C., Baldari, C., & Guidetti, L. (2007). Mental training in rhythmic gymnastics: Actual training habits and effectiveness of practice on technical learning. *Medicine and Science in Sports and Exercise, 39*, S217.

Caird, S. J., McKenzie, A. D., & Sleivert, G. G. (1999). Biofeedback and relaxation techniques improve running economy in sub-elite long distance runners. *Medicine and Science in Sports and Exercise, 31*, 717–722.

Calfas, K. J., & Taylor, W. C. (1994). Effects of physical activity on psychological variable in adolescents. *Pediatric Exercise Science, 6,* 406–423.

Caprio, S., & Tamborlane, W. V. (1999). Metabolic impact of obesity in childhood. *Endocrinology and Metabolism Clinics of North America, 28,* 731–747.

Carrel, A. L., Clark, R. R., Peterson, S. E., Nemeth, B. A., Sullivan, J., & Allen, D. B. (2005). Improvement of fitness, body composition, and insulin sensitivity in overweight children in a school-based exercise program: A randomized, controlled study. *Archives of Pediatrics & Adolescent Medicine, 159,* 963–968.

Casey, B., & Terbizan, D. (2006). Improving lower body flexibility, comparing the use of yoga and a static stretching program. *Medicine and Science in Sports and Exercise, 38,* S279.

Conley, D., & Krahenbuhl, G. (1980). Running economy and distance running performance of highly trained athletes. *Medicine and Science in Sports and Exercise, 12,* 357–360.

Cook, S., Weitzman, M., & Auinger, P. (2003). Prevalence of a metabolic syndrome phenotype in adolescents: Findings from the third National Health and Nutrition Examination Survey, 1988–1994. *Archives of Pediatrics & Adolescent Medicine, 157,* 821–827.

Daley, A. J., Copeland, R. J., Wright, N. P., & Roalfe, A., & Wales, J. K. H. (2006). Exercise therapy as a treatment for psychopathologic conditions in obese and morbidly obese adolescents: A randomized, controlled trial. *Pediatrics, 118,* 2126–2134.

Davis, M. M., Gance-Cleveland, B., Hassink, S., Johnson, R., Paradis, G., & Resnicow K. (2007). Recommendations for prevention of childhood obesity. *Pediatrics, 120,* S229–S253.

Diabetes Prevention Program Research Group. (2002). Reduction in the incidence of type 2 diabetes with lifestyle intervention or metformin. *The New England Journal of Medicine, 346,* 393–403.

Dietz, W. D., & Robinson, T. N. (2005). Overweight children and adolescents. *The New England Journal of Medicine, 35,* 2100–2109.

Donohue, B., Miller, A., Beisecker, M., Houser, D., Valdez, R., Tiller, S., et al. (2005). Effects of brief yoga exercises and motivational preparatory interventions in distance runners: Space results of a controlled trial. *British Journal of Sports Medicine,* 60–63.

Epstein, L. H., Wing, R. R., Koeske, R., & Valoski, A. (1984). Effects of diet plus exercise on weight change in parents and children. *Journal of Consulting and Clinical Psychology, 52,* 429–437.

Epstein, L. H., Wing, R. R., Penner, B. C., & Dress, M. J. (1985). Effect of diet and controlled exercise on weight loss in obese children. *The Journal of Pediatrics, 107,* 358–361.

Epstein, L. H., Valoski, A. M., Vara, L. S., McCurley, J., Wisniewski L, Dalarchian MA, et al. (1995). Effects of decreasing sedentary behavior and increasing activity on weight change in obese children. *Health Psychology, 14,* 109–115.

Ernst, E. (1998). The "Hoddle Moddle": Using faith healers and other complementary therapists in sports medicine. *British Journal of Sports Medicine, 32,* 195.

Ernst, E., Willoughby, M., & Weihmayr, T. H. (1995). Nine possible reasons for choosing complementary medicine. *Perfusion, 8,* 356–358.

Farmer, M. E., Locke, B. Z., & Mocicki, E. K. (1988). Physical activity and depressive symptoms: The NHANES I Epidemiologic Follow-up study. *American Journal of Epidemiology, 128,* 1340–1351.

Feltz, D. L., & Landers, D. M. (1983). The effects of mental practice on motor skill learning and performance: A meta-analysis. *Journal of Sport Psychology, 5,* 25–57.

Fixler, D. E., Laird, W. P., & Fitzgerald, V. (1979). Hypertension screening in schools: Results of the Dallas study. *Pediatrics, 64,* 579–583.

Flynn, J. T. (2005). Hypertension in adolescents. *Adolescent Medicine, 16,* 11–29.

Freedman, D. S., Khan, L. K., Dietz, W. H., Srinivasan, S. R., & Berenson, G. S. (2001). Relationship of childhood obesity to coronary heart disease risk factors in adulthood: The Bogalusa Heart Study. *Pediatrics, 108*, 712–718.

Gungor, N., Hannon, T., Libman, I., Bacha, F., & Arslanina, S. (2005). Type 2 diabetes mellitus in youth: The complete picture to date. *Pediatric Clinics of North America, 52*, 1579–1609.

Gustaven, G. P., Claraco, A. E., Edelist, D. D., Chambers, C. V., Diamon, J. J., Besser, M., et al. (2003). A Single Segmental Electro-acupuncture treatment improves neuromuscular deficits in chronic functional ankle instability. *Medicine and Science in Sports and Exercise, 35*, S357.

Gutin, B., Barbeau, P., Owens, S., Lemmon, C. R., Bauman, M, Allison, J., et al. (2002). Effects of exercise intensity on cardiovascular fitness, total body composition and visceral adiposity of obese adolescents. *The American Journal of Clinical Nutrition,75*, 818–882.

Hansen, H. S., Froberg, K., Hyldebrandt, N., & Nielsen, J. R. (1991). A controlled study of eights months of physical training and reduction of blood pressure in children: The Odense school child study. *BMJ, 303*, 682–685.

Heinonen, A., Sievanen, H., Kannus, P., Oia, P., Pasanen, M., & Vuori, I. (2000). High-impact exercise and bones of growing girls: A 9-month controlled trial. *Osteoporosis International, 11*, 1010–1017.

Hilbert, J. E., Sforzo, G. A., & Swensen, T. (2001). The effects of massage on delayed onset muscle soreness. *Medicine and Science in Sports and Exercise, 33*, S123.

Hilbert, J. E., Sforzo, G. A., & Swensen, T. (2003). The effects of massage on delayed onset muscle soreness. *British Journal of Sports Medicine, 37*, 72–75.

Jenner, M. S., Spruijt-Metz, D., Bassin, S., & Cooper, D. M. (2004). A controlled evaluation of a school-based intervention to promote physical activity among sedentary adolescent females: Project FAB. *The Journal of Adolescent Health, 34*, 279–289.

Jastrow, J. (1892). Study of involuntary movements. *The American Journal of Psychology*, 398–407.

Jowdy, Murphy, Durschi, unpublished. Cited in Murphy S.

Karvelas, B. R., & Hoffman, M. D., & Zeni, A. I. (1996). Acute effects of acupuncture on physiological and psychological responses to cycle ergometry. *Archives of Physical Medicine & Rehabilitation, 77*, 1256–1259.

Kaufman, F. R. (2005). Type 2 diabetes in children and youth. *Endocrinology and Metabolism Clinics of North America, 34*, 659–676.

Kruisselbrink, D., & MacKinnon, D. D. (2006). Influence of positive and negative outcome images on the putting success of skilled amateur golfers. *Medicine and Science in Sports and Exercise, 38*, S229.

Kohrt, W. M., Bloomfield, S. A., Little, K. D., Nelson, M. E., & Yingling, V. R. (2004). Physical activity and bone health. *Medicine and Science in Sports and Exercise, 36*, 1985–1996.

Ludwig, D. S., Peterson, K. E., & Gortmaker, S. L. (2001). Relation between consumption of sugar-sweetened drinks and childhood obesity: A prospective observational analysis. *Lancet, 357*, 505–508.

Luepker, R. B., Jacobs, D. R., & Prineas, R. J. (1999). Secular trends of blood pressure and body size in a multi-ethnic adolescent population: 1986–1996. *The Journal of Pediatrics, 134*, 668–674.

Luma, G. B., & Spiotta, R. T. (2006). Hypertension in children and adolescents. *American Family Physician, 73*, 1158–1168.

Mancinelli, C. A., & Misty, B., Hendershot, A., Smith, C., & Stuchell, A. (2004). Effects of massage on delayed onset muscle sorenss and physical performance in female college athletes. *Medicine and Science in Sports and Exercise, 36*, S168.

Marcus, R. (2001). Role of exercise in prevention and treating osteoporosis. *Rheumatic Diseases Clinics of North America, 27*, 131–141.

Miller, A., & Donohue, B. (2003). The development and controlled evaluation of athletic mental preparation strategies in high school distance runners. *Journal of Applied Sport Psychology, 15,* 321–334.

Miyamoto, T. Acupuncture treatment for muscle injury. *Japanese Journal of Physical Fitness and Sports Medicine,* 1997, *43,* 39–41.

Moraska, A. (2005). Sports massage: A comprehensive review. *The Journal of Sports Medicine and Physical Fitness, 45,* 370–380.

Morgan, W. P., & Pollock, M. (1977). Psychologic characterization of the elite distance runner. *Annals of the New York Academy of Sciences, 301,* 382–403.

Morrison, J. A., Sprecher, D. L., & Barton, B. A. (1999). Overweight, fat patterning and cardiovascular disease risk factors in black and white girls: The National Heart, Lung and Blood Institute Growth and Health Study. *The Journal of Pediatrics, 114,* 963–967.

Murphy, S. M. (1994). Imagery interventions in sport. *Medicine and Science in Sports and Exercise, 26,* 486–494.

Must, A., & Strauss, R. S. (1999). Risks and consequences of childhood and adolescent obesity. *Journal of International Association for the Study of Obesity, 23,* S2–S11.

Nabkasorn, C., Miyai, N., Sootmongkol, A., Junprasert, S., Yamamoto, H., Arita, M., et al. (2006). Effects of physical exercise on depression, neuroendocrine stress hormones and physiological fitness in adolescent females with depressive symptoms. *European Journal of Public Health, 16,* 179–184.

National High Blood Pressure Education Program. (2004). The fourth report on the diagnosis, evaluation and treatment of high blood pressure in children and adolescents. Bethesda: National Heart, Lung and Blood Institute.

Nichols, A. W., & Harrigan, R. (2006). Complementary and alternative medicine usage by intercollegiate athletes. *Clinical Journal of Sport Medicine, 3,* 232–237.

Ogden, C. L., Carroll, M. D., Curtin, L. R., McDowell, M. A., Tabak, C. J., & Flegal, K. M. (2006). Prevalence of overweight and obesity in the United States, 1999–2004. *JAMA, 295,* 1549–1555.

Owens, S., Gutin, B., Allison, J., Riggs, S., Fergusion, M., Litaker, M., & Thompson, W. (1999). Effect of physical training on total and visceral fat in obese children. *Medicine and Science in Sports and Exercise, 31,* 143–148.

Pan, X. R., Li, G. W., & Hu, Y. H. (1997). Effects of diet and exercise in preventing NIDDM in people with impaired glucose tolerance: The DaQuing IGT and Diabetes Study. *Diabetes Care, 20,* 537–544.

Petersen, K., Silverstein, J., Kaufman, F., & Warren-Boulton, E. Management of type 2 diabetes in youth: An update. *American Family Physician, 76,* 658–664.

Pratt, H. D., & Tsitsika, A. K. (2007). Fetal, childhood, and adolescence interventions leading to adult disease prevention. *Primary Care, 34,* 203–217.

Psychological Issues Related to Injury in Athletes and the Team Physician: A Consensus Statement. (2006) *Medicine and Science in Sports and Exercise, 38*(11), 2034.

Richardson, A. (1969). *Mental imagery.* New York: Springer.

Riddoch, C., & Boreham, C. (2000). Physical activity, physical fitness and children's health: Current concepts. In N. Armstrong, W. van Mechelen (Eds.), *Pediatric exercise science and medicine* (pp. 243–252). Oxford: Oxford University Press.

Ritchie, L. D., Crawford, P. B., Hoelscher, D. M., & Sothern, M. S. (2006). Position of the American dietetic association: Individual-, family-, school, and community-based interventions for pediatric overweight *Journal of the American Dietetic Association, 106,* 925–945.

Rosenbloom, A. L., Joe, J. R., & Young, R. S. (1999). Emerging epidemic of type 2 diabetes in youth. *Diabetes Care, 22,* 345–354.

Sallis, J. (1993). Epidemiology of physical activity and fitness in children and adolescents. *Critical Reviews in Food Science and Nutrition, 33,* 403–408.

Shephard, R. J. (2004). Role of the physician in childhood obesity. *Clinical Journal of Sport Medicine, 14,* 161–168.

Sinaiko, A. R. Gomez-Marion. O., & Prineas, R. J. (1989). Prevalence of "significant" hypertension in junior high school-aged children. The children and adolescent blood pressure program. *The Journal of Pediatrics, 114,* 664–669.

Soroff, J. M., Poffenbarger, T., & Franco, K. (2002). Isolates systolic hypertension, obesity and hyperkinetic hemodynamic states in children. *The Journal of Pediatrics, 140,* 660–666.

Sothern, M. S., Loftin, J. M., Udall, J. N., Susking, R. M., Ewing, T. L., Tand, S. C., et al. (2000). Weight loss and growth velocity in obese children after very low calorie diet, exercise and behavior modification. *Acta Paediatrica, 89,* 1036–1043.

Strong, W. B., Malina, R. M., Bumkie, C. J., Daniels, S. R., Dishman, R. K., & Butin, B., et al. (2005). Evidence based physical activity for school-age youth. *The Journal of Pediatrics, 146,* 732–737.

Strong, J. P., Malcolm, G. T., & McMahan, C. A. (1999). Prevalence and extent of atherosclerosis in adolescents and young adults: Implications for prevention from the Pathobiological Determinants of Atherosclerosis in Youth Study. *JAMA, 281,* 727–735.

Suinn, R. M. (1983). Imagery and sports. In A. A. Sheikh (Ed.), *Imagery: Current theory, research, and applications* (pp. 507–534). New York: John Wiley and Sons.

Weiss, R., Dufour, S., & Falk-Petersen, K. (2002). Increased intramyocellular lipid content in obese adolescents with impared glucose tolerance. *Diabetes, 51*(suppl 2), A68.

Whitaker, R. C., Wright, J. A., Pepe, M. S., Seidel, K. D., & Dieta, W. H. (1997). Predicting obesity in young adulthood from childhood and parental obesity. N Engl J Med.; *337,* 869–873.

Woo, K. S., Chook, P., Yu, C. W., Sung, R. Y. T., Qiao, M., & Leung, S. S. F. (2004). Effects of diet and exercise on obesity-related vascular dysfunction in children. *Circulation, 109,* 1981–1986.

11

A Pediatric Perspective on Herbals and Supplements

PAULA GARDINER AND TIERAONA LOW DOG

KEY CONCEPTS

- Ask all your patients and their parents about herbal medicine use. (Provide examples of types of products, teas, foods, etc.)
- Advise parents and patients about the safety and effectiveness of the products they are using or are considering using.
- Dietary supplements (just like drugs) may have beneficial effects as well as expected and sometimes unanticipated toxicity.
- When you uncover a possible adverse effect associated with an herb, report it to the manufacturer and the FDA Medwatch Program.

■

Trends in Pediatric Herbal Medicine Use

Although recent national surveys indicate that the most common dietary supplement used by children is multivitamins, the prevalence of herbal medicine use by children and adolescents is not clear (Eichenberger Gilmore, Hong, Broffitt, & Levy, 2005; Ervin, Wright, & Reed-Gillette, 2004; Wilson et al., 2006). Several small regional and clinical surveys have reported on herbal medicine use. For example, among parents who report using complementary and alternative medicine (CAM), 40–45% gave their child an herbal product (Lanski, Greenwald, Perkins, & Simon, 2003; Ottolini et al., 2001; Sawni-Sikand, Schubiner, & Thomas, 2002). Several surveys have found that children with chronic conditions such as attention deficit hyperactivity disorder (ADHD), asthma, atopic dermatitis, allergic rhinitis, cancer, inflammatory bowel disease, and headache use herbal medicine (Angsten, 2000; Ball, Kertesz, & Moyer-Mileur, 2005; Chan, Rappaport, & Kemper, 2003; Gardiner, Dvorkin, & Kemper, 2004;

Heuschkel et al., 2002; Johnston, 2003; Mazur, De Ybarrondo, Miller, & Colasurdo, 2001; Orhan et al., 2003; Ottolini et al., 2001; Sinha & Efron, 2005a, 2005b; Slader, Reddel, Jenkins, Armour, & Bosnic-Anticevich, 2006). Reports from an inpatient holistic pediatric consultation service noted out of 70 consultations, 80% of patients had at least one question about a particular herb or dietary supplement (Kemper & Wornham, 2001). Lin et al. reported in a survey of 1021 pediatric patients undergoing surgery that 29.5% had indicated that they had tried one or more CAM therapies in the past year, and 12.8% had used herbal remedies prior to surgery. The most popular herbs included Echinacea, aloe, cranberry, St. John's wort, and goldenseal (Lin, Bioteau, Ferrari, & Berde, 2004).

It has also been noted that adolescents are consumers of herbal medicine and dietary supplements. One on-line survey of teens reported that ginseng, zinc, Echinacea, ginkgo, weight-loss supplements, and creatine were commonly used by the respondents (Wilson et al., 2006).

Many children and teens might be taking an over-the-counter or prescription medication concurrently with an herbal remedy. Despite the prevalence of patient use of herbal products, fewer than half of patients who use herbs typically discuss their use with their clinicians (Blendon, DesRoches, Benson, Brodie, & Altman, 2001; Leung, Dzankic, Manku, & Yuan, 2001). Therefore, it is critical to have an approach to discussing herb use with patients and/or their parents.

DESCRIPTION OF HERBAL MEDICINE

Herbal medicine, also known as phytotherapy, is a clinical modality that utilizes botanical remedies as part of a therapeutic approach. Since many herbal remedies have their origins in traditional medical systems that are hundreds, if not thousands of years old, the vast majority of evidence for their therapeutic activity has originated from direct human experience and observation. However, this picture is changing, due to rapidly expanding growth in the pharmacological research of plants and an increasing number of randomized, controlled clinical trials. Clinical trials are generally conducted on one individual herb, or phytopharmaceutical, that has been standardized to a particular marker compound and then studied for its effectiveness in a given condition. Examples of highly concentrated and standardized phytopharmaceuticals that have undergone considerable research include ginkgo (*Ginkgo biloba*), saw palmetto (*Serenoa repens*), and milk thistle (*Silybum marianum*).

While this is certainly a valid approach to studying botanical remedies, it could be easily argued that it does not truly reflect *the practice of herbal medicine*. Many herbalists object to the "standardized" approach of using one herb for one medical condition, claiming that each person must be individually treated according to their particular presentation and/or constitution. Indeed, one of the fundamental tenets of medical systems such as traditional Chinese medicine and Ayurveda is the individualization of treatment based upon the practitioner's differential diagnosis, that is, assessment of pulse, tongue, body type, and so forth. Each botanical preparation is then individually prepared for the patient's constitutional type and presenting complaint. This individual-ization of therapy generally extends beyond the choice of an herb or herbal formulation to a more generalized multi-modal approach to supporting the body's journey towards health. Dietary recommendations, exercise, lifestyle modifications, and stress manage-ment strategies are often recommended in addition to herbal therapy by most providers who use botanicals in their practice.

DEFINITIONS

With the recent marketing explosion of dietary supplements in North America, the majority of commercial herbal products are sold in solid dosage forms, such as tab-lets and capsules, though teas, tinctures and liquid extracts remain popular (Rotblatt, 1999). Teas (water extracts) have a long history of use but are often limited by taste and rapid spoilage (they have to be made fresh every day, or every 2–3 days if refrigerated). Hydroethanolic extracts, such as tinctures and fluid extracts are more concentrated and easier to administer, however, the alcohol content can be a problem for some children and many parents prefer glycerites. Herbal baths and lotions also have a long tradition of use with children (Table 11-1).

History of Herbal Medicine

The history of herbal medicine is universal, as plants have been used to heal the sick by peoples from all around the globe across the span of human time. Early humans learned which plants provided nourishment and could treat disease, as well as those that could harm or kill. Plants have been the primary source of medicine for millennia, and for this reason, one cannot discuss "herbal medicine" as if it existed outside the common medicine of a particular time in any given region.

From the formal, written treatises of Egypt, Greece, Rome, India, China, and the Middle East, to the rich oral traditions of Africa, Australia, and the Americas—plants have formed the basis of our pharmacopoeias and contributed greatly to our knowledge and understanding of illness and treatment. Herbal medicine gave rise to the fields of pharmacology, pharmacognosy and botany and up until the past 75 years, it provided the basis of the physician's apothecary.

How botanical medicines are viewed in the modern age depends, in part, upon which area of the world is being discussed. We can see the resurgence of herbal medicine as part of the complementary and alternative medicine movement in Europe, Canada, Australia, and the United States, while many in Asia, Africa, and South America still rely heavily upon local plants as a primary source of traditional medicine.

BRIEF REVIEW OF COMMON PEDIATRIC HERBS

There are few clinical trials and systematic reviews on the use of herbs with chil-dren (Charrois, Hrudey, & Vohra, 2006; Charrois, Sadler, & Vohra, 2007; Charrois,

Table 11-1. Types of Herbal Products

Pills, capsules, and tablets

An herb can be ground into a powder or made into a dried extract and placed in a pill, capsule, or tablet.

Teas, tisanes, infusions, or decoctions

An extraction prepared from fresh or dried flowers, leaves, or seeds that are steeped in hot water for 5–10 minutes. A decoction is simply a preparation made by simmering, instead of steeping the herbs.

Tinctures

An extraction of plant compounds (fresh or dried herb) in a calculated ratio of alcohol and water. Alcohol is a superior solvent to water. Alcohol content varies.

Glycerites and syrups

An extraction of plant compounds in a solution of glycerin. Glycerin is less efficient a solvent than alcohol but is often preferable in children's preparations.

Syrups are extracts, either tincture or strong infusions, that are typically sweetened and preserved with honey or sugar.

Foot, hand, or full body baths

Essentially, strong herbal infusions that are added to a pan or bath of water. Typically used to treat dermatological conditions or soothe an irritable child.

Skin Products such as balm, salve, ointments, creams

Salves and ointments are lipid-based preparations that are used for minor skin irritations and abrasions.

Lotions and creams are primarily water-based preparations making them more appropriate for weepy, irritated types of conditions.

Poultice/Compress

Poultices are moistened herbs that are applied directly to the skin or are wrapped in a cloth and applied. Compresses are prepared by soaking a cloth in a strong infusion and then applying the cloth to the affected part of the body.

Sandhu, & Vohra, 2006; Gardiner, 2007; Hrastinger, Dietz, Bauer, Sagraves, & Mahady, 2005; Shamseer, Charrois, & Vohra, 2006). Table 11-2 reviews commonly used herbs and their mechanism and recent trials in children.

It is worth mentioning that there is an increasing number of systematic reviews and meta-analyses where the data on both adults and children is combined. For example: the Cochrane collaboration and many other authors have published the following reviews: including Echinacea, garlic, gingko, ginger, and peppermint (Ackermann et al., 2001; Bhasale & Lissiman, 2007; Carlisle & Stevenson, 2007; Centre for Reviews and D., 2001, 2003, 2007a, 2007b, 2007c; Del-Rio-Navarro, Espinosa Rosales, Flenady, & Sienra-Monge, 2007; Huertas-Ceballos, Macarthur, & Logan, 2007; Jewell & Young, 2007; Linde, Barrett, Wolkart, Bauer, & Melchart, 2007; Liu, Yang, Liu, Wei, & Grimsgaard, 2007; Melchart, Linde, Fischer, & Kaesmayr, 2000; Pittler, Vogler, & Ernst, 2000; Quartero, Meineche-Schmidt, Muris, Rubin, & de Wit, 2007). While recognizing

Table 11-2. Commonly Used Pediatric Herbs

Herb	Mechanism of Action or Classification	Evidence based on Clinical Trials in Children and Adolescents
Aloe vera	Anti-inflammatory Antimicrobial Vulnerary	Effective topical vulnerary in treating leg ulcers, frostbite, and burn wounds.
Butterbur (*Petasites hybridus*)	Antispasmodic Anti-inflammatory Anti-histamine	Open label study showed reduction in migraine frequency in children and adolescents (6–17 years). Open trial of children and adults with asthma showed improvement of FEV1 and peak flow and reduction in medication use (Danesch, 2004; Pothmann, & Danesch, 2005).
German Chamomile (*Matricaria recutita*)	anti-inflammatory Antispasmodic Carminative Nervine Sedative Vulnerary	Chamomile/pectin combination has positive effects on diarrhea (Becker, Kuhn, & Hardewig-Budny, 2006; de la Motte, Bose-O'Reilly, Heinisch, & Harrison, 1997). Chamomile in combination with other herbs is effective for treating colic (Savino, Cresi, Castagno, Silvestro, & Oggero, 2005; Weizman, Alkrinawi, Goldfarb, & Bitran, 1993).
Garlic (*Allium sativum*)	Anti-inflammatory Antimicrobial Diaphoretic Diuretic Expectorant Hypoglycemic Hypotensive Lipid lowering	A randomized double-blind placebo controlled clinical trial found no change in cardiovascular risk factors compared to placebo in children with familial hyperlipidemia (McCrindle, Helden, & Conner, 1998).
Ginger (*Zingiber officinale*)	Antiemetic Antispasmodic Anti-viral Carminative Stimulates digestion	Clinical trials had mixed results for ginger as a treatment for motion sickness.
Ivy (*Hedera helix*)	Antispasmodic Expectorant Anticatarrhal	Small open studies show improved respiratory function in children with asthma. Large post-marketing surveillance study shows ivy leaf extract well tolerated in children (Hofmann, Hecker, & Volp, 2003).
Lemon balm (*Melissa officinalis*)	Antispasmodic Anxiolytic Calmative Digestive aid	One study showed a sleep promoting effect of the combination valerian and lemon balm (Fazio, Pouso, & Dolinsky, 2006; Muller & Klement, 2006).

(continued)

Table 11-2. (Continued)

Herb	Mechanism of Action or Classification	Evidence based on Clinical Trials in Children and Adolescents
Peppermint (*Mentha piperita*)	Antimicrobial Digestive aid Carminative Antispasmodic	Enteric-coated peppermint oil capsules appear helpful in the treatment of irritable bowel syndrome/spastic colon (Kline, Kline, Di Palma, & Barbero, 2001).
Purple Cone Flower (*Echinacea angustifolia* or *E. purpurea*)	Anti-inflammatory Antimicrobial Antiseptic Immune modulator	A recent randomized placebo controlled trial of 524 children with upper respiratory tract infection found no significant difference in duration or symptoms of those receiving Echinacea purpurea (Taylor et al., 2003).

the value of meta-analyses in the medical literature, it is important to point out one potential problem with this approach in the field of herbal medicine—the "pooling" of different products to reach a specific conclusion about a particular plant. For example, when comparing products that differ in extraction technique, plant part, delivery system, and dose—it makes the question of equivalency a very valid one. So what does the conclusion of a systematic review or meta-analysis of all clinical trials of Echinacea mean when the pooled studies include products containing *Echinacea purpurea*, fresh-pressed juice from the aerial parts of the plant, *Echinacea purpurea* root, *Echinacea pallida* root, *Echinacea angustifolia* root, or any combination thereof, using different solvents in differing doses. When one evaluates these products from an analytical perspective, there are clearly significant differences between *E. purpurea* fresh-pressed juice and *E. angustifolia* root hydroethanolic extract. This makes any conclusion about efficacy (or lack thereof) questionable.

Safety Considerations in Pediatric Herb Use

INTRODUCTION

There are definite reasons to be cautious in the use of medicine, including herbal medicine, in children and adolescents. Children and adolescents are undergoing formative physical and neurological development and their metabolism and clearance of drug and botanical compounds are not the same as adults. When recommending an herb for any age group, it is important to review the safety profile, looking specifically for adverse effects, contraindications, mechanism of action (if known), safety in pregnancy and lactation, interactions with medications, and history of contamination or adulteration.

Like any chemically active substance, whether an herb is safe or toxic depends on the dose, form of product, what it is taken with, and the underlying constitution of the child or adolescent. Overall, most herbs in general commerce in the United States have relatively good safety profiles, and the incidence of herbal adverse events are infrequent. In a 6-month survey of 1183 telephone calls to a California poison control center on dietary supplement exposures, half the calls involved children. Dietary supplement-related adverse events (including all supplements, not just botanicals) were reported in 134 children (28%) (Dennehy, Tsourounis, & Horn, 2005).

There are a few herbs to be aware of, such as mistletoe, lobelia, digitalis, ephedra and pennyroyal essential oil, which can cause severe, potentially life-threatening adverse effects. The chronic use of other herbs, such as comfrey, chaparral, and licorice can cause severe hepatic, renal, or electrolyte abnormalities. As with medications, even when an herb is safe when used correctly, it can cause mild or severe toxicity when used incorrectly. For example, tea tree essential oil is quite safe when used topically for minor infections of the skin but if taken orally, it can cause unconsciousness in small children (Morris, Donoghue, Markowitz, & Osterhoudt, 2003).

CONTAMINATION AND MISIDENTIFICATION

The World Health Organization noted that there were approximately 8000 case reports of adverse effects from herbs from 1968 to 1997. One hundred of these were in children under 10 years of age and 100 were adolescents (Ernst, 2003). Most of the evidence is anecdotal in nature, and frequently adverse effects are caused not by the supplements themselves, but rather by contaminants. The issue of contamination and adulteration is a real concern as more and more case reports on pediatric poisonings arise in the literature (Ko, 2006; Roche, Florkowski, & Walmsley, 2005; Woolf & Woolf, 2005).

Herbal products may be unintentionally or intentionally contaminated with bacteria, heavy metals, pesticides, herbicides, medications, or the other supplements (Ernst, 2003; Ize-Ludlow et al., 2004; Moore & Adler, 2000; Sas, Enrione, & Schwartz, 2004). For example, concern has been raised regarding the adulteration of Chinese star anise (*Illicium verum*), a popular colic remedy, with Japanese star anise *I anisatum*), which has led to recalls in Spain, France, Scotland, China, Japan, and Netherlands (Ize-Ludlow et al., 2004). Japanese star anise (*Illicium anisatum*) is well-documented to cause both neurologic and gastrointestinal toxicities. These effects are thought to be caused by secondary metabolites that act as potent neurotoxins, such as anisatin, neoanisatin, and pseudoanisatin.

Several studies and case reports have shown products with toxic levels of mercury, cadmium, or lead, either from unintentional contamination during manufacturing or from intentional additions by producers who believe these metals have therapeutic value (Kauffman et al., 2007; Linke, 2004; Raman, Patino, & Nair, 2004; Roche, Florkowski, & Walmsley, 2005; Saper et al., 2004; Woolf & Woolf, 2005). Additionally, even small amounts of heavy metals that would not affect the health of an adult can be toxic to the developing brain of an infant or toddler.

In the future, concerns of contamination or adulteration of pediatric products could be less of a concern. In June of 2007, the US Food and Drug Administration (FDA) released long-awaited "good manufacturing practices" (GMPs) for the dietary supplement industry in the United States.

The rule ensures that dietary supplements are produced in a quality manner, do not contain contaminants or impurities, and are accurately labeled. GMPs will do the following:

- Ensure quality throughout the manufacturing, packaging, labeling, and storing of dietary supplements.
- Put in place quality control procedures and guidelines for testing ingredients and the finished product.
- Require recordkeeping and handling consumer product complaints (FDA, 2007).

When discussing safety of herbs for children and adolescents, it is important to look at the framework of the Dietary Supplement and Health Education Act (DSHEA), which influences how herbal products are sold and marketed to parents and adolescents (FDA). Unlike pediatric prescription medications, DSHEA allows herbal supplements which entered the market prior to 1994, to be marketed without prior approval of their efficacy and safety by the Food and Drug Administration (FDA). Manufacturers are permitted to claim that the product affects the structure or function of the body, as long as there is no claim of effectiveness for the prevention or treatment of a specific disease. If the claim is to "enhance gastrointestinal health of a baby," it can be sold on the market. There need not be any infant colic clinical trials for the gastrointestinal health claims or trials on dosing for infants.

To report a drug herb interaction or an adverse effect contact MedWatch, a program administered by the FDA. Another excellent resource is to contact your local poison control centers; the new nationwide toll-free number for poison control is 800-222-1222.

PRESCRIPTION MEDICATIONS

Very little is known about the safety of combining herbs with pharmaceutical drugs in the pediatric population. It is common for children taking prescription or over-the-counter medication to use dietary supplements including herbals. A survey of 117 parents of children and adolescents with ADHD or depression, demonstrated that 15% had used herbal medicine in the last year. Almost 83% of caregivers gave herbal medicines alone and 13% gave them with prescription drugs. Most caregivers (78%) supervised the administration of herbal therapy in their children; the children's psychiatrists (70%), pediatricians (56%), or pharmacists (74%) typically were not aware of use (Cala, Crismon, & Baumgartner, 2003).

While there is limited evidence of harm from this practice in the adult population, certain herbs and drugs are known to interact. Thus, it is best to follow safety guidelines similar to those for adults to avoid potentially harmful herb–drug interactions.

Training/Accreditation/Licensure

Naturopathic physicians and acupuncturists can prescribe herbal therapies under their licensure; however unlike Europe, and specifically Great Britain, there is no standard training or credentialing program for herbalists in the United States. The American Herbalist Guild (AHG) is the only peer-reviewed organization in the United States for professional herbalists specializing in the medicinal use of plants. To attain status as a professional member, an individual must successfully undergo an admissions review process by a group of peers to assure that a relatively high level of competency, education, and experience has been attained. AHG members have specific continuing education requirements and must adhere to a code of ethics. Professional AHG members can be identified by the term "Herbalist AHG" or simply "AHG" after their name. Like many groups, herbalists are a diverse group of professionals, with differing views on a number of topics that deal with both philosophical and practical concerns. While the science of phytomedicine is growing, the practice of herbal medicine is often empirical and art-based.

Dosing

The type of herbal preparation a clinician chooses to use depends upon a variety of considerations including the patient, acute or chronic nature of the medical problem, personal preferences and medicinal properties of the herb. For example, valerian tea can be unpleasant tasting for many children—a tincture or capsule may represent a better chance of adherence to therapy.

When it comes to dosing of herbal therapies, there is little consistency across the myriad of products found in the marketplace. This leaves consumers confused about how much to take and practitioners confused about how much to recommend. Unless one is familiar with using herbal medicines, it is probably best to start by looking at the clinical trials that have been conducted on an herbal product, whether it was conducted in children or adults or both in children and adults. Here you can find out the product studied, the dose used, and side effects reported in the trials. The majority of herbal clinical trials have been conducted on standardized extracts in solid dosage forms (capsules and tablets). There are also some resources on line that can help you find a recommended dose range for herbs, especially those that have not been subjected to clinical trials but are in common usage.

Talking with Families about Herbal Medicine

There are many reasons why parents might choose to give their children herbal medicine. In some families there may be a strong cultural or folk medicine use of herbs in children. Other reasons may include socioeconomic status, parental beliefs surrounding healing and wellness, or dissatisfaction with conventional approaches, especially with chronic medical conditions. Most parents are self-prescribers for their families and obtain their information about herbs from friends, family, lay healers, the popular press, and the Internet (Lanski, Greenwald, Perkins, & Simon, 2003). Most parents do not get information about herbal therapies from their providers and surveys consistently show that few parents even discuss their children's use of herbs with their physicians (Martin, Jordan, Vassar, & White, 2002; Sawni-Sikand, Schubiner, & Thomas, 2002).

Healthcare providers must be able to engage in dialogue with parents and patients about a wide variety of treatment options, including herbal medicine. Because there is the potential for both benefit and harm, it is important that providers approach the topic of herb usage in an open and non-judgmental way. By asking a few open-ended questions, a provider should be able to assess the parents' and patient's beliefs and cultural practices regarding their use of herbal medicines.

- When you were growing up, did you or your family ever use any medicinal plants or herbal remedies? For example: did your parents or grandparents make teas, soups, rubs, or baths?
- How do you use herbal remedies in with your children?
- Are you using any herbs or herbal medicines for your child now? If so, what are you trying to treat and do you think the herbs are working?

A FEW CASE EXAMPLES OF HERBAL MEDICINE IN PEDIATRICS

CASE #1

Karen is a 10-year-old with a 3-year history of recurrent abdominal pain that has gotten worse over the past 4 months. She complains of peri-umbilical abdominal pain that is dull and crampy, not accompanied by nausea or vomiting but sometimes she has diarrhea; occurring 4 to 5 days per week and lasting up to 2 to 3 hours. The pain sometimes makes her stop what she is doing so that she can lie down. The timing is not related just to school days, but also to social events that she looks forward to attending. She has good grades, though she has missed quite a few days due to pain. She has a good appetite, normal bowel movements and has not had any weight loss or inappropriate weight gain. After speaking with Karen and her parents, there is no evidence to suggest that she is malingering or manipulating the situation for secondary gain.

Three months ago Karen underwent an endoscopy and colonoscopy, both of which were entirely normal. Celiac antibody panel, food allergy testing and other routine screening labs were also normal. After a 1-month trial of lansoprazole had no effect, Karen was started on tegaserod, which has also had no effect.

This is an excellent example of a case that would likely respond well to an integrative approach that could include botanicals. We will not discuss mind-body approaches or nutrition since these are covered in other chapters of this text.

Enteric-coated peppermint oil capsules may help Karen, as one study in children (ages 8–17) with recurrent abdominal pain/irritable bowel syndrome showed decreased pain compared to placebo (Kline et al., 2001). Capsules generally come in 0.2 ml of oil and the dose is 1 capsule taken 3 times daily for those >45 kg. The clinical trial used 0.1 ml 3 times daily for children under 45 kg, A systematic review of peppermint oil capsules (mostly in adults) showed the herb to be superior to placebo in 8 of 12 studies and equivalent to smooth muscle relaxants in 3 trials (Grigoleit, 2005). Other essential oils with excellent gut anti-spasmodic activity include thyme and caraway, which are often combined with peppermint oil.

Chamomile (Matricaria recutita) is considered by most herbal practitioners to be the premiere herb for functional abdominal pain and soothing an anxious child. Two studies have shown chamomile with pectin to relieve diarrhea in children, which might be of benefit for Karen. Lemon balm (Melissa officinalis) is another herb commonly used in pediatrics for functional abdominal pain, colic, and to relieve anxiety. Though both of these herbs have a long history of use in children, other than basic science, one study in infantile colic (using a combination of herbs) and the two studies of chamomile/pectin for diarrhea, there is little contemporary research to validate their effectiveness. They have excellent safety profiles (other than extremely rare allergic reactions to chamomile) and can be used as tea or glycerites. Products containing chamomile and pectin are available for purchase in the United States.

CASE #2

Juan is a 5-year-old boy who presents to your office with his mother today because of frequent upper respiratory infections. He started kindergarten

6 months ago and has had 4 to 5 colds "running from one to the next" ever since. Mom says he has a persistently runny nose and sometimes coughs at night. She has not noticed any wheezing or difficulty running or playing. He has a history of middle ear infections (2–3 per year) since he was about 1 year old. Juan lives with non-smoking parents and his 9-year-old brother who had a tonsillectomy last year for "chronic sore throats." There are no pets in the house because his mom has asthma and is allergic to pet dander. Juan eats cereal with milk for breakfast, peanut butter/jelly sandwich, cookies and chocolate milk for lunch, and some form of meat with vegetables for dinner. He takes no supplements and is not currently on any medication. On physical exam his TMs are dull but mobile; turbinates inflamed, moderate yellow discharge. No sinus tenderness. Small, firm cervical nodes. Mom is frustrated with the repeated rounds of antibiotics and wants to try "a more natural approach."

Again, this is an example of a child that could be helped considerably with an integrative approach, with particular attention being paid to his diet (i.e., food allergies/sensitivities), recommending a multivitamin and Omega-3 fatty acid, and so forth. Again, though, we will limit our comments to botanical medicines.

The most commonly used herbal medicine for URI in children is Echinacea (Echinacea spp). This native North American herb has a long history in treating respiratory ailments in both adults and children. There have been numerous studies in adults demonstrating that Echinacea purpurea can shorten the duration and reduce the severity of the common cold. The study of E. purpurea in children ages 2 to 11 years (Tayler 2003) did not show any affect on acute URI compared to placebo; however, the use of Echinacea was associated with a 28% decreased risk of subsequent URI suggesting a possible protective effect (Weber et al., 2005). There were no significant adverse events, though there were more cases of rash in the Echinacea than placebo group. Most herbal practitioners consider Echinacea to be a safe and highly effective herb for the treatment of acute URI in children. Glycerites are available, many of them pleasantly flavored.

Thyme (Thymus vulgaris) is perhaps one of the most respected herbs for the treatment of upper respiratory infection, cough, and congestion, being approved for such by the German health authorities. While there are no studies looking at thyme as a monotherapy for colds, it has some data showing that the combination with ivy is effective in children (2–17 years) with acute bronchitis and productive cough (Marzian, 2007). Ivy (Hedera helix) has a number of small trials and a large post-marketing surveillance study indicating that it has good safety in children 4 years and older (Hecker, Runkel, & Voelp, 2002). Syrups of thyme and ivy are available in the United States.

Other herbs that might be considered by herbalists in this case, given his mother's history of asthma and allergies, include Chinese skullcap (Scutellaria baicalensis), an herb that is often used for the treatment of eczema, hay fever, and allergic rhinitis; and nettles (Urtica dioica), which has one small study in adults showing relief of allergic rhinitis but is often used in children due to its excellent safety profile (Mittman, 1990).

And finally, the use of hypertonic nasal saline irrigation is considered mainstay by many conventional practitioners today. Sometimes a few drops of tea tree essential oil are added to the mixture as an anti-bacterial agent, especially in those with recurrent sinus infections.

Hypertonic Nasal Saline Irrigation

1 pint clean jar with lid

Fill jar with bottled water

Add 1½ tsp of salt

Add ½ tsp baking soda

Add 5 drops tea tree oil.

Store at room temperature and shake before each use.

REFERENCES

Ackermann, R. T., Mulrow, C. D., Ramirez, G., Gardner, C. D., Morbidoni, L., & Lawrence, VA. (2001, March). Garlic shows promise for improving some cardiovascular risk factors [see comment]. *Archives of Internal Medicine, 161*(6), 813–824.

Angsten, J. M. (2000, October). Use of complementary and alternative medicine in the treatment of asthma. *Adolescent Medicine, 11*(3), 535–546.

Ball, S. D., Kertesz, D., & Moyer-Mileur, L. J. (2005, January). Dietary supplement use is prevalent among children with a chronic illness. *Journal of the American Dietetic Association, 105*(1), 78–84.

Becker, B., Kuhn, U., & Hardewig-Budny, B. (2006). Double-blind, randomized evaluation of clinical efficacy and tolerability of an apple pectin-chamomile extract in children with unspecific diarrhea. *Arzneimittel-Forschung, 56*(6), 387–393.

Bhasale, A., & Lissiman, E. (2007). Garlic for the common cold [Protocol]. *Cochrane Database of Systematic Reviews, 2007*(3).

Blendon, R. J., DesRoches, C. M., Benson, J. M., Brodie, M., & Altman, D. E. (2001, March). Americans' views on the use and regulation of dietary supplements. *Archives of Internal Medicine, 161*(6), 805–810.

Cala, S., Crismon, M. L., & Baumgartner, J. (2003, February). A survey of herbal use in children with attention-deficit-hyperactivity disorder or depression. *Pharmacotherapy, 23*(2), 222–230.

Carlisle, J. B., & Stevenson, C. A. (2007). Drugs for preventing postoperative nausea and vomiting [Systematic Review]. *Cochrane Database of Systematic Reviews, 2007*(3).

Centre for Reviews and D. (2001). Review: Herbal preparations may improve FEV_1 and symptoms in asthma [Therapeutics] The efficacy of ginseng: A systematic review of randomised clinical trials (Structured abstract). *ACP Journal Club, 134*(3), 96.

Centre for Reviews and D. (2003). Review: Herbal medicinal products seem to be effective and safe in nonulcer dyspepsia [Therapeutics] Peppermint oil for irritable bowel syndrome: A critical review and metaanalysis (Structured abstract). *ACP Journal Club, 139*(2), 43.

Centre for Reviews and D. (2007a). A meta-analysis of intervention effectiveness for symptom management in oncology nursing research (Structured abstract). *Database of Abstracts of Reviews of Effects.* 2007(3).

Centre for Reviews and D. (2007b). Efficacy of ginger for nausea and vomiting: A systematic review of randomized clinical trials (Structured abstract). *Database of Abstracts of Reviews of Effects,* 2007(3).

Centre for Reviews and D. (2007c). The efficacy of ginger for the prevention of postoperative nausea and vomiting: A meta-analysis (Structured abstract). *Database of Abstracts of Reviews of Effects,* 2007(3).

Chan, E., Rappaport, L. A., & Kemper, K. J. (2003, February). Complementary and alternative therapies in childhood attention and hyperactivity problems. *Journal of Developmental and Behavioral Pediatrics, 24*(1), 4–8.

Charrois, T. L., Hrudey, J., & Vohra, S. (2006, October). American Academy of Pediatrics Provisional Section on Complementary HaIM. Echinacea. *Pediatrics in Review, 27*(10), 385–387.

Charrois, T. L., Sadler, C., & Vohra, S. (2007, February). American Academy of Pediatrics Provisional Section on Complementary HaIM. Complementary, holistic, and integrative medicine: St. John's wort. *Pediatrics in Review, 28*(2), 69–72.

Charrois, T. L., Sandhu, G., & Vohra, S. (2006, April). Probiotics. *Pediatrics in Review, 27*(4), 137–139.

Danesch U. (2004). Petasites hybridus (Butterbur root) extract in the treatment of asthma—an open trial. *Alternative Medicine Review, 9,* 54–62.

de la Motte, S., Bose-O'Reilly, S., Heinisch, M., & Harrison, F. (1997, November). [Double-blind comparison of an apple pectin-chamomile extract preparation with placebo in children with diarrhea]. *Arzneimittel-Forschung, 47*(11), 1247–1249.

Del-Rio-Navarro, B. E., Espinosa Rosales, F., Flenady, V., & Sienra-Monge, J. J. L. (2007). Immunostimulants for preventing respiratory tract infection in children [Systematic Review]. *Cochrane Database of Systematic Reviews,* 2007(3).

Dennehy, C. E., Tsourounis, C., & Horn, A. J. (2005, July). Dietary supplement-related adverse events reported to the California Poison Control System. *American Journal of Health-System Pharmacy, 62*(14), 1476–1482.

Eichenberger Gilmore. J. M., Hong, L., Broffitt, B., & Levy, S. M. (2005, May). Longitudinal patterns of vitamin and mineral supplement use in young white children. *Journal of the American Dietetic Association, 105*(5), 763–772; quiz 773–764.

Ernst, E. (2003, February). Serious adverse effects of unconventional therapies for children and adolescents: A systematic review of recent evidence. *European Journal of Pediatrics, 162*(2), 72–80.

Ervin, R. B., Wright, J. D., & Reed-Gillette, D. (2004). Prevalence of leading types of dietary supplements used in the Third National Health and Nutrition Examination Survey, 1988–94. *Advance Data, 349,* 1–7.

Fazio, S., Pouso, J., & Dolinsky, D. (2006, July). Tolerance, safety and efficacy of Hedera helix extract in inflammatory bronchial diseases under clinical practice conditions: A prospective, open, multicentre postmarketing study in 9657 patients. *Phytomedicine, 20.*

FDA. (2007, June). Dietary Supplement Current Good Manufacturing Practices and Interim Final Rule Facts. http://www.cfsan.fda.gov/~dms/dscgmps6.html

FDA. Dietary Supplement Health and Education Act.

Gardiner, P. (2007, April). Complementary, holistic, and integrative medicine: Chamomile. *Pediatrics in Review, 28*(4), e16–e18.

Gardiner, P., Dvorkin, L., & Kemper, K. J. (2004, April). Supplement use growing among children and adolescents. *Pediatric Annals, 33*(4), 227–232.

Grigoleit, H. (2005). Peppermint oil in irritable bowel syndrome. *Phytomedicine, 12*(8), 601–606.

Hecker, M., Runkel, F., & Voelp, A. (2002, April). [Treatment of chronic bronchitis with ivy leaf special extract—multicenter post-marketing surveillance study in 1,350 patients]. *Forsch Komplementarmed Klass Naturheilkd, 9*(2), 77–84.

Heuschkel, R., Afzal, N., Wuerth, A., Zurakowski, D., Leichtner, A., Kemper, K., et al. (2002, February). Complementary medicine use in children and young adults with inflammatory bowel disease. *The American Journal of Gastroenterology, 97*(2), 382–388.

Hofmann, D., Hecker, M., & Volp, A. (2003, March). Efficacy of dry extract of ivy leaves in children with bronchial asthma—a review of randomized controlled trials. *Phytomedicine, 10*(2–3), 213–220.

Hrastinger, A., Dietz, B., Bauer, R., Sagraves, R., & Mahady, G. (2005, March). Is there clinical evidence supporting the use of botanical dietary supplements in children? *The Journal of Pediatrics, 146*(3), 311–317.

Huertas-Ceballos, A., Macarthur, C., & Logan, S. (2007). Pharmacological interventions for recurrent abdominal pain (RAP) in childhood [Systematic Review]. *Cochrane Database of Systematic Reviews.* 2007(3).

Ize-Ludlow, D., Ragone, S., Bruck, I. S., Bernstein, J. N., Duchowny, M., & Pena, B. M. (2004, Novemeber). Neurotoxicities in infants seen with the consumption of star anise tea. *Pediatrics, 114*(5), e653–e656.

Jewell, D., & Young, G. (2007). Interventions for nausea and vomiting in early pregnancy [Systematic Review]. *Cochrane Database of Systematic Reviews,* 2007(3).

Johnston, G. (2003). The use of complementary medicine in children with atopic dermatitis in secondary care in Leicester. *The British Journal of Dermatology, 149*(3), 566.

Kauffman, J. F., Westenberger, B. J., Robertson, J. D., Guthrie, J., Jacobs, A., & Cummins, S. K. (2007, July). Lead in pharmaceutical products and dietary supplements. *Regulatory Toxicology and Pharmacology, 48*(2), 128–134.

Kemper, K. J., & Wornham, W. L. (2001, April). Consultations for holistic pediatric services for inpatients and outpatient oncology patients at a children's hospital. *Archives of Pediatrics & Adolescent Medicine, 155*(4), 449–454.

Kline, R. M., Kline, J. J., Di Palma, J., & Barbero, G. J. (2001, January). Enteric-coated, pH-dependent peppermint oil capsules for the treatment of irritable bowel syndrome in children. *Journal of Pediatrics, 138*(1), 125–128.

Ko, R. (2006). Safety of ethnic & imported herbal and dietary supplements. *Clinical Toxicology: The Official Journal of the American Academy of Clinical Toxicology & European Association of Poisons Centres & Clinical Toxicologists, 44*(5), 611–616.

Lanski, S. L., Greenwald, M., Perkins, A., & Simon, H. K. (2003, May). Herbal therapy use in a pediatric emergency department population: Expect the unexpected. *Pediatrics, 111*(5 Pt 1), 981–985.

Leung, J. M., Dzankic, S., Manku, K., & Yuan, S. (2001, October). The prevalence and predictors of the use of alternative medicine in pre-surgical patients in five California hospitals. *Anesthesia and Analgesia, 93*(4), 1062–1068.

Lin, Y.C., Bioteau, A. B., Ferrari, L. R., & Berde, C. B. (2004, February). The use of herbs and complementary and alternative medicine in pediatric preoperative patients. *Journal of Clinical Anesthesia, 16*(1), 4–6.

Linde, K., Barrett, B., Wolkart, K., Bauer, R., & Melchart, D. (2007). Echinacea for preventing and treating the common cold [Systematic Review]. *Cochrane Database of Systematic Reviews, 2007*(2).

Linke, S. (2004, April). [Chronic lead poisoning caused by Ayurvedic health pills]. *Deutsche Medizinische Wochenschrift, 129*(16), 910; author reply 910.

Liu, J. P., Yang, M., Liu, Y. X., Wei, M. L., & Grimsgaard, S. (2007). Herbal medicines for treatment of irritable bowel syndrome [Systematic Review]. *Cochrane Database of Systematic Reviews, 2007*(3).

Martin, K. J., Jordan, T. R., Vassar, A. D., & White, D. B. (2002, Decemeber). Herbal and non-herbal alternative medicine use in Northwest Ohio. *The Annals of Pharmacotherapy, 36*(12), 1862–1869.

Marzian, O. (2007). Treatment of acute bronchitis in children and adolescents. Non-interventional postmarketing surveillance study confirms the benefit and safety of a syrup made of extracts from thyme and ivy leaves. *MMW Fortschritte der Medizin, 149*(11), 69–74.

Mazur, L. J., De Ybarrondo, L., Miller, J., & Colasurdo, G. (2001, June). Use of alternative and complementary therapies for pediatric asthma. *Texas Medicine, 97*(6), 64–68.

McCrindle, B. W., Helden, E., & Conner, W. T. (1998, November). Garlic extract therapy in children with hypercholesterolemia. *Archives of Pediatrics & Adolescent Medicine, 152*(11), 1089–1094.

Melchart, D., Linde, K., Fischer, P., & Kaesmayr, J. (2000). Echinacea for preventing and treating the common cold. *Cochrane Database of Systematic Reviews, 2000*(2), CD000530.

Mittman, P. (1990). Randomized, double-blind study of freeze-dried Urtica dioica in the treatment of allergic rhinitis. *Planta Medica, 56*(1), 44–47.

Moore, C., & Adler, R. (2000, September). Herbal vitamins: Lead toxicity and developmental delay. *Pediatrics, 106*(3), 600–602.

Morris, M. C., Donoghue, A., Markowitz, J. A., & Osterhoudt, K. C. (2003, June). Ingestion of tea tree oil (Melaleuca oil) by a 4-year-old boy. *Pediatric Emergency Care, 19*(3), 169–171.

Muller, S. F., & Klement, S. (2006, June). A combination of valerian and lemon balm is effective in the treatment of restlessness and dyssomnia in children. *Phytomedicine, 13*(6), 383–387.

Orhan, F., Sekerel, B. E., Kocabas, C. N., Sackesen, C., Adalioglu, G., & Tuncer A. (2003, June). Complementary and alternative medicine in children with asthma. *Annals of Allergy, Asthma & Immunology, 90*(6), 611–615.

Ottolini, M. C., Hamburger, E. K., Loprieato, J. O., Coleman, R. H., Sachs, H. C., Madden, R., et al. (2001, March–April). Complementary and alternative medicine use among children in the Washington, DC area. *Ambulatory Pediatrics, 1*(2), 122–125.

Pittler, M. H., Vogler, B. K., & Ernst, E. (2000). Feverfew for preventing migraine. *Cochrane Database of Systematic Reviews, 2000*(3):CD002286.

Pothmann, R., & Danesch, U. (2005, March). Migraine prevention in children and adolescents: Results of an open study with a special butterbur root extract. *Headache, 45*(3), 196–203.

Quartero, A. O., Meineche-Schmidt, V., Muris, J., Rubin, G., & de Wit, N. (2007). Bulking agents, antispasmodic and antidepressant medication for the treatment of irritable bowel syndrome [Systematic Review]. *Cochrane Database of Systematic Reviews, 2007*(3).

Raman, P., Patino, L. C., & Nair, M. G. (2004, December). Evaluation of metal and microbial contamination in botanical supplements. *Journal of Agricultural and Food Chemistry, 52*(26), 7822–7827.

Roche, A., Florkowski, C., & Walmsley, T. (2005, July). Lead poisoning due to ingestion of Indian herbal remedies. *The New Zealand Medical Journal, 118*(1219), U1587.

Rotblatt, M. D. (1999, September). Cranberry, feverfew, horse chestnut, and kava. *The Western Journal of Medicine, 171*(3), 195–198.

Saper, R. B., Kales, S. N., Paquin, J., Burns, M. J., Eisenberg, D. M., & Davis, R.B., et al. (2004). Heavy metal content of ayurvedic herbal medicine products. *JAMA, 292*(23), 2868.

Sas, D., Enrione, M. A., & Schwartz, R. H. (2004, February). Pseudomonas aeruginosa septic shock secondary to "gripe water" ingestion. *The Pediatric Infectious Disease Journal, 23*(2), 176–177.

Savino, F., Cresi, F., Castagno, E., Silvestro, L., & Oggero, R. (2005, April). A randomized double-blind placebo-controlled trial of a standardized extract of Matricariae recutita, Foeniculum vulgare and Melissa officinalis (ColiMil) in the treatment of breastfed colicky infants. *Phytotherapy Research, 19*(4), 335–340.

Sawni-Sikand, A., Schubiner, H., & Thomas, R. L. (2002, Mar–April). Use of complementary/alternative therapies among children in primary care pediatrics. *Ambulatory Pediatrics, 2*(2), 99–103.

Shamseer, L., Charrois, T. L., & Vohra, S. (2006, December). American Academy of Pediatrics Provisional Section on Complementary HaIM. Complementary, holistic, and integrative medicine: Garlic. *Pediatrics in Review, 27*(12), e77–e80.

Sinha, D., & Efron, D. (2005a). Complementary and alternative medicine use in children with attention deficit hyperactivity disorder. *Journal of Paediatrics and Child Health.* Blackwell Publishing, Melbourne, Australia (1/2, 23–26).

Sinha, D., & Efron, D. (2005b, January–February). Complementary and alternative medicine use in children with attention deficit hyperactivity disorder. *Journal of Paediatrics and Child Health, 41*(1–2), 23–26.

Slader, C. A., Reddel, H. K., Jenkins, C. R., Armour, C. L., & Bosnic-Anticevich, S. Z. (2006, July). Complementary and alternative medicine use in asthma: Who is using what? *Respirology, 11*(4), 373–387.

Taylor, J. A., Weber, W., Standish, L., Quinn, H., Goesling, J., McGann, M., et al. (2003, December). Efficacy and safety of echinacea in treating upper respiratory tract infections in children: A randomized controlled trial. *JAMA, 290*(21), 2824–2830.

Weber, W., Taylor, J. A., Stoep, A. V., Weiss, N. S., Standish, L. J., & Calabrese, C. (2005, December). Echinacea purpurea for prevention of upper respiratory tract infections in children [see comment]. *Journal of Alternative & Complementary Medicine, 11*(6), 1021–1026.

Weizman, Z., Alkrinawi, S., Goldfarb, D., & Bitran, C. (1993). Efficacy of herbal tea preparation in infantile colic [see comments]. *The Journal of Pediatrics, 122*(4), 650–652.

Wilson, K. M., Klein, J. D., Sesselberg, T. S., Yussman, S. M., Markow, D. B., Green, A. E., et al. (2006, April). Use of complementary medicine and dietary supplements among U.S. adolescents. *The Journal of Adolescent Health, 38*(4), 385–394.

Woolf, A. D., & Woolf, N. T. (2005, August). Childhood lead poisoning in 2 families associated with spices used in food preparation. *Pediatrics, 116*(2), e314–e318.

12

A Pediatric Perspective on Homeopathy

DAVID RILEY, MENACHEM OBERBAUM, AND
SHEPHERD ROEE SINGER

KEY CONCEPTS

- The discipline of homeopathy identifes three key principles: law of Similars, individualization of therapy, and the minimum dose.
- Homeopathic medicines (single remedies or combination remedies) are prepared by a unique pharmaceutical production process involving serial dilutions alternating with vigorous shaking or succussion.
- Homeopathy is regulated as drug therapy by the FDA and has been since the 1938 Food, Drug, and Cosmetic Act (FDCA).
- There are several main styles of homeopathic practice; one dispenses primarily a single homeopathic medicine based on the total symptom picture of a patient. Another involves using single or complex homeopathic medicines administered for clinical situations related to conventional diagnoses.
- There is a small but robust research portfolio for homeopathy ranging from basic science to clinical research and it is continuing to grow today around the world.

■

Introduction

Homeopathy is a 200-year-old system of medicine based on the principle of "*Similia similibus curentur*," treating like with like. Homeopathy employs high dilutions of natural substances with the intention of inducing a healing response. The source of these "remedies" is chiefly botanical, mineral, or animal. Homeopathy is generally safe, as might be expected, considering the miniscule doses employed.

Homeopathy is used widely in the United States, by both adults and children. It is estimated that more than 20,000 healthcare providers either prescribe or recommend homeopathy for their patients. In spite of this widespread use, homeopathy remains controversial, particularly in the conventional medical community. This stems primarily from the lack of a plausible mechanism to explain its biological activity. That said, a small but growing body of research supports the activity of homeopathic dilutions, in cellular and animal models, as well as in humans.

Background

THE PRINCIPLES OF HOMEOPATHY

Homeopathy is based upon three primary principles. The first is the *Principle of Similarity*: "Similia similibus curentur" ("Let like be cured by like"). First stated by the German physician Samuel Hahnemann in 1796, this principle implies that substances capable of causing signs and symptoms in healthy subjects are capable of curing sick individuals expressing those same signs and symptoms. Hippocrates recognized the importance of "like-things" in pathogenesis and cure (Hippocrates), but never converted the concept into practice. Likewise, the concept is mentioned in the traditional medical systems of India and China. Homeopathy is a holistic form of medicine that views health as a dynamic process. Homeopathic medicines are purported to stimulate the body's self-regulatory mechanisms and cure, not only the patients chief complaint, but also underlying malaise and maladies, which the patient may have forgotten or ignored.

The second homeopathic principle is that of *individualization of treatment*. In homeopathy, particularly in the "classic" form (see below), great effort is invested in gleaning the finer characteristics of the patient, in health and illness, in order to prescribe a medicine as similar as possible to his/her current state. In its most exacting form This individualization may take place at the level of the "whole person," taking account of the signs and symptoms of disease, the patient's physical build, personality, temperament, and genetic predispositions. However, this level of individualization is not always required. In acute conditions, "similarity" at a more specific, physical level, may suffice.

The third principle central to the practice of homeopathy is that of the *minimum dose*. Homeopaths may infrequently employ "crude" (undiluted) doses of indicated remedies, but the hallmark of homeopathy is the use of high dilutions. Homeopathic dilutions may in fact range from 1/100 of the initial solution to dilutions far beyond Avogadro's number, that is, unlikely to contain a single molecule of the initial substance. These may be termed "ultra-molecular" dilutions. Though considered by many the "hallmark" of homeopathy, these high dilutions were, in fact, an afterthought of Hahnemann's, intended to minimize the side effects of the large doses in use in his era.

No comprehensive explanation yet exists for the ostensible effect of these dilutions. This apparent lack of plausibility no doubt hinders homeopathy's broader acceptance.

HOMEOPATHIC PHARMACOLOGY

Homeopathic medicines, termed remedies, are derived predominantly from botanical, mineral, or animal sources. Details of their preparation, first delineated by Hahnemann in the early 1800s, are precisely defined in the FDA-recognized "Homeopathic Pharmacopoeia of the United States" (HPUS). Remedy production begins with a concentrated "mother tincture" for soluble substances, or a "triturate," for insoluble ones. A triturate is prepared by successively grinding the desired substance (e.g., a metal) with lactose powder, until sufficiently "dissolved" to allow suspension in a liquid medium. In either case, the resulting solution is subject to serial dilutions alternating with vigorous shaking (succussion). This process is known as potentization, and the resulting product, potencies. Once the initial substance has been chosen, (in accordance with the principle of individualization), two factors remain to be determined: the dilution scale, and the number of repetitions. The most commonly employed dilution scales are the decimal (1:10) and centesimal (1:100), designated "D" and "C," respectively. The initial solution is diluted with water by 1:10 or 1:100 and vigorously shaken (succussed). The resulting dilute is diluted by the same factor and again shaken. This process is repeated until the predetermined "potency" (i.e., number of repetitions) has been reached. Once a dilution scale has been chosen, that scale is maintained throughout preparation of the remedy. Homeopathic potencies are designated by a number and letter, referring to the number of repetitions and dilution scale. The mother tincture (denoted "Ø") may be administered undiluted. More commonly it is "potentiated." Typical dilutions are 3D, 6D, 9D, up to 30D (decimal dilutions typically being used for the lower potencies) whereas typical centesimal potencies are 30C, 200C, 1000C, and above. Avogadro's number (6.02×10^{23}), that is, the statistical probability that even a single molecule of the initial substance remains in the dilute, is surpassed at 12C or 24D. If the entire universe were put in a test tube and diluted to 40C, a milliliter of the dilute would be unlikely to contain a single atom.

Homeopathic medicines are marketed under two broad categories: "single" and "complex." Single homeopathic medicines are composed from an individual initial substance. Complex homeopathic medicines are fixed combinations of homeopathic medicines, potentiated separately but later combined, typically for a given clinical indication (i.e., Asthma or headache).

HOMEOPATHIC PRESCRIBING

There are several distinct styles of homeopathic practice. The two main types are "classical" and "clinical." In classical homeopathy, a single homeopathic medicine is commonly selected on the basis of the total symptom picture of a patient, including mental, general, and constitutional features. This is then prescribed in ultra-dilution, and repeated infrequently. In clinical homeopathy, one or more single or complex homeopathic medicines are administered for clinical situations pertaining to conventional diagnoses. Potencies are generally lower and often repeated several times a day. Homeopathic complexes are prescribed or purchased OTC for specific conventional diagnoses and are commonly used in clinical homeopathy. In addition to their strictly "homeopathic" use, homeopathic medicines are employed in other therapeutic approaches such as anthroposophic medicine and homotoxicology.

"Isopathy" is a distinct but related modality. By this method, the medicine prescribed is not "similar" but *exactly the same*. For example, a case of streptococcal pharyngitis might be treated with the streptococcus bacteria, denatured and highly diluted. This is not strictly in accordance with the "law of similars," which prescribes based upon *similarity of signs and symptoms*. Various types of herbal or natural healing modalities borrow the term homeopathy, though they employ none of homeopathy's basic principles (law of similars, dilution, and individualization).

SAFETY

Homeopathy is considered one of the safest modalities in complementary and alternative medicine (CAM). The medical literature contains no reference to adverse effects of remedies diluted beyond 6C. There are isolated instances of adverse reactions to lower dilutions (i.e., crude or nearly crude substances), however these were always due to substandard quality of care. Homeopathy may cause an initial aggravation of symptoms, but this is generally regarded as a favorable early response, and subsides over time.

While there are challenges relating to under-reporting and mistaken identity (i.e., herbal medicines identified as homeopathic), the level of direct risk resulting from the use of homeopathic medicinal products is probably extremely low (Dantas & Rampes, 2000).

Use of Homeopathy

GLOBAL USE

Homeopathy and other CAM therapies have enjoyed sustained growth since the early 1960s. Homeopathy is among the five most widely used CAM therapies in the United States, and enjoys popularity in high-, medium-, and low-income countries. India boasts over 200,000 registered practitioners, more than 150 homeopathic universities and over 300 homeopathic hospitals (Department of Ayush, 2007). Homeopathy is widely practiced in Europe, North, Central, and South America, and has been integrated into the national healthcare systems in many of these countries (WHO, 2001).

Use in the United States

Children, adolescents, and their families use homeopathy. Their use of homeopathy depends on characteristics of the population in question: age, state of health, socio-economic background or ethnic background. Recent national surveys in the United States have revealed that more than 20%–40% of all children and 20%–30% of adolescents in the United States have used or are using alternative medicine products (Ervin, 1999, 2004; Yu, 1997). The 1999–2000 NHANES reported that approximately 1 in 4 adolescents ages 12 to 15 used CAM products, with higher rates for those between the age of 16 and 19 (Briefel, 2004).

In 1996 Vincent identified reasons that patients seek complementary therapies, including homeopathy. These included a positive value associated with complementary treatment, the ineffectiveness of orthodox treatment for their complaint, concern about the adverse effects of orthodox medicine, concerns about communication with doctors and, finally, the availability of complementary medicine. Homeopathy patients were most strongly influenced by the ineffectiveness of orthodox medicine for their complaints. Astin (Jain, 2001) found that people are less likely to use CAM, including homeopathy, if they believe that the therapies are in general ineffective or inferior to conventional methods or if they perceive that their conventional physician does not support the use of CAM.

There are many reasons why parents give their children homeopathic remedies, including maintaining health, preventing disease, and treating a chronic or acute disease. Additionally, several clinical surveys have demonstrated a strong cultural or folk medicine use in children (Pachter, 1998). It is important to be aware of why families and patients are using these homeopathic preparations, in order to make effective recommendations. Parents get their information from numerous places: friends, family, popular press, the Internet, and finally, healthcare professionals. In 2003, of the 142 families surveyed in an ER, 45% of these caregivers reported giving their child an herbal product. Of those who used CAM therapies, 80% reported either friends or relatives as their primary source of information. Only 45% of those giving their children CAM products reported discussing the use with their child's primary health care provider (Lanski, 2004). This low rate of disclosure of CAM use has been noted repeatedly.

Regulation of Homeopathy

Homeopathy is not a recognized medical profession in the United States. Three states, Arizona, Connecticut, and Nevada, license physicians to practice homeopathy.

Nationwide, most practitioners are not physicians, and their medical training is variable. Dozens of schools teach homeopathy, but the level of training is not uniform. A few national organizations offer voluntary certification, but no literature exists comparing the proficiency of certified versus uncertified practitioners.

Homeopathic remedies in the United States are regulated as drugs under the 1938 Federal Food Drug and Cosmetic Act (FFDCA), which defines "drugs" as "articles recognized in...the official Homeopathic Pharmacopeia of the United States (HPUS); and articles intended for use in the diagnosis, cure, mitigation, treatment, or the prevention of disease in man.... Whether or not they are official homeopathic remedies, those products offered for the cure, mitigation, prevention, or treatment of disease conditions are regarded as drugs within the meaning of Section 201(g)(l) of the FFDCA. Homeopathic drugs must also comply with the labeling provisions of Sections 502 and 503 of the [FFDCA] and Part 201 Title 21 of the Code of Federal Regulations (CFR)...." In practice, homeopathic medicines can be obtained OTC in most states.

Homeopathic Training

Homeopathic training among licensed health care providers in the United States is most commonly pursued as a post-graduate training activity and varies considerable in content and quality. The physician practice of homeopathy is directly regulated in three states (Arizona, Connecticut, and Nevada) and naturopathic physicians receive training in homeopathy in their medical school curriculum. Schools and organizations that provide post-graduate training in various aspects of homeopathy for a variety of licensed health care providers included: the Arizona Medical College of Homeopathy, the International Academy for Homotoxicology (IAH), the New England School of Homeopathy, and the Seattle School of Homeopathy.

Efficacy

In light of the questionable physical plausibility of such extreme dilutions inducing a physiological response, the burden of evidence would appear to rest firmly at the feet of the homeopathic community. Historically, homeopathy has employed internal measures of efficacy, and has not invested itself in objective scientific evaluation. Few homeopaths or supporters of homeopathy are trained in scientific research methods. Furthermore, because most homeopathic medicines are derived from natural sources and have been known for decades, they are un-patentable, therefore undermining the financial incentive to support research. Finally, editors of respectable medical journals have historically been reluctant to publish positive homeopathic findings, possibly for fear of being marginalized. In spite of these limitations, a growing number of clinical and basic science trails have demonstrated a statistically significant effect of homeopathic medications. We will discuss the realm of homeopathic research in the following pages.

Table 12-1. Levels of Scientific Evidence, as Recognized by the WHO (2001)

Evidence Category	Source of Evidence
Ia	Systematic review of randomized controlled trials
Ib	At least one randomized controlled trial
IIa	At least one well-designed, quasi-experimental trial
IIb	At least one type of well-designed quasi-experimental study
III	Well-designed non-experimental descriptive studies (e.g., comparative studies, correlation studies)
IV	Expert committee reports from respected authorities

Homeopathic Research

The call to arms of medical research at the turn of the millennium has become "evidence-based medicine" (EBM). EBM ranks scientific research by type, allocating the greatest value to randomized controlled trials (RCTs) and systematic reviews based thereupon. "Lesser" forms of research are evoked when these are unavailable. The World Health Organization and many regulatory agencies use the following guidelines for evaluating evidence (WHO, 2001; Table 12-1).

While homeopathy is still far from being able to claim itself a "proven therapy," much work has been done, and moderate success attained, in moving a previously esoteric treatment modality closer to the scientific limelight. We will discuss the status of homeopathic research in the area of basic science and clinical research, particularly in relationship to pediatric medicine.

BASIC SCIENCE RESEARCH

Basic science research in homeopathy has advanced in two main areas: physical research on ultra-molecular dilutions, and in vitro or in vivo biological models of the action of ultra-molecular dilutions and their potential mechanisms of action. A comprehensive database of basic research in homeopathy, the Homeopathy Basic Research Experiments ("HomBRex") Database, is available at http://www.carstens-stiftung.de/hombrex/index.php (Albrecht, van Wijk, & Dittloff, 2002). This database contains information on experiments on biological systems in vivo and in vitro, in healthy or diseased states, ranging from the intact organism to the subcellular level, with measures of effect ranging from viability to molecular processes; and research on physico-chemical effects of serial dilution and succussion (potentization).

CLINICAL RESEARCH

Some 200 randomized controlled clinical trials on homeopathy have been published in the peer-reviewed medical literature. Of those, about 15 have focused on the pediatric population.

Pediatric indications for which objective research exists supporting a role for homeopathy include: ADHD, otitis, influenza, radiation-induced stomatitis. It should be noted at this point that, while homeopathy is commonly employed for a wide range of pediatric indications, only a selected few are supported by evidence other than anecdotal.

Clinical Trials in Homeopathy

Homeopathy is frequently prescribed for children with behavioral disorders. However, research to support the practice is very new. In a study of children suffering from ADHD, patients received homeopathy or placebo for 6 weeks, and then crossed over to receive placebo or verum for a second period of 6 weeks (Frei et al., 2005). A standard rating scale was used, and the results showed a significant improvement in the homeopathic treatment group.

One of the most common pediatric indications seen in homeopathic clinics is otitis media. A placebo-controlled trial of homeopathy for otitis media in children (Jacobs, 2001) demonstrated a significant effect in the homeopathic treatment group at 24 and 64 hours. In a related trial, children suffering from chronic serous otitis media were randomized to receive either homeopathy or standard care. A significantly higher proportion of children receiving homeopathy had normal tympanograms at 12 months than in the standard care group (Harrison, 1999). Friese (1997) compared homoeopathic and conventional medicines in 103 children with acute otitis media. Median duration of pain was 2 days in the homeopathy group, as compared with 3 days in the conventional group. Seventy percent of the homeopathy group were free of recurrence in the following year, as compared with 56% of those treated conventionally.

It should be noted that in all of these studies, homeopathic treatment was individualized; thus, it is not possible to state "such-and-such" remedy is effective for the given indication. It can only be stated that *homeopathy as a method* was superior to placebo or conventional care.

The following studies investigated *complex* homeopathy; in these trials, a single complex was administered to all "verum" recipients. Homeopathy in the treatment of influenza has been investigated in two large randomized controlled clinical trials of *Anas barbariae hepatis et cordis extractum* (*Oscillococcinum*®) (Ferley, 1989; Papp, 1998). Symptoms were significantly reduced in the verum group at 48 hours as compared with placebo.

Oberbaum (2001) has demonstrated a statistically significant reduction in chemotherapy-induced stomatitis in children using *Traumeel S*® liquid during stem cell transplantation (p <0.01), and this therapy is currently under investigation in a second clinical trial conducted under the auspices of the National Cancer Institute. Zell (1988) evaluated the same homeopathic remedy, Traumeel, applied topically for ankle sprains, and found that by day 10 ankle had normalized in 51.5% of patients in the verum group as compared with 25.0% in the placebo group (p = 0.03).

Systematic Reviews

Four major meta-analyses to date have purported to review all available research to evaluate the effectiveness of homeopathy as a system. *The Lancet* published a meta-analysis (Linde et al., 1997) analyzing 89 placebo-controlled studies of homeopathy. The overall mean odds ratio for these 89 clinical trials was 2.45 (95% confidence interval 2.05–2.93) in favor of homeopathy. This indicated that the chance of homeopathy being useful was 2–3 times greater than placebo. Even after correction for several potential confounders the results remained statistically significant. The authors concluded that the results "were not compatible with the hypothesis that the effects of homoeopathy are completely due to placebo." Several systematic reviews have been positive for homeopathy with relevance for the pediatric population. They include childhood diarrhea (Jacobs, 2003), influenza (Vickers, 2006), post-operative ileus (Barnes, 1997), seasonal allergic rhinitis (Taylor, 2000), vertigo (Schneider, 2005), and rheumatic diseases (Jonas, 2000).

Four meta-analyses of the available homeopathic research performed over the last two decades, have reached conflicting conclusions; however, these appear to reflect more about the article inclusion criteria than any over-arching conclusion.

RESEARCH CHALLENGES IN HOMEOPATHY

Patient Preference

The use of homeopathy, particularly in clinical research, is often associated with strong patient preference issues. The challenges of recruitment where subjects refuse to be randomized can, to some extent, be controlled statistically, however homeopathy, already under intense scientific scrutiny, can ill afford to rely upon assailable study designs.

Specific and Non-specific Effects

It is near-axiomatic in many conventional circles that any benefit of CAM therapies can be attributable only to "non-specific" effects. A major line of criticism of homeopathy, as with other CAM modalities, is that any salubrious effect these methods may have is likely due to these "agent-independent" effects. Many conventional physicians attribute the surge in interest in CAM to the "longer time spent with patients," "greater attention to the individual," and "having someone who really listens." These criticisms may sound particularly appropriate for homeopathy, with its long visits, individualized interviews, and penchant for minutiae. It is not unreasonable to wonder if any apparent effects of homeopathy, or other CAM modalities, are merely non-specific responses to the personable nature of these modalities. Teasing apart the specific from the non-specific remains a major challenge facing homeopathic research.

Chronic Illness

Many patients seeking herbal or homeopathic treatment suffer from chronic illnesses, and hope for long-term cure rather than short-lived symptom control. In chronic illness, any change is likely to be slow. Studies focused on short-term improvement will to miss long-term effects. However, long-term follow up is expensive, even by conventional medical standards, and is thus rarely performed as part of an RCT.

Individualization

Therapeutic intervention using dietary supplements and homeopathic medicines are often individualized. Homeopathy in particular is often highly individualized: the same homeopathic remedies are not prescribed for all patients with the same clinical diagnosis. Therefore, some of the better homeopathic studies can compare only "homeopathy-as-a-method" with control. Conventional clinicians (and editors) will find it frustrating that after a long a drawn-out trail, the researchers cannot present a single remedy as "effective" for a given indication.

Funding and Skepticism

In common with many other forms of CAM/TM, homeopathy lacks research funding and infrastructure. This is due, in part, to the fact that most dietary supplements and homeopathic medicines are generic and there are no intellectual property rights or patents available. Few practitioners of homeopathy have interest or training in conventional research techniques. Finally skepticism limits academic collaboration and editor willingness to publish.

INTERACTIONS WITH CONVENTIONAL MEDICINE

Homeopathic medicines are not known to interact, chemically or pharmacologically, with conventional pharmacological agents. This would be unlikely, given the extreme dilutions employed. That stated, homeopathic treatment may "interact" with conventional medical therapy in several important ways. It therefore behooves physicians to be versed in and inquire about patient use of CAM.

Homeopathy may employ any of more than 3000 natural substances as the basis for treatment. However, because these agents do not interact chemically or pharmacologically with conventional drugs, it is not necessary for the physician to be familiar with the action of any agent specifically.

Patients undergoing homeopathic treatment often undergo an "initial aggravation," that is, the patients' symptoms may worsen transitorily. In the eyes of the homeopath,

Homeopathy in Practice

The various homeopathic interactions differ greatly one from the other, and from conventional medical interactions.

"Modern" homeopathy is the branch of homeopathy most similar to conventional medicine, and indeed the most frequently intermingled with it. Most practitioners of this branch of homeopathy are conventionally trained physicians who employ homeopathy in their daily practice. Modern homeopathy employs conventional medical diagnoses, and prescribes one or several homeopathic remedies, in conjunction with, or in lieu of, conventional medicines. The potencies used are typically low, in the 3D–12C range, and repetition is usually tid or qid. Though no literature has clearly addressed the question, it is presumed that modern homeopathy is more appropriate for acute indications, and less so for chronic.

"Complex" homeopathy is most reminiscent of OTC self-care, though there are practitioners who deal in this form of homeopathy. "Complexes" are combinations of homeopathic remedies considered effective for a given indication. These may be pre-packaged and sold under propriety trade names, or prescribed by practitioner. In the latter instance, the "complex" can be tailored to meet the patient's outstanding diagnostic characteristics.

Classical homeopathy is the form farthest removed from convention medical practice. In most western nations, the large majority of classical homeopaths are not physicians. Patients are seen for an initial visit, typically 60 to 90 minutes long, during which the homeopath investigates various aspects of the patient's illness and characteristics, with emphasis on the idiosyncratic. The prescription may entail a single dose of medicine. Follow-up visits may occur once every month or two, at which a new prescription is likely to be made. The length of treatment is, of course, proportional to the severity of the disease. Many common pediatric problems (recurrent otitis media, asthma, recurrent streptococcal pharyngitis), may be cured within a period of 3–6 months.

this is viewed as a desirable "healing crisis." However, the physician, unaware that his patient is undergoing homeopathic treatment, may be alarmed at a sudden and unexplained exacerbation of symptoms. Open communication with the patient and/or his/her homeopath would likely assuage such concerns.

Lay homeopaths may perceive that conventional medications interfere with the action of the homeopathic prescription. Unversed in the power of these medications, they may be tempted to reduce or eliminate prescribed medications before undertaking homeopathic prescribing. This is both dangerous and illegal, and should be vehemently proscribed. Open disclosure by patients would help avert such transgressions.

Finally, on a hopeful note, if, as many perceive, homeopathy is indeed effective, patients may be cured or symptoms significantly ameliorated, beyond the expectations the physician may have from his own treatment. Physicians should be alert to the possibility of reducing or discontinuing medications as they become superfluous.

Conclusion

Use of homeopathy among the many CAM modalities is on the rise. Many pediatric patients and their families, especially those with chronic or recurrent conditions, turn to homeopathy for hope of cure, avoidance of side-effects, or the appeal of the holistic approach. Primary care physicians, the first who should know of such choices, are not always informed. Homeopathy is generally safe, and some evidence exists to support its use in certain pediatric indications. Some problems may arise from lack of communication with patient and practitioner. Health care practitioners should be encouraged to question their patients about CAM usage, and to help their patients balance the level of evidence of efficacy with safety, personal preference or belief, and the medical condition under treatment.

REFERENCES

Albrecht, van Wijk, & Dittloff. (2002). Homeopathy Basic Research Experiments ('HomBRex') Database http://www.carstens-stiftung.de/hombrex/index.php

Barnes, J., Resch, K.-L., & Ernst, E. (1997). Homeopathy for postoperative ileus? A meta-analysis. *Journal of Clinical Gastroenterology, 25*, 628–633.

Briefel, R. R., & Johnson. C. L. (2004). Secular trends in dietary intake in the United States. *Annual Review of Nutrition, 24*, 401.

Dantas, F., & Rampes, H. (2000). Do homeopathic medicines provoke adverse effects? A systematic review. *British Homeopathic Journal, 89*(Suppl 1), S35–S38.

Department of AYUSH (Ayurveda, Yoga & Naturopathy, Unani, Siddha and Homoeopathy). Ministry of Health & Family Welfare, Government of India.

Ferley, J. P., Poutignat, A., Azzopardi, Y., Charrel, M., & Zmirou, D. (1987). Evaluation in ambulatory medicine of the effect of a homeopathic complex remedy in the prevention of flu and flu-like syndromes. *Immunologie Médicale, 20*, 22–28.

Ferley, J. P., Zmirou, D., D'Adhemar, D., & Balducci, F. (1989). A controlled evaluation of a homoeopathic preparation in the treatment of influenza like syndromes. *British Journal of Clinical Pharmacology, 27*, 329–335.

Friese, K.-H., Kruse, S., Lüdtke, R., & Moeller, H. (1997). The homoeopathic treatment of otitis media in children—comparisons with conventional therapy. *International Journal of Clinical Pharmacology and Therapeutics, 35*, 296–301.

Hippocrates: On the place of things which regard man. Basel, Froben: 1538, p. 72.

Jacobs, J., Jimenez, L. M., Gloyd. S. S., Gale, J. L., & Crothers, D. (1994). Treatment of acute childhood diarrhea with homoeopathic medicine—A randomized clinical trial in Nicaragua. *Pediatrics, 93,* 719–725.

Jacobs, J., Jonas, W. B., Jimenez-Perez, M., & Crothers, D. (2003). Homeopathy for childhood diarrhea: Combined results and metaanalysis from three randomized, controlled clinical trials. *Pediatric Infectious Disease Journal, 22,* 229–234.

Jacobs, J., Springer, D., & Crothers, D. (2001). Homeopathic treatment of acute otitis media in children: A preliminary randomized placebo-controlled trial. *Pediatric Infectious Disease Journal, 20,* 177–183.

Jain, N., & Astin, J. A. (2001). Barriers to acceptance: an exploratory study of complementary/alternative medicine disuse. *Journal of Alternative and Complementary Medicine, 7,* 689–696.

Jonas, W. B., Kaptchuk, T. J., & Linde, K. (2003). A critical overview of homeopathy. *Annals of Internal Medicine, 138,* 393–399.

Jonas, W. B., Linde. K., & Ramirez, G. (2000). Homeopathy and rheumatic disease. *Rheumatic Disease Clinics of North America, 26,* 117–123.

Lanski, S. L., Greenwald, M., Perkins, A., et al. (2003). Herbal therapy use in a pediatric emergency department population: Expect the unexpected. *Pediatrics, 111,* 981.

Lewith, G. T., Watkins, A. D., Hyland, M. E., Shaw, S., Broomfield, J. A., Dolan, G., et al. (2002). Use of ultramolecular potencies of allergen to treat asthmatic people allergic to house dust mite: Double blind randomized controlled clinical trial. *British Medical Journal, 324,* 520–523.

Linde, K., Clausius, N., Ramirez, G., Melchart, D., Eitel, F., Hedges, L. V., et al. (1997). Are the clinical effects of homeopathy placebo effects? A meta-analysis of placebo-controlled trials. *Lancet, 350,* 834–843.

Linde, K., Jonas, W. B., Melchart, D., Worku, F., Wagner, H., & Eitel, F. (1994). Critical review and meta-analysis of serial agitated dilutions in experimental toxicology. *Human & Experimental Toxicology, 13,* 481–492.

Linde, K., Scholz, M., Ramirez, G., Clausius, N., Melchart, D., & Jonas, W. B. (1999). Impact of study quality on outcome in placebo controlled trials of homeopathy. *Journal of Clinical Epidemiology, 52,* 631–636.

Mathie, R. T. (2003). The research evidence base for homeopathy: A fresh assessment of the literature. *Homeopathy, 92,* 84–91.

Oberbaum, M., Yaniv, I., Ben-Gal, Y., Stein, J., Ben-Zvi, N., Freedman, L. S., et al. (2001). A randomized, controlled clinical trial of the homeopathic medication Traumeel S in the treatment of chemotherapy-induced stomatitis in children undergoing stem cell transplantation. *Cancer, 92,* 684–690.

Pachter, L. M., Sumner, T., Fontan, A., et al. Home-based therapies for the common cold among European American and ethnic minority families: the interface between alternative and complementary and folk medicine. *Archives of Pediatrics & Adolescent Medicine, 152*(11), 1083–1088.

Papp, R., Schuback, G., Beck, E., Burkard, G., Bengel, J., Lehrl, S., et al. (1998). Oscillococcinum® in patients with influenza-like syndromes: A placebo controlled double-blind evaluation. *British Homeopathic Journal, 87,* 69–76.

Reilly, D. T., Taylor, M. A., Beattie, N. G. M, & Campbell, J. H. (1994). Is evidence for homeopathy reproducible? *Lancet, 344,* 1601–1606.

Reilly, D. T., Taylor, M. A., McSharry, C., & Aitchison, T. (1986). Is Homeopathy a placebo response? Controlled trial of homoeopathic potency—with pollen in hay fever as model. *Lancet, ii,* 881–886.

Riley, D., Fisher, M., Sigh, B., Haidvogl, M., & Heger, M. (2001). Homeopathy and conventional medicine: An outcomes study comparing effectiveness in a primary care setting. *Journal of Alternative and Complementary Medicine, 7*, 149–159.

Schneider, B., Klein, P., & Weiser, M. (2005). Treatment of vertigo with a homeopathic complex remedy compared with usual treatments: A meta-analysis of clinical trials. *Arzneimittel-Forschung, 55*, 23–29.

Steinsbekk, A., Bentzen, N., Fønnebø, V., & Lewith, G. (2005). Self treatment with one of three self selected, ultramolecular homeopathic medicines for the prevention of upper respiratory tract infections in children. A double-blind randomized placebo controlled trial. *British Journal of Clinical Pharmacology, 59*, 447–455.

Steinsbekk, A., Fønnebø, V., Lewith, G., & Bentzen, N. (2005). Homeopathic care for the prevention of upper respiratory tract infections in children: A pragmatic, randomized, controlled trial comparing randomized homeopathic care and waiting-list controls. *Complementary Therapies in Medicine, 13*, 231–238.

Taylor, M. A., Reilly, D., Llewellyn-Jones, R. H., McSharry, C., & Aitchison, T. C. (2000). Randomized controlled trials of homeopathy versus placebo in perennial allergic rhinitis with overview of four trial series. *British Medical Journal, 321*, 471–476.

Vincent, C., & Furnham, A. (1996). Why do patients turn to complementary medicine? An empirical study. *British Journal of Clinical Psychology, 35*, 37–48.

Weiser, M., Gegenheimer, L., & Klein, P. (1999). A randomized equivalence trial comparing the efficacy and safety of Luffa comp.-Heel nasal spray with cromolyn sodium spray in the treatment of seasonal allergic rhinitis. *Forschende Komplementärmedizin, 6*, 142–148.

Weiser, M., Strösser, W., & Klein, P. (1998). Homeopathic vs conventional treatment of vertigo—A randomized double-blind controlled clinical study. *Archives of Otolaryngology, 124*, 879–885.

Wiesenauer, M., & Lüdtke, R. (1996). A meta-analysis of the homeopathic treatment of pollinosis with Galphimia glauca. *Forschende Komplementärmedizin und Klassische Naturheilkunde, 3*, 230–236.

Wiesenauer, M., Gaus, W., & Häussler, S. (1990). Treatment of pollinosis with Galphimia glauca. A double-blind trial in clinical practice. *Allergologie, 13*, 359–363.

World Health Organization. (2001). *Legal Status of Traditional Medicine and Complementary/Alternative Medicine: a Worldwide Review.* Geneva, World Health Organization (document reference WHO/EDM/TRM/2001.2)

Zell, J., Connert, W. D., Mau, J., & Feuerstake, G. (1988). Treatment of acute sprains of the ankle. Controlled double-blind trial to test the effectiveness of a homeopathic ointment. *Fortschritte der Medizin, 106*, 96–100.

13

A Pediatric Perspective on Massage

SHAY BEIDER, ERIN T. O'CALLAGHAN, AND JEFFREY I. GOLD

KEY CONCEPTS

- Massage is one of the oldest treatment modalities in existence and has been used cross culturally for thousands of years.
- Touch and massage are widely used in the general population and are increasing in popularity.
- Health care professionals and those they treat will benefit from a fundamental understanding of massage and its clinical applications in order to educate, advise, and consult with their patients.
- There are a variety of massage techniques, each with unique guiding principles, methodologies, and outcomes.
- Touch and massage have been shown to have a role in neurobiological and immune alterations, with recent interest focused on the psychoneuroimmunologic response.
- Massage is used for a variety of health-related purposes including the treatment of specific conditions/diseases and general health and wellness.
- There appear to be few risks associated with massage if it is appropriately applied and provided by a trained massage professional.

■

Introduction

Massage therapy (MT) is part of a growing trend in integrative medicine use in the United States and represents one of the most widely used complementary and alternative medicine (CAM) therapies. Almost one quarter of adults in the United States have reported that they had a massage at least once in the last 12 months (American Massage Therapy Association [AMTA] Massage Therapy Industry

Fact Sheet, 2008). Nineteen percent of adults in the United States report discussing MT with their doctors or health care providers and 58% of those said that their physician strongly recommended or encouraged MT (AMTA Consumer Survey, 2007). MT usage in hospitals is also increasing in popularity. From 2004 to 2006, the number of hospitals offering MT increased by 30% (American Hospital Association, 2006). Hospital-based programs indicate that they offer MT for patient stress management and comfort (71%) and for pain management (67%) (American Hospital Association, 2006). According to the Rosenthal Center for Complementary and Alternative Medicine (June, 2007), 36 states offer CAM courses at U.S. medical schools, undergraduate, postgraduate, and continuing medical education programs. As MT use has increased in adult populations, it has similarly increased in pediatric populations. A study on the use of CAM practices among children found that 33% of parents reported using CAM for their child within the past year and that MT was one of the most popular therapies selected (Loman, 2003). A study of CAM use among families of children with special health care needs found that these families are almost twice as likely to have used CAM for their child (Sanders et al., 2003). Clearly, there is a growing interest in the field of pediatric MT that is likely to increase over time.

SCOPE OF CHAPTER

This chapter will provide an overview of pediatric MT. The goal is for the reader to gain insight and understanding into the current state of MT for children and adolescents. This chapter aims to provide (1) a history of MT, (2) definitions of MT/therapeutic techniques, (3) professional standards, training, and licensure, (4) theories and proposed mechanisms of action, (5) current research evidence, (6) clinical applications, (7) safety, and (8) conclusions.

History of Massage

Massage and healing touch have existed in various cultures across the world for thousands of years.[1] Archaeological evidence suggests that the practice of MT existed as early as 15,000 BC when European cave paintings and artifacts from this period depict the practice. On the basis of this evidence, it is likely that MT was used for healing purposes. The first written records of the practice of MT were from Chinese and Egyptian records dating around 3000 BC. When Chinese medicine developed between 200 BC and AD 100, MT was used along with other methods to treat illnesses. By AD 500, MT was a well-established method of treatment and a variety of massage techniques were used. During this time, MT was also being used in other Asian cultures, such as Japan and India.

---

[1] The following brief history of MT was collected from a variety of sources, including several web sites that are cited in the reference section and Susan G. Salvo's textbook, *MT Principles and Practice, 3rd edition.*

In the Western world, MT was used for healing purposes in Greece beginning around 700 BC and in Rome beginning around 200 BC. In Greece, the "Father of Western Medicine", Hippocrates (460–374 BC), promoted MT as one of the key ways to maintain health. On the basis of Hippocrates' beliefs about the healing properties of MT, the ancient Greek physician, Galen (AD 130–200), also wrote about and encouraged the use of MT for healing purposes. During this era, MT was very popular in the Roman culture and physicians frequently provided massages to Romans in their homes or in public bathhouses. In the middle ages, medical professionals preferred other treatments; however, midwives and folk healers continued to use MT regularly as part of their repertoire of treatments.

Interest in MT for healing purposes was revived in the Western world during the European Renaissance and Enlightenment. During the Renaissance, major discoveries were made in the field of medicine. The foundations of modern anatomy, pharmacology, and surgery all originated in this period. Several physicians from this time were advocates of MT for therapeutic and medical purposes.

The modern era of MT began in the early nineteenth century with the publication of a variety of new books promoting MT and the development of individual therapeutic systems. One of the most important authors during this period was Pehr Henrik Ling (1776–1839), a Swedish physiologist and gymnastics instructor who developed the Swedish Movements system, which included massage techniques. Swedish Movements were introduced to the United States in 1856. Throughout the late nineteenth and early twentieth centuries, several publications about the history and benefits of MT were written. Notable examples include *Swedish Movement and Massage* (1888) by Hartvig Nissen and *A Treatise on Massage, Its History, Mode of Application and Effects* (1902) by Douglas O. Graham. These important texts were among the first to present the effectiveness of MT in the United States. In the early twentieth century, a variety of historical events led to increased use of MT. World War I and the development of physical therapy resulted in the use of MT to treat injured soldiers. It was during this period that standardization and training of massage therapists began to emerge in the Western world. The first massage association in the United States was the New York State Society of Medical Massage Therapists, initiated in 1927.

The middle-late twentieth century was a time of increasing prevalence of MT in the United States. Many city and state-wide MT associations were founded. Membership steadily increased as the popularity of the profession increased and led to the development of national organizations, such as the AMTA. As a result, numerous MT periodicals, magazines, and books were published and interest in the benefits of MT boomed. In 1992, a national certification and licensing process was initiated. Various subtypes of MT were defined and MT became an increasingly common way to achieve relaxation in spas and health care centers across the country.

At present, there is a significant trend toward integrating MT in Western medical practices. Massage therapists are being employed in hospital and hospice settings throughout the United States and MT is often used as an adjunct treatment for a variety of medical conditions. The rise of research on the health benefits of MT reflects the integration of MT into health care and the increasing acceptance of this therapy in medical settings. In fact, the White House Commission on Complementary and Alternative Medicine Policy (U.S. Department of Health and Human Services, 2002) called for further research examining the effectiveness and mechanisms of action for CAM therapies, including MT. This is an exciting time for MT. Current research and clinical trends indicate MT will continue to expand as a field well into the future.

Definition of Massage and Therapeutic Techniques

Massage therapy is a growing field and there are an increasing number of new modalities and subspecialties being offered. The term MT covers a group of practices and techniques. There are thought to be more than 250 types of massage, bodywork, and somatic therapies currently available (www.massagetherapy.com/glossary/index.php). In applying these modalities, therapists use a variety of pressing, rubbing, and stroking motions to manipulate the muscles and other soft tissues of the body. Pressure, movement, site restrictions, and variations are common. Most techniques are applied using the hands and fingers, but certain modalities incorporate a variety of other body parts including the forearms, elbows, knees, and feet. The intention of MT is most often to relax the soft tissues, increase delivery of blood and oxygen to the massaged areas, warm the massaged areas, and decrease pain. However, there are other physiological, psychological, and spiritual therapeutic effects that are sought as well.

The following definitions provide brief descriptions of a few of the most popular techniques currently in practice:

- *Aromatherapy massage* incorporates one or more scented plant oils called essential oils to address specific needs.
- *Asian bodywork* is a form of bodywork that monitors the flow of the vital life energy—known as chi, ki, prana, or qi. Using manipulation and pressure, the practitioner evaluates and modulates the energy flow to facilitate a balanced state. Popular modalities include shiatsu, amma, Jin Shin Do, Thai massage, and tui na.
- *Cranio-Sacral* is a gentle touch technique for evaluating and optimizing the functioning of the cranio-sacral system—comprised of the membranes and cerebrospinal fluid that surround and protect the brain and spinal cord.
- *Deep tissue* is a technique designed to release patterns of tension in the body through slow, deep strokes and finger pressure in contracted, tense areas.
- *Myofascial release* is a technique using long stretching strokes to rebalance the body by releasing tension in the fascia/connective tissue.
- *Reflexology* is a technique which uses pressure points on the feet, hands, and ears that are thought to correspond to specific areas of the body.

- *Sports massage* is a style of massage focusing on the muscle systems relevant to a particular sport. Modifications are made for training, sporting events, and post-sporting activities.
- *Swedish massage* is a system of massage that uses long strokes, kneading, and friction techniques combined with active and passive joint movements.
- *Trigger point therapy, myotherapy, or neuromuscular therapy* is a method that applies finger pressure to trigger points to break down patterns of pain and relieve spasms.

Massage therapy can be applied with a wide range of pressure, site, position, and dis-ease-specific restrictions. This will result in tremendous variability in terms of applied pressure, speed of delivery, and the manual techniques selected. The success of the MT is dependent on the massage therapist's ability to make these necessary therapeutic adjust-ments. While there is an increased understanding of the specific effects of MT, the treat-ments themselves still contain an artfulness that predates evidence-based studies. The most expert massage therapists combine knowledge and art in their practice of MT.

Pediatric MT has been generally described as the manual manipulation of soft tis-sue intended to promote health and well-being in children and adolescents (Beider & Moyer, 2006). Massage for children varies substantially from MT for adults. Children are typically more actively engaged during the therapeutic session and enjoy partici-pating in a variety of ways. This can include the incorporation of storytelling, games, discussion, objects, or toys. Children will often direct the MT session, change position, desire more direct eye contact, and request that the massage therapist shift from one area of the body to another.

Children with medical conditions require that the massage therapist make appro-priate position, pressure, site, and disease-specific adjustments and modifications. Although Classic Swedish or circulatory MT is most commonly provided, it may not be therapeutically appropriate for children with certain medical conditions. MT prac-ticed in a hospital or hospice environment presents unique demands, and for some the term "massage" can be misleading. As a result, therapists who specialize in pediatric hospital-based MT are developing new terminology to describe their treatments. Terms such as Integrative Touch™ and Compassionate Touch˙ have been developed to address these concerns. Integrative Touch™ is a gentle form of MT that is sensitive to the med-ical needs of patients who are hospitalized or in hospice care (www.integrativetouch. org). Integrative Touch™ takes into consideration the whole patient—mind, body, and spirit—and uses gentle, noncirculatory techniques. Compassionate Touch˙ is a term that has been used to describe a therapeutic modality created for the elderly, ill, or dying (www.compassionate-touch.org). Compassionate Touch˙ involves one-on-one focused attention, intentional touch, and sensitive massage with specialized communication skills to help enhance quality of life. This new linguistic development highlights the evolution of MT.

Professional Standards, Training, and Licensure

An individual who professionally provides MT is most often called a massage therapist, although there are other health care providers, such as physical and occupational therapists, who also have massage training. It is increasingly common for nurses and allied health care providers to seek education and training in MT. It is estimated that there are 265,000 to 300,000 massage therapists and students in the United States (AMTA Massage Therapy Industry Fact Sheet, 2008). Significantly smaller numbers have training or experience working with pediatric populations—particularly children with special health care needs. This requires advanced training and pediatric experience beyond what is provided in basic MT training programs. However, to date, there are a limited number of programs or continuing education courses available nationally offering pediatric specific MT (e.g., www.massageforchildren.com and http://marybettssinclair.com/). Employment for massage therapists is expected to increase 20% from 2006 to 2016 according to the U.S. Department of Labor (AMTA Massage Therapy Industry Fact Sheet, 2008). On the basis of a comparison of results of an AMTA Industry Survey (2007) and the U.S. Department of Labor Bureau of Labor (2008), today's massage therapists are predominately female (85%), most likely enter MT as a second profession, and are likely to provide MT in a number of different settings (e.g., the home, spa/salon, office, health care setting, health club, or MT franchise or chain). Swedish massage is the most commonly used modality provided by 82% of practitioners, followed by deep tissue massage (70%), trigger point (43%), and sports massage (40%). Sole practitioners or independent contractors account for the largest percentage of practicing massage therapists (AMTA Industry Survey, 2007). As of December 2007, massage therapists have an average of 688 hours of initial training (AMTA, 2007). There are roughly 1500 MT postsecondary schools, college programs, and training programs throughout the country according to U.S. Department of Labor, Bureau of Labor Statistics (2008). The vast majority of massage therapists agree that MT should be integrated into health care.

At present, 38 states and the District of Columbia regulate massage therapists. In states that do not regulate massage therapists, local municipalities often take on this role. The minimum number of hours of MT training is typically 500 hours, although there are some exceptions—especially in states that do not mandate state licensure. Written, oral, and/or hands on examinations are typically required. The majority of states have continuing education requirements for renewal of licensure. Licenses or certifications for massage therapists include the following designations: LMT (licensed massage therapist), LMP (licensed massage practitioner), CMT (certified massage therapist), and two national certifications NCTMB (National Certification in Therapeutic Massage and Bodywork), and NCTM (National Certification in Therapeutic Massage). Certifications for infant and pediatric massage therapists include the following designations: CEIM (Certified Educator of Infant Massage), CIIM (Certified Instructor of Infant Massage), CIMI (Certified Infant Massage Instructor), CPMP (Certified

Pediatric Massage Practitioner), CPMS (Certified Pediatric Massage Specialist), and CPMT (Certified Pediatric Massage Therapist). These certifications vary in terms of the number of training hours, expected level of expertise, and examination or assessment required for certification.

The National Certification Board for Therapeutic Massage and Bodywork (NCBTMB) upholds a national standard of excellence (www.ncbtmb.com). More than 89,000 massage therapists and bodyworkers have been certified by NCBTMB since their inception. To become nationally certified, practitioners must complete a minimum of 500 hours of instruction, demonstrate mastery of core skills, abilities and knowledge, pass a standardized examination, and uphold NCBTMB's Standards of Practice and Code of Ethics. Massage therapists in a professional setting practice codes of ethics, which are established either by NCBTMB or by the association to which they belong (e.g., AMTA, Association of Bodywork and Massage Professionals).

Standards of practice are maintained in the areas of professionalism, legal and ethical requirements, confidentiality, business practices, roles and boundaries, and the prevention of sexual misconduct. Codes of ethics include ethical considerations such as honest representation, practicing safely within the boundaries of known indications/contraindications, providing treatment when there is expected client benefit, maintaining competence, meeting professional expectations, safeguarding confidentiality, obtaining consent, respecting the client's right of refusal, maintaining a healthy professional relationship, avoiding conflicts of interest, and following procedures, guidelines, regulations and professional codes and requirements.

The skills of massage therapists are often divided into two categories: hard skills and soft skills. Hard skills include knowledge of physiology, pathology, anatomy, tactile technique, and massage acumen. Soft skills include management of the therapeutic relationship (e.g., communication, professionalism, managing healthy boundaries), an often overlooked and understudied aspect of MT. The therapeutic relationship is comprised of several important factors including trust, compassion, client-centered care, safety, respect, and a recognition of the perceived power differential between the client and practitioner. This is particularly important when working with pediatric clients and especially those who are medically vulnerable. By recognizing that children are inherently more susceptible to adult influence and often overwhelmed by the medical environment, it is crucial to maintain these soft skills while providing pediatric MT.

Massage therapy treatments usually last 30 to 60 minutes; however, treatments may be as short as 10 to 15 minutes or as long as 2 hours. For pediatric clients, shorter sessions are often indicated. A series of appointments is usually recommended, particularly for children with medical conditions. An effort is made on the part of the massage therapist to create an environment that is calm and soothing, although this is not always possible in certain settings. The use of dim lighting, soothing music, and a calm, quiet, and relaxed environment are all thought to contribute to the overall experience of MT and healing.

Theories and Proposed Mechanisms of Action

From the beginning, MT was practiced as a healing method. Later it was used as an adjunct therapy to well-established methods of treatment and promoted as one of the key ways to maintain health. During the Renaissance period, physicians supported the use of massage for therapeutic and medical purposes. It was at this point that the medical profession began to explore mechanistic actions associated with MT. To date, there continues to be a split between those who view MT as a mode of symptom management and those who view MT as enhancing overall well-being. Theorized by Beider, Mahrer, and Gold (2007), MT can be viewed as creating enhanced well-being through multisystem integration (MSI) and organization, which can lead to an optimal healing experience. The authors explain that MSI has an emphasis on balance, homeostasis, healing, well-being, and a shift away from symptom abatement alone.

While the effectiveness of MT in Western Medicine is often measured in terms of reduced symptom distress, holistically, MT may work through MSI, targeting the interactions between the immune, muscular, cardiovascular, endocrine, and nervous systems. For example, some theorists have proposed explanations for the effects of MT on weight gain (e.g., the role of increased vagal activity and the release of hormones in the gastrointestinal tract to promote more efficient food absorption) (Field, 2002), while others have reflected on the synergistic effects of vagal activity and stress reduction on weight gain (Scafidi & Field, 1996; Vickers, Ohlsson, Lacy, & Horsley, 2004). Fortunately, investigators are beginning to embrace a more holistic or MSI approach for understanding the mechanisms of action of MT.

Clinicians have long noted some of the effects they see associated with MT, which include (1) enhanced relaxation and stress reduction, (2) therapeutic benefit from the interaction between the therapist and patient, (3) reduction in pain signals sent to the brain, (4) the release of certain chemicals in the body, such as serotonin or endorphins, creating feelings of enhanced well-being, and (5) improved sleep, which is known to have a role in affecting both pain and healing. MT also appears to promote a shift in the central nervous system toward a parasympathetic state. The parasympathetic nervous system creates what some call the "rest and digest" response (heart rate and breathing rate slow down, blood vessels dilate, and activity increases in many parts of the digestive tract). The parasympathetic response supports rest and healing for the MT recipient.

Psychoneuroimmunology (PNI) is a multidisciplinary field of research that may help to explain the effectiveness of MT in chronically ill patients. PNI examines the interactions between the behavioral science, neuroscience, endocrinology, and immunology fields in order to understand how the convergence of these disciplines influences health and disease (Ader, 2007). Only a handful of studies have specifically examined the impact of pediatric MT on immune, neuroendocrine, and psychological functioning in chronically ill children and adolescents. These studies have found some improvements in immune, neuroendocrine, and psychological functioning after a period of MT (e.g., Diego et al., 2001; Field, 2006; Shor-Posner et al., 2006). Although there is a paucity of research examining the PNI response and MT in pediatric populations, overall, these results are promising and indicate that MT may result in improved immune and endocrine functioning, which consequently can result in decreases in disease progression and improved functional status. Future research needs to further examine the role of PNI in pediatric MT in order to more fully understand the mechanisms by which MT improves physiological and psychological functioning.

Current Research Evidence

Massage therapy has been widely practiced for thousands of years. Clients and massage therapists have noted many anecdotal benefits. In fact, most of what is known about the effects of MT is experiential in nature. Following pediatric MT, patients and massage therapists have reported experiencing such benefits as an increase in overall relaxation, decrease in pain and soreness, improved sleep, stress relief, and a greater connection to the body. Research is just beginning to examine the physiological and psychological benefits of MT. Thus far this research has been limited in scope. To date, the majority of randomized controlled clinical trials examining the effects of MT have utilized Swedish massage techniques. The effects of other popular MT modalities (e.g., Asian bodywork techniques, deep tissue, trigger point therapies) have not been adequately researched. As the field grows, research needs to incorporate a range of massage modalities. Although research in pediatric MT is more limited than studies in adults, there have been some studies specifically examining the physiological and psychological benefits of MT in pediatric populations. A review article of randomized controlled trials of pediatric MT summarizes the state of the literature (Beider & Moyer, 2006). More recently, a clinical overview by Beider, Mahrer, and Gold (2007) reviewed the pediatric MT literature and reported on proven and promising effects.

Research has shown there are physiological benefits to the patient and psychological benefits to both the patient and caregiver following MT sessions. In infants, examples of potential physiological benefits include increased weight gain and shorter hospital stays in premature/low birth weight infants (Vickers et al., 2004) and improved sleep, increased relaxation, and decreased crying (Underdown, 2006). Research has demonstrated various physiological benefits following MT including improved muscle tone, increased airflow in children with pulmonary disorders, reductions in chronic pain associated with specific areas of the body (i.e., the lower back, neck, and shoulder) and particular conditions such as, headaches, fibromyalgia, carpal tunnel syndrome, and juvenile rheumatoid arthritis (Beider & Moyer, 2007; Tsao, 2007).

Research on caregiver-provided MT to infants suggests that caregivers may experience psychological benefits such as greater satisfaction, improved infant/caregiver interaction, improved overall mood, and declines in depressive symptoms (Fujita et al., 2006; Livingston et al., 2007; Underdown et al., 2006; Vickers et al., 2004).

In addition, children have been shown to experience psychological benefits as a result of MT including decreases in anxiety, dysthymia, depression, negative mood, and disruptive behavioral problems (Beider & Moyer, 2007; Zebracki et al., 2007). Although research examining the physiological and psychological outcomes of MT is in the early stages, there is increasing interest in this area.

A search on the National Institutes of Health (NIH) Computer Retrieval of Information on Scientific Projects (CRISP) database (http://crisp.cit.nih.gov) revealed several ongoing NIH-funded research projects investigating the physiological and psychological effects of MT in pediatric populations. One study being conducted by Sheila Wang, Ph.D., at Children's Memorial Hospital is comparing the immune, autonomic, hormonal, and behavioral effects of MT versus relaxation training in unmedicated adolescents with HIV. Sean Phipps, Ph.D., of St. Jude's Children's Research Hospital, is conducting a randomized intervention trial comparing the psychological and medical outcomes of a child-targeted intervention that includes MT and humor therapy and a parent-targeted intervention which involves MT and relaxation therapy compared to standard care. Finally, Cynthia Myers, Ph.D., was funded to study the effectiveness of MT versus superficial heat application in controlling pain intensity and pain-related negative affect in children with advanced cancer.

Clinical Applications

In this section, the clinical effects of massage will be reviewed. An emphasis on clinical anecdotes and evidence-based practice in the well child, as well as the effects of MT in children with system-specific dysregulations will be discussed.

GENERAL EFFECTS IN THE WELL CHILD

Massage for children can have many health benefits. These benefits include enhanced self-esteem, body image, and well-being. MT can also support children in developing healthy lifestyle habits and boundaries in their personal relationships. Communication and sociability seem to be enhanced with MT, and children's mental alertness and academic performance may improve following therapy. Touch aversion and touch sensitivity can be minimized and feelings of acceptance and nurturing are often reported. When practiced within the family context, massage can enhance intimate relationships and support children in developing a sense of connection to their bodies and respect for their loved ones. Siblings are often able to work out some of their differences and engage in less aggressive physical behaviors when they have a positive outlet for touch through massage. The field is a long way from discerning the mechanisms of action for each of these reported outcomes; however, it is important to note that MT may enhance MSI and function, which would explain the breadth and scope of previously reported findings.

There are specific conditions that well children may experience in daily life for which massage can be beneficial. When children feel intestinal discomfort or constipation, a stomach massage routine similar to the colic routine widely used in infant massage can be helpful. Abdominal massage promotes elimination and decreases feelings of pain and discomfort. When children are experiencing growth spurts and growing pains, massage can lessen the associated discomfort. If a child has sleep difficulties, a night time massage ritual can help promote relaxation and improve sleep. Children who experience worries surrounding school examinations, extracurricular activities, or peer relationships may find that massage helps relieve some of their stress and concern.

EFFECTS ON THE SKIN

Clinical observations have shown that massage increases skin temperature, improves skin condition, and stimulates oil gland production. As circulation increases with MT, more nutrients become available and there is an improvement in the overall texture and appearance of the skin. MT has been shown to reduce skin itching, redness, and flakiness (Schachner, Field, Hernandez-Reif, Duarte, & Krasnegor, 1998). This can be particularly helpful for conditions such as eczema and psoriasis so long as the skin is not susceptible to infection. When the skin is not intact, MT is locally contraindicated but the surrounding tissue can be touched and this can expedite the healing process. In addition, the oil or lotion that is applied with MT can help improve skin condition. MT has also been beneficial in treating burns in the subacute stage. MT can be useful for rehabilitating the skin by positively affecting pruritus and scar status (Roh, Cho, Oh, & Yoon, 2007), and minimizing the stress, anxiety, and pain associated with skin debridement (Field, 2005). For children with special health care needs who may develop pressure sores, massage can promote enhanced circulation and healing and prevent the development of new pressure sores.

EFFECTS ON THE MUSCULOSKELETAL SYSTEM

Clinical observations reveal that MT relieves muscle tightness, restrictions, stiffness, and spasms. It is thought that MT may reduce muscle excitability. Promising effects for pain reduction as mediated by the sympathetic nervous system have been observed, leading to muscle relaxation. MT manually separates muscle fibers and lengthens muscles, which increases flexibility. It is theorized that MT tones weak muscles by increasing muscle spindle activity and minute muscle contractions. This has beneficial effects for individuals experiencing flaccidity, atrophy, or prolonged periods of inactivity. Because MT increases the amount of oxygen and nutrients available to muscles via improved blood circulation, muscle fatigue, and soreness are reduced and waste products are eliminated more quickly. Evidence suggests that postexercise massage may be helpful in reducing delayed onset muscle soreness (Hilbert, Sforzo, & Swenson, 2003). Field and colleagues found that after 30 days of daily 15 minute massages in 10 children with mild to moderate JRA, that child-, parent-, and physician-report all indicated decreased pain (Field et al., 1997). Although this study is limited by its small sample size, the results are promising and demonstrate the potential effects of MT in children with JRA.

Massage therapy can provide release of muscular, tendinous, and ligamentous tension that is found with postural deviations and lumbar or thoracic curves. When MT is carefully applied to the surrounding areas of a broken or fractured bone, it can reduce the development of compensation patterns, improve muscle tone and circulation, and reduce edema. In the subacute stage, sprains and tendonitis respond well to MT, which can minimize swelling and allow for increased joint mobility (Werner, 2002). Physical therapists and rehabilitation practitioners have often applied MT to treat contractures and edema (Vasudevan & Melvin, 1979). This can be helpful for a variety of different conditions including neurodevelopmental disorders, such as cerebral palsy. In general, the acute phase of musculoskeletal injury should be avoided but subacute and chronic injuries may respond well to MT.

EFFECTS ON THE NERVOUS AND ENDOCRINE SYSTEMS

Massage is thought to promote general relaxation through the activation of the relaxation response. It appears that beta brainwaves may be decreased during MT and delta brainwaves may be increased, encouraging sleep and relaxation. It has been proposed that dopamine and serotonin levels are increased leading to decreased stress and depression. Increased serotonin levels may consequently inhibit pain signals, thereby reducing the sensation of pain. For example, a study of adults with fibromyalgia indicated that following MT, sleep improved, pain decreased, and substance P decreased (Field et al., 2002). Researchers have also reported that MT is associated with increases in Stage III and Stage IV restorative sleep (Field, 2007). Some studies conducted by Field and colleagues at the Touch Research Institute, have reported a decrease in cortisol associated with MT. In a recent meta-analysis of randomized control trials in adults receiving MT, no significant decreases in cortisol were noted (Moyer, Rounds, & Hannum, 2004). This was corroborated by Beider and Moyer (2006) in a clinical review of pediatric MT studies. In a meta-analysis of MT for adults, significant reductions in depression and anxiety have been shown (Moyer et al., 2004). In a review of randomized controlled trials in pediatric MT, reductions in pain appear to be promising, although further study is needed (Beider & Moyer, 2006).

Massage therapy has shown clinical benefits for conditions where peripheral nerves have been impacted. It also appears to be useful for decreasing rigidity, contractures, and stiffness associated with neurological conditions such as multiple sclerosis (Salvo, 2004). Hypertonic muscles respond favorably to a relaxing massage, whereas hypotonic muscles respond better to increased stimulation. MT is particularly useful for stimulating blood circulation and increasing mobility, range of motion, and function. Massage can be a useful treatment for enhancing the benefits of physical and occupational therapy by increasing circulation and minimizing muscular degeneration, which is sometimes caused by proprioceptive misinformation (Werner, 2002).

EFFECTS ON THE CARDIOVASCULAR SYSTEM

There are several ways that massage is thought to affect the cardiovascular system. The most prominent belief is that MT creates an overall improvement in blood circulation (Salvo, 2007). Clinically, it is suggested that massage dilates blood vessels, decreases blood pressure, increases blood flow, replenishes nutrients and oxygen to cells and tissues, and removes waste products. MT is also thought to reduce heart and pulse rates through activation of the relaxation response. Other positive effects include an increase in stroke volume, red and white blood cell counts, platelets, and oxygen saturation. For children with conditions that involve compromised blood vessels, hypertension, or high blood pressure, circulatory MT is generally thought to be contraindicated but gentle holding or very light touch techniques such as Integrative Touch™ may be applied.

EFFECTS ON THE LYMPHATIC AND IMMUNE SYSTEMS

Similar to the circulatory effects described for the cardiovascular system, the effects of massage on the lymphatic system are thought to include enhanced lymph circulation. MT can cause fluid to be drawn into lymphatic capillaries and thereby increase lymphatic flow. This can reduce edema and the associated weight and swelling that accompany this condition. There may also be positive benefits to the functioning of the immune system through increased lymphocyte counts and an increase in the number and function of natural killer cells, CD4 cells, and the CD4/CD8 ratio. To date, two research studies have found enhanced HIV-related immune functioning in children and adolescents with HIV after receiving two massages a week for 12 weeks (Diego et al., 2001; Shor-Posner et al., 2006). Further, Diego and colleagues (2001) discovered that adolescents with HIV reported significantly less depressive and anxious symptoms following MT. Because HIV involves immune dysregulation, these findings are of extreme importance and indicate that following MT, children and adolescents with HIV may not only experience decreased psychological distress but may also experience an increase in immune functioning. This improvement in immune functioning could delay disease progression. As previously stated, further studies in this area are currently being conducted.

EFFECTS ON THE RESPIRATORY SYSTEM

Generally, MT is thought to reduce respiration rate, strengthen respiratory muscles, and improve pulmonary function. It is thought that respiration rate is decreased due to the activation of the relaxation response. MT can loosen tight respiratory muscles and fascia and mechanically help to loosen and discharge phlegm. Muscular relaxation in the back, chest, and neck combined with postural drainage can have a positive effect for children with chronic respiratory conditions. Early data on MT and pulmonary function have been promising and MT may be helpful for reducing allergies that irritate respiratory function (Beider & Moyer, 2006). Research also suggests that children with cystic fibrosis may have improved pulmonary function following MT (Hernandez-Reif et al., 1999).

EFFECTS ON THE DIGESTIVE AND URINARY SYSTEMS

Clinical observation and client reports have shown that MT promotes evacuation of the colon. This is thought to occur through an increase in peristaltic activity, which encourages movement and relieves constipation. For infants, MT improves the symptoms of colic and reduces intestinal gas. Because the relaxation response is stimulated during MT, digestion is activated. It has been postulated that MT facilitates the reabsorption of lymphatic fluids for filtration by the kidney and is thought to activate dormant capillary beds, which increase the amount of urine produced and the frequency of urination. Metabolic waste products are also released during MT. These include nitrogen, sodium chloride, and inorganic phosphorus (Salvo, 2007).

INDICATIONS FOR SPECIAL POPULATIONS

There are a variety of special medical conditions in children (e.g., cancer) for which massage has been shown to be beneficial. In addition, there are specific populations who are thought to benefit from MT (e.g., children who have been neglected or abused). Children that appear to respond favorably to MT based on clinical observation include patients with cancer, chronic pain, palliative care needs and children in hospice In addition, children who have been abused and neglected, hospitalized infants and children, children with psychological conditions (e.g., eating disorders, anxiety, depression), and chronic stress appear to respond favorably to MT. When MT is practiced as an integrative therapeutic intervention for children with special health conditions, it may be vital for managing symptoms and enhancing wellness. The multidimensional therapeutic aspects of MT can provide children with a sense of comfort, safety, and psychological well-being in addition to physiological improvement and/or symptom management.

Safety

Considering the popularity and wide use of MT, the number of reported adverse events has been minute (Ernst, 2003). Though adverse events are rare, safety remains a vital concern. A clinical review conducted by Ernst (2003) found 16 case reports and 4 case series where adverse events were reported as a result of MT. These events ranged from various pain syndromes and leg ulcers to more serious events such as cerebrovascular accidents, hematoma, ruptured uterus, and strangulation of the neck. However, it should be noted that in most cases, untrained massage therapists employed exotic massage techniques rather than circulatory massage techniques (Ernst, 2003). Corbin (2005) has investigated the safety of massage specifically in patients with cancer. She concluded that MT could safely be incorporated into conventional care for patients with cancer; however, patients may be at higher risk for rare adverse events. Because patients with cancer may be at a higher risk for rare adverse events, MT may require modification to maximize safety. To date, MT practice and research conducted with licensed massage therapists has demonstrated feasibility and safety. Nonetheless, practitioners need to consider the patient's overall health status and specific medical conditions in order to assign the appropriate massage restrictions and techniques.

CONTRAINDICATIONS AND MEDICATION CONSIDERATIONS

The two main categories of contraindication for MT are local and absolute contraindications. Local contraindications include specific regional areas of the body where MT must be avoided. This might be an area of inflammation or injury or the site of an intravenous line or surgical incision. Absolute contraindications include conditions for which MT is inappropriate, ill advised, or potentially harmful. Examples include widespread inflammation, infection, high fever, or medical emergencies. Endangerment sites are areas of the body that are delicate or relatively vulnerable and may necessitate caution or limitations. These include nerves, blood vessels, organs, and bony projections. Pressure and positioning restrictions are required when implementing MT in these areas.

Certain medications contraindicate some types of MT treatment. Analgesics can effect changes in tissue response, which in turn can alter the temperature, local blood flow, and muscle guarding (Uretsky, 2006). Therefore, therapists need to apply lighter pressure and a more conservative MT approach for pediatric clients on analgesics. Muscle relaxants can interfere with muscle reflexes, so stretching and deeper work should be avoided. Clot management medications, including anticoagulants and antiplatelets, can create an increased risk for bleeding and bruising. In these circumstances, gentle touch or holding is recommended (Ross-Flanigan, 2006). Some of the side effects from antidepressant medications, including dizziness and light-headedness, can be exaggerated following MT (Health A to Z, 2006), therefore children and adolescents need to be advised to move slowly and cautiously following treatment. Anxiolytic medications have a range of side effects including poor reflexes, CNS depression, and exhaustion (Health A to Z, 2006), which can substantially affect treatment. MT should be conducted with caution and practiced in close communication with the medical team. In all cases when medications are being administered to children, massage therapists need to be aware of their potential effects and maintain an open dialogue with the prescribing physician.

Conclusions

The field of integrative medicine is growing rapidly and pediatric MT is gaining significant attention in both clinical and research practice. Over the last several decades, MT has become a profession with national accreditation, local and state-wide licensing and organizations, and professional periodicals. Health professionals and family members continue to be increasingly educated about their health care choices and have begun to request more CAM approaches to their care. Owing to the recent surge in MT evidence-based research findings, which illuminate the benefits and potential mechanisms of action of MT, as well as its popularity in the general population, MT is now being incorporated into community and medical settings as an adjunct treatment for well children and children with a variety of medical conditions.

Despite the increased prevalence of pediatric MT, there are a limited number of massage therapists with the specialized training necessary to perform MT safely for children with medical conditions. Traditionally, massage school graduates in the United States receive little or no education in the areas of infant and pediatric MT. Currently, a limited number of high-quality continuing education programs exist nationally. Therefore, it is essential that more pediatric specific training programs are developed and that massage therapists participate in these specialized training programs. It is particularly important that massage therapists receive advanced training in pediatric MT for working with children in hospital- and hospice-based settings. Increased dialogue between massage therapists and other members of the health care team is necessary to promote collaborative trainings and clinical research investigations.

In many respects, the field of integrative pediatric MT is still in its infancy. The majority of perceived effects have been based on massage therapists' and their clients' clinical experience. However, randomized control trials have demonstrated decreases in anxiety and pain and revealed improvements in pulmonary function and muscle tone. Anecdotal evidence and clinical research indicate improved physiological and psychological states following MT. Clinicians have noted the effects associated with MT, which include enhanced relaxation, reduced stress, benefits from the therapeutic relationship, reductions in pain, the release of certain chemicals in the body that create feelings of enhanced well-being, and improvements in sleep. More recently, attention has been turned toward PNI, which examines the relationships between the behavioral sciences, neuroscience, endocrinology, and immunology fields in order to understand how their associated interactions influence health and disease (Ader, 2007), as a way to describe how MT affects physiological and psychological states.

This is an exciting time of growth for the field of pediatric MT. There are numerous cutting-edge studies currently being conducted with federal funding from the NIH to explore the mechanisms of action of MT. Furthermore, MT is more popular than ever before in society and is now being included in health care settings across the country. As research studies continue to include larger sample sizes, more diverse patient populations, and test a broader range of MT modalities, additional information regarding the effects of MT will be revealed.

Massage therapy is a vital CAM therapy within integrative medicine and is viewed as a holistic approach to health and healing. Concepts of healing beyond those practiced in Western medicine are being explored to maximize health outcomes and redefine the underlying principles of healing across multiple domains (i.e., mind–body–spirit). MT is used to maintain health and wellness and may also be utilized to manage symptoms and enhance MSI in infants and children with medical conditions. Future research employing state-of-the-art scientific techniques and study designs to evaluate ancient healing practices, such as MT, presents us with rare opportunities to formulate new health identities that surpass reductionistic models of disease and expand our concepts of healing and wellness. Integrating MT into routine child care and health care practice can deeply influence the way we think about health and healing for our children.

REFERENCES

Ader, R. (2007). Preface to the fourth edition. In R. Ader (Ed.), *Psychoneuroimmunology* (4th Ed., Vol. 1, p. xv). Elsevier.

American Massage Therapy Association (AMTA). (2008). Massage Therapy Industry Fact Sheet. Retrieved May 17 2008, from http://www.amtamassage.org/news/MTIndustryFactSheet.html

American Massage Therapy Association (AMTA). (2007). AMTA Consumer Survey. Retrieved May 10, 2008, from http://www.amtamassage.org/media/consumersurvey_factsheet.html

American Hospital Association. (2006). *2005 Health Forum Complementary and Alternative Medicine Survey Summary Report*: Ananth, S., & Martin, W.

Beider, S., Mahrer, N., & Gold, J.I. (2007). Pediatric massage therapy: An overview for clinicians. *Pediatric Clinics of North America: Complementary and Alternative Medicine, 54*(6), 1025–1042.

Beider, S., & Moyer, C. A. (2006). Randomized control trials of pediatric massage: A review. *Evidence-Based Complementary & Alternative Medicine, 4*(1), 23–34.

Corbin, L. (2005). Safety and efficacy of massage therapy for patients with cancer. *Cancer Control, 12*(3), 158–164.

Diego, M. A., Field, T., Hernandez-Reif, M., Shaw, K., Friedman, L., & Ironson, G. (2001). HIV adolescents show improved immune function following massage therapy. *International Journal of Neuroscience, 106*(1–2), 35–45.

Ernst, E. (2003). The safety of massage therapy. *Rheumatology, 42*, 1101–1106.

Field, T. (2002). Massage therapy. *Medical Clinics of North America, 86*, 163–171.

Field T. (2005). Massage therapy for skin conditions in young children. *Dermatology Clinics, 23*, 717–721.

Field T. (2007). *Touch therapy.* London: Churchill Livingston Press.

Field, T., Hernandez-Reif, M., Diego, M., Figueiredo, B., Schanberg, S., & Kuhn, C. (2006). Prenatal cortisol, prematurity and low birthweight. *Infant Behavior and Development, 29*(2), 268–275.

Field, T., Diego, M., Cullen, C., Hernandez-Reif, M., Sunshine W., & Douglas, S. (2002). Fibromyalgia, pain, and substance P decrease and sleep improves after massage therapy. *Journal of Clinical Rheumatology, 8*, 72–76.

Field, T., Hernandez-Reif, M., Seligman, S., Krasnegor, J., Sunshine, W., Rivas-Chacon, R., et al. (1997). Juvenile rheumatoid arthritis: Benefits from massage therapy. *Journal of Pediatric Psychology, 22*, 607–617.

Fujita, M., Endoh, Y., Saimon, N., & Yamaguchi, S. (2006). Effect of massaging babies on mothers: Pilot study on the changes in mood states and salivary cortisol level. *Complementary Therapies in Clinical Practice, 12*(3), 181–185.

Health A to Z. (2006). *Anti-anxiety medications.* Retrieved May 1, 2008, from http://www.healthatoz.com/healthatoz/Atoz/common/standard/transform.jsp?requestURI=/healthatoz/Atoz/dc/caz/ment/anxi/antianxiety.jsp

Health A to Z. (2006). *Antidepressant medications.* Retrieved May 1, 2008, from http://www. healthatoz.com/healthatoz/Atoz/common/standard/transform.jsp?requestURI=/healthatoz/Atoz/dc/caz/ment/depr/antidepressant.jsp

Hernandez-Reif, M., Field, T., Krasnegor, J., Martinez, E., Schwartzman, M., & Mavunda, K. (1999). Children with cystic fibrosis benefit from massage therapy. *Journal of Pediatric Psychology, 24,* 175–181.

Hilbert, J. E., Sforzo G. A., & Swenson T. (2003). The effects of massage on delayed onset muscle soreness. *British Journal of Sports Medicine, 37,* 72–74.

Livingston, L., Beider, S., Kant, A., Gallardo, C., Joseph, M. H., & Gold, J. I. (2007). Touch and massage for medically fragile infants. *Evidence-Based Complementary and Alternative Medicine (eCAM),* doi: 10.1093/ecam/nem076

Loman, D. G. (2003). The use of complementary and alternative health care practices among children. *Journal of Pediatric Health Care, 17,* 58–63.

Moyer, C. A., Rounds, J., & Hannum, J. W. (2004). A meta-analysis of massage therapy research. *Psychological Bulletin, 130*(1), 3–18.

Onofrio, J. The history of massage, bodywork and related modalities. Retrieved August 1, 2007 from, http://www.thebodyworker.com/history.htm

Roh, Y. S., Cho, H., Oh, J. O., & Yoon, C. J. (2007). Effects of skin rehabilitation massage therapy on pruritus, skin status, and depression in burn survivors. *Taehan Kanho Hakhoe Chi, 37,* 221–226.

Rosenthal Center for Complementary and Alternative Medicine. Retrieved March 28, 2008, from www.rosenthal.hs.columbia.edu/MD_Courses.html

Ross-Flanigan, N. (2006). *Antidepressant medications.* Retrieved July 24, 2007, from http://www. healthatoz.com/healthatoz/Atoz/common/standard/transform.jsp?requestURI=/healthatoz/Atoz/dc/caz/ment/depr/antidepressant.jsp

Salvo S. G. (2004). *Mosbys pathology for massage therapists.* Philadelphia: Elsevier Mosby.

Salvo, S. G. (2007). *Massage therapy: Principles & practice* (3rd ed.). Philadelphia: Elsevier Health Sciences.

Sanders, H., Davis, M. F., Duncan, B., Meaney, F. J., Haynes, J., & Barton, L. L. (2003). Use of complementary and alternative medical therapies among children with special health care needs in southern Arizona. *Pediatrics, 111*(3), 584–587.

Scafidi, F., & Field, T. (1996). Massage therapy improves behavior in neonates born to HIV-positive mothers. *Journal of Pediatric Psychology, 21,* 889–897.

Schachner, L., Field, T., Hernandez-Reif, M., Duarte, A. M., & Krasnegor, J. (1998). Atopic dermatitis symptoms decreased in children following massage therapy. *Pediatric Dermatology, 15,* 390–395.

Shor-Posner, G., Hernandez-Reif, M., Miguez, M. J., Fletcher, M., Quintero, N., Baez, J., et al. (2006). Impact of a massage therapy clinical trial on immune status in young Dominican children infected with HIV-1. *The Journal of Alternative and Complementary Medicine, 12*(6), 511–516.

Tsao, J. C. (2007). Effectiveness of massage therapy for chronic, non-malignant pain: A review. *Evidence-Based Complementary and Alternative Medicine : ECAM, 4*(2), 165–179.

Underdown, A., Barlow, J., Chung, V., & Stewart-Brown, S. (2006). Massage intervention for promoting mental and physical health in infants aged under six months. *Cochrane Database System Review, 4,* 1–28.

United States Department of Health and Human Services. (2002, March). *White House Commission on Complementary and Alternative Medicine Policy: Final Report.* Retrieved May 7, 2008, from http://www.whccamp.hhs.gov/pdfs/fr2002_document.pdf

Uretsky, S. (2006). *Anelgesics*. Retrieved January 28, 2009, from http://www.healthline.com/galecontent/analgesics

U.S. Department of Labor, Bureau of Labor Statistics. (2008). *Occupational Outlook Handbook 2008-2009 Edition*. Retrieved May 19, 2008, from http://www.bls.gov/oco/

Vasudevan, S. V., & Melvin, J. L. (1979). Upper extremity edema control: Rationale of the techniques. *American Journal of Occupational Therapy, 33*, 520–523.

Vickers, A., Ohlsson, A., Lacy, J. B., & Horsley, A. (2004). Massage for promoting growth and development of preterm/or low birth weight infants. *Cochrane Review, 2*, 1–33.

Werner, R. (2002). *A massage therapists' guide to pathology* (2nd ed.). Philadelphia: Lippincott, Williams & Wilkins.

Zebracki, K., Holzman, K., Bitter, K. J., Feehan, K., & Miller, M. L. (2007). Brief report: Use of complementary and alternative medicine and psychological functioning in Latino children with juvenile idiopathic arthritis or arthralgia. *Journal of Pediatric Psychology, 32*(8), 1006–1110.

14

A Pediatric Perspective on Mind-Body Medicine

DANIEL P. KOHEN

KEY CONCEPTS

- The mind and body are in constant bidirectional communication through neurologic, biochemical, immunological, and energetic pathways.
- There are many mind/body skills that children and teens can learn and apply throughout life.
- All hypnosis is self-hypnosis.
- Hypnosis involves the cultivation of imagination.
- Increasingly sophisticated biofeedback allows a "real-time" glimpse of mind-body interaction.
- The mind-body is its own best biofeedback "machine."
- Goals of mind/body skills training include "balancing" of the ANS as well as the cultivation of positive emotional states and self-directed therapeutic suggestions.

■

Introduction

relationship between the mind and body has been debated, acknowledged, described, and refuted for millennia. In modern times the medical world and the broader community were re-introduced to this relationship (and debate) by Norman Cousins who wrote of his personal success with laughter as a means to his own healing (1979) and the value of emotions, belief, and attitude in his recovery from a severe heart attack (1983). Cousins' experiences, writings, and subsequent teaching were amongst several catalysts to both the emergence of, and attention to, a "field" of mind-body medicine, beginning to emerge in the 1960s. Others included the at once exciting, provocative, and controversial work of O. Carl Simonton (1978) and others in promoting the use of imagery as a means toward curing of cancer, and Bill Moyers' book and television series *Healing and the Mind* (Moyers, 1993) which sought to bring an up-to-date awareness to us of "where are we now?" in understanding the connections between mind, body, and health. With a specific focus on The Mind/Body Connection (Moyers, 1993, Section III, pp. 177–256), Moyers work also explored The Art of Healing (pp. 7–70), Healing from Within (pp. 71–176), The Mystery of Chi (pp. 256–322), and Wounded Healers (pp. 323–364).

In the seventeenth century Rene Descartes suggested that the body works like a machine, that it has the material properties of extension and motion, and that it follows the laws of physics. The mind (or soul) was described as a nonmaterial entity that lacks extension and motion, and does not follow the laws of physics. Descartes argued that only humans have minds, and that the mind interacts with the body at the pineal gland. This form of dualism proposed that the mind controls the body, but that the body can also influence the otherwise rational mind, such as when people act out of passion. Most of the previous accounts of the relationship between mind and body had been uni-directional. Descartes dualism evolved into a split between mind and body, resulting in science and medicine emphasizing the body, largely to the exclusion of the mind or its influence. The philosophical question continued for hundreds of years...asking how a nonmaterial mind can influence a material body without invoking supernatural explanations (Cottingham, Stoothoff, Murdock, & Kenny, 1991).

With the gradual but growing willingness of medicine and science to re-address, re-investigate, and re-confront the question, new answers have emerged toward understanding and resolution of what had been an enduring enigma.

Proposed Mechanisms of Change: How Thinking and Emotion Trigger Physiologic Change

In the 1980s molecular biologists and other scientists began to identify endorphins and other peptides, not only in the brain, but in the endocrine and immune systems and throughout the body, involved in a kind of psychosomatic communicating network. Dr. Candace Pert described this as "Information is flowing. These molecules are being released from one place, they're diffusing all over the body, and they're tickling the receptors that are on the surface of every cell in your body...these peptides appear to mediate intercellular communication throughout the brain and body...these neuropeptides and their receptors are the biochemical correlates of emotions" (Moyers, 1993, p. 178).

And, "... emotions...are the bridge between the mental and the physical, or the physical and the mental.... It's either way" (Pert, 1997).

Throughout the 1980s and early 1990s, pioneer Dr. Robert Ader, developed the field of psychoneuroimmunology, largely with animal research, offering the observation in 1991 that

> There [are] now abundant data documenting neuroanatomical, neuroendocrine, and neurochemical links to the immune system... The existence of *bidirectional pathways of communication between nervous and immune systems* provides an experimental foundation for the observation of *behavioral and stress-induced influences on immune function and, conversely, the effects of immune processes on behavior.* [italics added]) (Ader, 1991, p. xxvi)

In the late 1970s, Olness began her work with psychoneuroimmunology research with children (Olness & Kohen, 1996, p. 334) and studies of self-regulation, conditioning, and mind-body healing continued with a variety of inquiries into the self-healing capacities of young people (Hall, Minnes, & Olness, 1993; Lee & Olness, 1996; Olness & Conroy, 1985; Olness & Rusin, 1990a; Olness, 1990b).

A 4-year consortium study of nonpharmacological treatment of warts in children 6–12 years old (Felt et al., 1998) compared the effects of self-hypnosis training with conventional topical treatment and attention-control treatment. Group data analysis found no significant differences among groups, though evidence of wart regression was present in each group and some children in the self-hypnosis group had dramatic wart regression. Dramatic wart regression with self-hypnosis training has been described in many clinical reports (Olness & Kohen, 1996, pp. 340–341) and also has been described in a deaf child (Kohen, Mann-Rinehart, Schmitz, & Wills, 1998). While the precise mechanisms of these self-cures have been elusive, new perspectives on relationships between our emotions, our genes and their expression, and psychobiology offer promise for clarity of understanding the development and cultivation of self-regulation.

Self-Regulation in Children

In a recent review, Bell and Deater-Deckard (2007) describe self-regulation in children as operating at "the physiological, attentional, emotional, cognitive, and behavioral levels; and define self-regulation as the ability to control inner states or responses with respects to thoughts, emotions, attention, and performance... our conceptualization of self-regulation could be described as cognitive control and emotion control." They begin from the premise that psychophysiological processes (attention, cognition, and emotion) are intermediaries between gene expression and complex psychological behaviors; and posit that self-regulation includes complex interactions of various mechanisms, including serotonin and dopamine neurotransmitter system genes, central and peripheral nervous system connectivity, and activation involving prefrontal cortical and limbic regions of the brain (Bell & Deater-Deckard, 2007, p. 409). In their examination and discussion of genetic and psychophysiologic aspects of self-regulatory behavior in early development, Bell and Deater-Deckard amplify the influence of temperament on behavior, the differences in working memory capacity as mediators of differences in executive function, and the importance of both working memory and emotional related regulation to attention control (pp. 410–411). Much of the theory and application of these investigations describe the clinical impact in the arena of Attention Deficit Hyperactivity Disorder. Thus, Bell and Deater-Packard (2007, p. 415) note that a deficit in self-regulation is ADHD, the inattentive type of which may be the result of a child's inability to hold information active in memory and use that information to guide behavior. And, that "the neural systems implicated in self-regulatory problems associated with ADHD may be involved in both cognitive and emotional control." Beyond the significance of these considerations for the behavioral problems and challenges of common disorders like ADHD and the broader group of disruptive behavior disorders as considered by Deater-Packard and Bell (2007), Ernest Rossi (2002) challenges us to explore and understand that "nature and nurture are cooperative partners that coordinate gene expression and neurogenesis to create our life experiences and continually update our memories in fresh ways, whether we are aware of it or not." In *The Psychobiology of Gene Expression: Neuroscience and Neurogenesis in Hypnosis and the Healing Arts* (2002) Rossi describes how significant life experiences turn on gene expression and neurogenesis to continually update the brain and body to modulate our consciousness, memory, learning and behavior in health and illness. Rossi's (2002) compelling considerations of the relational research between genetics, neurobiology, psychology, and the healing arts at once remind us of the reality and validity of the mind-body methodologies described herein, and of the need for continuing research to truly understand the precise mechanisms that allow them to "really work!"

Hypnosis

HISTORICAL PERSPECTIVES

Hypnosis with children has been documented since ancient times. Many cultures have rich histories of healing, religious, and/or initiation rites which involve trance or trance-like phenomena in children. Biblical stories recount healing of children in response to faith beliefs and suggestion (I Kings XVII: 17–24; Mark IX: 17–27). In more modern times, Dr. Franz Mesmer's application of *animal magnetism* was used in the treatment of children as well as adults (Tinterow, 1970). While the Franklin Commission's investigation of Mesmer in 1784 concluded that the described clinical effects were not due to *magnetism*, it also specifically attributed their observations to "imagination," (Tinterow, 1970, p. 114) now recognized as a critical operative ingredient in child hypnosis.

Prior to the development of chemical anesthesia, Braid and Elliotson successfully applied hypnotic strategies with many children to facilitate their comfort during major surgery. (Elliotson, 1843a,b) At the end of the nineteenth century, French physicians Liebault and Bernheim reported the use of hypnotic techniques for childhood habit problems and also reported on child hypnotic susceptibility (Bramwell, 1903/1956; Tinterow, 1970). In his hypnosis textbook of 1903, J. Milne Bramwell, an English psychotherapist, reported the successful use of hypnotherapy with habits such as nail biting enuresis, eczema, night terrors, stammering, and recurrent headaches (Bramwell, 1903/1956).

Little attention was paid to the use of hypnosis with children in North America during the first half of the twentieth century. In the late 1950s the use of hypnosis with children was promoted by Drs. Milton Erickson (Erickson, 1958) and M. Erik Wright (Wright & Wright, 1987, pp. 100, 170). In the 1960s the San Francisco pediatrician, Dr. Franz Baumann, amplified our understanding of the spectrum of applications of clinical hypnosis with children, by describing and teaching its efficacy for children with asthma, enuresis and encopresis, and substance abuse (Baumann, 1970; Erickson, 1958; Olness & Kohen 1996; Tinterow, 1970).

Hypnosis involves the cultivation of imagination.

Increased documentation of successful clinical applications of hypnosis with children (Gardner, 1976, 1978; Hilgard & Morgan, 1978; Olness, 1975) appeared in the 1970s. During the same time, research began to report both the clinical efficacy and psychophysiologic changes associated with self-hypnosis in children. And, the benefits of hypnosis training were recognized for children with chronic illnesses such as cancer, hemophilia, and asthma (Aronoff, Aronoff, & Peck, 1975; Diamond, 1959; Khan, 1977; Kohen & Wynne, 1988; Kohen, 1980, 1986a, 1986c, 1995c; LaBaw, 1975, 1973; Olness, 1981).

The numbers of child health professionals trained in hypnosis have increased substantially over the past 30 years. Increasing numbers of substantive research projects seek to understand the clinical effects of these self-regulation methods and to apply them with greater precision. In the largest series to date of children treated with hypnosis for a variety of different clinical problems, Kohen and associates reported that in 505 children treated with hypnosis over 83% were successful in reducing their problem by at least 50%, and demonstrated that success within four visits or less (Kohen, Olness, Colwell, & Heimel, 1984).

Hypnotherapeutic methods with and without other self-regulation training (e.g., biofeedback) (Culbert, Reaney, & Kohen, 1994) offer child health professionals opportunities to facilitate development of competency and a sense of personal mastery in children with whom they work. Successful applications of self-regulation include a focus on personal control and decision-making by the child, and specific attention to their preferences in using personal imagery skills. Ongoing research examining the characteristics of children's imagery (Kosslyn, Margolis, Barrett, Goldknopf, & Daly,

1990) will hopefully provide clinicians more precise guidelines in selecting individual hypnotherapeutic approaches for a given child.

DEFINITION AND THEORETICAL UNDERSTANDING

As a clinical tool, and different "state," hypnosis may well be best understood as the cultivation of imagination. While hypnosis has been defined in myriad ways and there is no universally accepted single definition (Lynn & Rhue, 1991), most child health clinicians agree that functionally, hypnosis in children can be defined as an alternative state of awareness and alertness (similar in *feeling* to daydreaming or imagination) in which an individual is selectively focused, absorbed, and concentrating upon a particular idea or image (with or without relaxation), with a specific purpose of achieving some goal or realizing some potential. Depending upon the child's development and individual needs and variations, the state as such may or may not involve physical relaxation (Olness & Kohen, 1996).

We probably are "doing" hypnosis work when we engage our young patients in conversation in which they are absorbed, paying attention, listening, and responding as requested. Most children move in and out of spontaneous hypnotic-like states as they focus their concentration, for example, on video games, "text-messaging" on cell-phones, favorite movies (e.g., The Lion King, The Little Mermaid), TV football, playing "house," listening to stories, enjoying puppet play, or otherwise engaging in fantasy. Kuttner (1988) has noted that especially young children have blurred boundaries, and move frequently, naturally, and easily from fantasy to reality.

These natural, spontaneous hypnotic states are usually positive, and are characterized, as are "induced" hypnotic states, by absorption in fantasy/imagination, focused attention, and heightened suggestibility. While relaxation facilitates children's hypnotic states some of the time, it is neither universal nor necessary for successful child hypnosis. While spontaneous stillness and the relaxation response may be observed with children as with adults, younger children (under 6 or 7 years) commonly do not visibly relax (and therefore should not be expected to) when in hypnosis. Younger children in hypnosis commonly move around as part of their absorption and engagement in fantasy. In such involved hypnotic experiences younger children often prefer to not close their eyes. Mindful of this, clinicians modify their approaches and language accordingly to facilitate this "active alert hypnosis."

There are many roads available to the thoughtful child health clinician to guide a child toward these states of focused concentration, whether toward solving a problem, controlling discomfort, easing or eliminating anxiety, alleviating a habit, or modulating disease processes. Paths available are limited only by the creativity and therapeutic relationship of the clinician and the child. Induction techniques and strategies to begin hypnosis are myriad, including virtually limitless iterations of relaxation and mental imagery (RMI), biofeedback, art therapy, music, drama, and movement therapy (Olness & Kohen, 1996).

Scales of hypnotic "susceptibility" or "suggestibility" were described early in the nineteenth century by Liebault and Bernheim, and more recently in 1963 in London's Children's Hypnotic Susceptibility Scale, and Morgan and Hilgard's Stanford Hypnotic Susceptibility Scale for Children in 1979 (Olness & Kohen, 1996). None have proven to be of predictive value in anticipating clinical success or failure of hypnosis for a given child or diagnosis. Most children score high on the Standard Hypnotic Susceptibility Scale for Children (Kohen, 2004). It remains the task of research regarding properties and characteristics of children's imagery (Kosslyn et al., 1990) and neurophysiologic correlates of hypnotic experiences (Raz, 2005) to provide clinical guidelines in selecting approaches for a given child. Continuing research ultimately must define and identify the ideal children's clinical hypnotic susceptibility scale. Such a scale would be

1. brief (e.g., 5 to 15 minutes long);
2. interesting and absorbing;
3. developmentally sensitive and specific;
4. learning style sensitive and specific;
5. multi-sensory and, perhaps, discriminating between senses;
6. free of cultural bias; and
7. predictive (i.e., would guide a clinician in determining what type of hypnotic strategy would be most helpful for a given child, learning style, level of development, with a given problem) (Kohen, 2001).

Although this ideal has not *yet* been realized, the ever-growing body of research and clinical knowledge of hypnosis with children allow a strong and informed position from which to depart. Positive expectations allow us to identify factors which may potentially affect outcome; that is, the child's personal history, and their desire, motivation, and expectation for positive outcome. Since we know that hypnosis is safe and effective and has no adverse side effects (Olness & Kohen, 1996), it is an important tool in adjunct and primary management of a wide variety of child healthcare issues.

In one of the earliest controlled studies of hypnosis, Goldie (1956) described the use of hypno-anesthesia in the emergency room for children 3–7 years old, reporting that with hypnosis there was a significant reduction in the percentage of patients requiring pharmacotherapeutic analgesia or anesthesia for reduction of fractures or for suturing. In a prospective, randomized controlled trial of hypnosis compared to propranolol and placebo, Olness et al. found hypnosis significantly more effective in reducing the frequency of headaches than either propranolol or placebo (Olness, Culbert, & MacDonald, 1987). In a recent report Kohen and Zajac described a large clinical population of 144 consecutive children and youth with recurrent headaches who with self-hypnosis training were able to significantly reduce frequency, intensity, and duration of headaches compared to before learning self-hypnosis (Kohen & Zajac, 2007). Butler et al. (2005) described hypnosis training for children undergoing VCUG radiographic procedures who had previously experienced distress with the same procedure. With brief training in hypnosis, and coaching by a trained therapist, children displayed less distress, were more compliant with the procedure, and required 14 fewer minutes to complete the VCUG compared to a control group who received standard behavioral intervention, but no formal training in hypnosis per se.

Sugarman and Kohen (2007) described the broad efficacy of clinical hypnosis in a general pediatric environment. Liossi et al. (2006) showed that children undergoing spinal taps had less anticipatory anxiety and procedure-associated pain when hypnosis was combined with topical EMLA cream than when children received only the EMLA cream, or when it was combined with a therapist's attention. Anbar and Hall (2004) recently demonstrated the value of hypnosis in helping children help themselves with chronic habit cough/paradoxical vocal cord spasm. Anbar (2001) has also suggested the efficacy of hypnotic approaches to functional recurrent abdominal pain. Kohen and Murray (2006) have described the clinical value of hypnotic strategies in helping young people manage depressed mood in its various forms, from adjustment disorder with depressed mood in children with chronic illness, to clinical depression and bipolar disorder.

In the day-to-day clinical practice of child healthcare we can and should make the assumption that all children (except those with moderate to severe mental retardation) have the potential for positive hypnotic responsiveness, and that with them we can indeed "find the hypnosis in the encounter" (Sugarman, 2007). Beginning with this positive expectation allows clinicians to identify those logical factors which may potentially affect outcome, including the child's (and family's) personal history, their motivation, desire, and expectation for change and positive outcome.

Brief Review of Common Adult and Pediatric Applications

The list of applications of clinical hypnosis in the health care of adults and children is extensive, and continues to grow as the number and diversity of clinicians applying hypnotic approaches grows. The range of applications is described in Tables 14-1 and 14-2.

In adults, one would add obstetrics and gynecology, but beyond the specificity and distinctions between those uniquely childhood disorders (e.g., nocturnal enuresis) and uniquely adult disorders (e.g., coronary artery disease), the spectrum of applications is quite similar. We wish to make the case for the greater significance of learning self-hypnosis during childhood because of the potential it provides for application as children mature into adolescents and adults. An analogous case could be made, however, for the value of self-hypnosis learning at *any* age toward contributing to the individual's continuing evolution, development, and comfort in their life.

CASE: Headache

[* Initially appeared as Kohen, DP "The Case of Anna-Headache and Heartache" in Cases of the New England Society of Clinical Hypnosis www.nesch.org No. 2.1, March 2000.]

Table 14-1. Applications of Hypnosis in Children

1. Habit disorders: e.g., thumb-sucking, nail-biting, hair-pulling, nocturnal enuresis, habit cough

2. Pain: acute, chronic, "constant", episodic (e.g., repeated medical procedures)

3. Psychological problems
   a. Anxiety disorders: separation anxiety, phobias, PTSD, performance anxiety, sleep onset insomnia, panic, OCD
   b. Depression: adjustment disorder with depressed mood, depression, dysthymia

4. Psychophysiologic disorders: e.g., asthma, migraine H.A., irritable bowel syndrome, inflammatory bowel disease, fibromyalgia, hypertension, eating disorders (obesity, anorexia)

5. Chronic illness: e.g., asthma, rheumatoid arthritis, cancer, cystic fibrosis, chronic renal disease, sickle cell disease, etc.

6. Palliative care—dying: grief and bereavement

Table 14-2. Applications of Hypnosis in Adults

1. Habit disorders: e.g., nailbiting, hair-pulling, smoking

2. Pain: acute, chronic, "constant," episodic (e.g., repeated medical procedures)

3. Psychological problems
   a. Anxiety disorders: separation anxiety, phobias, PTSD, performance anxiety, panic, OCD
   b. Depression: adjustment disorder with depressed mood, depression

4. Psychophysiologic disorders: e.g., asthma, migraine, irritable bowel syndrome, inflammatory bowel disease, hypertension, fibromyalgia, chronic fatigue syndrome

5. Chronic illness: e.g., asthma, COPD, arthritis, cancer, chronic renal disease, coronary artery disease, sickle cell disease

6. Obstetrics/gynecology—pelvic examination: menstrual cramps, hyperemesis gravidarum, labor and delivery

7. Palliative care—dying: grief and bereavement

Chief Complaint: 15 year old A presented with a history of chronic headaches for several years. There was no history of aura or associated sensory phenomena. A's history was positive for familial lipidemia and hypercholesterolemia. Evaluation by her pediatrician and neurologist revealed a normal MRI and a sleep-deprived EEG suggested "possible small seizures." She failed a series of medication trials, including Amitryptaline, Depakote and Tegretol, that is, all produced drowsiness with no significant relief. She was on no medication at the time of her referral for hypnosis. Her father "suffered from migraine" and familial lipidemia contributed to his death. Her father died when A. was 11 years old, and multiple deaths of extended family members occurred within a 16-month period surrounding his death. Although A's presenting complaint was headache, she gave the general impression of being depressed; but did not meet criteria for clinical depression. She was an average student with many friends, and was involved in extracurricular activities.

A. described two types of headache: daily tension headache, rated 7–8 on a 0–12 scale; and bi-temporal migraines twice monthly, with nausea, flushing, pallor, dizziness, and fatigue. She had a history of daily tension headaches during fourth grade. A variety of medications were tried without success, and the headaches remitted spontaneously. After her great-grandmother died (8/97), A. reportedly "fell apart," saying she "couldn't cope." Chronic tension headache and intermittent migraines began the following January, 1998. Migraines occurred on her father's birthday, on the anniversary of his death, and upon visiting their previous home. Assessment focused on the related problems of unresolved grief and chronic migraine headache.

Treatment: *First session: Self-monitoring leading to self-regulation* was introduced with a 0–12 scale for pain to be recorded each evening on a "headache calendar." Positive "waking suggestion" expectations were introduced: "I am 100% certain I can help you help yourself, provided you don't need the headaches for anything." Using humor and challenge to "think differently," the clinician pointed to the file cabinet, asking A. if she knew what was in there. She responded "files, papers, books, etc." The clinician added "right, of course, but also in there are *Headaches*, because I collect them. If you miss them, and want them back, I'll return them… *You can send me all past, present, and future headaches…*" A. was a bit perplexed. The clinician said "I know it sounds weird; just think about it." When the clinician asked A. to "tell me about your Dad?" she quietly shook her head no, but agreed when asked "perhaps some other time, then?" Tears welled up and she spoke much less thereafter.

Second session(2 weeks later): "A" was invited to differentiate psychological distress from physical pain by creating a 0–12 "paying attention to it" scale to be used along with the headache pain scale. Grief work was initiated by asking which death (of family members) she wanted to discuss first. She discussed these losses in the order she chose, ending with her father's death 3+ years earlier. When asked if she thought that being sad and missing her Dad had anything to do with headaches, she said "Yes!" She was told "sometimes people are very surprised…after they let difficult feelings out, that…the feelings don't have to come out 'sideways'…like through headaches or stomach aches." While a formal hypnotic trance was not induced, she clearly was in a spontaneous trance state throughout the grief work.

After appropriate education about what hypnosis is and is not, "A" was taught formally how to enter hypnosis. After hypnotic suggestion to "Picture in your mind a ruler of some kind to measure *those* headaches—I don't know what it will look like or where you'll see it in your mind, but you'll know, just notice it…" "A" reported seeing a blue ruler with black letters. Asked to notice what color and shape a headache was, she said "red" and said "no headache" was white.

Using story-telling metaphors, "A" was told how others had reduced headaches. These included an elevator metaphor ("this one kid I knew imagined he was on an elevator any time he had a headache. As he rode down from 8 to 7 to 6 and the elevator went down, his headache went down…sometimes he went down floor by floor, and other times he took the express elevator and zoomed down from 9 to 1 or 0.); and the *story of the girl* "who didn't like elevators: She used a water slide down into a cool swimming pool. Twelve was at the top and 0 was in the pool, happy and swimming around." "A" was instructed to practice self-hypnosis twice daily, by self-induction of "*imagining something fun,*" and reducing intensity of headache, using whatever images came to her mind. She was asked to track headaches and self-hypnosis practice.

Fourth visit (1 month later): A. was remarkably improved; headache ratings showed a 33% improvement in pain and distress over 2 weeks earlier. She practiced 20–30 minutes per night, using varying hypnotic images for pain reduction. When asked expectantly to speculate when the next 1/3 improvement would occur, she said "two months."

Fifth visit (2 months later): "A" had no further improvement. The session was audiotaped at her request. After providing details about her imagery at home, these details were integrated with open-ended suggestion into the hypnosis session which was audiorecorded. Direct suggestions were offered for "paying attention to the tension and how tension goes away and the way that you do that," and to be "surprised and proud at how good you are getting at this, how effective you are becoming…. Before you finish be sure to congratulate yourself for the gift of your own imagination and being the boss of your body and how you feel."

Sixth visit (1 month later): "A" reported no headaches since the last visit. She was taught rapid self-hypnosis as "stress immunization" throughout the school day. At a follow-up *seventh visit* 2.5 months later she remained headache-free. Termination was begun with the waking suggestion "I wonder how you'll know when the right time is to stop coming for appointments?"

Eighth and final visit: "A" reported continued absence of headaches. When asked, she said matter-of-factly "because of self-hypnosis … I do it before I get a headache…I know when I'm gonna get one because I can feel it in the back of my eyes." She was educated about aura. While this aura had occurred once a week, she would "just do my self-hypnosis and it goes away…!"

Years later, participating in a survey of headache patients (Kohen, 2007; Kohen & Zajac, 2007) she ("A") reported no headache over the preceding 6 years.

Case Commentary (original commentary: Max Shapiro, PhD, Cases of the New England Society of Hypnosis 2.3, March, 2000 www.nesch.org)

This case presents the significant gains achievable when hypnosis is an integrated part of a comprehensive healthcare intervention. A. was referred for hypnotherapy only after a full evaluation had been conducted by her pediatrician and a consulting neurologist. This sequence is important because attempts to modify physiological symptoms through hypnosis are generally limited unless the patient can be assured that *the symptom is not serving a valid physiological function*. Pain sensations that protect the individual, or that serve to alert her to an unrecognized problem are not likely to be modulated by hypnosis very much or for very long.

Secondly, the clinician assessed the possible psychological developmental functions of the headache. The history suggested a link between A's difficulty managing important family losses and her symptom course. Third, the focus was upon teaching A. how to achieve *active mastery*. While important for all hypnotic work, it is *essential* for work with adolescents for whom mastery is a key developmental issue. By presenting hypnosis as a way for A. to 'be the boss of the body' she was empowered to take charge of the headache."

The "waking suggestion" to "send me all your past, present, and future headaches" was an invitation to dissociate headache discomfort in the future *and also* to develop amnesia for previous headaches. This was likely very useful since the memory of previous pain serves as a trigger for stress and anxiety which inevitably increases suffering in people with recurrent pain.

Visualization of the discomfort by numerical ratings, shapes, and colors allowed A. to accept suggestions to manipulate— i.e. lower, eliminate—the symptom by strengthening the mind-body connection. This is a common and intriguing application of the hypnotic process.

CASE: Nocturnal Enuresis

JB was 9 years old when they were referred for hypnosis for longstanding primary nocturnal enuresis. He had never been dry at night. Before the appointment, the family began using a bed-wetting alarm (a kind of biofeedback device—see Biofeedback section below). Mother left a voice mail message asking if she should keep the scheduled appointment since the bed-wetting alarm "seemed to be working, but not 100%." JB was brought by his father for the initial visit. When the physician asked JB how come he had come over, he said he had no clue. In developing rapport, JB was able to talk about other things but the most he was willing to say early in the visit was "Diapers...I have problems...at bed!" and then he cried, hiding his face while wiping tears with his shirt. Reluctant to talk, he allowed his Dad to "start off the conversation." Reflecting the family's belief system, Dad said "He has a problem where he doesn't wake up, so he'll wet the bed." Until 3 weeks prior, he had been wearing diapers nightly. JB said, "I hate 'em!" His growth and development were normal. There was no constipation or soiling, daytime wetting, urinary tract infection, diabetes mellitus, allergies, enuresis in the family, or sleep disorders. JB reviewed their usual night-time routine. He said they were "done" with the buzzer (nighttime alarm). "It was supposed to wake me up to go to the bathroom but I didn't like it and Mom didn't like it..." Dad didn't hear it as he is a 'sound sleeper." They had high hopes for this alarm and were disappointed when it didn't work. He had briefly achieved 5 nights out of 7 (71%) dryness while using the alarm, but then reverted to nightly bed-wetting before the first appointment.

The last 2/3 of the first appointment focused on educating JB about how the body works, re-framing suggestions about mind-body interactions, and enthusiastic, positive expectations about the likelihood of being able to soon become dry every night. This was accomplished in the context of developing rapport, without mention of hypnosis or hypnotherapy. This is not to say that spontaneous hypnosis was not occurring. Indeed, as the task of the clinician was to "find the hypnosis in the encounter"; elements of absorption, intrigue, and focused concentration were key in utilizing naturalistic hypnotic behavior and context to teach positive expectancy and ways of thinking about solving the enuresis problem that "used to be there."

Concepts of mind-body relationships were introduced conversationally as JB readily discussed riding a bicycle, and muscles required to do so. He was invited to realize that at one time he had *not* known how to ride, and to describe how he learned. ("My Dad ran next to me. Then one time he let go and I rode for a while and then crashed . . . then I got back on and did it . . ."); and then how he got better ("I practiced . . ."). Asked how he knew how to ride the bike in the spring after several months of not riding in winter, JB said all of those different muscles (hands, arms, legs, feet, eyes, etc.) *remembered* how; *and* the brain could tell them *what to do* in just a few seconds. In the spring, therefore, he could take his bicycle out and just ride, without needing to say or think "Okay, hands hold the handle bars, feet push the pedals, eyes stay open, butt sit straight . . ." Without explaining the connecting metaphor, the pediatrician engaged JB in discussion of how the body works, by drawing a valentine (heart), kidneys, bladder, and the "nerve lines" connecting bladder and brain. A "mock conversation" on "imaginary cell-phones" followed: The bladder calls the brain to tell it when it's full. The brain instructs the bladder's muscle gate to stay closed until the brain tells the feet to walk to the bathroom and "get ready" and then tells the gate to open, letting the urine out in the toilet "where it belongs." Discussion followed that this is "exactly what happens all day without even thinking about it. That's why you don't pee in your pants" The so-called motivating, waking hypnotic suggestion that followed was almost a foregone conclusion, that is, "So, *since* the problem is already solved in the daytime (JB does not wet his pants), and *since* your brain and bladder already know each other and are friends, and *since* it's the same bladder and brain at night, all you need to do before you go to sleep is remind your brain and bladder to talk to each other at night *so that you can wake up in the morning in a nice warm, dry bed.* So, maybe you'll tell them something like this: "Bladder and brain, tonight I'm going to be asleep so please talk to each other 'cause I'm going to be busy having a nice dream: Bladder, your easy job is just to let the brain know when you're full, that's it. Brain, you'll get a message from the bladder when it's full. Then you have a *choice*: You could wake me up, I'll get out of bed, walk to the bathroom, open the gate, aim, let the urine out in the toilet, flush, wash and dry my hands, go back to my nice, comfortable, warm, dry bed: *or*, you know brain, I'm going to be cozy, having a nice dream, so instead *you could just tell the gate to stay closed and locked all night long*, sleep all night in my *nice, comfortable, warm, dry bed* and wake up in the morning in *my nice, comfortable, warm, dry bed* and *then* walk to the bathroom, open the gate, aim, let the urine out in the toilet, flush, wash and dry my hands, brush my teeth, get dressed, have breakfast and have a great day. I'll be so proud of myself waking up in a nice dry bed."

JB agreed to give these instructions each night and to use star stickers to keep track of dry beds on a calendar. They agreed to stop using diapers.

Two weeks later JB proudly showed his chart with a star on every day, that is, reflecting 100% dry in the interim 14 days! Asked "How did you *do* that?" he said "I don't know," *but* drew his own version of the picture drawn two weeks earlier, highlighting a smiley face, brain, heart, kidneys "to wash the blood and make pee," and bladder with the "door." He accurately described the "nerves" that help the bladder and brain talk to each other. JB was very proud, and acknowledged that his parents and I were also proud of him, though he was most proud. He and his parents decided that they did not need to come back for any further follow-up. A three months telephone follow-up indicated he remained 100% dry.

Case commentary: in this case, hypnosis took place naturalistically as [hypnotic] rapport evolved rapidly while coming to know JB in a child-centered, humor-based encounter at the first visit. Rapport developed as the focus was upon engaging him in giving the history—almost to the exclusion of the father—and was followed by interest in the child independent of the problem, engaging him in discussion of what he liked about school, what he did for fun, what he does "best." A description of genito-urinary anatomy and physiology was offered as an interactive educational drawing in which he was an active participant, focused narrowly, concentrating, and responding to suggestions for participation. Empowering suggestions, future positive expectations, and "how to do it at home" ended this "hypnotic conversation" and resulted in achievement of the desired goal, with 100% dryness achieved by the second visit, and sustained over the ensuing months. Precisely how this "works" is not clear, nor is it clear how or why this is so effective in some cases like JB, while in seemingly analogous situations there are slower, and/or less immediately successful outcomes.

Proposed Mechanism of Biological Effect

The precise mechanism for the biologic effects of hypnosis has not yet been precisely defined. Over the past 50 years we have been able to describe physiologic effects and changes which occur and are measurable during hypnosis. These have included lowering of blood pressure, slowing of pulse rate, slowing of respiratory rate, (Benson, 1975; See BFT section below) increase of electrodermal activity, skeletal muscle relaxation, increase of peripheral temperature, and the ability of children and adults to purposely evoke these and other physiologic alterations with the application of self-hypnosis skills (Kohen, 1995; Dikel & Olness, 1980; Kohen & Ondich, 2004; Kohen & Wynne, 1997;

Olness & Conroy, 1985). The mechanism of *how* these changes are effected has remained elusive. However, in recent years some very exciting research has begun to elucidate very precise central nervous system biological changes which are concurrent with observed and reported hypnotic behavior and phenomenology (Raz, Fan, & Posner, 2005; Raz, 2005).

Safety/Risks

Parental education about the application and efficacy of hypnosis in children and youth is essential, and fosters successful learning and mastery of hypnosis by young people. Since all hypnosis is self-hypnosis, most training and reinforcement sessions of hypnosis with children are conducted in private. Parents are encouraged to understand that, while practice of self-hypnosis is critical to its success in helping the problem, that practice should really be left up to the child and represent an understanding between the child and the clinician, who is their coach/teacher. Unlike practice of the piano, the clarinet, or school homework, parents should not provide reminders or scheduled time for self-hypnosis. Instead, this should be a decision and agreement between the child and their clinician/coach. Exceptions to this would be appropriate with children who ordinarily require reminders, encouragement, and support in their lives, like most children under the age of 5 or 6; or like children with significant problems with disorganization (e.g., some children with ADHD). Thus, as in all situations in childhood, where ongoing mastery is part of the natural developmental process, parents should be alerted to take a graded approach to their involvement in their child's self-hypnosis, and be less and less involved or directive as children "get older."

Key ingredients of effective clinical hypnosis: imaginative involvement and patients' positive expectations and motivation for success.

The key ingredients in effectiveness of hypnosis are expectations and motivation. Thus, *when* an individual has a problem which is known to be amenable to modulation/relief/elimination with hypnosis, *when* they are *motivated* to make that change, and *when* they come to *expect* that to be possible, *then* it is only a matter of time and practice before success is achieved. If parents interfere with that process (e.g., through reminders to practice which inadvertently convey lack of confidence in the child's ability and/or the parent's mistaken belief that they—and not the child—are "in charge"), this may delay or even obviate success. If there are concomitant psycho-emotional issues (e.g., anxiety or depression) which require therapy, these may require concurrent attention, with hypnosis and/or other therapeutic approaches.

Used appropriately, hypnosis is safe; and there are no risks (Olness & Kohen, 1996).

All hypnosis is self-hypnosis.

Training/Accreditation/Licensure

The American Society of Clinical Hypnosis (www.asch.net) has a certification of training process which defines the core content requirements for basic and advanced level
of expertise in clinical hypnosis. Successful completion of this training provides either
certification by ASCH (basic) or certification as an approved consultant in clinical hypnosis. Other countries have extensive curricular requirements for training in hypnosis
(Australian Society of Hypnosis: www.ozhypnosis.com.au, Dutch Society of Hypnosis:
www.nvvh.com, Israel Society of Hypnosis: www.hypno.co.il/english.asp).

The American Boards of Clinical Hypnosis (American Board of Medical Hypnosis,
American Board of Psychological Hypnosis, American Board of Hypnosis in Clinical
Social Work, American Board of Dental Hypnosis, and the emerging American Board
of Hypnosis in Nursing) offer certification of competency in clinical hypnosis within
one's clinical specialty. Each Board requires an application process and submission of
case example(s) of one's clinical work with hypnosis, and conducts an examination process. The American Board of Medical Hypnosis examination includes written, oral, and
practical (demonstration) examinations. Information regarding the examinations of
the respective boards is available on their respective websites (available through www.
asch.net).

Making a Referral

Individuals in North America seeking clinical hypnosis consultation may review the
American Society of Clinical Hypnosis (www.asch.net) website for a roster of clinicians
trained in clinical hypnosis, their areas of interest and expertise, and their geographic
location throughout the United States and Canada. Contact with regional "component
sections" of the ASCH is also available through this website. Additional information is
also available through the Society for Clinical and Experimental Hypnosis (www.sceh.us).

Biofeedback

INTRODUCTION

Biofeedback refers to provision of (self-generated) physiological information to people,
typically for using that information for their benefit, for example, to alter an undesirable
(psycho) physiological response. The word biofeedback was coined in the late 1960s
to describe laboratory procedures then being used to train subjects in experimental

research to alter brain activity, blood pressure, heart rate, and other bodily functions (then) typically not controlled voluntarily (Runck, 1983). Before the word biofeedback was created, everyday examples of what we understand to be equivalent, simple bio-feedback instruments and experiences (though they weren't called that) were bathroom scales giving people information about their weight, oral thermometers conveying information about body temperature, or a standard doctor's office sphygmomanometer, for measuring blood pressure. Most simply, biofeedback involves using mechanical or electronic equipment to measure and reveal information about physiologic functions, that is, what is going on in the body. Practically, biofeedback is employed to provide these kinds of information in response to individuals' psychological processes. Schwartz and Olson (2003, p. 5) observe, "An assumption of clinical biofeedback is that it can help persons improve the accuracy of their perceptions of their visceral events. The perceptions allow them to gain greater self-regulation of these processes. Indeed some professionals view some biofeedback as instrumental conditioning of visceral responses." The clinician aims to guide and direct this conditioning of psychophysiological reflexes in adaptive directions. Ultimately the goal—often unspoken—may be to generalize the originally targeted self-regulation to an overall sense of well-being, or whole body health.

> When mothers take children's temperatures, biofeedback is at work; we just don't call it that.

The development of biofeedback as a "therapy" is the result of a confluence of learning theory, behavioral psychology, psychophysiology, behavioral medicine, biomedical engineering and cybernetics (Schwartz & Olson, 2003). Arguably, applied psychophysiology has its roots in the stress research of Selye who elucidated the essentials of brain-body connections associated with homeostasis and an understanding of the role of stress in physical and mental diseases (Selye, 1974, 1976). This awareness led to the growth of relaxation strategies involving primarily physical (progressive muscle relaxation, hatha yoga) and mental (meditation, "relaxation response" and related techniques) (Schwartz & Olson, pp. 6–8). After World War II, technological developments allowed accurate and reliable physiological measurements to be represented as audio and visual feedback. While this evolution drew the mental and physical together, it is of significance historically to note the relationship of biofeedback and hypnosis, described and in a sense predicted by James Braid. Braid, a British physician who coined the word "hypnotism" and suggested that all hypnosis is self-hypnosis, wrote in *Physiology of Fascination* (1855): "My investigations have proved, beyond all controversy, that by these means the ordinary mental and physical functions may be changed...and *all* the natural functions may be excited or depressed with great uniformity, even in the waking condition, according to the dominant idea existing in the mind...whether that has arisen spontaneously, had been the result of previous associations, or of the suggestion of others...And, finally, as a generic term, comprising the *whole* of these phenomena which result from the reciprocal actions of mind and matter upon each other, I think no term could be more appropriate than *psychophysiology*."

Surface electromyography (sEMG or EMG), peripheral skin temperature (TEMP), respiratory rate and depth as pneumography (PNG), sweat gland activity as a function of skin conductance (also called electrodermal activity [EDA]), various electroencephalographic modalities (EEG), blood pressure (BP), and heart rate variability (HRV) have all been employed to provide individuals with insights about their physiology. These modalities provide a reflective interface that allows an individual to perceive, experience, and resonate with the physiological effects of their own mental processes. The choice of which interface, modality or combination of modalities is subject to the orientation of the therapist and is discussed in Section "Biofeedback Strategies."

The study of biofeedback began in 1969 when Miller (1969) described operant conditioning of autonomic nervous system functions, for example, blood pressure, heart rate, intestinal motility, and gastric and peripheral blood flow in the curarized rat. Subsequently, hundreds of studies have described the successful use of various types of biofeedback for varying types of clinical problems (Brown, 1974; Basmajian, 1989; Olton & Noonberg, 1980; Schwartz & Andrasik, 2003). Biofeedback with children began in the 1970s. Early prospective controlled studies with children naïve to biofeedback (or hypnosis) documented their ability to intentionally alter various autonomic responses. These included Dikel and Olness' study (1980) documenting children's ability to voluntarily alter peripheral temperature with a few minutes of focused mental effort, capacity to intentionally change auditory evoked potentials (Olness & Conroy, 1985), blood pressure (Kohen & Ondich, 2004), electrodermal activity (Olness & Rusin, 1990), and muscle responses including anorectal function (Hibi, Iwai, Kimura, Sasaki, & Tsuda, 2003; Olness, McParland, & Piper, 1980; Palsson, Heymen, & Whitehead, 2004). In the mid-1970s the work of Lubar (1991; Lubar & Bahler, 1976), reflected early and ongoing interest in and investigation of the possibility and promise of EEG biofeedback for various CNS disorders. These included reports regarding the value of biofeedback training of sensorimotor rhythm in control of epilepsy, and the investigation of neurofeedback for treatment of Attention Deficit Hyperactivity Disorder (Fox, Tharp, & Fox, 2005; Lubar, 1991). Following upon these foundational works, many clinical applications, clinical reports, and controlled studies have described the utility and efficacy of biofeedback strategies and approaches in children, and are summarized quite thoroughly by Culbert and Banez (2003).

BIOFEEDBACK TOOLS

The logarithmic growth of biomedical and interactive computer technologies has stimulated an increasingly sophisticated variety of computer-assisted biofeedback devices.

Since young people are accustomed to viewing high-quality video graphics, biofeedback training that employs computer-generated graphics to represent physiological functions are particularly engaging and motivating. Culbert and Banez have identified that three essential elements of videogames—fantasy, curiosity and challenge—can be integrated into biofeedback software to render the clinical application "a computer game for the body" (Culbert & Banez, 2003, p. 701).

The variety of interactive formats include the NeXus-10 platform with user-friendly BioTrace software (Stens Corporation: www.Stens-biofeedback.com) that has state-of-the-art, engaging games and challenges for children as they move toward a physiological threshold. Heartmath (www.heartmath.com) via its Emwave PC HRV hardware/software package, challenges youngsters to colorize greytones, move a balloon over a landscape, and move along a rainbow to a pot of gold by reaching and regulating their heart rate variability (HRV), in the process gaining control of their emotional state and cultivating a lower state of arousal. Heartmath also has a nice hand-held device, the emWave PSR (personal stress reliever) which children enjoy and learn quickly. The Mind/Body Game (Performance Concepts, 8250 Tyler Blvd, Mentor OH 44050) invites children to create more positive facial expressions on their choice of four animals by lowering their own skin conductance while a narrator reinforces the message, "You *are* the boss of your body." Thought Technology's Biograph Software includes a changing sunset, a face than frowns or smiles with one's variability around a threshold and a range of musical, audio feedback that allows reinforcement for youngsters who may be visually impaired or who choose to close their eyes. This palette of interfaces allows the therapist to choose any combination of physiological measurements to be presented to the child or adolescent in ways that best fit their physiological reactivity and individual motivation.

While engaging and reinforcing, sophisticated and multifaceted biofeedback technologies are not necessary to provide young people with physiological feedback. Many devices not originally designed with clinical biofeedback in mind can be creatively recruited for that purpose. While watching a pulse oximeter display, both heart rate and percentage oxygen saturation, a young person with dyspnea due to asthma can be encouraged to "help *this* number [heart rate] go down so *that* number [percentage of oxygen saturation] will go up *as* your breathing gets more and more comfortable." Children enjoy listening to their own heart beat with a stethoscope and can learn even quite quickly to realize that they can vary it with their attention.

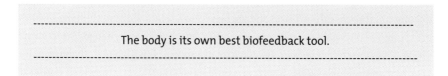

The body is its own best biofeedback tool.

Many children with primary nocturnal enuresis are offered the opportunity of "dry night training" through an alarm system designed to sense the smallest amount of moisture (urine) and then awaken them to go to the bathroom to urinate rather than wetting their bed. These conditioning alarms are reviewed and described by Mellon and McGrath (2000) as not only effective, but even as "necessary" in the treatment of enuresis. We disagree that they are "necessary." Indeed, as in the foregoing case, (pages 278–279) many children solve the problem of nocturnal enuresis once they understand how their body works, and have learned ways, such as self-hypnosis, to instruct their mind and body to work together. It is clear, however, that when they are used, conditioning alarms are functioning as "biofeedback" devices, though few studies and none of the alarm systems/products mention the word "biofeedback." A simple mirror may become a biofeedback device to allow youngsters to literally picture the expressive effects of their emotional states, or, for example, to note the degree/presence/absence of tic behaviors in response to affective changes. Analogously, a youngster with a tic disorder (e.g., Tourette's Syndrome) may benefit from viewing a DVD recording of him/herself having tics and then having them dissipate while doing self-hypnosis or relaxation. *Viewing* this process on a DVD provides "feedback" and, therefore, reinforcement that the desired and now observed change is, in fact, possible.

Liquid crystals that vary color (on "Dermatherms," Sharn, Inc., 4801 George Road, Tampa, FL 33634; "Temp Dots," "Stress Cards") with surface temperature are available to monitor peripheral perfusion as a manifestation of sympathetic nervous system arousal, and can be applied to the hand or wrist and provide feedback during therapy or throughout the day. In carefully selected, defined situations, even physiological displays in inpatient settings (e.g., postoperative recovery and intensive care units) when presented with care and sensitivity, can be made visibly accessible to the patient so that they can begin to see and learn to regulate their autonomic responses.

BIOFEEDBACK STRATEGIES

The fundamental notion that feedback reinforces behavior and can be used to change behavior derives from learning theory and cybernetics. (Schwarz & Olson, 2003, pp. 4–10) Biofeedback builds on these principles by using physiological feedback about maladaptive behavior that is less voluntarily determined to promote therapeutic, adaptive change. Culbert and Banez (2003, p. 700) offer the "Discern-Control-Generalize" model to characterize a general approach to the patient. In the "discern" phase, children learn to notice specific mind-body links (e.g., rapid, often dramatic increased skin conductance in response to surprise) and are helped to see how shifts in thinking, images, breathing and physical relaxation cause a physiological variable to change. The "control" phase allows the child to master their control of a specific function (e.g., diaphragmatic breathing, muscle relaxation, lowering skin conductance) over a specified period of time and toward a threshold level. Most importantly, the child learns to "generalize" this adaptive physiological self-regulation into their life outside of the biofeedback room. This phase necessarily involves identification of external cues that remind them to use their new skills and maintaining the newly acquired internal sensitivity to a state of lowered arousal. Whether this generalization and adaptive self-regulation represents "biofeedback" at home, or "self-hypnosis" or some combination is discussed further below, and may indeed be moot.

The choice of which physiological functions to use for a given clinical situation remains controversial. One extreme supports the notion of "specificity." "Specificity" involves the degree of correlation between a given physiological parameter (e.g., hand warming) and a given symptom complex (e.g., migraine headaches); and that this correlation holds for large populations of individuals. This means one would always do peripheral temperature biofeedback for a child or adolescent with migraine headaches. The other extreme might be labeled "sensitivity." This perspective holds that individual proclivities and resources best determine the modality of biofeedback and that biofeedback is primarily a metaphor for autonomic control. (Olness & Kohen, 1996, pp. 320–321). In this view, the clinician would use a given child's most engaging and reactive physiological function(s) regardless of the presenting problem. The role of expectancy in both situations is likely very strong, and continues to be an area of important, and as yet inadequate, investigation.

THE HYPNOSIS/BIOFEEDBACK INTERFACE

Hypnosis and biofeedback are strategies directed at evoking innate experiential resources to alter psycho-physiological responses which have become maladaptive. Hypnosis relies on the resonance and rapport of a therapeutic relationship and the language of positive expectancy to cultivate the imagination. Biofeedback provides an external, somatic focus as a proxy for internal psycho-physiological change. Both involve narrowly focused, intensified attention and heightened responsiveness to new ideas and associations. This "trance" state can be reinforced by the clinician's therapeutic language as described earlier. It is generally agreed that positive expectancy, permissive (as opposed to directive), patient-centered approaches that stimulate curiosity and imagination promote success in both strategies, at least in part through intensification of the trance experience characterizing the encounter. For example, someone who practices self-hypnosis to reduce frequency and intensity of migraine headaches can receive validation of what they are learning at a follow up visit involving biofeedback. They can learn that they actually lower electrodermal activity (state of autonomic arousal) and raise peripheral temperature *while rehearsing self-hypnosis* (hypnosis-assisted biofeedback). By contrast, another child with a migraine headache problem may be hesitant to believe that the mind effects change in the body, and *their* biofeedback/self-hypnosis training may occur in the opposite direction. Thus, through absorption and increased attention to the engaging nature of a computerized biofeedback game, the hypnotic trance may be achieved (biofeedback-assisted hypnosis) *while* they experience increase in peripheral temperature, reduction in electrodermal activity, or reduction in muscle tension. Experiencing this change as evidence that their mind can create bodily changes may allow this child to begin to believe and expect success, and foster their motivation to practice "biofeedback" at home.

Unless the child has an external device for measuring, for example, peripheral temperature or electrodermal activity, at home, when they are practicing "biofeedback" at home, we believe they are, in fact, practicing self-hypnosis. Even when connected to computerized biofeedback, we believe little, if anything, "happens" without the child concurrently accessing that alternative state of consciousness we have come to call ' "trance," ' that is, the hypnotic state. Ultimately, the name does not matter, especially as the goal is kept clearly in mind to facilitate resolution of a problem, effect a positive change, or maximize some potential; and credit is given appropriately to the child whose self-regulation rehearsal has created and allowed the change to come about.

When utilized and understood together, biofeedback and self-hypnosis can commonly facilitate change which may be greater than either could achieve alone. Credence for this was understood in the 1970s when Beata Jencks described the body as its own best biofeedback device in *Your Body—Biofeedback at its Best* (Jencks, 1977); and Silver and Blanchard (1978) compared biofeedback with relaxation training in assessing the efficacy of treatment for psycho-physiological disorders. In assessing preference for a given approach (e.g., relaxation or biofeedback), Silver and Blanchard suggested consideration of efficacy (Which works better?), efficiency (Which works faster?), durability (Which benefits last longer?), generality (Which benefits the most, i.e., greater percentage of a given sample?), convenience, and cost. They concluded that relaxation may be the critical variable in the success of treatment, and that biofeedback is one way of producing relaxation. Underlying this conclusion is the concept that many psycho-physiological disorders may be due to excessive sympathetic arousal and, as described by Gellhorn and Kiely (1972) and Benson (1975), meditation, progressive relaxation, autogenic training produce a shift toward decreased sympathetic arousal with decrease in heart rate, blood pressure, muscle activity. Analogous changes have been described with biofeedback (Culbert & Banez, 2003; Schandler & Grings, 1976) and hypnosis (Kohen & Ondich, 2004; Lee & Olness, 1996), and summarized by Benson (1975).

INTEGRATING BIOFEEDBACK INTO PRACTICE

Biofeedback may be easily introduced into any clinical practice setting with the use of "Biodots," "Dermatherm," or other "Stress Cards." These liquid crystals vary color and monitor peripheral perfusion as a reflection of sympathetic nervous system arousal. They can be applied to the hand to provide ongoing feedback during a clinical session, and may serve as a quick, simple introduction to the concept that the mind and body are "constantly working together." Analogously, in the office, simple, portable peripheral temperature monitors may be affixed to a fingertip to provide "evidence" that change in mind can effect change in some part of our physiology (e.g., skin temperature). While individual clinicians must do this in their own personal style, an example of introducing simple peripheral temperature biofeedback or electrodermal activity follows.

Taking clear advantage of children's natural curiosity and eagerness to learn new things, one might say at a propitious moment: "Would you like to learn something cool and do an experiment at the same time? This is a thermometer. It measures temperature, right? This one doesn't go in your mouth or your ear. This goes easily on your (fingertip, wrist, hand) like this (attaching). It doesn't bother. Taking it off feels like it feels to take off a band-aid.

See how (the color is changing, or the numbers are changing)…it's taking your temperature (or measuring how calm you feel).

For temperature: "So, what would happen if we put some snow on your hand? Right, it would go down. If I turned up the heat in the room? Right, it'd go up. If we put a warm cloth on your hand? Right, it would go up. If I turned up the air conditioning? Right, it would get cooler. If we did nothing? Right, it would stay the same. *What if you changed your thinking?*" Most children say they don't know. Some speculate (incorrectly): "If I got mad it would go up 'cause I feel hot if I get mad!" Typically with the agitation and arousal associated with anger, peripheral temperature *decreases* (Dikel & Olness, 1980). Once understanding has been established one can begin by suggesting simply "Let's do an experiment…" After an "okay" the clinician may suggest "Okay, just close your eyes and 'pretend' (or 'daydream' for an older child, or 'imagine' for an adolescent) that you're not here" (note: With eye closure and suggestions for imagery, this becomes a rather easily, quickly conducted hypnotic experience—and depending on the individual patient/family, this may or may not be important to discuss as such): "Just imagine that you are somewhere where you are having a great time, enjoying what you're doing—with friends or family or maybe you're alone…wherever you want, you're the boss of your imagination—notice what you're doing, how much fun it is! Notice the sounds—maybe talking or laughing or music, or sounds of the weather…and you can even experiment with making the sounds really loud in your mind, or pretend you have the volume controller and turn them down or all the way off. Maybe you'll imagine having a snack, some favorite food and you can smell the smells of that food 'cause you're the boss of it…" This kind of open-ended, multi-sensory imagery is readily acceptable to children and adults alike, and within a few minutes facilitates development of a nice, relaxed hypnotic trance. For purposes of introducing biofeedback, this is all that is necessary as the clinician can, by monitoring the biofeedback device, notice change that has occurred, and within a few minutes say something reinforcing: "When you're ready in a moment open your eyes, check the (peripheral temperature) and notice what it says *now*…when you open your eyes and come back to the room, bring your relaxed feelings with you. Most children are pleasantly surprised, often even"astonished!" to see that their skin temperature has changed "THAT MUCH!" in but a few minutes. The clinician might appropriately marvel at the change, saying "Wow! Look ... just from changing what you were imagining, the temperature went (e.g., up from 92°F to 96°F)! Amazing! What do you think about that?? How did you DO that??"

(Even after over 30 years of doing this work, I never cease to enjoy and become excited at the changes children create and evoke in these experiences!) With allowances for obvious differences between patients, the clinician can easily build on this positive mind-body experience to ask questions, give clinical "homework," move into more sophisticated biofeedback and/or hypnosis training, etc. Ways of doing that might be to say:

- "So, I *wonder* what *this experiment* might have to do with *those headaches you've been having*?" and invite the 11–12 year-old to write down a few ideas/answers to discuss at future visits.
- Or, "Now that you've seen that the mind and body work together without really knowing it, next time we can learn about biofeedback with a computer, and figure out together ways to help you help that worry that was bothering you so much."
- Or, "When kids learn this stuff they usually discover what the next step might be to using their minds to help their bodies feel better. Maybe we can talk about that next time?"
- Or, "I wonder what two times each day you will practice this (raising your temperature, calming your mind) for ten minutes each time, and see how that affects your (anger, headache, habits, sadness etc.)."

TRAINING/ACCREDITATION/LICENSURE

Formal training in biofeedback is strongly recommended for anyone wishing to develop skills and incorporate this useful modality into clinical practice. Training is available through the Association for Applied Psychophysiology and Biofeedback (AAPB), 10200 West 44th Ave, #304 Wheat Ridge, CO 80033-2840; www.aapb.org.

Making a referral:

The AAPB (www.aapb.org) provides contact information about their members who provide clinical biofeedback services, and who meet and adhere to prescribed professional and ethical standards of care.

MEDITATION

Dean Ornish says, "Meditation is the art of paying attention, of listening to your heart" (Kabat-Zinn, 1994).

For most people unfamiliar with meditation, the term evokes an image of someone sitting calmly in the lotus position with their eyes closed and apparently concentrating. Often when asked "Have you ever heard of meditation?" children—in playful or even mocking fashion—will quickly sit cross-legged, close their eyes, extend their arms and, forming a ring with their thumbs and index fingers, chant "Ohmmm" with no real knowledge of what they are doing. Their usual explanation is to say that they saw this depicted in a cartoon on TV. Like many adults, that is the extent of their knowledge, beyond that it is somehow mysterious or mystical.

Most generally, meditation amounts to thinking in a very controlled fashion, that is, deciding consciously how to direct the mind for a period of time, and then doing so (Kaplan, 1985). This is far from easy if one has had no experience or training; but, like most things, improves steadily with training and rehearsal. Indeed "thought-stopping" takes considerable practice and is the first and major goal of the various meditative traditions. For most traditional forms of meditation, a singular goal seems to be the achievement of a higher state of consciousness and is commonly associated with a sense of spirituality. Thus, through various forms of meditation one is able to reach a "higher," more spiritual state of being, one in which one may feel more fulfilled, more "at one" with the universe, "closer to God," in a greater, more peaceful, more harmonious state of being. One of the goals of meditation is to develop influence/control of the subconscious (= unconscious) part of the mind toward a sense of mastery. Focused concentration, enhanced awareness, and perception are all goals of meditation and are accomplished by quieting the mind, not concentrating on the immediate experience (e.g., of appreciating the beauty of a flower), thus eliminating interference with focus, and by focusing more of the mind on the target (the flower) at hand.

In Bill Moyers *The Healing Mind*, Jon Kabat-Zinn notes that "The essence of the discipline [of meditation] … has to do with cultivating awareness and a deep understanding of what it means to be human" (Moyers, 1993, p. 135).

Though various forms of meditation have been associated with many ancient traditions (Kabat-Zinn, 1994, 2005; Kaplan, 1985;), so-called medical meditation has only recently made its way into mainstream medicine.

Kabat-Zinn's work with mindfulness in a healthcare environment eschews even the use of the word meditation out of recognition/fear that a misconception may indeed interfere with the process of mindfulness, enhanced focus and awareness, and the ultimate goal of improved health through the cultivated use of this modality (Moyers, 1993).

Like the interconnectedness of hypnosis and biofeedback, it seems clear to us that the process of [medical] meditation is similar, if not identical, to the process we describe here as hypnosis. Certainly shared characteristics of hypnosis (and biofeedback) and meditation include narrowed, focused concentration, "turning inward," sustained concentration and relaxation, and often stillness—of mind and body. In so-called traditional—or transcendental—meditation the purpose of this is indeed spiritual, reaching a higher plane of consciousness, closer to holiness or oneness; whereas in hypnosis the purpose is not so much or only the achievement of that state, as it is what one does with it, that is, relieving pain, reversing an undesired habit, reducing anxiety, etc.

Curiously, just as Kabat-Zinn avoided the use of the word meditation in the beginning of his mindfulness meditation groups, so Garth in the nineties (1991, 1992, 1997) specifically *used* the word meditation in the books she wrote, for example, *Meditations for Children*, and did not use the word "hypnosis." A review of these stories, like other therapeutic storytelling books for helping children (Brett, 1986, 1992; Mills & Crowley, 1986; Thomson, 2005), reveals that the essential ingredients of the "meditations" and "storytelling" are indeed the same as those of hypnosis, that is, imagery and relaxation, characterized by focused, narrowed attention, absorption with some idea or imagery, with the explicit purpose of solving a problem, reducing a discomfort, or maximizing a potential.

A search on *Google* (www.google.com) of "Children's Meditation" returned 594,000 citations! No research was identified. Citations typically provide websites with information and often books, tapes/CDs, and classes for children and/or for parents to learn to guide their children with meditation practices. A random sampling of dozens of these citations revealed recurrent themes: children can use and learn meditation easily and effectively. Meditation is promoted for its value in general relaxation, reduction of stress, relief of anxiety, facilitation of sleep, and relief of discomfort. Perhaps most importantly, each site reviewed characterized meditation by its significant and critical ingredients as we have discussed here, that is, relaxation, imagery or imagination, an inward focus of attention, and positive expectancy. These remain the critical, functional ingredients of *all* mind-body techniques.

Many of these reviewed sites, as with the work of Thomson (2005), Brett (1986, 1992), and Garth (1991, 1992, 1997) emphasize appropriately that the effectiveness of "meditation" in children is often best facilitated through guidance by the parent functioning as the storyteller or guide, certainly at least in the beginning of learning the how-to and potential value of the meditation. This *important role for parents*, as with the learning of self-hypnosis, is emphasized especially for young children, under the age of about 7 or 8, who developmentally and appropriately rely on their parents to facilitate, guide, and reinforce their learning and behavior. As children mature and in most aspects of their lives are developing increasing mastery and autonomy with decreasing involvement of parents, so it is and should be that parental involvement in storytelling, guided meditation, guided hypnosis, guided biofeedback decrease in favor of encouraging and facilitating their children's autonomous application and development of these self-regulation skills.

PROGRESSIVE RELAXATION/"BREATH WORK"

Description/Definitions/History

The tightness of muscles and muscle group asymmetries can contribute to discomfort in a variety of acute and chronic conditions of pain and associated anxiety. Learning to relax muscles helps children become more aware of their bodies in general and specific muscles/muscle groups in particular, and in turn to learn about the value of focusing and re-focusing (e.g., on muscles) and how that contributes to relaxation of the mind.

Some clinicians teach that alternating between tension and relaxation of muscle groups sequentially down (or up) the body allows children to learn discrimination and control of areas of muscle tension, learning in time to discharge excessive nervous and muscle tension and improve comfort (Culbert, Friedrichsdorf, & Kuttner, 2007). This approach likely had its origins with Jacobsonian Relaxation which was first described in 1924 with the publication of "The Technic of Progressive Relaxation" in which Dr. Edmund Jacobson first described his didactic approach. This was followed soon thereafter by the first edition of his book *Progressive Relaxation* (Gessel, 1989).

In the originally described Jacobsonian relaxation and so-called traditional progressive relaxation, the concept of first tensing the designated muscle and then allowing it to relax was emphasized. Jacobson's "Method" begins with a brief description of the mechanics of the motor system, followed by a series of studies that demonstrate the basic technical skills. The instructions start simply:

> 1. Lying in a quiet place, bend the hand back at the wrist and study the sensation arising from the act (the sensation in the forearm). This first item of instruction is not relaxation, but observation, the all important ability to monitor tension, the basic element of action and behavior.
>
> 2. Discontinue that activity, and observe the changes in sensation. Practice relaxing, under the direction of awareness.
>
> This manoeuvre is repeated twice more, allowing several minutes between each contraction. The remainder of the recommended hour of practice is spent lying quietly, essentially doing nothing. This doing of nothing is also a highly technical matter, including maintaining a light concentration, a slight focus of awareness on the proprioceptive senses, mainly on the muscle being studied in that session. (Gessel, 1989, p. 3)

The intention was to teach and demonstrate to the learning patient the obvious, discernible, distinct difference between the "very tight" of tension and the "very loose" of relaxation, making the state of relaxation that much more attractive, and desirable. We see in addition, the un-discussed but clearly significant ingredients of clearing of the mind, focused attention, and curiosity, analogous to the ingredients of the other mind-body methodologies described. The described and prescribed goal is to gradually move the tension–relaxation down the body, successively tensing and relaxation each next muscle group until all muscles are relaxed. The focus of the person's attention *on* the tension, and then *on* the relaxation not only allows for physical relaxation to be experienced dramatically and to build with each next muscle group relaxing, but also relaxes the mind through the narrowed focus of attention [on muscles relaxing] familiar to the other self-regulation methods described.

While Jacobson may not have mentioned hypnosis or "mind and body" per se, there is no doubt that his work provided important foundational concepts for mind-body understanding. "He began his work by adapting 19th Century introspective techniques to study the nature of the mind and gradually adding the training in relaxation to provide a treatment process for stress-induced disorders…and the result was a concept of a functional interaction of the mental and motor systems" (Gessel, 1989), and what we now understand as mind-body interaction. Thus, the phenomenology of so-called progressive relaxation is indeed that of mind-body narrowed, focused attention for the explicit, defined purpose of achieving a goal (relaxation) and/or solving a problem (such as anxiety or insomnia). As such, we might just as easily name the "mind-body technique" of progressive relaxation a hypnotic strategy.

A less arduous, and often just as easily accepted method of progressive relaxation is easily accomplished by asking children to "just notice what *happens* (= effortless) to your shoulders *when* you take a deep breath in…and out. Your shoulders go *down*, don't they? That's nature's way of relaxing automatically (= effortlessly!) just by *breathing naturally*." In this way the natural relaxation response (Benson, 1975) is easily taught, learned, and experienced and youth are concurrently taught the natural mind-body connection between breathing and muscle relaxation. In a "standard" procedure the child is invited to "Just *notice* how the relaxing feeling naturally moves down your body at the right speed for you each time that you breathe….out…." And, "…signal to yourself, perhaps by nodding your head or saying 'yes' inside of your thinking when you notice that the relaxation has moved down your upper arms, around the bend at the elbow, and then…down to your forearms, wrists, and even the little muscles of your fingers can become loose and soft and relaxed *because* it feels so good to do that." This is continued down through successive muscle groups through the chest, abdomen, hips, legs, ankles, feet, toes. Alternatively, one may offer progressive relaxation in an analogous manner moving UP the body, beginning with feet and toes relaxing.

So-called Breath Work is often described as a methodology of focused breathing which in and of itself allows for the occurrence of relaxation of mind and body (and spirit). As with progressive relaxation, however, breath work is not easily separated as a distinct "therapy" as much as, like progressive relaxation, it has clear and distinct elements which make it a form and/or integral part of hypnosis or kind of hypnotic strategy. These ingredients, that is, focused attention (on the breath), associated body relaxation and comfort that evolves, and the sense of mind calming that accompanies this work, combine to generate the desired outcome of slowed respirations, relaxed body, and relaxed mind, much as a hypnotic procedure does, and is a major stated goal of hypnosis, biofeedback, meditation. From a clinical hypnosis perspective, "breath work" is indeed considered one very useful and effective type of hypnotic induction strategy.

Sighing is nature's built-in biofeedback, self-hypnosis, relaxation, and breath-work... we do it to help ourselves feel better in the moment.

Brief Review of Common Adult and Pediatric Applications

The most commonly described applications for progressive relaxation or "relaxation techniques" in general have been for various forms of anxiety, both in adults and children.

Susie, age 9, was brought to her pediatrician with a complaint of difficulty falling asleep. Even though she was tired, when bedtime came Susie would cooperatively get ready for bed, enjoy conversation and a story with her parent, say prayers, get kisses and hugs, and say goodnight. Beginning as soon as 10–15 minutes later, however, Susie typically called to her Mom or Dad "I can't sleep..." asking for a drink of water, or to come to her parents' bed. Eventually she'd say "I'm scared...!" and would cry. In response, her parents would often allow her to come to bed with them, where she'd usually fall asleep in minutes. Her parents later took her back to her own bed. Usually she remained asleep, but sometimes she'd awaken in her own bed, be frightened, and the going-to-bed anxiety would repeat itself. This went on for months before the family sought help. After reviewing the history, the pediatrician met privately with Susie. The pediatrician learned that Susie was afraid of the dark and that she worried about someone breaking in and hurting her or her parents ever since a few months ago when she saw a TV news report about a break-in and robbery in their neighborhood. Susie also told the pediatrician that her mind "won't stop thinking about that or about all the things that happened at school or are supposed to happen tomorrow at school... and she said "It's like a TV that's broken and won't turn off." She said when her mind is racing around, she "can't get comfortable" in bed and "squirms around a lot and just get up and walk around the room." The pediatrician asked her "Did you know that you can teach your body to relax and your mind will kind of relax automatically at the same time?" Susie said she didn't know that but was intrigued and willing to learn. The pediatrician said "Just pretend that you're in your bed at home, and if you want to close your eyes you can, or you can keep them open until they close." She then instructed Susie in progressive muscle relaxation, first tensing her forehead and face muscles and then letting them relax as she breathed out; and then doing the same with her neck muscles, and then her shoulders, and gradually down her body, from upper arms, to forearms, wrists, fingers, chest, abdomen, thighs, legs, ankles, feet, and toes. Susie was encouraged to practice doing this after school every day and again at bedtime. When she came back the following week she and her parents were ecstatic, and reported that she had no further difficulty falling asleep, had not come into her parents' bed, and in fact was a little frustrated that she didn't "do it right" because she fell asleep " before I even got down to my legs!"

Proposed Mechanism of Biological Effect

Relaxation "works" through the decrease of sympathetic arousal and associated parasympathetic relaxation, with slowing of the heart rate upon slowing of the respiratory rate which accompanies the relaxation response. The fact that this is naturally occurring (as in the common everyday SIGH which changes the breath, the respiratory rate, relaxes the muscles, notably the shoulders and neck, and reduces anxiety) allows for its ease of accessibility to children and adults alike as a "very easy to learn technique, because you already know how, you just may not know that you knew."

Training/Accreditation/Licensure

While one needs no particular formal training in doing relaxation (because we all know how), training is recommended in order to learn a context and the best practices of how to teach relaxation strategies. Hypnosis training is recommended. Those who may learn "relaxation training" or "visualization" or "breath work" without learning a framework in which to understand unconscious processes are at risk for mis-use of powerful techniques which have their effects in both the conscious and unconscious mind. A solid foundation of knowledge about hypnosis—and these either "sub-forms" or closely related mind-body strategies—will obviate misunderstandings, misguided applications, and inappropriate utilization of these techniques.

Conclusion

Beyond understanding that what we are doing are "mind-body techniques," as clinicians helping young people to help themselves, it is less important what we "name" or "call" what we do, than the confidence, competence, manner, and context within which we seek to teach and promote self-regulation. Fundamental to the provision of any clinical intervention, of course, is the development and evolution of a careful and comprehensive history (and physical examination) in the context of a thoughtful and purposeful cultivation of rapport with the patient. Whether one then teaches and applies "biofeedback-assisted hypnosis" or "hypnosis-assisted biofeedback" or "meditation" or "visualization and breath work" should, accordingly, be a function of that unique relationship.

Factors influencing the decision to move ahead with hypnosis (in the absence of biofeedback) may derive quickly from a given patient's/family's orientation and expectation communicated even before arrival e.g., "I heard that Dr. _____ has success in treating _____with teaching self-hypnosis" or "My neighbor said that biofeedback really helped her daughter with stomach aches and we wonder if it can help our child…but we really don't know what it is …". Or, in the context of an evolving history, the clinician may learn that the patient is fascinated and facile with computer games and may opt accordingly to introduce self-regulation with biofeedback by asking the child "Would you like to learn a cool computer game for your body? It's called biofeedback…come on, I'll show you in the room down the hall…you're going to think this is really amazing!" Or, another family may find a discussion of the value of self-hypnosis to be "hard to believe" but upon observing biofeedback " in action" with, that is, peripheral temperature increases or electrodermal decreases in association with calming and a relaxed state, they may well appropriately conclude that "seeing is believing."

Being facile with doing self-hypnosis (or meditation, or breath work, or biofeedback) ourselves goes a long way toward reinforcing our authenticity when offering a sharing of these techniques with the children and families with whom we work. When we are comfortable, competent, and confident, so will be our patients as they learn. And, then, as Milton Erickson advised, we should and will "Go with the child…" (Haley, 1973).

REFERENCES

Ader, R. (Ed.). (1981). *Psychoneuroimmunology.* New York: Academic Press.

Ader, R. (1989). Conditioned immune responses and pharmacotherapy. *Arthritis Care Research, 2,* S58–S64.

Ader, R. (Ed.). (1991). *Psychoneuroimmunolgy* (2nd ed.). New York: Academic Press.

Anbar, R. D. (2001). Self-hypnosis for treatment of functional abdominal pain in childhood. *Clinical Pediatrics, 40,* 447–451.

Anbar, R. D., & Hall, H. H. (2004). Childhood habit cough treated with self-hypnosis *The Journal of Pediatrics, 144*(2), 213–217

Aronoff, G. M., Aronoff, S., & Peck L.W. (1975). Hypnotherapy in the treatment of bronchial asthma. *Annals of Allergy, 34,* 356–362.

Basmajian, J. V. (1989). *Biofeedback: Principles and practice for clinicians.* Baltimore, MD: Williams & Wilkins.

Baumann F. (1970). Hypnosis and the adolescent drug abuser. *The American Journal of Clinical Hypnosis, 13,* 17–21.

Bell, M. A. & Deater-Deckard, K. (2007). Biological systems and the development of self-regulation: Integrating behavior, genetics, and psychophysiology. *Journal of Developmental and Behavioral Pediatrics 28,* 409–420.

Benson, H. (1975). *The relaxation response.* New York: Harper Torch.

Braid, J. (1855). *The physiology of fascination and the critics criticized.* Manchester, UK: Grant and Co, Corporation Street.

Bramwell, J. M. (1956). *Hypnotism: Its history, practice and theory.* (Reissued with new introduction). New York: Julian Press. (Original work published 1903).

Brett, D. (1986). *Annie stories.* Victoria, Australia: McPhee Gribble/Penguin Books.

Brett, D. (1992). *More Annie stories: Therapeutic storytelling techniques.* New York: Magination Press.

Brown, B. (1974). *New mind: New body.* New York: Harper & Row.

Butler, L., Spiegel, D. et al (2005). Hypnosis reduces distress and duration of an invasive medical procedure for children. *Pediatrics*, 115, e77–e85.

Cottingham, Stoothoff, Murdock, Kenny (Transl.). (1991). *The philosophical writings of descartes.*

Cousins, N. (1979). *Anatomy of an illness.* New York: W.W. Norton and Company.

Cousins, N. (1983). *The healing heart: Antidotes to panic and helplessness.* New York: W.W. Norton and Company.

Culbert, T., & Banez, G. A. (2003). Pediatric applications other than headache. In M. S. Schwartz & F. Andrasik, (Eds.), *Biofeedback: A practitioner's guide.* New York: The Guilford Press.

Culbert, T., Reaney. J., & Kohen, D. P. (1994). Cyber-physiologic strategies in children: The biofeedback-hypnosis interface. *The International Journal of Clinical and Experimental Hypnosis,* 42(2), 97–117.

Culbert, T., Reaney, J., & Kohen, D. P. (1996). Uses of hypnosis and biofeedback for children with dysphagia. *Journal of Developmental and Behavioral Pediatrics,* 17(5), 335–341.

Culbert, T., Friedrichsdorf, S., & Kuttner, L. (2007). Mind/body skills for children in pain. In H. Breivik, C. Campbell, & C. Eccleston (Eds.), *Clinical pain management: Practical applications and procedures.* (2nd ed., Chapter 163). Part of the Clinical Pain Management Series. A. Rice, C.Warfield, D. Justins and C. Eccleston London, UK: Arnold Publishing.

Diamond, H. H. (1959). Hypnosis in children: The complete cure of forty cases of asthma. *American Journal of Clinical Hypnosis,* 1, 124–129.

Dikel, W., & Olness, K. (1980). Self hypnosis, biofeedback, and voluntary peripheral temperature control in children. *Pediatrics,* 66, 335–340.

Elliotson, J. (1843a). Cases of cures by mesmerism. *The Zoist,* 1, 161–208.

Elliotson, J. (1843b). *Numerous cases of surgical operations without pain in the mesmeric state.* Philadelphia, PA: Lea & Blanchard.

Erickson, M. H. (1958b). Pediatric hypnotherapy. *American Journal of Clinical Hypnosis,* 1, 25–29.

Felt, B. T., Berman, B., Broffman, G., Coury, D., Dattner, A., French, G., et al. (1998). Wart regression in children: Comparison of relaxation-imagery to topical treatment and equal time interventions. *American Journal of Clinical Hypnosis,* 41, 2, 130–138.

Fox, D. J., Tharp, D., & Fox, L. C. (2005). Neurofeedback: An alternative and efficacious treatment for attention deficit hyperactivity disorder. *Applied Psychophysiology and Biofeedback, 30*(4), 365–373.

Gardner, G. G. (1976b). Childhood, death, and human dignity: Hypnotherapy for David. *International Journal of Clinical and Experimental Hypnosis,* 24, 122–139.

Gardner, G. G. (1977a). Hypnosis with infants and preschool children. *American Journal of Clinical Hypnosis,* 19, 158–162.

Garth, M. (1991). *Starbright. Meditations for children.* New York: HarperCollins Publishers.

Garth, M. (1992). *Moonbeam. A book of meditations for children.* Australia: HarperCollins Publishers.

Garth, M. (1997). *Earthlight. New meditations for children.* Australia: HarperCollins Publishers.

Gellhorn, E., & Kiely, W. F. (1972). Mystical states of consciousness: Neurophysiological and clinical aspects. *The Journal of Nervous and Mental Disease,,* 154, 399–405.

Gessel, A. H. (1989). Edmund Jacobson, M.D., Ph.D.; the founder of scientific relaxation. *International Journal of Psychosomatics,* 36, 1–4.

Goldie, C. (1956). Hypnosis in the casualty department. *British Medical Journal,* 2, 1340–1342.

Haley, J. (1973). *Uncommon therapy—the psychiatric techniques of Milton H. Erickson M.D.* New York: W.W. Norton Co.

Hall, H. H. Minnes, L., & Olness, K. N. (1993). The Psychophysiology of voluntary immunomodulation. *The International Journal of Neuroscience,* 69, 221–234.

Hibi, M., Iwai, N., Kimura O., Sasaki, Y., & Tsuda, T. (2003). Results of biofeedback therapy for fecal incontinence in children with encopresis and following surgery for anorectal malformations. *Diseases of the Colon and Rectum, 46*(Suppl), S54–S58.

Hilgard, J. R., & Morgan, A. H. (1978). Treatment of anxiety and pain in childhood cancer through hypnosis. In F. H. Frankel & H. S. Zamansky (Eds.), *Hypnosis at its bicentennial: Selected papers.* New York: Plenum Press.

Jencks, B. (1977). *Your body—biofeedback at its best.* Chicago, IL: Nelson-Hall Publisher.

Kabat-Zinn, J. (1994). *Wherever you go, there you are. Mindfulness meditation in everyday life.* New York: Hyperion.

Kabat-Zinn, J. (2005). *Coming to our senses. Healing ourselves and the world through mindfulness.* New York: Hyperion.

Kaplan, A. (1985). *Jewish meditation.* New York: Schocken Books.

Khan, A. U., Staerk, M., & Bonk, C. (1974). Hypnotic suggestibility compared with other methods of isolating emotionally-prone asthmatic children. *American Journal of Clinical Hypnosis, 17,* 50–53.

Kohen, D. P. (1980a). Hypnotherapy in a child with asthma. Videotape presented at the annual meeting of the Ambulatory Pediatric Association, San Antonio, TX.

Kohen, D. P. (1982). Use of relaxation/mental imagery in an 11-1/2 y.o. boy with asthma. Videotape presented to the American Society of Clinical Hypnosis. Denver, CO.

Kohen, D. P. (1986). The value of relaxation/mental imagery (self-hypnosis) to the management of children with asthma: A cyberphysiologic approach. *Topics in Pediatrics, 4*(1), 11–18.

Kohen, D. P. (1986). Applications of relaxation/mental imagery (self-hypnosis) in pediatric emergencies. *International Journal of Clinical and Experimental Hypnosis, 34*(4), 283–294.

Kohen, D. P. (1995). Relaxation/mental imagery (self-hypnosis) for childhood asthma: Behavioral outcomes in a prospective, controlled study. *Hypnos-Swedish Journal of Hypnosis in Psychotherapy and Psychosomatic Medicine and the Journal of the European Society of Hypnosis in Psychotherapy and Psychosomatic Medicine, 22,* 132–144.

Kohen, D. P., Colwell, S. O., Heimel, A., & Olness, K. N. (1984). The use of relaxation-mental imagery (self-hypnosis) in the management of 505 pediatric behavioral encounters. *Journal of Developmental and Behavioral Pediatrics, 51,* 21–25.

Kohen, D. P. (1997). Teaching children with asthma to help themselves with relaxation/mental imagery (self-hypnosis). In W. J. Matthews & J. H. Edgette (Eds.), *Current thinking and research in brief therapy: Solutions, strategies, narratives—annual publication of the M.H. Erickson foundation* (pp. 169–191). New York: Brunner/Mazel.

Kohen, D. P., Mann-Rinehart, P., Schmitz, D., & Wills, L. M. (1998). Using hypnosis to help deaf children help themselves: Report of two cases. *The American Journal of Clinical Hypnosis, 40*(4), 288–296.

Kohen, D. P. & Murray, K. (2006). Depression in children and youth: Applications of hypnosis to help young people help themselves. In M. D. Yapko (Ed.), *Applying hypnosis in treating depression: Innovations in clinical practice* (pp. 189–216). New York: Routledge Press.

Kohen, D. P., & Wynne, E. (1997). Applying hypnosis in a preschool family asthma education program: Uses of storytelling, imagery and relaxation. *American Journal of Clinical Hypnosis, 39*(3), 2–14.

Kohen, D. P. (2000). The case of Anna-headache and heartache. In *Cases of the New England society of clinical hypnosis* www.nesch.org No. 2.1

Kohen, D. P. (2001). Applications of clinical hypnosis with children. In G. D. Burrows, R. O. Stanley, & P. B. Bloom (Eds.), *International handbook of clinical hypnosis.* Chichester, NY: John Wiley & Sons, LTD.

Kohen, D. P., & Ondich, S. K. W. (2004). Children's Self-regulation of Cardiovascular function with relaxation/mental imagery (self-hypnosis): Report of a controlled study. *HYPNOS - The Journal of European Society of Hypnosis in Psychotherapy and Psychosomatic Medicine, 31*(2), 61–74.

Kohen, D. P. (2007). *Hypnosis for Headaches in Children: Long-Term Follow-up and What the Children Say.* Presentation at ASCH/SCEH 49th Annual Scientific Meeting, Dallas, TX.

Kohen, D. P., & Zajac, R. (2007). Self-hypnosis training for headaches in children and adolescents. *The Journal of Pediatrics, 150,* 635–639.

Kosslyn, S. M., Margolis, J. A., Barrett, A. M., Goldknopf, E. J., & Daly, P. F. (1990). Age differences in imagery abilities. *Child Development, 61,* 995–1010.

Kuttner, L. (1988). Favorite stories: A hypnotic pain reducing technique for children in acute pain. *American Journal of Clinical Hypnosis, 30*(4), 289–295.

LaBaw, W. L. (1973). Adjunctive trance therapy with several burned children. *International Journal of Child Psychotherapy, 2,* 80–92.

LaBaw, W. L. (1975). Autohypnosis in hemophilia. *Haematologia 9,* 103–110.

Langer, E. J. (1989). *Mindfulness.* New York: Addison-Wesley Publishing Company, Inc.

Lee, L., & Olness, K. (1996). Effects of self-induced mental imagery on autonomic reactivity in children. *Journal of Developmental and Behavioral Pediatrics, 17,* 323–327.

Liossi, C., White, P., & Hatira, P. (2006). Randomized clinical trial of local anesthetic versus combination of local anesthetic with self-hypnosis in the management of pediatric procedure-related pain. *Health Psychology, 25,* 307–315.

Lubar, J., & Bahler, W. (1976). Behavioral management of epileptic seizures following EEG biofeedback training of the sensorimotor rhythm. *Biofeedback and Self-Regulation, 1,* 77–104.

Lubar, J. F. (1991). Discourse on the development of EEG diagnostics and biofeedback for attention-deficit/hyperactivity disorders. *Biofeedback and Self-Regulation, 16,* 201–226.

Lynn, S. J., & Rhue, J. W. (Eds.). (1991). *Theories of hypnosis: Current models and perspectives.* New York: The Guilford Press.

Miller, N. E. (1969). Learning of visceral and glandular responses. *Science, 163,* 434–445.

Mills, J. C., & Crowley, R. J. (1986). *Therapeutic metaphors for children and the child within.* New York: Brunner/Mazel.

Moyers, B. (1993). *Healing and the mind.* New York: Doubleday.

Olness, K. (1975). The use of self-hypnosis in the treatment of childhood nocturnal enuresis: A report on forty patients. *Clinical Pediatrics, 14,* 273–279.

Olness, K. (1976). Autohypnosis in functional megacolon in children. *American Journal of Clinical Hypnosis, 19,* 28–32.

Olness, K., McParland, F. A., & Piper, J. (1980). Biofeedback: A new modality in the management of children with fecal soiling. *Journal of Pediatrics, 96,* 505–509.

Olness, K. (1981a). Hypnosis in pediatric practice (Monograph). *Current Problems in Pediatrics, 12,* 3–47.

Olness, K (1981b). Imagery (self-hypnosis) as adjunct care in childhood cancer: Clinical experience with 25 patients. *American Journal of Pediatric Hematology/Oncology, 3,* 313–321.

Olness, K., & Conroy, M. (1985). A pilot study of voluntary control of transcutaneous po2 by children. *International Journal of Clinical and Experimental Hypnosis, 33,* 1–5.

Olness, K., MacDonald, J., & Uden, D. (1987). A prospective study comparing self-hypnosis, propranolol, and placebo in management of juvenile migraine. *Pediatrics, 79,* 593–597.

Olness, K. N., Culbert, T. C., & Uden, D. (1989). Self-regulation of salivary immunoglobulin A by children. *Pediatrics, 83,* 66–71.

Olness, K., & Rusin, W. (1990a). Cyberphysiology in children and its relationship to self-regulatory control. In L. P. Lipsitt & L. I. Mitnick (Eds.), *Loss of self-regulatory control: Its causes and
consequences* (pp. 241–256). Norwood, NJ: Ablex Press.

Olness K. (1990b). Pediatric psychoneurimmunology: Hypnosis as a possible mediator: Potentials
and problems. In *Hypnosis: Current therapy, research and practice.* VU University Press:
Amsterdam.

Olness, K. N., & Kohen, D. P. (1996). *Hypnosis and hypnotherapy with children* (3rd ed.) New York:
The Guilford Press.

Olton, D. S., & Noonberg, A. R. (1980). *Biofeedback: Clinical applications in behavioral medicine.*

Palsson, O. S., Heymen, S., & Whitehead, W. E. (2004). Biofeedback treatment for functional anorectal disorders: A comprehensive efficacy review. *Applied Psychophysiology and Biofeedback,*
29(3), 153–174.

Pert, C. (1997). *Molecules of emotion.* New York: Touchstone.

Raz, A. (2005). Attention and hypnosis: Neural substrates and genetic associations of two converg-
ing processes. *International Journal of Clinical and Experimental Hypnosis, 53*(3), 237–258.

Raz, A., Fan, J., & Posner, M. I. (2005). Hypnotic suggestion reduces conflict in the human brain.
Proceedings of the National Academy of Sciences, 102(28), 9978–9983.

Rhue, J. W., Lynn, S. J., & Kirsch I. (Eds.). (1993). *Handbook of clinical hypnosis.* Washington, DC:
American Psychological Association.

Rossi, E. L. (2002) *The psychobiology of gene expression.* New York: W.W. Norton & Company.

Rock, B. (1983). *Biofeedback.* Washington, DC: NIMH—DHHS Publication No. (ADM) 83-1273.

Schandler, S. L., & Grings, W. W. (1976). An examination of methods for producing relaxation
during short term laboratory sessions. *Behaviour Research and Therapy, 14,* 419–426.

Schwartz, M. S., & Olson, R. P. (2003). History, entering and definitions. In M.S. Schwartz & F.
Andrasik (Eds.), *Biofeedback: A practitioner's guide.* New York: The Guilford Press.

Schwartz, M. S., & Andrasik, F. (Eds.), *Biofeedback: A practitioner's guide.* New York: The Guilford
Press.

Selye, H. (1974). *Stress without distress.* Philadelphia, PA: Lippincott.

Selye, H. (1976). *The stress of life* (rev ed). New York: McGraw-Hill.

Silver, B. V., & Blanchard, E. B. (1978). Biofeedback and relaxation training in the treatment of
psychophysiological disorders: Or are the machines really necessary? *Journal of Behavioral
Medicine, 1*(2), 217–239.

Simonton, O. C, Matthews-Simonton, S., & Creighton, J. (1978). *Getting well again.* New York: J.P.
Tarcher Co.

Sugarman, L. I., & Kohen, D. P. (2007). Integrating hypnosis into acute care settings. In W. C.
Wester & L. I. Sugarman (Eds.), *Therapeutic hypnosis with children and adolescents* (Chapter
14). Wales, UK: Crown House Publishing.

Tansey, M. A. (1990). Righting the rhythms of reason: EEG Biofeedback training as a therapeutic
modality in a clinical office setting. *Medical Psychotherapy, 3,* 57–68.

Thomson, L. (2005). *Harry the hypno-potamus: Metaphorical tales for the treatment of children.*
Carmarthen, Wales, UK: Crown House Publishing Ltd.

Tinterow, M. M. (1970). *Foundations of hypnosis: From Mesmer to Freud.* Springfield, IL: Charles
C Thomas.

Wester, W. C., & Sugarman, L. I. (Eds.). (2007). *Therapeutic hypnosis with children and adolescents.*
Wales, UK: Crown House Publishers.

Wright, M. E., & Wright, B. A. (1987). *Clinical practice of hypnotherapy.* New York: The Guilford
Press.

15

A Pediatric Perspective on
Naturopathic Medicine

MATTHEW I. BARAL, WENDY WEBER, AND JESSICA MITCHELL

KEY CONCEPTS

- A licensed naturopathic physician receives a degree from an accredited 4-year naturopathic medical program.
- Licensed naturopathic physicians complete a minimum of 4100 hours of training in basic and clinical sciences.
- Naturopathic physicians are required to take two national board exams for licensure.
- A naturopathic physician has been trained in many different natural therapies including botanical medicine, homeopathy, physical medicine, mind-body medicine, nutritional therapy, and diet and lifestyle recommendations.
- Naturopathic medicine stems from the "Nature Cure" movement in Europe in the nineteenth century.
- Naturopathic medicine was significantly popular in the United States in the early part of the twentieth century.
- Naturopathic medicine experienced a dramatic resurgence in the late twentieth century.
- A portion of naturopathic physicians treat children on a regular basis, in some cases serving as the primary healthcare provider for children.
- Naturopathic physicians treat children for a wide variety of medical conditions including coughs, colds, and ear infections; skin disorders; gastrointestinal complaints; psychiatric or behavioral problems; allergies; and respiratory conditions.

■

Introduction

Naturopathic medicine is a profession deeply rooted in philosophy. A naturopathic physician (also known as naturopathic doctor/ND or naturopathic medical doctor/NMD) has been trained to utilize many different natural forms of therapies with patients. Depending on the individual state licensure in which they practice, a naturopathic physician may use botanical medicine, oriental medicine, homeopathy, physical medicine, mind-body medicine, nutritional therapy, or diet and lifestyle changes to treat patients. In addition, some states grant naturopathic physicians pharmaceutical prescribing privileges. The accredited naturopathic medical schools in North America prepare their students as family practitioners, yet there are graduates that gravitate towards specific areas of medicine such as pediatrics, cardiology, women's health, men's health, endocrinology, and gastroenterology. Other naturopathic physicians prefer to concentrate on individual treatment modalities such as nutrition, homeopathy, herbal medicine, hydrotherapy, counseling, or physical medicine. Although it can be a diverse group, the majority of the profession concurs on the common doctrine of naturopathic medicine.

History

Naturopathy emerged from what has been referred to as the "Nature Cure" movement that was popular in Europe in the early nineteenth century. Vincent Priessnitz is recognized as one of the first practitioners of what is known today as naturopathic medicine. His treatments consisted of using baths and hot and cold compresses (otherwise known as water cure and later termed hydrotherapy), outdoor exposure, exercise, and nutrition to treat patients from children to the elderly. This was the impetus of today's European and American spas. Priessnitz's treatment of childhood diseases would likely be viewed today as unorthodox. However, at the time, it was cutting edge and quite effective. An example of a case is described in the book *Nature Doctors* (Kirchfeld & Boyle, 1994):

> The Syndie's five children all took scarlet fever and were treated by an ordinary doctor. Three died. The father then begged the aid of Priessnitz, who said he would help only if the doctors were dismissed. To this the father could not agree and a fourth child died. The father then put the last child wholly in the hands of Priessnitz, who plunged it into ice-water for a minute or so, felt the body carefully all over, repeated the plunge four or five times, and then allowed the child to fall asleep. When it woke, the fever was gone.

Practitioners of the nature cure enjoyed much popularity in the nineteenth century. Father Sebastian Kneipp (1824–1897), a practitioner partly responsible for the wide recognition of the nature cure in Germany, was reported by an American newspaper to be the third-most popular person in the world—behind the US president and the German chancellor (Burghardt, 1988). His influence eventually spread throughout Europe and North America.

Benedict Lust (1872–1945), a student and past patient of Father Kneipp, is considered the father of American Nature Cure. Responsible for bringing it to North America, he would later coin the term "Naturopathy" to describe the use of the water cure and the application of botanical medicine, homeopathy, nutrition, diet therapy, and sun therapy. In time, physical medicine modalities such as massage and manual manipulation, similar to chiropractic and osteopathic techniques, were added to the practice of naturopathy.

Naturopathic medicine thrived in the United States in the early twentieth century. There were many training programs, and licensure existed in the majority of states. However, by the middle of the century, the movement was significantly impeded due to political issues within medicine, and all naturopathic medical programs were eliminated. In 1908, The Carnegie Foundation funded the Flexner Report. It was designed to evaluate medical schools in America, and headed by Abraham Flexner and prominent members of the American Medical Association. Prior to the report, naturopathic, homeopathic, and even conventional medical schools had very differing standards for what represented adequate medical education. The duration of training varied greatly, and in some cases, degrees could be obtained by mail order and distance learning.

The Flexner report was preferential to 4-year programs, and it was preferred that the education was to be conducted by educators, not clinicians. The use of certain treatments was based on whether clinical research had been conducted on them, and most naturopathic schools did not meet the minimum standards developed. Much of the naturopathic treatment used was very successful, but based on empirical data and anecdotal evidence. The scientific method was becoming the preferred process for validating medicine, and the advent of drugs and antibiotics held the hope of eliminating all disease and symptoms. As a result, healthcare disciplines such as naturopathy that strayed from the "traditional" approach were shunned and practitioners of these therapies were labeled charlatans. When the results of the Flexner report were accepted by the government as the medical school standard, only those graduates of the "approved" schools were allowed to sit for the medical licensure exams. Both naturopathic and homeopathic schools suffered as a result and nearly all of them closed their doors eventually. The mid-twentieth century saw the elimination of most naturopathy programs and fewer and fewer states were licensing naturopathic physicians.

The desire for alternative therapies such as naturopathic medicine has increased greatly in the last 15 to 20 years for a number of reasons. Conventional treatments have proven to be quite effective in the treatment of acute disease, but in chronic illness the long-term effects of some medications have left parents seeking other options. In fact, there has been an increased use of complementary and alternative therapies in the disease management of children (Pitetti et al., 2001). Conventional medications may only provide short-term palliation of symptoms and lose their efficacy over time. This has led some to conclude that much of conventional medicine is symptom management and the true cause of disease is often not addressed.

Philosophy

The principles of naturopathic medicine form the basis for the naturopathic approach to healthcare.

PRINCIPLES OF NATUROPATHIC MEDICINE

- First, do no harm (*primum non-nocere*): naturopathic physicians and medical doctors share this common principle of practice. This means choosing the therapies that are least invasive and have the lowest potential for side effects that will be medically effective in treating the condition.
- The healing power of nature (*vis medicatrix naturae*): health is the natural state of the body, and when it is provided with the right tools, it will heal itself. In many cases, children seem to recover quicker than adults, as they have less time to accrue the effects of a toxic diet or environment.
- Identify and treat the cause (*tolle causam*): Naturopathic physicians see symptoms as the reflection of disease, not the disease itself. One of the most important beliefs in naturopathy is that the body has an inherent ability to heal itself, referred to as the *vis medicatrix naturae*, or *healing power of nature*. The *vis* can function best when the causes of disease are removed, which are referred to as "obstacles to cure." The use of naturopathic treatments can help to influence our healing capabilities. The conventional medical approach to the atopic diseases such as eczema, asthma, or allergic rhinitis focuses on symptom treatment as opposed to the symptom cause. In many cases, simply addressing the diet can have impressive results.
- Treat the whole person (*tolle totum*): disease can be the result of many factors. Nutrition, emotional stress, genetic predisposition, and environmental insults can all contribute to the development of disease. In order to truly be holistic in the care of a child, the physician must address all of these issues.
- Doctor as teacher (*docere*): the word doctor literally translates into *teacher*. A large part of any visit with a naturopathic physician involves education of the parents and if appropriate, the child. Teaching about how the body works and how it is affected by lifestyle is often just as helpful as providing treatment.
- Prevention (*prevenir*): preventing disease is much easier than its treatment. Having the opportunity to start preventative measures at an early age allows for greater effects in the future.

Jared Zeff, ND, Lac, and Pamela Snider, ND, developed the Therapeutic Order in 1999. It is a system designed to prioritize treatment approaches. It employs both the principles of naturopathic medicine and the use of conventional therapies at times when they are the appropriate options. The steps of treatment are to:

1. Re-establish the basis for health
    Remove obstacles to cure by establishing a healthy regimen, including healthy diet and appropriate exercise.
2. Stimulate the healing power of nature
    Use various systems of health such as botanical medicine, homeopathy, Chinese medicine, Ayurvedic medicine, nutrition, or psychospiritual medicine.
3. Tonify weakened systems
    Use modalities as needed to strengthen the immune system, decrease toxicity, normalize inflammatory function, optimize metabolic function, balance regulatory systems, enhance regeneration, and harmonize life forces.
4. Correct structural integrity
    Use therapeutic exercise, naturopathic spinal manipulation, massage, and cranio-sacral therapy to return the body to optimal structural condition.
5. Prescribe specific natural substances for pathology
    Use vitamins, minerals, and herbs to promote health.
6. Prescribe pharmacological substances for pathology
    Use pharmaceutical drugs to return patient to a healthy state.
7. Prescribe or refer patient for surgery, suppressive drugs, radiation and chemotherapy
    Use aggressive therapies to attempt to maintain health.

Training and Accreditation

Doctors of Naturopathic Medicine (ND) complete a 4-year graduate-level program with a minimum of 4100 hours of training. This program includes a basic science education with training in anatomy, physiology, pathology, biochemistry, environmental health, public health, pharmacology, and pharmacognosy. The clinical sciences curriculum includes clinical nutrition, homeopathy, botanical medicine, physical manipulation, counseling, hydrotherapy, and may include acupuncture. In addition to this course work, each student completes 1200 hours of clinical training (www. CNME.org).

The Council on Naturopathic Medical Education (CNME) regulates accreditation (www.naturopathic.org). The CNME is a member of the Association of Specialized and Professional Accreditors, which is recognized by the United States Secretary of Education (www.cnme.org). Once accepted into accreditation candidacy schools may confer ND degrees while full accreditation is pending. Preaccredited status has the effect of temporary accreditation. Currently six schools in North America are accredited or preaccredited (candidacy) to provide training in Naturopathic Medicine by the CNME:

Bastyr University (Kenmore, Washington)

Boucher Institute of Naturopathic Medicine (New Westminster, British Columbia)

Canadian College of Naturopathic Medicine (Toronto, Ontario)

National College of Natural Medicine (Portland, Oregon)

Southwest College of Naturopathic Medicine (Tempe, Arizona)

University of Bridgeport—College of Naturopathic Medicine (Bridgeport, Connecticut)

All of these schools are members of the Association of Accredited Naturopathic Medical Colleges (AANMC).

Licensing

Naturopathic Physician Licensing Examinations (NPLEX) are administered by the North American Board of Naturopathic Examiners (NABNE). After the first two years of school a student from a CNME-accredited school is eligible to take the first licensing board exam, known as *Basic Sciences*. This examination consists of five parts: anatomy, biochemistry, microbiology, physiology, and pathology. Upon completion of naturopathic medical school, a graduate takes the second licensing examination, or *Clinical Sciences*. This examination is a single, case-based assessment covering the following subjects: physical and clinical diagnosis; laboratory diagnosis and diagnostic imaging; botanical medicine; clinical nutrition; physical medicine; homeopathy; psychology; and emergency medicine and medical procedures; and pharmacology.

In addition, there are two clinical elective examinations—minor surgery and acupuncture. The requirements for passing the elective examinations vary by state. (www.nabne.org).

There are currently 14 states and two territories that license naturopathic physicians:

Alaska

Arizona

California

Connecticut

District of Columbia

Hawaii

Idaho

Kansas

Maine

Montana

New Hampshire
Oregon
Utah
Vermont
Washington
Puerto Rico, and the
Virgin Islands (www.naturopathic.org)

Four Canadian provinces regulate naturopathic physicians:
British Columbia
Saskatchewan
Manitoba
Ontario

Alberta regulations are expected to be complete by 2010 (www.cand.ca).

To apply for state or provincial licensure, a naturopathic physician must have graduated from a CNME-accredited naturopathic medical program and have achieved a passing score on the NPLEX. The scope of practice for a naturopathic physician varies by state and province and is defined by the state or provincial law. Mandatory annual continuing education requirements also vary by state or province (www.naturopathic. org).

It is important to mention that there are schools which offer naturopathic education and degrees through correspondence classes. These correspondence education-trained individuals receive no directly supervised clinical experience and are not required to take board exams. These correspondence training programs can be as short as 100 hours. Graduates from these schools refer to themselves as "naturopaths" and often use the title "ND" or "NMD." These schools are not recognized by the CNME as accredited to train students and grant the degree of doctorate in naturopathic medicine. The correspondence schools have created their own "accreditation process," but this accrediting body is not recognized by the United States Secretary of Education. Advice for parents who plan to take their child to see a naturopathic physician ask the provider about their training, and specifically if they went to one of the above-mentioned CNME-accredited naturopathic medical schools.

Characteristics of Naturopathic Medical Care

Several surveys have explored the characteristics of patients treated by naturopathic physicians and the naturopathic physicians providing this care. The majority of these studies report that nearly 60% of naturopathic physicians are female and the mean age of naturopathic physicians is approximately 44 years (Cherkin et al., 2002a; Weber et al., 2007). A random survey of naturopathic physicians in Connecticut and Washington State report that nearly 80% of patients treated by NDs are between the ages of 15 and 64 years and approximately 11% of patients are under the age of 15 years (Cherkin et al.,

2002b). Cherkin, et al. also report that nearly 75% of visits to naturopathic physicians were for chronic conditions, and that 75% of patients were female. Naturopathic physicians treat a broad range of conditions, with the top five conditions only representing 25% of their patient concerns. The most common conditions treated by naturopathic physicians included fatigue, headache, back symptoms, anxiety or depression, skin rashes, menopausal symptoms, and routine/special examinations (Cherkin et al., 2002b). Insurance covered the cost of 50–60% of visits to naturopathic physicians in this survey (Cherkin et al., 2002b). Contrary to reports of adult utilization of complementary and alternative medicine, which consistently find that women are more likely to use CAM treatments, pediatric studies have found that nearly equal numbers of girls and boys were seen by naturopathic physicians (Barnes, Powell-Griner, McFann, & Nahin, 2004; McMahon et al., 2003; Weber et al., 2007; Wilson et al., 2005).

A few studies have examined the frequency and reasons for visits to naturopathic physicians by children (Cherkin et al., 2002b; Lee and Kemper, 2000; Weber et al., 2007; Wilson et al., 2005). One survey reported that naturopathic physicians treat an average of five pediatric patients per week and that 19% of visits to a naturopathic physician were by children (Lee & Kemper, 2000). In a review of insurance claims data, Bellas, Lafferty, Lind, and Tyree (2005) found that 1.0% of children enrolled in two large insurance plans in Washington State had visited a naturopathic physician and that the children were treated by naturopathic physicians for a similar range of complaints as those treated by conventional physicians. Wilson et al. summarized the chief complaints reported by 482 parents bringing their child in for naturopathic care at a large academic naturopathic clinic in Toronto, Canada (Wilson et al., 2005). Weber et al. described the reasons children were seen by licensed naturopathic physicians in Washington state who treat more than five pediatric patients per week, and approximately 15% of naturopathic physicians in the state of Washington treat pediatric patients on a regular basis. Three studies have described the most common conditions treated by naturopathic physicians and they include: ear, nose, and throat conditions including coughs, colds, and ear infections (18.4%–22.6% of visits); administrative/general health supervision (12.3%–27.4% of visits); skin disorders (10.1%–23.4%); gastrointestinal complaints (8.9%–16.8%); psychiatric or behavioral concerns (7.4%–14.5%); allergies (6.2%–22.3%); and respiratory conditions (8.8%–11.4%) (Bellas et al., 2005; Weber et al., 2007; Wilson et al., 2005). The range of estimates for each condition is likely due to the differences in insurance coverage for naturopathic care which covers the majority of visits in the Bellas and Weber articles and the majority of out-of-pocket expenditures required for visits reported in the Wilson article.

Overview of Naturopathic Medicine's Approach to Treating Children

Naturopathic physicians pride themselves on treating the whole child, which means working with the family to address nutrition, lifestyle, and exercise, as well as specific

Table 15-1. Naturopathic Medicine Approach
to Treating Children

Whole foods diet with adequate protein intake
Balanced diet—Eat a Rainbow a Day
Appropriate water intake
Essential fatty acids (fish or flax oil)
Multivitamin/mineral
Remove food sensitivities
Specific treatments as needed

treatments for medical concerns when needed. As stated previously, naturopathic physicians treat patients based on the philosophy of the medicine. One of the first things naturopathic physicians do when they work with pediatric patients is learn more about the nutrition of the child to determine the adequacy of the diet. Naturopathic physicians are able to provide a great deal of nutritional education to the child and parent because visits to naturopathic physicians, are on average, 45 minutes in length (Cherkin et al., 2002b). These long visits allow the naturopathic physician an opportunity to really get to know their patients and the parents of their patients (Table 15-1).

The nutritional advice provided by naturopathic physicians often emphasizes a whole foods diet. A whole foods diet is one that contains primarily fruits, vegetables, whole grains, and animal protein sources. Patients are encouraged to limit processed foods such as breads, pasta, pizza, cookies, crackers, and other manufactured foods. One way to recognize a whole food is to read the label of the product if it lists only one ingredient, it is a whole food. Many whole foods do not need labels, such as chicken, broccoli, and bananas. If the food item has 10–20 ingredients, it is processed; The food contains a large amount of ingredients, usually including preservatives and food colorings.

Naturopathic physicians strongly encourage children to eat a variety of fruits and vegetables during the day. One strategy that can help children achieve this goal is to ask them to eat a rainbow of colors from fruits and vegetables. It is important to remind children that food coloring does not count as a color, so "Skittles" and "M&Ms" do not count as a rainbow. By encouraging children to eat a variety of fruits and vegetables, they increase their intake of necessary vitamins, minerals, and antioxidants which naturally occur in these foods. It is often a big challenge to get children to broaden their diet, and the reality is that many children eat a limited diet. In these cases, it is important that children get a daily multivitamin-mineral supplement. Vitamins and minerals play a key role in the way the human body functions, and they are essential for growth and development.

It is surprising how many children do not consume any water throughout the day. Water plays an important role in assisting the kidneys to eliminate properly. Encouraging pure water intake is another important approach in naturopathic medicine. A general rule of thumb is to have children consume 1/2–3/4 ounces of water per pound of body weight per day. It is important that a child not drink too much water, as this can cause a dangerous drop in potassium levels.

The majority of Americans do not get adequate intake of essential fatty acids in their diet on a regular basis, specifically omega-3 fatty acids. The reason for this is that the only food sources of omega-3 fatty acids are cold water fish, algae, ground flax seeds, walnuts, cashew nuts, and Brazil nuts. Unfortunately, due to the high content of mercury and other chemicals in seafood, children should not be encouraged to eat fish more than once or twice a week. Because of the difficulty getting adequate intake in the diet, many naturopathic physicians recommend supplementation of this key nutrient with either fish or flax oils. It is essential that the manufacturer of the fish oil test their product for mercury and other chemicals, and the label of the product should state the product contains less than the FDA limits of these contaminants. Children taking essential fatty acids need to inform all other medical providers about its use, especially prior to any surgery. Initial evidence suggested that omega-3 fatty acids may increase the risk for bleeding, yet controlled clinical trials have not been able to document this effect (Bays, 2007). However, it is still advised that patients taking essential fatty acids discontinue them at least 2 weeks prior to any planned surgery or dental extraction.

A somewhat unique approach in naturopathic medicine is working with families to determine if the medical conditions the child has may be related in some way to the food they consume. The term to describe this reaction is food sensitivity. Some children develop sensitivities to certain foods, and these sensitivities can be the root cause of a number of health concerns in children including eczema, asthma, abdominal pain, sinus congestion, hyperactivity, and headaches. Some naturopathic physicians will work with a family to conduct what is known as an elimination diet. The elimination diet removes foods that are suspected to be potential food sensitivity for a child. The food is generally removed for two to three weeks, and then the suspected foods are reintroduced into the diet one at a time. The child is then is observed for a reaction to each food. If the food causes no reaction, it can be adopted back into the diet. Foods that cause a reaction are generally kept out of the diet for a longer period of time (3–6 months) and then re-challenged to see if there is any reaction. If the food removed is a major source of a key nutrient, the naturopathic physician will work with the family to discuss how to be sure to get this key nutrient from other sources or from a dietary supplement. For example, if dairy products are found to exacerbate symptoms of eczema, the child would be advised to keep all dairy products out of the diet and to increase dark greens or add a calcium supplement to be sure the child consumes an adequate calcium intake. The most common foods associated with sensitivities include wheat, dairy, egg, corn, soy, yeast, and citrus, although any food can be a problem.

Once the naturopathic physician has worked with the family to get the child to eat a healthy diet and exercise adequately, the child has a foundation for optimal health.

In many cases correcting these issues may resolve the medical condition of the child. However, in some cases the concern may be more urgent, and making dietary changes may not be preferred by the family because it is a slow and sometimes difficult process to change. In these situations, the naturopathic physician will pull from the broad base of natural treatment modalities in which they have extensive training (see above). They may use botanical medicine, homeopathy, mind/body techniques, specific nutritional supplements, energy medicine, manual medicine, or nature cure. This chapter does not provide space to fully describe the naturopathic approach to treating all medical conditions, and much of what naturopathic physicians do to treat children with these different modalities is described in the chapters describing natural treatments for each of the specific conditions. Naturopathic physicians who treat children on a regular basis have excellent success working with children with chronic conditions such as asthma, ADHD, autism, allergies, eczema, chronic abdominal pain, headaches, irritable bowel syndrome, and recurrent otitis media. In addition, naturopathic physicians work with children during conditions such as acute upper respiratory infections and bronchitis. In some cases naturopathic physicians provide the primary care for children and in other situations they provide adjunct care for chronic pediatric conditions (Weber, Taylor, McCarty, & Johnson-Grass, 2007).

Referral to Naturopathic Physicians

The process of referral to a naturopathic physician should include a review of the provider's training to ensure that he or she graduated from an accredited naturopathic school and has a state or provincial license. Many Doctors of Naturopathic Medicine practicing in non-licensing states carry a license from another state. The American Association of Naturopathic Physician's website provides information on finding a Naturopathic Physician according to state and by practice emphasis.

Resources

- American Association of Naturopathic Physicians: www.naturopathic.org
- Association of Accredited Naturopathic Medical Colleges: www.anmc.org
- Canadian Association of Naturopathic Doctors: www.cand.org
- Council on Naturopathic Medical Education: www.cnme.org
- Federation of Naturopathic Physicians Licensing Authorities: www.fnpla.org
- North American Board of Naturopathic Examiners: www.nabne.org
- Bastyr University: www.bastyr.edu
- Boucher Institute of Naturopathic Medicine: www.binm.org
- Canadian College of Naturopathic Medicine: www.ccnm.edu
- National College of Natural Medicine: www.ncnm.edu
- Southwest College of Naturopathic Medicine: www.scnm.edu
- University of Bridgeport – College of Naturopathic Medicine: www.bridgeport.edu

REFERENCES

Barnes, P. M., Powell-Griner, E., McFann, K., & Nahin, R. L. (2004, May 27). Complementary and alternative medicine use among adults: United States, 2002. *Advance Data, 343*, 1–19.

Bays, H. E. (2007). Safety considerations with omega-3 fatty acid therapy. *The American Journal of Cardiology, 99*, 35C–43C.

Bellas, A., Lafferty, W. E., Lind, B., & Tyree, P. T. (2005). Frequency, predictors, and expenditures for pediatric insurance claims for complementary and alternative medical professionals in Washington State. *The American Journal of Cardiology, 159*, 367–372.

Burghardt, L. (1988). *Sebastian Kneipp: Helfer der Menschheit* (Sebastian Kneipp: Helper of Mankind). Bad Worishofen: Kneipp Verlag.

Cherkin, D. C., Deyo, R. A., Sherman, K. J., Hart, L. G., Street, J. H., Hrbek, A., et al. (2002a). Characteristics of licensed acupuncturists, chiropractors, massage therapists, and naturopathic physicians. *The Journal of the American Board of Family Practice, 15*, 378–390.

Cherkin, D. C., Deyo, R. A., Sherman, K. J., Hart, L. G., Street, J. H., Hrbek, A., et al. (2002b). Characteristics of visits to licensed acupuncturists, chiropractors, massage therapists, and naturopathic physicians. *The Journal of the American Board of Family Practice, 15*, 463–472.

CNME Accreditation Standards for Naturopathic Medicine Programs (excerpt from Part Two of the CNME Handbook). The Council on Naturopathic Medical Education website. Retrieved September 21, 2007, from www.cnme.org. Updated April 2006.

Description of the NPLEX Examinations. North American Board of Naturopathic Examiners website. Retrieved September 21, 2007, from www.nabne.org/nabne_page_23.php#Anchor5. Copyright 2006.

Education. American Association of Naturopathic Physicians website. Retrieved August 30, 2007, from http://www.naturopathic.org/viewbulletin.php?id=29. Copyright 2006.

Kirchfeld, F., & Boyle, W. (1994). *Nature doctors: Pioneers in naturopathic medicine.* Ohio: Buckeye Naturopathic Press.

Lee, A. C., & Kemper, K. J. (2000). Homeopathy and naturopathy: Practice characteristics and pediatric care. *Archives of Pediatrics & Adolescent Medicine, 154*, 75–80.

Licensing States and Authorities. American Association of Naturopathic Physicians website. Retrieved August 30, 2007, from http://www.naturopathic.org/viewbulletin.php?id=18. Copyright 2006.

McMahon, S. R., Iwamoto, M., Massoudi, M. S., Yusuf, H. R., Stevenson, J. M., David, F., et al. (2003) Comparison of e-mail, fax, and postal surveys of pediatricians. *Pediatrics, 111*, e299–e303.

Pitetti R., Singh S., Hornyak D., Garcia S.E., & Herr S. (2001). Complementary and alternative medicine use in children. *Pediatric Emergency Care, 17*(3), 165–169.

Questions. Education and Regulations. Canadian Association of Naturopathic Doctors website. Retrieved September 21, 2007, from www.cand.ca/index.php?40.

Weber, W., Taylor, J. A., McCarty, R. L., & Johnson-Grass, A. (2007). Frequency and characteristics of pediatric and adolescent visits in naturopathic medical practice. *Pediatrics, 120*, e142–e146.

Wilson, K., Busse, J. W., Gilchrist, A., Vohra, S., Boon, H., & Mills, E. (2005). Characteristics of pediatric and adolescent patients attending a naturopathic college clinic in Canada. *Pediatrics, 115*, e338–e343.

16

A Pediatric Perspective on Nutritional Therapeutics

BENJAMIN KLIGLER AND EMILIE SCOTT

KEY CONCEPTS

- For infants, the nutrition literature supports that breastfeeding is best; and that waiting until 6 months of age to introduce solids, reduces likelihood of food allergies and atopic conditions.
- Fish oil (specifically DHA/EPA) supplementation during pregnancy and breastfeeding has a positive impact on cognitive development.
- Supplements, including fish oil and probiotics, can be used safely in children for certain conditions.
- Choosing organic and/or locally grown foods when possible may have health benefits and is critical in helping preserve a safe and clean environment for our patients.
- The elimination diet can be an extremely useful tool in treating children with asthma, atopic dermatitis, juvenile migraine, and a number of other conditions.

■

INTRODUCTION

Perhaps the greatest challenge in describing the "integrative" approach to nutritional interventions in children is in delineating which nutritional recommendations are really an accepted part of routine pediatric practice and which are in fact untraditional or integrative. This is a moving target, since recommendations regarding healthy nutrition in both the conventional and "alternative" worlds seem to

314

shift from one day to the next, and a suggestion which would have been seen as "fringe" a short time ago is suddenly seen as "mainstream."

Rather than focus on these distinctions—and rather than provide a comprehensive guide to pediatric nutrition, which would require an entire textbook—this chapter will aim to provide clinically useful recommendations to complement the nutritional advice generally given by pediatricians and family physicians to young families. In particular, we will focus on prenatal nutrition and the safe and evidence-based use of nutritional supplements during pregnancy and early childhood; on food choices in infants and young children; and on the use of specific therapeutic diets, including the elimination diet. As a means to illustrate how these elements can come together in clinical practice, we will also discuss the nutritional therapeutics approach to several specific conditions, including asthma, recurrent upper respiratory infection and neurodevelopmental disorders.

Prenatal Nutrition

The importance of folic acid supplementation in the preconception period to prevent neural tube defects is well established. Most women are prescribed prenatal vitamins and advised to maintain calcium intake during pregnancy at 1000–1200 mg per day. In addition to the general advice most women receive regarding eating a generally varied diet and maintaining weight gain within a reasonable range during pregnancy, there are several specific suggestions from the "integrative nutrition" perspective which can be helpful. One area which many find challenging is how to advise pregnant women on intake of fish and essential fatty acids (EFA), given the tension between potentially contaminated fish supplies and mounting evidence for benefit from maternal intake of DHA and EPA during pregnancy.

FISH CONSUMPTION

The dangers of mercury toxicity from eating fish have been widely publicized now in the United States, to the point where many women of childbearing years are fearful regarding eating any fish at all. These fears may be somewhat justified: a NY DOH study in 2007 found that one in four women aged 20–49 in New York had serum mercury levels greater than 5 mcg/L, the reportable level for mercury toxicity (NYC Department of Health, 2007).

Mercury is not the only contaminant to be concerned about in fish. In one study of children born to women who ate Lake Michigan fish during pregnancy and lactation, exposure to PCBs in utero was linked to significantly lower IQ scores and reading comprehension at age 11. Although larger concentrations of PCBs were transferred in breast milk than in utero, there was no impairment in children who were only exposed via lactation—possibly suggesting a unique susceptibility of the developing fetal brain to PCBs (Jacobson, 1996). Farm-raised fish are often high in PCBs and other contaminants (Figure 16-1).

CHEC's Safe Fish Chart

Frequent Consumption 2 to 3 times per week	Once a Week (with no other fish)	Once a Month or Less (with no other fish)	Avoid Highly Contaminated	Overfished Wild Species
Anchovies	Catfish (Farmed)	Bullheads	Bass, Freshwater	Caviar (Sturgeon
Clams (Farmed)	Cod, Atlantic	Mackerel, Jack	Bass, Largemouth	Roe)
Crawfish	Cod, Pacific	and Spanish	Bass, Sea	Cod, Atlantic
Fish Sticks	Crab (except Blue from	Mussels (Farmed)	Bluefish	Flounder, Atlantic
Flounder, Atlantic	Gulf of Mexico)	Oysters (Farmed in	Carp	Flounder, Pacific
(Summer or Fluke,	Crappie	Gulf of Mexico)	Catfish, Wild Channel	Grouper
Winter or Sole)	Haddock	Pollock, Atlantic	Blue Crab, Gulf Of	Hake, Atlantic
Flounder, Pacific (Starry)	Hake, Atlantic	Salmon, Farmed	Mexico	Halibut, Atlantic
Rainbow Trout (Farmed)	Hake, Pacific	(Includes All	Great Lakes Fish	Lingcod
Shrimp (Farmed)	Herring	Atlantic Salmon)	Grouper	Lobster
Shrimp (Trap-Caught,	Mahi Mahi (Hook-And-		Halibut, Pacific	Monkfish
i.e., California Spot	Line Caught)		Halibut, Atlantic	Orange Roughy
Prawns, Atlantic	Mackerel, Atlantic		Lobster	Pollock, Atlantic
or Northern Pin Shrimp)	or Boston		King Mackerel	Red Snapper
	Oysters (Farmed, and		Orange Roughy	Salmon, Wild Atlantic
	Not from Gulf		Pike	Sea Bass, Chilean
	Of Mexico)		Red Snapper	(aka Patagonian
	Perch		Shark	Toothfish)
	Pollock, Pacific		Swordfish	Shark
	Salmon, Wild Alaskan		Tilefish	Sole, Atlantic
	and Pacific		Tuna, Steaks	Sole, Pacific
	Sardines		Tuna, Canned White	Sturgeon
	Sea Bass, Striped		(Albacore)	Swordfish
	(Farmed)		Walleye	Tilefish
	Scallops, Bay		White Croaker	Tuna, Bluefin
	Scallops, Sea (Farmed)			
	Smelt			
	Sunfish			
	Tilapia (Farmed)			
	Tuna, Canned Chunk			
	Light (Not White)			

OR OR BUT NOT

FIGURE 16-1. CHEC safe fish chart.

Choose wild-caught instead of farmed for most species

Avoid large predatory species

Keep portions modest and vary type of seafood you choose

Use cooking methods that reduce PCBs/dioxins, such as trimming skin, fat and dark meat, avoiding frying, removing mustard from crabs and tomalley from lobsters

Choose small fish, low in fat, non-bottom dwellers

Be aware of state-by-state fish advisories if eating fish you or someone else has caught

Source: **Children's Health Environmental Coalition HealtheHouse website www.checnet.org/healtheHouse**

On the other side of this debate is the mounting evidence of benefits to infants whose mothers supplement with fish oil during pregnancy. For example, in one randomized, double-blinded study, a total of 341 pregnant women were recruited in week 18 of pregnancy and randomized to take either 10 mL of cod liver oil daily or a corn oil placebo until 3 months after delivery. Children who were born to mothers who had taken cod liver oil during pregnancy and lactation scored significantly higher on the Mental Processing Composite of the K-ABC at 4 years of age as compared with children whose mothers had taken corn oil (106.4 [7.4] versus 102.3 [11.3]). The children's mental processing scores at 4 years of age correlated significantly with maternal intake of DHA and EPA during pregnancy.

The dose of fish oil used in this study contained approximately 1200 mg of DHA and 800 mg of EPA per day (Helland, 2003). Given the challenges of maintaining this level of omega-3 EFA intake during pregnancy and lactation in the face of all the current concerns regarding mercury and PCB contamination, adding a fish-oil supplement to the diet of pregnant mothers would appear to be important.

Early Nutrition

BREASTFEEDING

The benefits of breastfeeding are clearly established and do not need review here. Among other benefits exclusive breastfeeding for the "first months" leads to reduced risk (OR = 0.73) for asthma, which is even more pronounced in children with a family history of atopy (OR = 0.52) (Gdalevich, 2001). Similar benefits are found in the frequency of otitis media and other respiratory infection (Chantry, 2006). The American Academy of Pediatrics currently recommends breastfeeding for the first 12 months of life.

Despite the fact that most physicians are aware of these benefits, they are often not as active as they might be in supporting women who may be experiencing difficulty in breastfeeding. For example, the impact of maternal stress on breast milk production, and the potential role of the pediatrician or family physician in helping identify and address this barrier, are factors often overlooked (O'Connor, 1998). Mothers who are overly stressed by the demands of parenting, or who experience early problems with breast milk supply or delivery, often fall into a self-fulfilling negative cycle of increased self-doubt, decreased self-esteem, and consequent further decrease in breast milk supply. Maternal anxiety is sometimes also communicated to the newborn non-verbally and can complicate latching problems, particularly in a high-need baby. Sometimes just the recognition and acknowledgement of this problem by the physician, and some simple suggestions for reducing stress wherever possible—putting on music at home, having food or meals delivered, a foot massage for the new mom—can be critical in helping prevent this cycle, particularly in first-time mothers.

A crucial and underutilized resource available to physicians is the board-certified lactation consultant (BCLC), a specialty health professional focused specifically on breastfeeding support. Many women do not have access to the kind of experience and knowledge regarding the common problems encountered in breastfeeding which were once provided by their mothers and grandmothers. BCLCs are highly trained specialists who can fill this niche; in our practice many women who would otherwise have given up breastfeeding early because of production or latching problems have managed to continue nursing with the support of lactation consultants. Given the strong evidence for benefit of breastfeeding, this could be a very useful intervention for many families.

STARTING SOLIDS

In the past, there has been some debate regarding whether 4 or 6 months of age is the proper time to start solid foods; at this point—although different cultures have drastically different beliefs on this subject—there is general consensus among physicians that waiting until 6 months is probably best. A 17-year nonrandomized study reported that, compared with short or no breastfeeding, 6 months of exclusive breastfeeding is associated with less eczema and food allergy at ages 1 and 3 years and a long-term allergy protective effect on the respiratory allergy during adolescence (Saarinen, 1995). Solid food avoidance until 4 months has been clearly shown to decrease the incidence of atopic disease and atopic sensitization; however delaying until 6 months has not been clearly shown to add additional benefit (Schoetzau, 2002; Zutavern, 2006). Nevertheless, in children who are growing well, waiting until 6 months remains probably the most commonly accepted recommendation.

ORGANIC VERSUS CONVENTIONAL FOODS

As the young child starts on solids, one of the major issues which confronts physicians and families committed to an integrative approach is the question of whether choosing organic foods for the child will promote better health. Surprisingly, the answer to this question is not totally clear. Certainly far more people in the United States are now choosing organic; but to date, at least, there are no significant studies showing that any specific health outcomes are better in patients eating an organic diet when compared to those eating more conventional foods (Magkos, 2006).

What we do know is that there are a tremendous number of chemicals in our conventional food chain now which were not there two or three decades ago. These include pesticide residues, by-products from manufacturing processes, flame retardants, antibiotics, growth hormones, and many others. We also know that these chemicals are being absorbed into our children's bodies: when children ages two to five eat a diet that is more than 75% conventional foods, they have concentrations of organophosphate pesticide metabolites in their blood which are six times higher than that found in children eating a diet of >75% organic foods (Curl, 2003). We also know that organophosphates are potentially neurotoxic in animal studies.

The question of what might be long-term risks for neurological consequences from these exposures is harder to answer. One recent, large, long-term study of household rather than dietary exposure in New York did find that children exposed prenatally and in early childhood to the organophosphate chlorpyrifos via household pesticide use may have increased risk of developmental delay. In this study of 254 children over the first three years of life, researchers found that children with the highest blood levels of chlorpyrifos had five times the risk of developmental delay compared to children with the lowest blood levels (Rauh, 2006). Although this study examined household exposure rather than exposure from foods, these findings are potentially groundbreaking in providing validation for limiting exposure of children to potential neurotoxins.

One of the most compelling concepts to emerge in recent years in the public and environmental health arenas is the Precautionary Principle which states, among other things, that "no evidence of harm does not equal evidence of no harm." This is probably the best and safest position for us as healthcare practitioners to take in counseling families on children's exposure to potentially toxic chemicals, whether through food choices, household products, or environmental pollution. This principle, as well as common sense, would dictate that wherever possible, even if risk has only been definitively demonstrated in vitro or in animal studies, we avoid exposing our children to untested chemicals.

The final important aspect of the organic question, if we are committed to an integrative approach which takes into account not only the individual and the family but their relationship to and interdependence with the natural world, is the potential impact of our food choices on the health of the environment. If we had raised our awareness and our standards regarding mercury emissions from power plants two or three decades ago, we would not now have to avoid many fish species—and the potential health benefits of a diet high in fish oils—because of environmental pollution. By the same token, if we start to more actively choose organic foods, we may prevent a future in which the soil and water supply are so heavily contaminated with antibiotic and endocrine-disrupting residues that we can no longer safely eat food grown in certain areas.

Although organic food production does put far fewer toxic chemicals into the environment, there are significant environmental problems associated with how organic foods are now being transported and marketed in the United States. The advent of large-scale organic agri-business has meant that many organic foods are now shipped long distances, requiring tremendous fuel consumption for transport and refrigeration. The potential consequences of this energy use on the future health of our children should also not be ignored. Many environmental advocates are now suggesting that at least as important as choosing organic foods is choosing, when possible, locally produced foods produced from sustainably managed farms, even if those farms are not entirely organic.

Although these issues of environmental health may seem unrelated to the specific details of our day-to-day work with our patients, we need only remember the mercury disaster to remind ourselves of the potential cost to our patients' future health if we do not begin to incorporate this type of education into our work with patients.

ORGANIC FOODS: 10 fruits and vegetables to buy organic

Peaches—iprodione and methyl parathion	Grapes—methyl parathion, methomyl
Apples—methyl parathion, chlorpyrifos	Strawberries—captan
Pear—methyl parathion, Ops	Raspberries—captan, iprodione, carbaryl
Winter squash—dieldrin, heptachlor	Spinach—permethrin, dimethoate, DDT
Green bean—neurotoxic OPs, endosulfan	Potatoes—dieldrin, methamidophos, aldicarb

Source: Consumers Union 1999

Use of Supplements in Infancy and Early Childhood

Despite all our efforts, it may be difficult for certain children to get all the nutrients they need from diet alone. There are a significant number of dietary supplements which can be used safely in children either for treatment of specific conditions, for prevention of such conditions in those at risk, or for overall health promotion. A few rules of thumb apply:

1. Where specific dosages have not been studied in clinical trials, dosages should be generally be adjusted by weight based on adult dosing.
2. Wherever possible, the use of a high-quality brand is important, since supplements are poorly regulated and there is a large degree of variation in quality. Consumerlabs.com, an independent laboratory, provides excellent information on specific supplements as to the quality of various brands.
3. Children with serious liver or kidney disease, in whom clearance of a particular supplement might be an issue, should be prescribed these with greater caution and at lower doses.

4. Children on multiple medications for serious illness, in whom interactions between supplements and medications might pose a problem, require special care and attention to dosing and interaction issues.

Because space here does not allow for a comprehensive discussion of the use of nutritional supplements in children, we will use two common supplements—fish oil and probiotics—to illustrate the potential utility of this approach in children.

FISH OIL

Fish oil has many potential applications in children, and studies of new applications appear in the literature on a regular basis. It can be used safely even in very young children; initial concerns regarding oil aspiration—based on several case reports from the 1950s and 1960s on mineral oil aspiration in young infants—have not been borne out by any published reports of fish oil aspiration despite its widespread use. Palatability can be an issue, and many preparations are available now with flavorings to encourage compliance. A comprehensive review of the literature on clinical applications of fish oil in children is beyond the scope of this chapter, but a few examples should suffice:

Cognitive Development

A randomized clinical trial ($n = 56$) of infant formula milk supplemented with DHA or with DHA plus arachidonic acid (AA), versus a control formula which provided no DHA or AA enrolled children in the first 5 days of life and fed them the assigned formula through 17 weeks of age. At 18 months of age both the cognitive and motor subscales of the Bayley Scales of Infant Development (BSID) showed a significant developmental age advantage for DHA⁻ and DHA+AA-supplemented groups compared to the control group. Neither the Psychomotor Development Index nor the Behavior Rating Scale of the BSID-II showed significant differences among diet groups, suggesting a specific effect of DHA supplementation on mental development. The plasma and RBC concentrations of DHA at 4 months of age—but not at 12 or 18 months—were significantly correlated with improved performance, suggesting that dietary availability of DHA early in infancy is most critical (Birch, 2000).

Crohn's Disease

Thirty-eight patients (20 male/18 females, mean age 10 years, range 5-16 years) with CD in remission were randomized into two groups and treated for 12 months. Group I (18 patients) received 5-ASA + omega-3 EFAs 3 g/d (EPA 1200 mg, DHA 600 mg). Group II (20 patients) received 5-ASA+olive oil placebo capsules. Patients were evaluated for fatty acid incorporation in red blood cell membranes by gas chromatography at baseline, and then at 6 and 12 months after the treatment. The number of patients who relapsed at 1 year was significantly lower in group I than in group II ($p < 0.001$). Patients in group I had a significant increase in the incorporation of EPA and DHA ($p < 0.001$) into cell membranes and a decrease in the presence of AA (Romano, 2005).

Depression

Twenty-eight patients were randomized to fish oil (400 mg EPA/ 200 mg DHA) versus placebo, and 20 completed at least 1 month's ratings. Analysis of variance showed highly significant effects of omega-3 on symptoms using the Children's Depression Rating Scale (CDRS), Children's Depression Inventory (CDI), and Clinical Global Impression (CGI). Although this was a short duration study only, it suggests that omega-3 fatty acids may have therapeutic benefits in childhood depression (Nemets, 2006) (Figure 16-2).

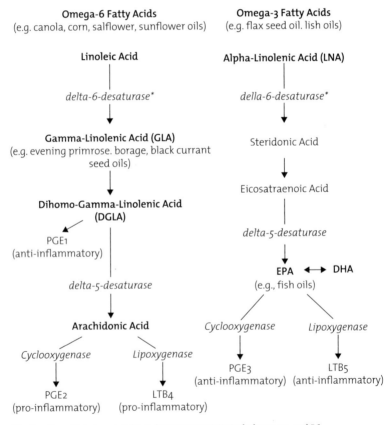

* Factors thought to impair delta-6-desaturase activity include mg, zn, and B6 deficiency; aging: alcohol; *trans* fatty acids: and high cholesterol levels.

FIGURE 16-2. Metabolic pathways of essential fatty acids.

PROBIOTICS

Probiotics are defined as "live microorganisms which, when administered in adequate amounts, confer a health benefit on the host" (Kligler, 2007). In children, the gut flora are enormously important in the development of the immune system, and a disturbed gut flora can predispose to a wide range of problems. Healthy gut flora in children apparently facilitates systemic down-regulation of inflammatory processes by balancing the generation of pro and anti-inflammatory cytokines. In addition, these bacteria reduce the dietary antigen load by degrading and modifying macromolecules in the gut, reverse the increased intestinal permeability characteristic of children with food allergy, and enhance specific IgA responses frequently defective in children with food allergy.

Indications examined in clinical trials to date include diarrhea (treatment and prevention), atopic dermatitis, irritable bowel syndrome, and inflammatory bowel disease. A large number of different organisms are now being used in clinical practice: the most widely used and thoroughly researched are *Lactobacillus* sp. (including *L. Acidophilus*, *L. rhamnosus*, *L. bulgaricus*, *L. reuteri*, and *L. casei* among others), *Bifidobacterium* sp., and *Saccharomyces boulardii*, a non-pathogenic yeast. The dose is generally in the 5–10 billion CFU/day range for children, though probiotics have an extremely wide safety margin and can be safely used at much higher doses as well. As is the case with fish oil, the clinical trials literature on probiotics in children is already quite large and is growing rapidly; a few examples are provided below.

Acute Diarrheal Illness (Treatment)

A systematic review and a recent meta-analysis both concluded that probiotics are probably effective in treatment of children with acute diarrhea. A Cochrane Review examined twenty-three studies of probiotic use for acute diarrhea in adults and children ($n = 1917$) in 2005, and found that in the subset of 12 studies performed in infants and children, mean duration of diarrhea was reduced by 29.2 hours in subjects taking probiotics (95% CI 25.1 to 33.2, $p < 0.00001$). The authors concluded that probiotics "appear to be a useful adjunct to rehydration therapy in treating acute, infectious diarrhea in adults and children [54]" (Allen, 2007). *S. boulardii* was also evaluated in a meta-analysis (four RCTs; $n = 619$) for treatment of acute gastroenteritis in children and found to produce a significant reduction in duration of diarrhea (–1.1 days, 95% CI –1.3 to –0.8.) in children taking *S. boulardii* when compared to placebo (Szajewska, 2007).

Prevention of Diarrheal Illness

A double-blind placebo controlled randomized trial at 14 childcare centers in Israel enrolled infants age 4 to 10 months old ($n = 201$) who received formula supplemented with either *L. reuteri*, *Bifidobacterium lactis*, or no probiotic for 12 weeks. Both probiotic groups had significantly fewer and shorter episodes of diarrheal illness than the control group, with no change in respiratory illness. Effects were more prominent in *L. reuteri* group, which also had less absences, clinic visits, and antibiotic prescriptions during the study period (Weizman, 2005).

Atopic Dermatitis

In an Australian trial, 53 children aged 6–18 months with moderate or severe AD were randomized either to a probiotic (*Lactobacillus fermentum*) or to a placebo and followed for 16 weeks. The treatment group had a significant decrease on a standardized measure of AD severity (SCORAD) ($p = 0.03$) that was not seen in the placebo group. Ninety-two percent of children receiving probiotics had a SCORAD index that was better than baseline at week 16 compared with 63% of the placebo group (Weston, 2005). In a sub-analysis of this trial the administration of probiotics was associated with a significant increase in T-helper type 1(Th1-type) cytokine IFN-gamma responses at the end of the supplementation period (week 8: P = 0.004 and 0.046) as well as 8 weeks after ceasing supplementation (week 16: P = 0.005 and 0.021) relative to baseline levels. No significant changes in Th1 responses were seen in the placebo group. The increase in IFN-gamma responses was directly proportional to the decrease in the severity of AD ($r = -0.445$, P = 0.026) over the intervention period, and this change persisted 2 months after supplementation was ended (Prescott, 2005).

Antibiotic-Associated Diarrhea

A meta-analysis by Szajewska et al. (2006) of six RCTs ($n = 766$) concluded that probiotics reduced the risk of AAD in children from 28.5% to 11.9% (RR 0.44, 95% CI 0.25–0.77) when compared with placebo. The risk reduction was similar regardless of the type of probiotic used (*Lactobacillus GG, S. boulardii,* or *Bifidobacterium lactis* plus *Streptococcus thermophilus*). The number needed to treat in this analysis was 7, suggesting that for every 7 patients that would develop diarrhea while being treated with antibiotics, one fewer will develop AAD if also receiving probiotics (Szajewska, 2006).

Therapeutic Diets

There are many therapeutic diets potentially applicable to the treatment of specific conditions or disorders in children. Here we discuss the elimination or food sensitivity diet; the gluten-free casein-free diet; and the specific carbohydrate diet (SCF).

ELIMINATION DIET

The elimination diet, which is based on the concept of food sensitivities, is one of the most frequently used interventions in the clinical practice of integrative nutrition. The concept underlying this diet is that some children have specific reactions to specific foods which are not necessarily detectable by traditional allergy testing, but which nevertheless can provoke profound systemic symptoms. The range of conditions for which

---

The reason the elimination diet is such an important tool is that, despite the potentially profound impact of food sensitivity on systemic conditions, conventional allergy testing—whether IgE RAST testing or skin testing—does not generally identify these foods as problematic. This may be because the systemic reactions causes by this type of sensitivity are mediated not by specific antibodies or by T-cell responses but rather by exposure of the gut-associated lymphoid tissue (GALT) to particular food antigens and the consequent discharge of inflammatory cytokines, interleukin, and TNF—which are not easily tested for outside of a research setting. Thus the process of food elimination with careful symptom monitoring is not only an important therapeutic maneuver but also the definitive diagnostic test for food sensitivity. The potential role of IgG food antibody testing in identifying potential cause of food sensitivity is controversial, with some recent studies suggesting that this test may have a role (Atkinson, 2004).

---

this diet is potentially applicable is huge, and includes eczema, asthma, migraine syndromes, irritable bowel syndrome, fibromyalgia, allergic rhinitis, and numerous others, as well as many poorly defined symptoms not fitting a specific diagnostic category. If a specific cause of food sensitivity can be identified and removed, children with these conditions will sometimes experience a dramatic decrease in symptoms.

The elimination diet consists of an elimination/exclusion phase, and a reintroduction/ provocation (or food testing) phase. During the elimination period, the patient eats an extremely simplified diet, with a number of foods which are common causes of food sensitivity excluded: dairy, soy, eggs, corn, wheat, citrus, nuts, shellfish, pork, and chocolate (Baker, 2000). This stage ideally lasts 3–4 weeks, during which the target symptom—whether chronic cough in a child with asthma, severity of eczema, or abdominal distress in a child with IBS—is closely monitored daily by the parent, generally using a 1 to 10 type of scoring system which will allow the detection of changes which may not be evident subjectively from day to day. If food sensitivity is in fact a problem in a given child, some change in scores or a subjective impression of improvement will be evident by the end of the elimination phase. If no such change is apparent, food sensitivity is probably not a major cause, and proceeding to the testing phase is not likely to be helpful.

In the classic model of this approach, the "testing" phase—in which each of the excluded food groups is introduced singly and then eaten regularly for 3–5 days with close monitoring of symptoms—follows the elimination phase. During this stage it is critical to reintroduce only one suspected food at a time so that if symptoms recur it is clear what food is responsible. If there is no reaction after 5 days, another food may be reintroduced. If a "positive" reaction occurs as evidenced by worsening of symptoms, then that food should be removed again and at least a 4-day period be allowed to pass before the next food is reintroduced. During the testing phase it is generally easiest to start with the foods eaten most frequently, as these are the ones most likely to be responsible for causing symptoms. Foods which are eaten only rarely are not likely to be the cause of an ongoing symptom.

The elimination approach described above may not be practical in certain children, especially those six or under who are often much more limited in their food choices and less willing to adjust those choices than a motivated older child. In particular, parents often worry that the children will be under-nourished during the elimination phase, and in some case this is a legitimate concern. In this situation we recommend a modified approach, which eliminates the potential culprit foods sequentially rather than in one comprehensive elimination phase. Foods are removed one at a time, each for a 2-week period, with symptom monitoring; for example dairy foods would be eliminated for 2 weeks, while the rest of the diet remains unchanged. If there is no change, dairy would be returned to the diet, and a second food group would be eliminated. If parents are not certain at the end of a given 2-week period if they see any change, they should reintroduce that food with close symptom monitoring in a 1–2 week "provocation test" of that food group.

The disadvantages of this modified approach are that it generally takes significantly longer than the classical approach, which can be a barrier to family motivation. Also, if a child is sensitive to two or more of the food groups, as many are, eliminating them one at a time may not produce a marked enough decrease in symptoms to be detected, potentially resulting in a "false negative" elimination diet test. Nevertheless, in young children and in those with particularly limited diets, this approach is practical and can be very useful.

One important caveat when considering the elimination diet as a tool in adolescents is that a thorough screening for eating disorders must be part of the process. For a child with a history of anorexia, or with an undiagnosed body image disorder or tendency to eating disorder, the elimination diet—which requires a fairly rigid discipline be applied to food choices—could be the wrong approach.

GLUTEN- AND CASEIN-FREE DIET

The GFCF diet, in which all foods containing gluten and casein are eliminated, has become very popular in autism and other neuro-behavioral disorders. The theory behind this approach is that in certain genetically susceptible individuals, gluten and casein are incompletely metabolized in the gut, leading to the presence of excess levels of certain peptides which are subsequently absorbed into the blood stream. These peptides, including casomorphines and gluten exorphines, which are chemically similar to opiate peptides, may exert an opiate-type effect in such susceptible people, leading to disturbances in brain development with consequent neurobehavioral difficulties.

The GFCF diet requires a significant commitment from the family, as it involves removing all sources of gluten—which include wheat, rye, barley, and sometimes oats—as well as all products containing casein. The latter is present not only in milk and cheese, but in many processed foods which contain non-fat milk solids as well as other foods which include casein as a means to provide texture. Whey protein, which is also derived from milk, is acceptable on the GFCF diet. The amount of time generally recommended for a trial of such a diet can range from 1 to 2 months to as long as 1 year.

Many parents subjectively report significant improvements in behavior and social functioning on the GFCF diet. To date, though, clinical trials have been quite small and have not been able to clearly confirm such an effect. A small study ($n = 15$) by Elder et al. (2006) used a double-blind crossover design to examine the impact of a GFCF diet in treating autism spectrum disorder in children aged 2 to 16. Outcomes examined included data on autistic symptoms and urinary peptide levels over the course of 12 weeks on the diet. No statistically significant findings were reported, although several parents reported subjective improvement in behavior. Another small study ($n = 20$), which was randomized but single-blind only, compared the GFCF diet to a control group over a period of 1 year. These investigators did report a significant difference on development in the treatment group as compared to controls (Knivsberg, 2002). Millward et al(2008) reviewed available trials of gluten/casein diets in children with ASD. Of seven trials reviewed, six were uncontrolled and one used a single-blind design. All reported efficacy in reducing some autism symptoms, and two groups of investigators also reported improvement in nonverbal cognition; however these reviewers felt that all of the studies suffered from significant methodological flaws which made it difficult to interpret their conclusions with confidence. A long-term double-blind clinical trial sponsored by the National Institute of Mental Health is ongoing; preliminary results are not yet available.

SPECIFIC CARBOHYDRATE DIET

As is the case with many pharmaceuticals, some of the dietary interventions which have begun to be shown to benefit adults with certain conditions have not yet been adequately tested in children. The SCD, which can be extremely helpful in both adults and children with Crohn's Disease and ulcerative colitis, is one such approach. The SCD is a diet extremely low in disaccharides and polysaccharides, based on the premise that these foods can lead to imbalances in the gut flora, which in turn can trigger in susceptible individuals a hypersensitive cellular immune response in the gut. Monosaccharides, which are much more easily digested and absorbed, do not leave behind the same type of residue as the more complex carbohydrates, and thus do not lead to an overgrowth of the potentially pathogenic bacteria which trigger this type of response. This diet, described in detail in Elaine Gottschall's book "Breaking the Vicious Cycle" (Gottschall, 1994) eliminates lactose-containing dairy, all grains, and all legumes. Certain fruits and starchy vegetables, as well as sucrose, are also restricted.

Several studies in adults have supported the use of dietary carbohydrate restriction in patients with CD. In one study of 204 patients with CD, 69 were randomized to a low-carbohydrate diet (84 g/day). Fifty-four percent of these benefited significantly for as long as they maintained the diet (Lorenz-Meyer, 1996). Elemental and exclusion diets have also been shown to be effective in some patients with CD (Sanderson, 1987). Another small study of 33 patients with CD reported that 29 had specific food intolerances, with 21 of these remaining in remission on dietary measures alone (elimination diet or elemental diet). The average duration of remission in this study was 15.2 months, and the most commonly reported causes of sensitivity were wheat and dairy products (Workman, 1984). In another study, a group of 20 patients with CD were followed for several years using variations on the SCD approach; all of these patients demonstrated a decrease in symptoms and reduction in medication use (Galland, 1999), and six patients experienced complete clinical remission, discontinued all medication, and maintained in remission for 5 to 80 months.

Specific Carbohydrate Diet Guidelines

Method: The only carbs allowed are the simple sugars—fructose, glucose, and galactose. Disaccharide sugars, made up of two molecules are not allowed, because they do not break down easily. Sucrose, or table sugar is a disaccharide, so is lactose in milk.

As well, certain starch molecules, called amylose starch, are easily broken down and are completely digested. Amylose is found in most vegetables. Another type of starch, amylopectin, is found in grains. It is much more difficult to digest, and any food containing it is not allowed.

The diet is kept natural and unrefined as much as possible, since sugars and starches are added to just about everything that has been processed.

All natural meats, fish, fowl, eggs, cheese, nuts, fats, butter, and oils are allowed and fish canned in water or oil. As well, home-made yogurt is encouraged for its benefit to bowel health. Non-starchy vegetables, and whole fruits (no juices) are allowed. Honey may be used, if obesity is not a concern. Zero-carb sweeteners may be used, without filler (maltodextrin is made from corn or barley), or stevia.

Not allowed: grains, not even rice, sucrose sugar including molasses, liquid milk, some beans including soy, white potatoes, corn, margarine, malt, fructose crystals (made from corn). The lists here are incomplete. There are extensive lists of allowed and not-allowed foods in the book. The book includes recipes, as well as suitable infant foods and formulas.

Typical Menu

Breakfast: baked apple, sweetened with honey if allowed, scrambled eggs, muffin made from almond flour.

Lunch: tuna salad w. home-made mayonnaise, dill pickle, radishes, chives on a bed of lettuce, pumpkin custard, beverage.

Dinner: home-made spaghetti sauce w. mushrooms & meat, on a bed of steamed spaghetti squash, green salad w. oil & vinegar dressing, fresh fruit, tea.

Source: From http://www.lowcarb.ca/atkins-diet-and-low-carb-plans/specific-carbohydrate-diet.html

---

Although to date, a significant body of research evidence for the SCD in the management of IBD is lacking—and no studies support its use specifically in children—anecdotal evidence is positive. Particularly in an older child who is motivated by the possibility of decreasing symptoms and medication requirement, this diet can be applied safely and may be effective. Generally a 6-week trial of the diet is adequate to determine if it is going to be helpful in a given patient.

Specific Conditions

RECURRENT URI

Some children suffer what seem like excessively frequent upper respiratory infections, often complicated by recurrent otitis. Prevention is perhaps the best nutritional medicine in this case: the duration of breast-feeding has been found to have a significant effect on the future development of recurrent otitis media/upper respiratory infections, with infants who were breastfed for over 6 months having a decreased risk of developing recurrent otitis media, upper respiratory infections, and pneumonia (Chantry, 2006). This emphasizes the recommendation that infants receive breast milk for at least the first 6 months of life.

Nutritional intervention holds promise for some of these children though as in all of the conditions discussed here determining exactly which children will respond can be difficult. Allergy testing can be helpful, though as discussed above, the testing may miss more subtle food sensitivities which are, in fact, contributing. Some studies have found a higher prevalence of food allergies—over 50% at times—in children with recurrent ear infections (McMahan, 1981). In one study of children with documented food allergies, elimination of the offending foods for 16 weeks led to significant improvement in serous otitis in 86% of the children (Nsouli, 1994). Based on these results, it is important for the clinician to consider food allergy as a possible contributing factor in recurrent otitis media. Although challenging to implement, especially in younger children, the elimination diet is the best tool available to determine if food sensitivities are a contributing factor.

Fish oil supplementation may also have a role in reducing frequency of URI. In a recent study, two private pediatric offices with similar demographics in upper Manhattan were randomized to a supplementation site and a medical records control site. Ninety-four children (47 at each site), 6 months to 5 years of age (mean age 2 years) were enrolled. Children ≤1 year of age in the supplementation group received 1 teaspoon of lemon-flavored cod liver oil per day (460–500 EPA/500–550 DHA) and one half-tablet of a children's multivitamin-mineral; the starting dose was halved for children <1 year of age.

The supplementation group had a statistically significant decrease in the mean number of upper respiratory tract visits over time, whereas the medical records control group had no change in this parameter. The supplements were well tolerated; per parental report, 70% of children completed the 5- to 6-month course of cod liver oil. Since use of these nutritional supplements was acceptable to the inner-city Latino families and their young children, and was associated with a decrease in upper respiratory tract pediatric visits over time, this strategy deserves further research and attention (Linday, 2004).

ATOPIC DERMATITIS

As always, prevention is the best approach to this condition, and physicians can advise families at high risk for atopic disease on several possible strategies. There is some evidence that maternal supplementation with fish oil (Denburg, 2005) and with probiotics during pregnancy may reduce the likelihood of atopic dermatitis developing in a child at increased risk. One double-blind randomized placebo-controlled trial (n = 132) of children with a strong family history of atopic disease administered Lactobacillus GG (1X 1010 CFUs) to mothers for 2–4 weeks prenatally and then to infants postnatally for 6 months. Atopic eczema was diagnosed by age 2 in 23% (15/64) of the probiotic group versus 46% (31/68) in the placebo group (RR 0.51 95% CI 0.32–0.84). This benefit persisted at 4 years of age as well (Kalliomaki, 2001, 2003). A more recent placebo controlled study of *Lactobacillus acidophilus* (n = 231) administration to newborns at high risk for AD failed to replicate this finding (Taylor, 2007), and additional studies are in progress. Exclusive breastfeeding for 4–6 months has also been associated with a lower risk of developing atopic dermatitis (Kull, 2005).

The question of whether maternal dietary manipulation can be useful in infants with either elevated risk or with established eczema who are exclusively breastfed has not been sufficiently studied to date, though there is some limited evidence to support maternal antigen avoidance during lactation as a means to improve atopic dermatitis in the infant (Hays, 2005; Zeiger, 1995). Families should be given careful guidance so as to avoid nutritional deficiencies that may be detrimental to the developing infant.

For example, avoidance of dairy foods, soy-based foods, eggs, nuts, wheat, and shellfish may create deficiencies in folic acid, calcium, or iron. For patients at high risk, the American Academy of Pediatrics does advise maternal avoidance of peanuts and tree nuts during lactation; however the European Society for Pediatric Allergology and Clinical Immunology does not support this recommendation (Zeiger, 2003).

Hypoallergenic, hydrolyzed, and elemental formulas are often recommended in non-breastfed children who are either at high risk for eczema or manifesting early signs of atopy, although the effectiveness of this strategy has not been clearly documented. For infants in whom exclusive breastfeeding is not possible, a trial of a hydrolyzed protein formula may be beneficial (Hays, 2005). There is general agreement among experts that because soy is an "allergenic" food soy formulas should be avoided in infants with atopic dermatitis (Zeiger, 2003); however soy formulas are more palatable than hydrolyzed formulas and have only a 14%–40% cross reactivity with cow's milk, so they may be an appropriate alternative when hydrolyzed proteins formulas are not an option (Hill, 1984; Zeiger, 1995). Other mammalian milks (goat and sheep milks) were shown to have 80%–90% cross reactivity with cow's milk, and so are not generally recommended as alternatives in infants with eczema who are suspected to have a cow's milk sensitivity (Belloni-Buscino, 1999). If no improvement is seen with any of these less allergenic formulas over a 1- to 2-week period, it is generally recommended to resume a standard cow's milk formula diet.

The timing of the introduction of solid foods into an infant's diet may have some effect on symptoms of atopic dermatitis. One study showed solid food introduction past the first 4 months of life decreased the odds of developing symptomatic atopic dermatitis (Zutavern, 2006). The American College of Allergy, Asthma, and Immunology recommends adding foods one at a time to an infant's diet (Fiocchi, 2006). This is especially important in children at high risk for atopic dermatitis or allergies. Waiting 2–3 days between new food introductions should be ample time to observe a negative response to the food if it exists. If a reaction is observed, the parent should be advised to avoid this food product in the diet for 6–12 months, then try reintroducing the food into the diet to assess if the child has outgrown his/her sensitivity.

Both food allergy and food sensitivity can play a role in children with eczema. Approximately 40% of infants and young children with moderate to severe atopic dermatitis have food allergy (Sicherer, 1999). In older children food allergy is a less common cause of atopic dermatitis, as most children outgrow their food allergies in early childhood. The hypersensitivities most likely to persist in older children are those to egg, milk, soy, wheat, and peanut (Sampson, 1989). A number of studies have shown that identification of hypersensitivities and elimination of the offending food leads to improvement in symptoms of atopic dermatitis (Atherton, 1978; Lever, 1998; Sampson, 1986; Sloper, 1991), and thus allergy consultation and testing is an accepted component in the mainstream medical management of eczema.

Identifying food sensitivities (as opposed to food allergies) is a more challenging prospect since these reactions will not manifest with positive serological or skin prick test results. Food-sensitive children may react to as little as 100 mg or less of a given food, and the dose causing a reaction and the severity of reaction is not predicted by the skin prick or food specific IgE RAST testing (Sicherer, 2000). The use of an elimination or avoidance diet is the most effective strategy for identifying this type of reaction, and several studies using the gold standard double blind placebo controlled food challenge, have found a positive response to an avoidance diet in some children with eczema (Fiocchi, 2004). This approach has been found to be most effective in children under 2 years of age with more severe or refractory forms of eczema (Sicherer, 2000). It is important to remind parents that are pursuing a strict elimination diet that most children outgrow their sensitivities and that reintroduction of foods in 6 to 12 months is generally advised.

As public awareness of the potential role of food reactions in childhood eczema has grown, the proportion of parents excluding foods from their child's diet for treatment of atopic dermatitis has increased, along with the number of patient's reporting that unsupervised dietary manipulation is beneficial (Johnston, 2004). However elimination diets are not free of risk—children in whom dairy and soy are excluded for long periods will need other sources of calcium and protein for example, or will need supplementation—and some studies have shown that avoidance diets are being utilized excessively (Sinagra, 2007). Further, the beneficial effect of skin care as a first step in the treatment of eczema should not be neglected and may obviate the need to proceed with an avoidance diet even in food-sensitive patients (Norman, 2005).

NEURO-DEVELOPMENTAL DISORDERS

There is widespread use of dietary manipulation as a therapeutic approach to neuro-developmental or behavioral problems in children in primary care settings (Chan 2003). Dietary modification holds considerable appeal for parents as it augments their sense of control and aligns well with the desire to promote a healthy lifestyle for their child (Cormier, 2007). To date, there is very little hard evidence supporting using a restrictive diet in the general population for attention deficit hyperactivity disorder (ADHD) or autism (Goldberg, 2004). However, there may be subsets of children who will respond to an elimination diet and subsequent removal of a specific food to which they may be sensitive or intolerant (Schnoll, 2003; Christison & Ivan 2006). As with any restrictive diet, care must be taken to avoid nutritional deficiencies. One study showed a trend for children with autism who were on restrictive diets to have an increased prevalence of essential amino acid deficiencies and lower plasma levels of essential acids when compared to children with autism on unrestricted diets (Arnold, 2003). Further, restrictive diets can lead to substantial emotional and financial burdens on families and children. This should not be taken lightly when considering that autism and ADHD already lead to significant social isolation. There are several restrictive diets that are particularly popular in autism and ADHD that primary care physicians should be aware of in order to address concerned parents' questions about their potential benefit.

The additive-free diet, sometimes referred to as the Feingold diet, is based on the idea that food additives (artificial colors and flavors and naturally occurring salicylates) are associated with behavioral problems in children and hyperactivity. Although several studies in the late 1970s and early 1980s, including several reviews (Mattes, 1983; Wender, 1986; Williams, 1978) and one meta-analysis (Kavale, 1983), concluded that the Feingold diet is not an effective treatment for hyperactivity, many parents nevertheless report some positive change with this approach. One recent meta-analysis did support the hypothesis that artificial food coloring can contribute to symptoms of childhood hyperactivity in some children (Sehab, 2004).

Another common dietary approach in hyperactive children is to limit sugar intake. Certainly many parents can testify to the erratic behavior that can follow a large sugar load even in non-hyperactive children. Here again though, a meta-analysis did not find a relationship between sugar and hyperactivity, attention span, or cognitive performance; however the possibility of a subset of children with sugar sensitivity could not be ruled out (Wolraich, 1995). As always, placebo effect and parental expectation play a large role in the evaluation of whether eliminating sugar actually is effective: one study showed that parents who thought that their child was receiving real sugar when it was actually artificial sweetener, rated the child's behavior as significantly worse and more demanding than parents who rightly expected their child to receive an artificial sweetener (Hoover, 1994).

The GFCF diet, sometimes also with soy restriction added, is also popular among parents of children with autism and ADHD. As discussed above, the data are very limited regarding effectiveness (Millward, 2008), but anecdotal reports of success abound. If possible, since in these children this will be a long-term intervention with the risk of possible nutritional deficiencies, this diet should be implemented with guidance from a nutritionist.

ASTHMA

Food allergies or sensitivities have been implicated in the development and severity of asthma. Two recent Cochrane reviews suggest that allergy avoidance during pregnancy and during early infancy may reduce the risk of developing asthma, especially cow's milk avoidance in patients with cow's milk allergy (Kramer, 2003; Ram, 2002). Both reviews conclude that further research is needed, though, to clarify the strength of these associations. In children with suspected food allergy, especially cow's milk allergy, a trial of an avoidance diet may be helpful; however special attention needs to be given to the overall nutritional value of the diet so as to assure the child is not at risk of developing malnutrition. The literature on asthma provides a number of studies on the use of elimination diet in children with asthma (Bock, 1987; James, 1994; Pelikan, 1987). Results are equivocal, and some authors feel that the role of food sensitivities has been overstated, and that most reported sensitivities do not stand up to the "gold-standard" test of randomized double-blind food challenge (Manteleone, 1997). However, in clinical practice, the elimination diet remains a useful tool in the treatment of asthma. Common causes of food sensitivity in children include dairy foods, eggs, citrus, peanuts, soy, wheat, and chocolate.

Vitamin D may also play role in asthma prevention. Low maternal dietary Vitamin D intakes during pregnancy in women from low-sun areas has been associated with increased wheezing symptoms in children at ages 3–5 years (Camargo, 2007; Devereux, 2007). Pregnant women who are from colder climates or who do not spend time in the sun should be encouraged to eat plenty of Vitamin D rich foods. Some examples of major food sources of Vitamin D include: Vitamin D-fortified dairy products, egg yolks, saltwater fish, and liver. There is also epidemiological data suggesting that children with a lower Vitamin C intake or lower serum levels of Vitamin C have a higher risk for asthma (Harik Khan, 2004; Huang, 2001). One study showed an association between the early introduction of daily fresh fruits and vegetables and a decreased risk of developing asthma after one year of age (Nja, 2005). This supports the idea of encouraging families to provide their children with a well-balanced diet with an emphasis on fresh fruits and vegetables which have adequate levels of Vitamin C.

Obesity or elevated BMI may also be a risk factor for asthma in children (Oddy, 2004). Therefore, encouraging parents of obese children to develop a weight loss plan is paramount, especially in families with significant asthma histories.

Despite the appealing notion that the impact of omega-3 EFAs on the production of inflammatory mediators should lead to a decrease in asthma symptoms, a recent Cochrane Systematic Review found that there is little evidence to recommend that people with asthma supplement or modify their dietary intake of marine n-3 fatty acids (fish oil) in order to improve their asthma control. There is at least some evidence that a modest benefit may be seen in children with asthma when food elimination is combined with the use of omega-threes, but further research on this approach is needed (Woods, 2002).

Conclusion

Nutritional medicine has tremendous potential to make our pediatric patients healthier and happier, both as a preventive strategy and as a therapeutic modality for established conditions. Counseling on healthy food choices, the judicious and evidence-based use of specific supplements, and the application of therapeutic diets should be part of the repertoire of every integrative pediatric practitioner.

REFERENCES

Allen, S. J., Okoko, B., Martinez, E., Gregorio G., & Dans LF. (2004). Probiotics for treating infectious diarrhoea. *Cochrane Database of Systematic Reviews, 2*:CD003048.

Arnold, G. L., Hyman, S. L., Mooney, R. A., & Kirby, R. S. (2003). Plasma amino acids profiles in children with autism: Potential risk of nutritional deficiencies. *Journal of Autism and Developmental Disorders, 33*(4), 449–454.

Atherton, D. J., Sewell, M., Soothill, J. F.,Wells, R. S., & Chilvers, C. E. (1978). A double-blind controlled crossover trial of an antigen-avoidance diet in atopic eczema. *Lancet, 1*(8061), 401–403.

Atkinson, W., Sheldon, T. A., Shaath, N., & Whorwell, P. J. (2004). Food elimination based on IgG antibodies in irritable bowel syndrome: A randomized controlled trial. *Gut, 53*(10), 1459–1464.

Baker, J. C., & Ayres, J. G. (2000). Diet and asthma. *Respiratory Medicine, 94,* 925–934.

Bellioni-Businco, B., Paganelli, R., Lucenti, P., Giampietro, P. G., Perborn, H., & Buscinco, L. (1999). Allergenicity of goat's milk in children with cow's milk allergy. *Journal of Allergy and Clinical Immunology, 103,* 191–194.

Birch, E. E., Garfield, S., Hoffman, D R., Uauy, R., & Birch, D. G. (2000). A randomized controlled trial of early dietary supply of long-chain polyunsaturated fatty acids and mental development in term infants. *Developmental Medicine & Child Neurology, 42*(3), 174–181.

Bock, S. A. (1987). Prospective appraisal of complaints of adverse reactions to foods in children during the first 3 years of life. *Pediatrics, 79,* 683–688.

Camargo, C. A. Jr., Rifas-Shiman, S. L., & Litonjua, A. A., (2007). Maternal intake of vitamin D during pregnancy and risk of recurrent wheeze in children at 3 y of age. *The American Journal of Clinical Nutrition, 85,* 788.

Chan E., Rappaport L. A., & Kemper KJ. (2003) Complementary and alternative therapies in childhood attention and hyperactivity problems. *Journal of Developmental & Behavioral Pediatrics, 24*(1):4–8.

Chantry, C. J., Howard, C. R., & Auinger, P. (2006). Full breastfeeding duration and associated decrease in respiratory tract infection in US children. *Pediatrics, 117*(2), 425–432.

Christison, G. W., & Ivan, K. (2006). Elimination diets in autism spectrum disorders: Any wheat amidst the chaff? *Journal of Developmental & Behavioral Pediatrics, 2,* S162–S171.

Cormier, E., & Elder, J. H. (2007). Diet and child behavior problems: Fact or fiction? *Pediatric Nursing, 33*(2), 138–143.

Curl, L. C., Fenske, R. A., & Elgethun, K. (2003). Organophosphorus pesticide exposure of urban and suburban preschool children with organic and conventional diets. *Environmental Health Perspectives, 111*(3):377–382.

Denburg, J. A., Hatfield, H. M., Cyr, M. M., et al. (2005). Fish oil supplementation in pregnancy modifies neonatal progenitors at birth in infants at risk of atopy. *Pediatric Research, 57,* 276–281.

Devereux, G., Litonjua, A. A., Turner, S. W., et al. (2007). Maternal vitamin D intake during pregnancy and early childhood wheezing. *The American Journal of Clinical Nutrition, 85,* 853.

Elder, J. H., Shankar, M., Shuster, J., Theriaque, D., Burns, S., & Sherrill, L. (2006). The gluten-free, casein-free diet in autism: Results of a preliminary double blind clinical trial. *Journal of Autism and Developmental Disorders, 36*(3), 413–420.

Evans, R. W., Fergusson, D. M., Allardyce, R. A., & Taylor, B. (1981). Maternal diet and infantile colic in breast-fed infants. *Lancet, 1,* 1340.

Fiocchi, A., Assa'ad, A., & Bahna, S.; Adverse Reactions to Foods Committee, American College of Allergy, Asthma, and Immunology. (2006). Food allergy and the introduction of solid foods to infants: A consensus document. *Annals of Allergy, Asthma & Immunology, 97*, 10–20

Fiocchi, A., Bouygue, G. R., Martelli, A., Terracciano, L., & Sarratud, T. (2004). Dietary treatment of childhood atopic eczema/dermatitis syndrome (AEDS). *Allergy, 59*(Suppl 78), 78–85.

Galland, L. *Dietary Approach to Inflammatory Bowel Disease.* Poster presentation at the Fourth Annual Symposium on Alternative Therapies at the New York Marriott World Trade Center March 28, 1999 by Leo Galland, M.D.

Garrison, M. M., & Christakis, D. A. (2000). A systematic review of treatments for infant colic. *Pediatrics, 106*(1 Pt 2), 184–190.

Gdalevich, M. et al. (2001). Breastfeeding and the risk of bronchial asthma in childhood: A systematic review with meta-analysis. *The Journal of Pediatrics, 139*, 261–266

Goldberg, E. A. (2004). The link between gastroenterology and autism. *Gastroenterology Nursing, 27*(1), 16–19.

Gottschall, E. G. (1994). *Breaking the vicious cycle: Intestinal health through diet.* Kirkson Press, Baltimore, Ontario, Canada..

Hays, T., & Wood, R. A. (2005). A Systematic review of the role of hydrolyzed infant formulas for allergy prevention. *Archives of Pediatrics & Adolescent Medicine, 159*, 810–816.

Harik Khan, R. I., Muller, D. C., & Wise, R. A. (2004). Serum vitamin levels and the risk of asthma in children. *American Journal of Epidemiology, 159*, 351–357

Helland, I., Smith, L., Saarem, K, & Saugstad, O. (2003). Drevon C Maternal supplementation with very-long-chain n-3 fatty acids during pregnancy and lactation augments children's IQ at 4 years of age. *Pediatrics, 111*(1), e39–44.

Hill, D. J., Ford, RP. K., Selton, M. J., & Hosking, C. S. (1984). A study of 100 infants and young children with cow's milk allergy. *Clinical Reviews in Allergy, 2*, 125–131.

Hill, D. J., Hudson, I. L., Sheffield, L. J., Shelton, M. J., Menahem, S., & Hosking, C. S. J. (1995). A low allergen diet is a significant intervention in infantile colic: Results of a community-based study. *Journal of Allergy and Clinical Immunology, 96*(6 Pt 1), 886–892.

Hoover, D. W., & Milich, R. (1994). Effects of sugar ingestion expectancies on mother-child interactions. *Journal of Abnormal Child Psychology, 22*, 501–515.

Host, A., Dreborg, S., Muraro, A., et al. (1999). Dietary products used in infants for treatment and prevention of food allergy. *Archives of Disease in Childhood, 81*, 80–84.

Huang, S. L., & Pan, W. H. (2001). Dietary fats and asthma in teenagers: Analyses of the first Nutrition and Health Survey in Taiwan (NAHSIT). *Clinical & Experimental Allergy, 31*(12), 1875–1880.

Jacobson, J. L., & Jacobson, S. W. (1996). Intellectual impairment in children exposed to polychlorinated biphenyls in utero. *The New England Journal of Medicine, 335*(11), 783–789.

James, J. M., Bernhisel-Broadbent, J., & Sampson, H. A. (1994). Respiratory reactions provoked by double-blind food challenges in children. *American Journal of Respiratory and Critical Care Medicine, 149*, 59–64.

Kalliomaki, M. et al. (2001). Probiotics in primary prevention of atopic disease: A randomised placebo-controlled trial. *Lancet, 357*, 1076–1079.

Kalliomaki, M., Salminen, S., Poussa, T., et al. (2003). Probiotics and prevention of atopic disease: 4-year follow-up of a randomized placebo-controlled trial. *Lancet, 361*, 1869–1871.

Kavale, K. A., & Forness, S. R. (1983). Hyperactivity and diet treatment: A meta-analysis of the Feingold hypothesis. *Journal of Learning Disabilities, 16*, 324–330.

Kligler B. Hanaway P., & Cohrssen A. (2007). Probiotics in children. *Pediatric Clinics of North America, 54*(6):949–967.

Knivsberg, A. M. et al. (2002). *A randomized, controlled study of dietary intervention in autistic syndromes. Nutritional Neuroscience, 5(4),* 251–261.

Kramer, M. S., & Kakuma, R. (2003). Maternal dietary antigen avoidance during pregnancy and/or lactation for preventing or treating atopic disease in the child. *The Cochrane Database of Systematic Reviews,* Issue 4. Art No.:CD000133. DOI: 10.1002/14651858.

Kull, I., Bohme, M., Wahlgren, C. F., et al. (2005). Breast-feeding reduces the risk for childhood eczema. *The Journal of Allergy and Clinical Immunology, 116,* 657–661.

Johnston, G. A., Bilbao, R. M., & Graham-Brown, R. A. (2004). The use of dietary manipulation by parents of children with atopic dermatitis. *British Journal of Dermatology, 150(6),* 1186–1189.

Lever, R., MacDonald, C., Waugh, P., & Aitchison, T. (1988). Randomized controlled trial of advice on an egg exclusion diet in young children with atopic eczema and sensitivity to eggs. *Pediatric allergy and immunology: Official publication of the European Society of Pediatric Allergy and Immunology, 9(1),* 13–19.

Linday, L. A., Shindledecker, R. D., Tapia-Mendoza, J., & Dolitsky, J. N. (2004). Effect of daily cod liver oil and a multivitamin-mineral supplement with selenium on upper respiratory tract pediatric visits by young, inner-city, Latino children: Randomized pediatric sites. *Annals of Otology, Rhinology & Laryngology, 113(11),* 891–901.

Lorenz-Meyer, H., Bauer, P., Nicolay, C., Schulz, B., Purrmann, J., Fleig, W. E., et al. (1996). Omega-3 fatty acids and low carbohydrate diet for maintenance of remission in Crohn's disease. A randomized controlled multicenter trial. *Scandinavian Journal of Gastroenterology, 31(8),* 778–785.

McMahan, J. T., Calenoff, E., Croft, J., et al. (1981). Chronic otitis media with effusion and allergy: Modified RAST analysis of 119 cases. *Otolaryngology And Head And Neck Surgery, 89,* 427–431.

Magkos, F., Arvaniti, F., & Zampelas, A. (2006). Organic food: Buying more safety or just peace of mind? A Critical review of the literature. *Critical Reviews in Food Science and Nutrition, 46,* 23–56.

Manteleone, C. A., & Sherman, A. R. (1997). Nutrition and asthma. *Archives of Internal Medicine, 157(1),* 23–34.

Mattes, J. A. (1983). The Feingold diet; a current reappraisal. *Journal of Learning Disabilities, 16,* 319–323.

Millward, C., Ferriter, M., Calver, S., & Connell-Jones, G. (2008). Gluten- and casein-free diets for autistic spectrum disorder Cochrane Database of Systematic Reviews CD003498.pub2

Nemets, H., Nemets, B., Apter, A., Bracha, Z., & Belmaker R. H. (2006). Omega-3 treatment of childhood depression: A controlled, double-blind pilot study. *American Journal of Psychiatry, 163(6),* 1098–1100.

Nja, F., Nystad, W., Lodrup Carlsen, K. C., Hetlevik, O., & Carlsen, K. H. (2005). Effects of early intake of fruit or vegetables in relation to later asthma and allergic sensitization in school-age children. *Acta Paediatrica, 94(2),* 147–154.

Norrman, G., Tomici, S., Bottcher, M. F., Oldaeus, G., Stromberg, L., & Falth-Magnusson, K. (2005). Significant improvement of eczema with skin care and food elimination in small children. *Acta Paediatrica, 94(10),* 1384–388.

Nsouli, T. M., Nsouli, S. M., Linde, R. E., et al. (1994). Role of food allergy in serous otitis media. *Annals of Allergy, 73,* 215–219.

NYC Department of Health and Mental Hygiene: One in Four NYC Adults Has Elevated Blood Mercury. Retrieved October 27, 2007, from http://www.nyc.gov/html/doh/html/pr2007/pr059-07.shtml

O'Connor, M. E., Schmidt, W., Carroll-Pankhurst, C., & Olness K. N. (1998). Relaxation training and breast milk secretory IgA. Archives of Pediatrics & Adolescent Medicine, 152, 1065–1070.

Oddy, W. H., Sherriff, J. L., de Klerk, N. H., Kendall, G. E., Sly P. D., Beilin L. J., et al. (2004). The relation of breastfeeding and body mass index to asthma and atopy in children: A prospective cohort study to age 6 years. American Journal of Public Health, 94(9), 1531–1537.

Pelikan, Z., & Pelikan-Filipek, M. (1987). Bronchial response to the food ingestion challenge. Ann Allergy, 58, 164–172.

Prescott, S. L., Dunstan, J. A., Hale, J., Breckler, L., Lehmann, H. ,Weston, S., et al. (2005). Clinical effects of probiotics are associated with increased interferon-gamma responses in very young children with atopic dermatitis. Clinical & Experimental Allergy, 35(12), 1557–1564.

Ram, F. S. F., Ducharme, F. M., & Scarlett, J. (2002). Cow's milk protein avoidance and development of childhood wheeze in children with a family history of atopy. The Cochrane Database of Systematic Reviews, (1) Art No.: CD003795. DOI: 10.1002/14651858. CD003795.

Rauh, V. A., Garfinkel, R., Perera, F. P., & Andrews, H. F. (2006). Impact of prenatal chlorpyrifos exposure on neurodevelopment in the first 3 years of life among inner-city children. Pediatrics, 118(6) 1845–1859.

Romano, C., Cucchiara, S., Barabino, A., Annese, V., & Sferlazzas, C. (2005). Usefulness of omega-3 fatty acid supplementation in addition to mesalazine in maintaining remission in pediatric Crohn's disease: A double-blind, randomized, placebo-controlled study. World Journal of Gastroenterology, 11(45), 7118–7121.

Saarinen, U. M., & Kajosaari, M. (1995). Breastfeeding as prophylaxis against atopic disease: Prospective follow-up study until 17 years old. Lancet, 346, 1065–1069.

Sampson, H. A. (1989). Scanlon SM Natural history of food hypersensitivity in children with atopic dermatitis. Journal of Pediatrics, 115(1), 23–27.

Sampson, H. A. (1986). Food hypersensitivity as a pathogenic factor in atopic dermatitis. New England and Regional Allergy Proceedings, 7(6), 511–519.

Sanderson, I. R., Boulton, P., Menzies, I., & Walker-Smith, J. A. (1987). Improvement of abnormal lactulose/rhamnose permeability in active Crohn's disease of the small bowel by an elemental diet. Gut, 28(9), 1073–1076.

Schnoll, R., Burshteyn, D., & Cea-Aravena, J. (2003). Nutrition in the treatment of attention-deficit hyperactivity disorder: A neglected but important aspect. Applied Psychobiology and Biofeedback, 28(1), 63–72.

Schoetzau, A. et al. (2002). Effect of exclusive breastfeeding and early solid food avoidance on the incidence of atopic dermatitis in high-risk infants at 1 year of age. Pediatric Allergy & Immunology, 13(4), 234–242

Sehab, D. W., & Trinh. N. T. (2004). Do artificial food colors promote hyperactivity in children with hyperactive syndromes? A meta-analysis of double-blind placebo controlled trials. Developmental and Behavioral Pediatrics, 25(6), 423–434.

Sicherer, S. H., & Sampson, H. A. (1999). Food hypersensitivity and atopic dermatitis: Pathophysiology, epidemiology, diagnosis, and management. The Journal of Allergy and Clinical Immunology, 104(3 Pt 2), S114–122.

Sicherer, S. H., Morrow, E. H., & Sampson, H. A. (2000). Dose-response in double-blind, placebo-controlled oral food challenges in children with atopic dermatitis. The Journal of Allergy and Clinical Immunology, 105, 582–586.

Sinagra J. L., Bordignon, V., Ferraro, C., Cristaudo, A., Di Rocco, M., Amorosi, B., et al. (2007). Unnecessary milk elimination diets in children with atopic dermatitis. Pediatric Dermatology, 24(1), 1–6.

Sloper, K. S., Wadsworth, J., & Brostoff, J. (1991). Children with atopic eczema. I: Clinical response to food elimination and subsequent double-blind food challenge. *The Quarterly Journal of Medicine, 80*(292), 677–693.

Stahlberg, M. R., & Savilahti, E. (1986). Infantile colic and feeding. *Archives of Disease in Childhood, 61*(12), 1232–1233.

Szajewska, H., Ruszczynski, M., & Radzikowski, A. (2006). Probiotics in the prevention of antibiotic-associated diarrhea in children: A meta-analysis of randomized controlled trials. *Journal of Pediatrics, 149*(3), 367–372.

Szajewska, H., Skorka, A., & Dylag, M. (2007). Meta-analysis: Saccharomyces boulardii for treating acute diarrhoea in children. Aliment Pharmacol Ther, *25*(3), 257–264.

Taylor, A. L., Dunstan, J. A., & Prescott, S. L. (2007). Probiotic supplementation for the first six months of life fails to reduce the risk of atopic dermatitis and increases the risk of allergen sensitization in high-risk children: A randomized controlled trial. *Journal of Allergy and Clinical Immunology, 119*(1),184–191.

Weizman, Z., Asli, G., & Alsheikh, A. (2005). Effect of a probiotic formula on infections in child care centers: Comparison of two probiotic agents. *Pediatrics, 115,* 5–9.

Wender, E. H. (1986). The food additive-free diet in the treatment of behavior disorders: A review. *Journal of Developmental Pediatrics and Behavioral Pediatrics, 7,* 35–42.

Weston, S., Halbert, A., Richmond, P., & Prescott, S. L. (2005). Effects of probiotics on atopic dermatitis: A randomized controlled trial. *Archives of Disease in Childhood, 90*(9), 892–897.

Williams, J. I., & Cram, D. M. (1978). Diet in the management of hyperkinesis: A review of the tests of the Feingold hypotheses. *Canadian Psychiatric Association Journal, 23,* 241–248.

Wolraich, M. L., Wilson, D. B., & White, J. W. (1995). The effect of sugar on the behavior or cognition in children: A meta-analysis. *Journal of the American Medical Association, 274,* 1617–1621.

Woods, R. K., & Thien, F. C., Abramson, M. J. (2002). Dietary marine fatty acids (fish oil) for asthma in adults and children. *Cochrane Database of Systematic Reviews,* (3), CD001283.

Workman, E. M., Alun Jones, V., Wilson, A. J., & Hunter, J. O. (1984). Diet in the management of Crohn's disease. *Human Nutrition—Applied Nutrition, 38*(6), 469–473.

Zeiger, R. S., & Heller, S. (1995). The development and prediction of atopy in high risk children: Follow up at age 7 years in a prospective randomized study of combined maternal and infant food allergen avoidance. *Journal of Allergy and Clinical Immunology, 95,* 1179–1190.

Zeiger, R. S. (2003). Food allergen avoidance in the prevention of food allergy in infants and children. *Pediatrics, 111,* 1662–1671.

Zutavern, A. et al. (2006). Timing of solid food introduction in relation to atopic dermatitis and atopic sensitization: Results from a prospective birth cohort study. *Pediatrics, 117,* 401–411.

17

A Pediatric Perspective on Osteopathic Medicine

ALI CARINE, MIRIAM MILLS, AND VIOLA FRYMANN

KEY CONCEPTS

- Osteopathic medicine, as founded by A.T. Still, has developed into a comprehensive, integrative approach to medicine. Doctors of osteopathic medicine (DO) apply the principles of osteopathy across all medical specialties.
- Rational treatment is based upon an understanding of the basic principles of body unity, self-regulation, and the interrelationship of structure and function.
- Osteopathic medicine utilizes any available treatment, nutritional interventions, surgery, medicine, or therapies, however, they are best known for their use of osteopathic manipulative treatments (OMT).
- Osteopathic physicians have developed a wide range of OMT modalities including, but not limited to, high velocity low amplitude, muscle energy, counterstrain, cranial osteopathy, and many variations of indirect techniques. Osteopathic treatments preferred by children include indirect techniques such as balanced ligamentous tension, myofascial release, and cranial osteopathy.
- Research into osteopathic medicine has traditionally focused on proof of principle studies, and those studies have lead to a better understanding into the physiologic mechanisms at work with OMT. Increased funding has now become available, and future studies will be looking into specific disease states and treatments.
- Pediatric osteopathic medicine is frequently used to treat infant colic, upper respiratory infections, recurrent otitis media, plagiocephaly, headaches, scoliosis, overuse injuries, and neurologic diseases such as cerebral palsy, autism, and seizures.

American osteopathic physicians pioneered the concept of "integrative" medicine. Throughout their existence they have utilized the benefits of the "mainstream" (allopathic) medicine of their time and incorporated the healing benefits of osteopathic manipulative treatment (OMT), and healthy lifestyle choices, especially nutrition. They are a minority group of physicians, and such, are often poorly understood. Any discussion of osteopathic medicine must start with an explanation of its current state of practice and a review of the historical roots.

Osteopathic physicians (DOs) have a philosophy of health woven throughout their training that shapes the way they practice medicine. OMT is based on well-recognized anatomic and physiologic principles involving the structural components of the body, and their relationship, particularly to the autonomic nervous system, but osteopathic philosophy encompasses more than manipulation alone.

The authors both regularly incorporate OMT into their practices of general pediatrics, and have found that the applications for its use are myriad, based on observations of often dramatic individual patient responses, as well as changes in the natural course of various pediatric conundrums in their patient populations over the years. Their experiences mirror those described in the literature and of others who have taught these principles, though well-designed prospective, blinded, placebo-controlled studies are in short supply.

Children provide a unique opportunity for OMT to shine. It has been said "as the twig is bent, so will be the tree" (Magoun, 1976). The ever developing and changing body and mind of a child is easily adaptable. Optimizing the health of a child is the best protection for health in the future. The nervous system is continually laying down new pathways, enabling the child to learn skills that it will rely on for the remainder of its life. Physicians who utilize osteopathy in children report that they need fewer treatments to achieve results than with adults, and often with dramatic results.

The remarkable and sometimes immediate response to manipulative treatment is believed to happen, at least partly, because physical restrictions (called "somatic dysfunction") around nerves, arteries, veins, and lymph flow are relieved. Neonates with borderline respiratory insufficiency otherwise not at risk for sepsis or other systemic problems, in a matter of a few minutes, are observed to take fuller, more relaxed breaths, and increase their oxygenation. Infants with intractable colic suddenly fall asleep with a deep sigh, and continue to sleep and eat without distress for weeks afterward. Children crying with ear pain, may yawn and soothe suddenly at the moment of a "release" in the tissues, and swallow or cough from the drainage just released down their throat. A fifteen month old who has always banged her head suddenly stops after being treated. A 5-year-old with recent onset of dizziness, at the moment of release of the tissues, no longer felt dizzy and simultaneously recalled having fallen off the bunk bed, hitting her head on the side of the dresser. These clinical responses are often associated with objective changes such as normalization of tympanograms, or changes in pulmonary function, but are not yet reported in the literature. While the placebo effect of any intervention is important to recognize, these dramatic immediate responses are important to note.

Not all responses are so immediate. Children with torticollis and plagiocephaly and chronic congestion, or older children with early scoliosis, tend to take longer to see results, and the later manipulation is started, the longer it takes. However, considering the rise in the use of helmet therapy for plagiocephaly, it seems to be an appropriate alternative to this approach (Mills, 2006).

Osteopathic History

A physician named Andrew Taylor Still was frustrated with the state of medicine in the 1860s, a time when medical practice included leeches and arsenic. He wrote about a time when he spent much time in prayer asking how he could better help mankind. He decided that if God had designed a perfect body, then it must possess its own capacity for health, and Still felt that his job was to understand how to support the body's efforts to heal itself. Although his most noted contribution lies in his development of manipulative medicine, he was also interested in nutrition and spiritual health. He then began the process of developing a school that would train physicians to treat their patients in this new system of medicine. Over the years, the schools have changed to meet the standards set by the larger medical community, so that osteopathic physicians could remain fully licensed physicians. This is something the profession felt was of key importance, to provide complete, holistic care. Now, osteopathic physicians practice in all fields of medicine and surgery. In thriving osteopathic cities like Columbus, Ohio, the attitude "caring for patients from birth to death," is a common motto of the osteopathic community. The network of physicians there is extensive, encompassing the full range of specialties. Across the country, osteopathic schools have a higher percentage of their graduates entering primary care fields. This reflects the idea that holistic, preventive care is best provided by physicians who can build an ongoing relationship with their patients. The field of manipulative medicine itself has grown dramatically, to include many different forms of manipulation that we will review later in the chapter. In addition to the refinement of osteopathic techniques by their own profession, osteopaths have benefited from the expansion of basic scientific knowledge of nutrition and mind-body health.

In addition to keeping strides with the advances in medicine, they are also now building bridges with their MD counterparts. Over half of all DO graduates enter ACGME residency programs. While training next to their MD colleagues, the divide between them is falling away, to the benefit of both professions. The depth of the *Accreditation Council for Graduate Medical Education (ACGME)* program's academic training benefits osteopathic physicians, while the facility of the DO graduates in patient interactions and holistic care is not going unnoticed: many programs are looking to their DO colleagues to help incorporate those skills into their residencies. Currently, the AAP (American Academy of Pediatrics) and the ACOP (American College of Osteopathic Pediatricians) hold joint conferences every other year; the first of these joint meetings was held in 2007 in Orlando, Florida, where the ACOP introduced a nine-module CD-ROM entitled "Pediatric Osteopathic Manipulative Treatment" (POMT). Also at that meeting, one of the authors (AC) led a hands-on workshop, which sparked considerable interest, even among the allopathic pediatricians (Schierhorn, 2007).

All around the globe, scientists and clinicians from all fields of medicine and science are collaborating more often. A recent international conference on fascia in 2007 in Boston provided an opportunity for scientists from many different disciplines to share their clinical experience and experimental findings. In addition, The International Symposium on Back Pain united physicians, chiropractors, scientists, and more in a common goal of information sharing (LeMoon, 2007).

For the purposes of this chapter however, we will focus the rest of our time on the use of manipulative medicine, as osteopathic physicians are best known for their use of OMT. Although manual medicine has been embraced by the lay public in various forms (e.g., massage, physical therapy, Reiki, and chiropractic), allopathic medical practitioners are only recently taking notice in larger numbers, as they confront the limitations of their usual modalities with challenges such as antibiotic-resistant bacteria and chronic illnesses. Throughout medical history, various cultures have realized the benefits to overall health that come from a well-functioning musculoskeletal system. In America, the fields of osteopathy and chiropractic developed near the same time, and Dr. Still and Dr. Palmer did know each other. These fields evolved somewhat independently, but have many similarities. The major difference between chiropractors and DOs is that osteopathic physicians have chosen to be fully licensed physicians and embrace the full spectrum of medical options. Osteopathic physicians have also developed a wide variety of other treatment modalities, some of which have now carried over into other musculoskeletal fields, like chiropractic and physical therapy.

Tenets of Osteopathic Medicine

To understand osteopathy, the reader must look closely at this equation.

$$host + disease = illness$$

All illness arises out of a combination of these two factors, the host and the disease. The host encompasses all the underlying homeostatic tendencies a person possesses: nutrition, social environment, spiritual health, anatomic function and autonomic regulation. The disease entity encompasses the known pathologic processes that contributed to the patient's illness: viruses, bacteria, genetic mutations and toxic exposures. These factors interact to produce the symptoms of illness. Different people exposed to the same disease process will manifest the illness with large variations. Most alternative and traditional therapies focus on strengthening the host. Most of mainstream allopathic medicine focuses on eradicating disease, using vaccinations, antibiotics, public health, chemotherapy, and now gene therapy. A well-trained osteopathic physician utilizes both of these approaches to accomplish alleviation of illness for the patient (Table 17-1).

Table 17-1. Some Simple Illustrations of This Principle

Host + disease = illness

HIV + candida = disseminated disease

Asthma + flu virus = hospitalization

Genetic predisposition + viral triggers = autism, diabetes

Weakened homeostasis + EBV = chronic fatigue

Somatic dysfunction + varicella = shingles

What follows is a consensus statement by the profession reflecting the core tenets of osteopathic medicine. Health is the adaptive and optimal attainment of physical, mental, emotional, and spiritual wellbeing. It is based on our natural capacity to meet, with adequate reserves, the usual stresses of daily life and the occasional severe stresses imposed by extremes of environment and activity. It includes our ability to resist and combat noxious influences in our environment and to compensate for their effects. One's health at any given time depends on many factors including his or her polygenetic inheritance, environmental influences, and adaptive response to stressors (Seffinger, 1997).

Four guiding principles

1. The body is a unit; the person is a unit of body, mind, and spirit.
2. The body is capable of self regulation, self-healing, and health maintenance.
3. Structure and function are reciprocally interrelated.
4. Rational treatment is based upon an understanding of the basic principles of body unity, self-regulation, and the interrelationship of structure and function.

Osteopathic physicians focus their treatment on areas of the body that display somatic dysfunction (SD). Trained palpation identifies alterations in homeostasis. It is the recognition, and subsequent treatment of SD, that is the hallmark of manipulative therapy. It is the improvement in the structure of these areas that then leads to better adaptive response and hence improved ability to ward off disease.

Somatic dysfunction is described as having four characteristics:

1. Changes is tissue texture;
2. Increased sensitivity to touch, termed hyperalgesia;
3. Altered ranges of motion, sometimes subtle; and
4. Anatomic asymmetry of the affected region (Brooks, 1997).

Basic Science of Manipulation

Osteopathic research is conducted and designed around osteopathic philosophy. The field carries the assumption that improvements in a person's anatomy and physiology lead to improvements in health. Research has focused on understanding these complicated interactions, and how manipulative therapy can lead to improvements in homeostasis. Most osteopathic research dollars are not spent on "randomized controlled trials" (RCT) of specific diseases and specific treatments. Instead, traditionally, studies have focused on proof of concept studies. The difference in medical paradigms is reflected in the type of literature that is published.

One of the earliest reports of the benefits of OMT, presented at the annual convention of the American Association of Clinical Research (Heath & Kelso, 1998) was from data obtained from 2445 DOs about the outcomes of victims of the influenza epidemic of 1918, showing a death rate of 1/40 that of patients treated by allopathic physicians among those who contracted pneumonia-complicating influenza. The profession just completed a multicenter, RCT to study the affects of OMT on hospitalized pneumonia patients, results of that study should reach publication by the end of 2009. Pneumonia is an excellent example of how OMT focused at the somatic system can afford positive effects on the body's ability to defend and heal.

Osteopathy is a clinical field that has evolved in its skills because of the benefit given to patients. The clinical application of this field has developed far past the basic science research into it, but more recently, research has been trying to document what the practitioners are experiencing. One of the challenges is that much of OMT research has not been well-represented in the allopathic medical literature, partly because the osteopathic approach is difficult to fit into the traditional prospective, randomized, placebo-controlled study paradigm, and partly because of inadequate funding for such research heretofore. With funding available for more "alternative" approaches to health, more RCTs can be undertaken.

Let us first look at the physiologic models that the profession uses to understand the body and its response to manipulative therapy. Jane Carreiro, DO has a well-written synopsis of this in the foreword of her book "An Osteopathic Approach to Children," where she details the anatomy and physiologic mechanisms at work in the pediatric patient. In addition, throughout this chapter there are numerous references to "The Foundations of Osteopathic Medicine," a very comprehensive text, which overviews all aspects of osteopathic medicine.

SOMATO-VISCERAL CONNECTIONS

Research now has demonstrated that the health of the musculoskeletal system and the viscera are intimately related. Detailed studies of spinal cord reflex arcs have shown that afferent nerves coming from the viscera and the somatic systems interact with each other prior to ascending up the spinal cord to the brain. Because of these relationships, within a certain spinal segment, the viscera and skeletal components of that segment can affect the function of one another. Osteopathic treatment can alter those afferent stimuli entering the spinal cord, and therefore help regulate the efferent response to both the musculoskeletal system and the viscera.

NEUROENDOCRINE-IMMUNE CONNECTION

In recent years, the scientific community has begun to document the complex relationships between various organs in the body. Our body's response to stress and adaptive ability is orchestrated through chemical and neuronal interactions from the nervous, endocrine and immunological systems in our body (Williard, 2003). Dividing our body into physiologic "systems" serves only to simplify the study of the body. This division has been held onto too strongly by the medical community, and it has led to stumbling blocks in understanding complex diseases, such as cancer, autism and inflammatory bowel disease. Osteopathic principles teach that addressing the neurologic, nutritional, emotional, and somatic stressors, has a dramatic effect on the immunologic response to a disease process.

Despite the ever-growing body of research into this concept, hospitals still remain one of the least conducive places to find emotional, mental, or spiritual health. But it is not just that good emotional health aids in healing. When a person's somatic and nutritional health is improved, they also have dramatic benefits in their mental health. If a patient's autonomic nervous system is not functioning well or they are unable to synthesize the neurotransmitters needed for proper mental functioning, the person will manifest symptoms of mental illness. Too often, we assume that the "stressed" child is having somatic complaints that are manifested from the stress. Perhaps the child's poor physical health is the cause of the anxiety. We all know that people respond in large variations to what appears to be psychological stress, from seemingly unaffected to dramatic depression. In the osteopathic approach, the somatic and nutritional health are addressed, to see if improvements in that lead to resolution of the depression or anxiety. It is for this reason that parents of autistic, inattentive, depressed, and anxious children often seek osteopathic treatment. Parents report that OMT directed at the somatic system of the body has beneficial effects on their children's mental health.

POSTURAL/BIOMECHANICAL MODEL AND RESPIRATORY/ CIRCULATORY MODEL

One of the most basic tenets of osteopathy is that the body functions best when the fascia and musculature are moving optimally. Structure and function are intimately related. Any treatment, medical or manipulative, to be effective, provides benefit all the way to the cellular level. For example, we know that asthma is a complex cascade of events that happens at the cellular level with inflammation and smooth muscle excitability. Clinically, OMT is used for asthmatic patients and some small studies have shown benefit (Guiney, Chou, Vianna, & Lovenheim, 2005). By removing restrictive motion in the rib cage, the vascular and lymphatic flow to the tissues improves, helping to bring needed nutrients and remove inflammatory debris. In addition, treatment focused on the sympathetic and parasympathetic innervation to the tissue calms the excitability of the smooth muscle and associated chemical cascade that follows.

In addition to these physiologic models, there is growing interest into the effects of OMT mediated by the autonomic nervous system. The role of the autonomic nervous system as a factor in a number of related but ill-defined symptom complexes, has been largely under-investigated, and is not well-recognized or adequately addressed by the allopathic approach. Research addressing the mechanisms by which osteopathic medicine affects the homeostasis of the autonomic system is ongoing, and may help explain the observations of clinical benefit from OMT. The vagus nerve has far-reaching effects on the viscera, providing the parasympathetic innervation to those tissues. It is commonly thought that compression or dysregulation of the vagus nerve is a major contributor to GERD and colic. Therefore, treatment for those conditions always includes release of tissues at the base of the head, relieving compression on the vagus nerve. The sympathetic system has an entirely different anatomic distribution. When treating a specific area, osteopathic physicians take into account the parasympathetic, sympathetic, and somatic innervation to the area.

Treatment Principles and Modalities

Somatic dysfunction is localized by palpating the changes in tissue texture, pain, motion, and asymmetry of bony structures. The diagnostic nomenclature given to a specific dysfunction is based on the position of the affected area, often a joint. The position of any joint is, however, a reflection of the muscular and fascial attachments acting on it, so despite the attention placed on the joint position in naming the "lesion," it is actually the soft tissues acting on that joint that are in need of correction. Bony position is, therefore, the end symptom of more complex anatomical and physiologic interactions. Research into the cause and treatment of somatic dysfunction is focused on these interactions. Significant attention has been given to the organization of afferent and efferent nerves and their connections to each other in the CNS. We know that effective treatment of any kind appears to "reset" the reflex arcs that deliver efferent nerves to their respective somatic or visceral organs.

So to illustrate, in Figure 17-1, the muscle contraction of both opposing muscle groups are intended to be balanced, as the EMG readings reflect in the neutral group. In the strain group, muscle A is suffering from significant muscle spasm and B is reflexively hypotonic; this is the condition commonly recognized as a "sprain strain" in the allopathic community. The dysfunction pattern illustrates a similar but more subtle pattern of muscular imbalance. It is imbalances of this sort that are the hallmark of osteopathic somatic dysfunction. Treatments of any modality serve to calm the spasm of muscle A and increase the tone of muscle B.

The intervention of OMT involves working on one or several different tissue "levels" (bone, fluid, fascia, muscle, even bioenergetic) with force that is directed against the barrier (direct), or away from the barrier (indirect), or a combination of these forces. Indirect techniques may seem counterintuitive (exaggerating the "lesion,") but are often gentler and better tolerated in children, and are highly effective, working presumably

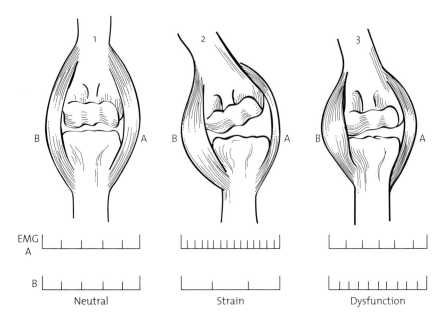

FIGURE 17-1. Jones neuromuscular model. (Modified from Jones, L.H.; Strain and Counterstrain, Newark, Ohio 1981, American Academy of Osteopathy.)

through resetting the balance of innervation to the area. Some examples of specific techniques are listed below.

High Velocity Low Amplitude (HVLA) Treatments

As the nomenclature implies, HVLA utilizes fast, short, and focused thrusts into a joint. Joints are taken toward the restrictive barrier; therefore, it is a direct treatment, and then the thrust moves it past the restrictive barrier. It is the modality many people have in their mind when they think of manual medicine as provided by DOs or chiropractors. It is an effective treatment, especially in regards to back pain. It is however, only one modality available to an osteopathic physician. In regards to children, HVLA is not commonly used. Their joints are still mostly cartilaginous, and comparatively lax. In addition, the children and parents prefer gentler techniques.

Muscle Energy (ME)

Muscle energy takes a joint toward the direction of restriction and is therefore a direct technique. The patient then provides an isometric contraction against the practitioner's resistance. Following treatment, EMGs indicate that the hypertonicity in the treated muscle group resolves and the joint returns to neutral. This modality is well tolerated by patients and provides excellent results, especially when applied to acute injuries that present to the primary care office. Older children and teenagers enjoy this modality and often view it as fun. Smaller children lack the cognitive ability to participate, so utilizing this modality with them is more difficult.

Counterstrain (CS)

This modality identifies CS points, small pea-sized tender points around the body in areas displaying somatic dysfunction. The practitioner then places the patient in a position that relieves the pain at the site of the tender point, usually away from the barrier to motion. It requires complete relaxation of the affected muscle groups, so cooperation by children is nearly impossible. It is, however, well tolerated by patients able to co-operate. It is a less common modality used by DOs; however, it is easy to learn and therefore, some massage therapists and physical therapists have begun utilizing it. CS is one form of indirect treatment, outlined below.

Indirect Techniques

There is a group of techniques that utilizes more subtle palpation and motion to achieve resolution of somatic dysfunction. Within this group are balanced ligamentous tension, myofascial release, functional technique, and visceral manipulation. Each of these techniques has their unique methodology. What they share in common is that a somatic dysfunction is moved away from the direction of restriction, held in a position that balances the fascial, ligamentous and muscular forces of the affected joint. The afferent fibers coming out of the region relax, and therefore the efferent response to the tissues calms down as well. The treatment allows the affected area to move back into the optimal position for health. These techniques take more focused palpation, and are therefore usually practiced by physicians that devote a higher proportion of their practice to OMT. They are the most popular techniques used by practitioners who treat children. These treatments require no effort by the patient and very little repositioning of the patient during an office visit. Many patients and observers when first exposed to these treatments feel the physician "isn't doing anything," because of the gentleness of them. Hesitation quickly subsides when the patient is provided relief.

Cranial Osteopathy

Cranial osteopathy is the modality most sought after by families of pediatric patients. It is imperative to note however, that proper osteopathic management includes addressing the entire patient. Cranial osteopathy is the application of osteopathic technique to the cranium, CNS, and sacrum. There has been significant attention in the public literature to the benefits of cranial-sacral therapy (CST). CST, is an example of a treatment modality that has been developed by the osteopathic community and is now being utilized in other fields of manual medicine. When utilized by non-physicians, it is termed "therapy" due to the less comprehensive approach that is taught to those practitioners.

Although the benefits of CST can be seen when performed by other practitioners, osteopathic physicians perform cranial osteopathy within the framework of a complete osteopathic evaluation and treatment plan.

Viola Frymann

Viola has dedicated her career to the osteopathic treatment of children. She runs the Osteopathic Center for Children in San Diego, California. There she treats children and educates physicians. Here is the description of how she began the study of cranial osteopathy of children after hearing a lecture by William Sutherland.

"The first lecture I heard from Sutherland concerned the common problem of the vomiting of the newborn. I had lost a baby after 3 months of recurrent uncontrollable vomiting despite the best medical advice. An autopsy revealed no anatomical reason for it. But Sutherland was describing the 'common condition' of compression of the occipital condylar parts from a long or difficult labor which disturbed the function of the vagus nerve (CN X). My baby had suffered a long and difficult labor, even intensified by a dose of castor oil. He then described a very simple, gentle technique that could relieve that compression and stop the vomiting. This seemed too simple. I had to satisfy myself that this was true. As soon as the opportunity presented itself, I began an 8-year study of newborn babies at the local osteopathic hospital and became satisfied that in patients of all ages, structure and function are interdependent (Frymann 1966).

Application of the osteopathic concept to the cranium was not extensively addressed by A.T. Still. It was William G. Sutherland that fully developed the principles behind treatment of the cranium, and its relationship to the sacrum through the dural attachments. As the basic understanding of this concept, it is believed that the sutures of the cranium are not completely solid, as once thought. Histological sections have now revealed some evidence that the movement palpated by DOs within the cranium is possible. It is, however, very subtle. In addition, the tissues of the CNS itself have rhythmic motion that is separate from the respiratory motion of the pulmonary system. It is this CNS motion that is believed to be the focus of evaluation and treatment when performing cranial osteopathy. This motion is referred to as the primary respiratory mechanism (PRM) because it is thought to be even more vital for life than the respiration of the pulmonary system. For this reason it is referred to as "the breath of life." (See Violas' description of the breath of life in two case studies, textbox) The same guiding principles that apply to the rest of the body are utilized during treatment of the CNS, cranium, and sacrum; movement of structures toward or away from restriction, in order to improve balance and symmetry. A treatment is considered successful if the PRM has a stronger amplitude and improved rhythm into the area. Some research has linked the PRM (as palpated by practitioners) to the Traube-Herring-Meyer wave, the small fluctuations in blood pressure seen during continuous monitoring by central arterial lines. This is fascinating research which may lead to a better understanding of the mechanisms of action at work during cranial treatments. Whatever the mechanism, the results can be dramatic. The clinical experience of practitioners utilizing this treatment and the dramatic improvements experienced by patients cannot be ignored. It is the fastest growing field of osteopathy, with demand by patients for treatment far outpacing the supply of talented practitioners.

Here Viola describes two cases that illustrate the breath of life

Case number 1: Prematurity

In 2007, I was invited to treat a number of tiny 25-week gestation neonates. Their connective tissues were translucent, their inherent vitality was almost imperceptible, and the cranial rhythmic impulse initially had to be believed even before it could be truly palpated. What could I do? What should I expect? Sutherland describes the Breath of Life. The breath of air is the pulmonary exchange of breathing, but the Breath of Life is that vital force that is activated at the moment life begins and persists until life in this physical realm ends. These little babies needed an infusion of this Breath of Life. Experience has taught us that by means of the temporal bones, resuscitation can be accomplished during an apneic spell. Tenderly and cautiously I placed pads of my index fingers on the little mastoid apophysis and suggested a tiny impulse toward external rotation, and I waited. At last that minute hand was lifted as if to wave. A little foot moved then I noted a very shallow gentle thoracic excursion of breathing. That was a most moving experience when the primary respiratory mechanism began to communicate with the secondary respiratory mechanism of breathing.

Case number 2: Spina Bifida

An 11-month-old infant with a spina bifida, surgically repaired meningomyelocele and accompanied by shunted hydrocephalus with bilateral convergent strabismus, complete paralytic paraplegia and marked hypotonicity, and inability to sit or move. What might I expect? I had little expectation but his grandfather was determined he should receive osteopathic treatment. I reluctantly agreed to a 3-month trial. My approach was with the cranial concept for I believed that the inherent therapeutic potency was the best chance he had. At the end of three months he could sit unsupported by himself. That was very gratifying but what next should I do or expect? His paralyzed legs provided little evidence of life. I placed one hand at the lowest level on his vertebral mechanism where I could feel a fluctuant wave of the PRM. I placed my other hand anterior to this hip joint—and I waited until I detected a small wave between my two hands. This was repeated regularly at every visit until my hands could be placed further and further apart. The climax of that story was his joyous achievement of standing on his fourth birthday. I later learned that this was indeed an awakening of axoplasmic flow. The work of Korr at the Kirksville College of Osteopathic Medicine described and further applied the concepts around 1967 (Korr 1979).

Cranial Osteopathy as Applied to Infants

When considering cranial osteopathy, the infant is particularly responsive to treatment due to the nature of its anatomy and the effect of the birth process on the infant skull. The literature does not yet adequately support this notion, but the authors have corroborated the clinical experience of practitioners of OMT worldwide over the last 100 years, in observing that certain symptoms are seen remarkably often following a history consistent with excessive compression of the baby's head. This may be due to prenatal intrauterine constraints (such as twin pregnancy or bicornuate uterus), or natal circumstances such as a long and difficult delivery, frequently augmented by exogenous stimulation of labor, sometimes associated with an atypical presentation of the head, or the use of forceps or suction to facilitate a difficult birth, or with a history of a very rapid tumultuous delivery, or a repeat C-section involving a difficult extraction through a stiff scar. The clinical manifestations (both physical asymmetries as well as symptoms) of perinatal strains related to head compression might not become apparent until later infancy, exacerbated by postnatal bone growth and the effects of position and gravity. However, data published in Pediatrics, indicates that when (Peitsch et al., 2002) carefully observed in the nursery, even the naked eye can see early signs of plagiocephaly. Follow-up with these children in the first two years of life often finds the condition worsening.

Given the anatomy of the infant skull, this should come as no surprise. The plasticity of the infant skull allows for passage through the birth canal, but also accounts for its vulnerability to compressive forces that do not always spontaneously normalize in the immediate postnatal period. Molding of the visually apparent skull (the vault) is only a hint of the deformation which may be manifested in the cranial base. The base serves as the point of emergence of the cranial nerves from the brain stem (especially the vagus), the carotids, jugulars, and the Eustachian tubes, as well as the entry point for the sympathetics, to name just a few vital structures. The experience of practitioners of cranial osteopathy is that when the somatic dysfunction is improved, there is a correlation with clinical improvement, be it a neonate with unexplained hypoventilation, an infant with colic, poor suck, recurrent vomiting, difficult defecation, or strabismus. The clinical effect of the OMT can be related anatomically to the site of the somatic dysfunction, and the changes are often coincident with the sensation of "release" in the tissues.

Viola Frymann described the effect that various patterns of cranial base distortion, if uncorrected, either spontaneously or with treatment, translates into a variety of deformations of the vault over time. She also recorded findings from the osteopathic examination of 1250 newborns (Frymann et al., 1966), and correlated the location of specific areas of compression with symptomatology in the newborn nursery. Infants with vasomotor instability tended to have more anterior compressions, and those with compression of the posterior skull tended to display more irritability. Frymann (1976) also postulated that children with learning problems are significantly more likely than those without such problems to have had difficult deliveries resulting in deformity of the infant's head severe enough for the mother to remember it.

Plagiocephaly

Prior to the back-to-sleep campaign in America, the incidence of serious, overt plagiocephaly was a rare condition. Nonetheless, osteopathic physicians could appreciate the more subtle findings of asymmetry, and have discussed in their literature the effects they were seeing in their patients (Sergueef, Nelson, & Glonek, 2006). As long ago as 1919, Mills related "cranial scoliosis" to strabismus, a finding which is still described in association with plagiocephaly. Now that the incidence has risen, there is evidence that even mild plagiocephaly can have clinical significance of an insidious and potentially chronic nature, beyond the cosmetic. Infants with plagiocephaly without synostosis demonstrate both cognitive and psychomotor developmental delays, according to two recent studies (Habal, Leimkuehler, Chambers, Scheuerle, & Guilford, 2003; Panchal et al., 2001). Another study found that infants with plagiocephaly exhibited diminished auditory event-related potential responses to tones, indicating dysfunction of central sound processing (Balan, Kushnerenko, Sahlin, Huotilainen, & Naatanen, 2002). Furthermore, infants who presented with plagiocephaly and who had no obvious signs of delay initially are felt to be at increased risk for developmental delay during the school-age years (Miller & Clarren, 2000). Strabismus has been documented as a late effect of plagiocephaly, especially involving vertical gaze (Habal, Leimkuehler, Chambers, Scheuerle, & Guilford, 2003). Another case reports dental problems later in life (Rout & Price, 1978–79). Some suggest that later-developing scoliosis is related to compensatory postural patterns originating from distortions of the cranial base ("intracranial scoliosis"), attempting to keep the eyes straight (Carreiro, 2003; Mills, 1919), or as a response to changes in a distorted cranial base with growth and weight-bearing (Magoun, 1976).

Although more commonly considered a separate diagnosis, osteopathic physicians see congenital torticollis and plagiocephaly as related syndromes, with the pattern of causality difficult to determine. They share similar histories in the prenatal, perinatal, and postnatal period. Magoun (1973) suggests that congenital torticollis is related to accessory nerve irritation secondary to stresses at the cranial base. Carreiro (2003) delineates primary plagiocephaly (from prenatal or natal causes), arising from pathology in the head, from secondary plagiocephaly (from postnatal influences.) She suggests how primary plagiocephaly can lead to torticollis and/or scoliosis, in an elegant description of the relation of posture, balance, movement, and vision.

A recent unpublished study (The Effect of OMT, 2003) on children who received OMT in the newborn nursery matched 58 treated patients with 58 control patients and reviewed their clinic charts for the first six months of life. The study yielded a few statistically significant differences between the two groups, in the direction of fewer health problems in the intervention patients. Primary care pediatricians that treat newborns regularly in primary care practices, cite early, thorough treatment of newborn plagiocephaly as the best example of preventative osteopathic care. When treated early, it is far easier for the practitioner to correct, and affords the newborn optimal structural health for growth and development. Their neurologic systems and adaptive responses are developing. Just as markedly hypotonic newborns may develop hypertonia over time, which sometimes necessitates physical therapy, so do these "shell-shocked" babies sometimes develop increasing fussiness and have gastrointestinal irritability in their early months, which often responds to manipulation. Furthermore, it appears that some of the same babies who did not have such intervention go on to develop chronic congestion, dacryostenosis, strabismus, or early onset of recurrent ear infections. Conversely, many of the children who have these latter conundrums, on close questioning, have a history of prior colic and feeding problems, often also with a history of a difficult delivery.

An osteopathic Approach to Colic

Colic or excessive crying is one of the most frequent problems presented to pediatricians by new parents. There is some evidence that colicky infants are temperamentally "different" from normal infants, but the osteopathic perspective is that this difference is often structural, and is usually amenable to treatment. Barr suggests that infants with colic have diminished regulatory capacity, and quiet for a shorter time in response to sucrose than normal infants (Barr & Young, 1997). He describes these infants as "dysregulated," possibly related to an atypical vagal responsiveness (Barr, 1998). This pattern is seen in children even four years old (DeGangi, Porges, Sickel, & Greenspan, 1993). This description sounds remarkably similar to the osteopathic view of autonomic dysregulation secondary to vagal compression at the cranial base.

Though A.T. Still (1910) first described using OMT for colic, the chiropractors Wiberg, Nordsteen, and Nillson (1999) showed a statistically significant difference in crying patterns, from day 5 on, in 25 children who were treated with manipulation, compared to 20 children who were not. Colic and gastro-esophageal reflux seem to be frequent co-morbid conditions, an observation that is not commonly discussed in the literature. Given the fact that the newborn occiput is in four parts at delivery, which may cause compression of the opening of the jugular with its proximity to the vagus, it should not be surprising that gastrointestinal motility and sphincter tone might be affected. In addition, the tone of the diaphragm can be affected by enervation from cervical nerves 3 to 5, and relief of spasm of the diaphragm has often been associated with improvement in reflux in infants, with and without formula changes.

Upper Respiratory Infections, Including Otitis Media

As with problems in the newborn, the anatomy of a child's ears helps explain its vulnerability to ear infections. The eustachian tube (ET) travels through the petrous portion of the temporal bone, emerging into a cartilaginous sheath, closely adherent to the base of the skull, nestled between the greater wing of the sphenoid and the petrous portion of the temporal bone, emerging into the posterior pharynx at the posterior edge of the medial pterygoid plate of the sphenoid (Bluestone, Stool, Alper, et al., 2003; Carreiro, 2003). The relationship of the tube to other contiguous structures, particularly the tensor veli palatini, the levator veli palatini, and the saplingopharyngeous muscles, and the difference between the characteristics of the cartilage between children and adults, may contribute to the relative dysfunction of the ET in young children.

In 1966, Purse performed a retrospective review of 4600 cases of URI and found a 17% complication rate in those treated with OMT as opposed to a 30%–35% rate described elsewhere in the literature. Schmidt (1982) in 1982 studied 100 cases of patients with URIs and found that application of OMT in the first day of symptoms showed a marked and early improvement and less need for antibiotics. Carreiro describes the finding of restrictions in the frontoethmoid-sphenoidal junction, or the ethmoid notch, and cranial base, in infants with persistent nasal congestion following difficult deliveries.

Degenhardt and Kuchera (2006) reported a pilot study of 8 children with recurrent otitis media who received OMT, five of which, after a year, had no recurrence, and only one of which required surgery for placement of ventilatory tubes. OMT has also been reported to show changes in tympanograms before and immediately after treatment (Carreiro, 2003). A national collaborative prospective randomized controlled study, was published in the Archives of Pediatrics and Adolescent Medicine in September 2003 (Mills, Henley, Barnes, Carreiro, & Degenhardt, 2003), on the use of OMT in children with recurrent acute otitis media, showing that intervention patients had fewer otitis episodes, more "surgery-free" months, and more frequently normal tympanogramps. Secondary analysis (Mills, Zaphiris, Wen, Jewell, & Boyer, 2004; Zaphiris, Mills, Jewell, & Boyce, 2004) of this study (not yet published) showed a marked difference in the pre- and post-study osteopathic examinations between the two groups, with a correlation between those osteopathic changes and changes in the tympanograms. The profession is currently working to expand this line of clinical research.

Neurologic Diseases

Children that suffer from a wide variety of neurological diseases seek care from osteopathic physicians, and frequently become very loyal patients. Common problems that these children have are autism, cerebral palsy, seizures, developmental delay, sensory integration, and ADHD. One similarity to almost all neurological disease states, is the idea of threshold. Commonly discussed in relation to seizures, every patient has a point of altered homeostasis that will result in neurological symptoms. Although the mechanism of action remains to be fully understood, it appears that OMT calms the neurological excitability and thereby raising that threshold. Frymann (2005) describes treating a number of children with seizures with OMT, of which 20 of 87 children had no more seizures off medication, and an additional 50 had marked improvement of their seizures.

The application of OMT in this population has so much promise. Neurology is a frustrating field of medicine, in its current state. Although we continue to understand the function of the brain more every year, effective treatment for many conditions remains difficult in the allopathic model. Approaching a patient with neurological compromise from the osteopathic perspective provides a safe, non-pharmaceutical way to improve functioning in these children. Viola Frymann compared two groups of children suffering from neurological delays over 3 years: one group comprised of children who were waiting to be treated in her clinic; and the second, a group of children who were admitted. She found that there was a significant improvement in neurologic performance, including school performance, in the children who had been treated, compared to those who were not (Frymann, 1992). Those differences then resolved once treatment began on the control group.

Beryl Arbuckel (1955, 1994) was one of the first osteopathic physicians to treat children with cerebral palsy, and set up a clinic focused on the care of these children. Clearly, OMT cannot reverse permanent nerve loss, but especially when begun at an early age, it can help with the formation of adaptive pathways (Arbuckle, 1955). Children with cerebral palsy, who benefit from physical therapy in strengthening and stretching, demonstrate noticeable and often immediate changes in overall muscle tone, presumably related to changes in descending cortical down-regulation of the abnormal spinal reflexes (Carreiro, 2003; Davis, Worden, Clawson, Meaney, & Duncan, 2007).

School performance, especially reading, can be related to visual perceptual problems, even without overt strabismus. There is an optimal age in which abnormalities in the visual system can be corrected, and most texts state that to be between 3 and 5 years old. This presents a "window of opportunity" (Carreiro, 2003) during which the somatic contributions to muscle imbalances might be reversed.

Autism is unfortunately a rising epidemic in our country. The complex interactions of environment, genetics and viral triggers, make the diagnosis particularly difficult. It is therefore, an excellent illustration of the tenets of osteopathy. Some children appear to be triggered by noxious insults of various types, suggesting an underlying weakness in

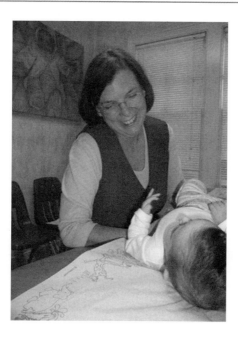

FIGURE 17-2. Gentle technique utilized by pediatric practitioners. This is a treatment of the pelvis area.

the child's homeostasis making them more vulnerable to the noxious stimuli than their peers. Our hope as primary care, osteopathic physicians, is to optimize a child's health to prevent the neurological damage in the first place, starting with intervention in the newborn period. That will be the challenge of ongoing research.

We have already observed that OMT can greatly benefit already-affected children, both in treating the CNS and other body regions. The relation of the intestines to autism has received significant attention. When treating these children, many osteopaths find somatic dysfunction in the mesenteric fascia and diaphragm. Treating this area helps to remove the congestion in the intestines that arises from chronic inflammation in that area. Treating the pelvic area also seems to help, as the parasympathetics to the lower intestines arise from there (Figure 17-2). Some of these children undergo biomedical treatments such as chelation and hyperbaric oxygen therapy, and OMT can augment those therapies. By improving blood flow and increasing lymphatic drainage, toxins can travel to the liver and kidneys without impedance, thereby reducing the side effects of these other interventions .

Unfortunately there is not sufficient time to discuss all of the clinical situations where OMT can be beneficial. Treatments are focused on the patients and their unique somatic findings. Therefore, at no time are treatments focused at a diagnosis. The application of this field is very far reaching. Patients seeking relief in osteopathic offices include those

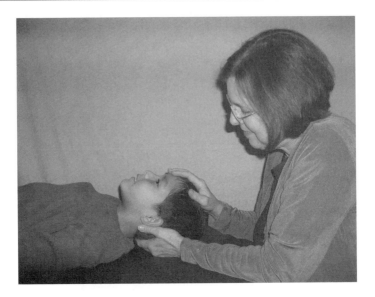

FIGURE 17-3. Gentle treatment of the cranium.

suffering from lacrimal duct stenosis, breastfeeding difficulties, constipation, nocturnal enuresis, speech delay, asthma, sports injuries, chronic sinusitis, and headaches. The application of OMT is limited only by the number of physicians trained to perform treatments and research in this field. As interest in integrative medicine grows in the medical community, hopefully more pediatricians will become trained to practice this way (Figure 17-3).

Finding a Pediatric Osteopathic Practitioner

Osteopathic treatments are not diagnosis- or specialty-specific, so it is not necessary to locate a physician that treats the specific diagnosis you are seeking the referral for. However, the treatment of children requires more specific palpation skills and an ounce of patience. Most physicians that utilize cranial osteopathy regularly are capable of treating children. When contacting an office to make a referral, be sure to ask how comfortable the physician is in treating children, and if they utilize cranial osteopathy.

There is a large variation in the skill level of practitioners, especially as it pertains to children. The profession has, in recent years, developed a board certification in osteopathic manipulation and neuromuscular medicine. Physicians with this designation devote most or all of their practice to the use of OMT and have demonstrated advanced skills through certification. As this is a recently formed board, there are many talented and experienced physicians that do not carry this certification. The American Academy of Osteopathy is the professional organization that represents physicians that utilize

OMT. They offer a referral database on their website, www.academyofosteopathy.org, and a listing of those certified through the board.

Training in Manipulative Medicine

Many physicians become interested in incorporating osteopathic treatments into their practice later in their careers. DO pediatricians often have not utilized OMT since their years of medical school, and recognize its many uses once they are in practice. These physicians must remediate the basic principles and then build on those with more advanced coursework. It is also possible for MDs interested in learning OMT to gain significant skill. One may notice that one of the authors of this chapter is a talented and respected practitioner of OMT. For both of these groups of physicians, coursework is offered by the same organizations.

The American Academy of Osteopathy offers CME coursework that varies from basic to more advanced. Their website www.Academyofosteopathy.org offers an extensive bookstore, CME calendar, and referral database.

Cranial osteopathy is an excellent starting point for pediatric physicians. The Sutherland Cranial Teaching Foundation (SCTF.com) and the Cranial Academy, (Cranialacademy.org), offer cranial osteopathy training for any licensed physician or dentist. At the basic courses they introduce the principles and anatomy of treating children. For those wishing to treat children, they are the most effective way to learn cranial osteopathy. Michigan State University offers Manipulative medicine courses for MDs and DOs in other modalities.

Osteopathic Medical Education

With one final note, the osteopathic community has been training physicians to be "integrative" for generations. The larger medical community now has interest in educating their graduates to think in a more "holistic" manner. Here are some highlights of priorities emphasized in the osteopathic education that are not as common in their allopathic counterparts.

CONNECTION

Even when an osteopathic physician does not utilize manipulative medicine, patients report a noticeable difference in the relationship they have with their DO physician. Because of having been trained in OMT, DO's have developed an "empathetic touch" which is both diagnostic, and potentially therapeutic, that most patients perceive intuitively and respond to positively. DOs are trained to touch their patients upon greeting them, look them in the eye, and consider family and psychological issues when gathering a history from a patient. These may seem to be just "good" medicine to most readers, but they are specifically emphasized in the osteopathic education in a way that produces a graduate that intentionally connects to their patients on many levels. This connection is a vital part of being able to treat a patient holistically. If a patient does not feel connected to their physician but instead feels there is a great divide between them, they are not able to share the numerous aspects of their life that contribute to their health. The physician can posses great knowledge, and give sound advice, but without a good connection with the patient, compliance is poor. As more patients and physicians become interested in the concept of integrative medicine, they must realize that the doctor patient relationship is the delivery system for that care. The routine doctor visit has to evolve.

INDIVIDUALISTIC CARE

Osteopathic physicians are more inclined to problem-solve cases that do not have a text-book diagnosis. "Evidence-based medicine" assumes that patients must have a definable disease, outlined in medical literature, with a defined treatment algorithm. One of the significant limitations of a medical system that calls for randomized controlled trials for any treatment, is that very few patients present in textbook fashion, allowing them to benefit from researched algorithms. Patients who seek "alternative" practitioners often do so after receiving no relief of their problem from the larger medical community. Osteopathic physicians are able to help patients by focusing on their overall health, utilizing manipulative medicine, nutrition and basic physiology to devise a treatment plan, even if the patient does not meet a definable condition. Because of their complete medical training and full licensure, they are able to utilize a full spectrum of medical, surgical and manipulative treatments to achieve their goals. All medical school training (MD and DO alike) is designed to educate physicians in the basic sciences, enabling them to problem-solve cases when an algorithm does not exist. We, as a nation, need to equip and challenge our future physicians to utilize the knowledge they have, and expand their comfort area to include the treatment of ill-defined ailments, in order to provide care for more of our patients.

STUDENT SELECTION

Osteopathic schools have a wider variation in the demography of their students. One of the areas in which they differ is in the value they see in the "non-traditional" student, one who has come to medical school following another career. These students often are more confident in their desire to be a physician, and have more life experience. In addition, osteopathic medical schools put an emphasis on the student's life outside the classroom prior to medical school, and how that impacts the student's ability to under-stand the people they will eventually serve. These qualities help them build a connection with their patients. A student that has spent all their time in the classroom will have even less in common with their patients once they graduate.

A Look into the Future

Pediatric medicine has endless potential in prevention of disease. Many years ago Irvin Korr, an osteopathic physiologist, wrote about the evolution of medicine.

In his well-articulated article, he put forth a challenge to osteopathic physicians. He acknowledged that medicine has existed in some form throughout time, but is in a constant state of change. The state of the art medicine of the day will be replaced by a new approach in the future. He asked, would the osteopathic profession mold itself with the status quo and therefore die as that status quo becomes extinct, or would they rather help to focus the medicine of the future? We think that is the challenge of integrative physicians everywhere. It is sometimes difficult to be the innovator, and not harmonize with the majority around oneself. It is those innovators however, that enjoy the benefit of knowing they are shaping the future.

REFERENCES

Arbuckle, B. E. (1955). The value of occupational and osteopathic manipulative therapy in the rehabilitation of the cerebral palsy victim. *The Journal of the American Osteopathic Association*, 55(4), 227–237.

Arbuckle, B. E. (1994). *The selective writings of beryl arbuckle, DO, FACOP.* Indianapolis, IN: American Academy of Osteopathy.

Balan, P., Kushnerenko, E., Sahlin, P., Huotilainen, M., & Naatanen, R. (2002). Auditory ERPs reveal brain dysfunction in infants with plagiocephaly. *Journal of Craniofacial Surgery*, 13(4), 520–526.

Barr R. G., & Young, S. N. (1997). A two phase model of the soothing taste response: implications for a taste probe of temperament and emotion regulation, In M. Lweris & D. Ramsay, (Eds.), *Soothing and stress*. Hillsdate, NJ: Lawrence Erlbaum Associates.

Barr, R. G. (1998). Colic and crying syndromes in infants. *Pediatrics*, 102(5), 1282–1286.

Bluestone, C. D., Stool, S. E., Alper, C. M. et al. (2003). *Pediatric otolaryngology*, (Vol 1., 3rd ed.). Philadelphia: Saunders—Elsevier Science.

Brooks, R. E. (1997). *Life in Motion, The Osteopathic Vision of Rollin Becker* (p. 61). DO, Runda Press Portland.

Carreiro J. A. (2003). *An osteopathic approach to children*. Edinburgh: Churchill Livingstone. Elsevier Science Limited.

Davis, M. F., Worden, K., Clawson, D., Meaney, F. J., & Duncan, B. (2007). Confirmatory factor analysis in osteopathic medicine: fascial and spinal motion restrictions as correlates of muscle spasticity in children with cerebral palsy. [Journal Article. Research Support, N.I.H., Extramural. Validation Studies] *Journal of the American Osteopathic Association*, 107(6), 226–232.

DeGangi G. A., Porges S. W., Sickel R. Z., & Greenspan, S. I. (1993). Four year follow-up of a sample of regulatory disordered infants. *Infant Mental Health Journal*, 14, 330–343.

Degenhardt, B. J., & Kuchera, M. L. (2006). Osteopathic evaluation and manipulative treatment in reducing the morbidity of otitis media: A pilot study. *Journal of the American Osteopathic Association*, 106(6), 327–334.

Frymann, V. M. (1976). Learning difficulties of children viewed in the light of the osteopathic concept. *Journal of the American Osteopathic Association*, 76, 46–61.

Frymann, V. M. (1992). Effect of osteopathic medical management on neurologic development of children. *Journal of the American Osteopathic Association*, 92(6), 729–738.

Frymann, V. M. (2005). The osteopathic approach to children with seizure disorders. Demos, New York. *Complementary and Alternative Therapies for Epilepsy*, 273–283.

Frymann, V. (1966). Relation of disturbance of craniosacral mechanism to symptomatology of the newborn: study of 1250 infants. *Journal of the American Osteopathic Association, 65,* 1059–1075.

Guiney, P. A., Chou, R., Vianna, A., & Lovenheim, J. (2005). Effects of osteopathic manipulative treatment on pediatric patients with asthma: A randomized controlled trial. *Journal of the American Osteopathic Association, 105*(1), 1–12.

Habal, M. B., Leimkuehler, T., Chambers, C., Scheuerle, J., & Guilford, A. M. (2003). Avoiding the sequela associated with deformational plagiocephaly. *Journal of Craniofacial Surgery, 14*(4), 430–437.

Heath, D., & Kelso, A. (1998). *AAO Journal.* originally published in JAOA (1920).

LeMoon, K. (2007). Fascia 2007: The First International Fascia Research Congress—A report. [Cited 2008 June 11] Available From: http://fascia2007.com/news/Article_YJBMT_596.pdf

Magoun, H. I. (1976). *Osteopathy in the cranial field* (3rd ed., p. 292). Kirksville, Mo: Journal Printing Co.

Magoun, H. I. S. (1973). Idiopathic adolescent spinal scoliosis. *The DO, 13*(6).

Miller, R. I., & Clarren, S. K. (2000). Long-term developmental outcomes in patients with deformational plagiocephaly. *Pediatrics, 105*(2), e26.

Mills, L. (1919). The effects of faulty cranio-spinal form and alignment upon the eyes. *American Journal of Ophthalmology, 2,* 493–499.

Mills, L. (1919). The effects of faulty cranio-spinal form and alignment upon the eyes. *American Journal of Ophthalmology, 2,* 493–499.

Mills, M. V. (2006). Consider osteopathic manipulative treatment in next research on positional plagiocephaly, Letter to Editor. *Journal of Pediatrics, 148*(5), 706–707.

Mills, M. V., Henley, C. E., Barnes, L. L. B., Carreiro, J. E., & Degenhardt, B. F. (2003). The use of osteopathic manipulative treatment as adjuvant therapy in children with recurrent acute otitis media. *Archives of Pediatrics & Adolescent Medicine, 157,* 861–866.

Mills, M. V., Zaphiris, A, Wen, F. K., Jewell, N. P., & Boyer, W. T. *Otitis media and osteopathic manipulative treatment: exploring structure and function.* Poster presented at International Conference on Advances in Osteopathic Research, September 2004.

Panchal, J., Amirsheybani, H., Gurwitch, R., Cook, V., Francel, P. et al. (2001). Neurodevelopment in children with single-suture craniosynostosis and plagiocephaly without synostosis. *Plastic and Reconstructive Surgery, 108*(6), 1492–1498.

Peitsch, W. K. et al. (2002). Incidence of cranial asymmetry in healthy newborns. *Pediatrics, 110*(6), 72.

Rout, P., & Price, P. (1978–79). Plagiocephaly. *British Journal of Oral Surgery, 16,* 163–168.

Schierhorn, C. (2007). DO's and MD's take fresh look at venerable OMT techniques for children. *The DO,* 24–30.

Schmidt, I. C. (1982). Osteopathic manipulative therapy in respiratory infections. *Journal of the American Osteopathic Association, 81*(6), 382–388.

Seffinger, M. A. (1997). Development of osteopathic philosophy. In R. C. Ward (Ed.), *Foundations for osteopathic medicine* (pp. 3–7). Baltimore: Williams & Wilkins.

Sergueef, N., Nelson, K. E., & Glonek, T. (2006). Palpatory diagnosis of plagiocephaly. *Complementary Therapies in Clinical Practice, 12,* 101–110.

Still A. T. (1910). *Osteopathy. Research and practice* (pp. 264–265). Kirksville, MO:.

The Effect of OMT as Newborns on the Health of Children in the First Six Months of Life. Poster presented in Osteopathic Collaborative Clinical Trials Initiatives Conference IV, Ottawa, Canada, March 2003.

Wiberg, M. M., Nordsteen, J., & Nilsson, N. (1999). The short-term effect of spinal manipulation in the treatment of infantile colic: a randomized controlled clinical trial with a blinded observer. *Journal of Manipulative and Physiological Therapeutics, 22*(8), 517–522.

Williard, F. (2003). *Nociception, the neuroendocrine immune system, and osteopathic medicine.* Ward, R. *Foundations for osteopathic medicine.* p. 137.

Zaphiris, A., Mills, M. V., Jewell, N. P., & Boyce, W. T. (2004). Osteopathic manipulative treatment and otitis media: Does improving somatic dysfunction improve clinical outcomes? (Abstract), *Journal of the American Osteopathic Association, 104*(1), 11.

III

Clinical Applications in Integrative Pediatrics

order to guarantee that the standards of care are met. The physical examination requires both recognition of the adolescent's need for privacy as well as additional skills in assessing pubertal development.

Adolescent development, despite its chaos, has been divided into three stages of psychological growth and development, each with separate attributes and developmental tasks.

- During *early adolescence*, a new body size and perception of this must occur for the 10- to 13-year olds. These youth are both shy and self-conscious and at the same time act as if the entire world is their stage. This is a time of concrete thinking, where black and white thinking is the norm. It is tempting for the parent and even the caregiver to be authoritarian and rigid, as compromise is not an option for the adolescent. For this reason, alternative forms of therapy such as mind-body interventions may be difficult for this population to accept.

- *Middle adolescents*, between 13 and 16 years, may exhibit risk-taking behaviors and can escalate separation from their families. They are heavily influenced by the need for acceptance by their peers. This age group is capable of thinking in abstract terms, yet their reasoning is often clouded by egocentrism and the concept that they are omnipotent. This is the time when they may be trying the newest supplement or ergogenic aid to promote weight loss and/or better athletic performance, despite risks inherent in their use. When they feel their invincibility is being questioned or their autonomy threatened, middle adolescents tend to become oppositional. With the strength of their peers behind them, they tend to revert to concrete thinking. Compromise is perceived as threatening, authoritarian counselling and parenting, although still tempting, is counterproductive during this developmental stage. The average age at which abstract reasoning occurs is 16. Many teens older and younger than this may have a modicum of abstract reasoning yet may appear physically mature. Without the abstract reasoning they may not be able to recognize side effects of medications and herbs. Sadly, many adults and care providers who work with this age group are unaware of this and may not know how crucial they are to help teens make sound choices and avoid dangerous decisions.

- In *late adolescents*, 18 to 21 years, the major goal is to acquire the ability to consider the needs of others, develop intimate and mutually respectful relationships and ultimately formulate a life plan for the future. Young adults at this stage tend to be less concerned about their bodies, identities, and peers' opinions. If they were able to pass through the experimental and risk-taking behaviors during middle adolescence relatively unscathed, they can mature psychosocially and lose most of their narcissistic feelings of personal omnipotence. They learn to reason abstractly and think causally as they look toward the future. The need for experimentation with newer forms of health interventions diminishes with the acquisition of cognitive skills and the ability to anticipate events. They are more likely to seek and follow healthcare advice on alternative forms of treatment when they are less concerned with a potential threat to their independence. Late adolescence is such a reprieve after middle adolescence that it is easy to overlook the fact that these youths can still revert to earlier adolescent behaviors

The majority of problems in the adolescent can be uncovered by the HEADSS (Home, Education, Activities, Drugs, Sexuality and Suicide) systematic interviewing method (Cohen, Mackenzie, & Yates, 1991). HEADSS organizes the important elements of a psychosocial history of adolescents in a natural pattern of progression in history taking. When using this method, the clinician should remember to consider the teen's developmental stage. Questions should be asked in a non-judgmental manner that can elicit useful and informative responses. The adolescent is more likely to feel comfortable, safe, and answer truthfully when the provider can reflect back knowledge on how other adolescents behave in the context of the question being asked.

If the provider worries that the adolescent will view questions as intrusive (particularly when they relate to risk-taking behaviors), the provider should explain, "I am asking these questions because it helps me determine what I need to do to help keep you healthy."

The following is a general description of the HEADSS mnemonic.

Home: Household composition, family dynamics, and relationships with family members are answered with this first series of questions. The clinician gains knowledge about the stability of the adolescent's household, the influence that her family has in her everyday life, who she relies on when she needs help, and any potential risks she may be exposed to.

Education: Topics covered include school attended and grades received; favorite/most difficult/best subject or class; attitudes toward school; goals and aspirations for the future.

Activities: These questions address physical activity, exercise, hobbies, sports participation, relationships with peers, and work experience. From these questions, the clinician learns about the types of individuals with whom the adolescent associates when he is not in school or at home and their influence on his values and decision-making. When questions relating to weight and diet are added to explore eating behaviors and disorders (anorexia and bulimia, the use of laxatives and diuretics, rigorous dietary restrictions), the clinician can gather additional information on body and self image.

Drugs: Questions in this category address cigarettes, alcohol and/or other drugs, use by friends, type of substance (i.e., beer, wine coolers), frequency and quantity used. From these questions, the clinician gains information about abuse that may be physically or psychologically damaging as well as the extent to which impaired judgment from the abuse puts the adolescent at further risk.

Sexuality: This covers sexual feelings toward the opposite or same sex; degree and types of sexual experiences and acts: age at first intercourse, number of lifetime and current partners, age of partners, and recent change in partners; knowledge and prevention of pregnancy and sexually transmitted infections; history of sexually transmitted infections, prior pregnancies, and abortions; and history of non-consensual intimate physical contact/sex.

Suicide/depression: Feelings about self, both positive and negative; vegetative signs of depression; other mental health problems, suicidal thoughts and prior attempts; preoccupation with death are explored with these questions; how these feelings are handled; and to whom the adolescent turns when she needs help.

Obtaining information on alternative forms of therapy care in the adolescent population is rewarding in that this group may be willing to try something that may be "outside the box." They are excited to talk about any success that they may have achieved with the use of CAM. Adolescents enjoy communicating to someone in authority such as their healthcare provider about something which may be a bit different and unique. They love to be listened to and respected. Talking about foraging into the world of CAM can be exciting for the teen and makes them feel a sense of autonomy when advocating for their own health. These discussions can be helpful when there is also a compelling need to discuss the prevention of high risk behavior such as drug use, unprotected sex, smoking, and violence.

Adolescent Case #1

Brain is a 14-year-old whose lifetime goal is to become an Olympic medallist in diving. He wakes up each morning at 4 AM and his parents take him to the pool where he dives with his coaches from 4:45 until 7 AM—then he showers and heads straight for his school where he is in the 8ᵗʰ grade and a straight-A student. His parents wonder if it is okay for them to start giving him Echinacea for URI prevention in addition to caffeine (green tea) to help his sports performance. Confidentially, he told you he is taking hoodia for weight loss and creatine for increased muscle mass.

Adolescent Case #2

Alicia is a 16-year-old who has been diagnosed with bipolar disease and is on Lithium and Welbutrin. She is having trouble falling asleep each night. Her parents want to try other remedies for her including St. John's wort and valerian. Before they do this. they want your support and any information you may have on these herbs.

Adolescent Case #3

Tyler is a 17-year-old with asthma who has confidentially told you that he has been using kava and ginseng every weekend to get "high" with his friends. He has also been drinking and smoking marijuana. How should you approach this patient? Should you tell his family? About what exactly?

Herbal Therapies and Nutritional Supplements

Adolescents frequently use herbal therapies and supplements for weight loss, depression and anxiety, upper respiratory tract infections, and the enhancement of athletic performance (Gardiner & Kemper, 2000). The following is a brief description of some of the herbal therapies and supplements used by adolescents.

EPHEDRA

Ephedra, or *Ma huang*, is used to suppress appetite, enhance sports performance, and increase vigor. Through its active ingredient ephedrine, ephedra increases the levels of norepinephrine, epinephrine, and dopamine, and also stimulates both alpha and beta adrenoreceptors. The combination of adrenergic and dopaminergic effects may synergistically cause increased alertness and less need for rest or sleep. Over time there may be increased anxiety and insomnia. Ephedrine and ephedra have been shown to promote modest short-term weight loss ($\approx$ 0.9 kg/mo compared to placebo), possibly due to either a decreased appetite or the thermogenic effect of ephedra (Shekelle et al., 2003).

In 2004, the FDA issued a temporary ban on the sale of dietary supplements containing ephedra due to reported serious adverse effects including associated deaths. The ban was rescinded. Nevertheless, ephedra use is not recommended under any circumstance. The combination of caffeine and ephedra may lead to euphoria, neurotic behavior, agitation, depressed mood, giddiness, and extreme irritability. Other side effects may include elevated blood pressure, palpitations, tachycardia, chest pain, coronary vasospasm, and possibly cardiomyopathy. Adolescents who use certain herbal therapies like ephedra may be more likely to abuse drugs (Yussman et al., 2002) and therefore, concern is warranted about ephedra use due its structural similarity to amphetamine.

CAFFEINE

Caffeine is easily and plentifully consumed by adolescents. Caffeine is found in pain relievers, diuretics, cold remedies, weight-control products, energy drinks, and sport supplements. In the younger child, ages 6–9, the mean daily caffeine intake is 20 mg compared to an adult where the average is 200 mg per day (Ahuja, 2001). Average daily caffeine intake was 18.9 mg, or 0.6 mg/kg, more than 50% of which was from carbonated beverages, reported in a survey of 8- to 11-year-olds (Ellison, 1993).

Caffeine, a member of the methylxanthine group, boosts norepinephrine and epinephrine secretion and obstructs central adenosine receptors. Caffeine can increase both the basal metabolic rate and the heart rate, and stimulate secretion of acid in the stomach. It acts as a diuretic, and promotes both vasoconstriction and vasodilatation. Caffeine improves attention and, important to the adolescent, can give them a terrific "buzz." The half-life of caffeine varies from several hours to days; the average in adults is 3–7 hours. In one clinical study comparing boys to adults after consuming caffeine, there were fewer omission errors on a continuous performance test in boys and a greater increase in motor activity including speech (Rapoport, Berg, Ismond, Zahn, & Neims, 1984). Studies have demonstrated that caffeine for ADHD has varied outcomes and in one report was found to be less effective than stimulant medication in treating ADHD symptoms (Huestis, Arnold, & Smeltzer, 1975; Stein, Krasowski, Leventhal, Phillips, & Bender, 1996).

Unfortunately caffeine withdrawal affects adolescents in much the same way as adults, and after only two weeks of daily consumption. Symptoms include irritability, depression, anxiety, fatigue, and headache. During caffeine withdrawal, children had a decrease in performance reaction time on a task requiring continued attention (Bernstein, 1998).

Importantly, because caffeine can interact with stimulant, analgesic, and other over-the-counter medications containing caffeine, it is not recommended for use in those who take prescribed stimulant medications.

Other concerns regard the increaced urinary calcium excretion when caffeine is ingested and the subsequent potential long-term effect on growth in adolescent bones. This was not substantiated in one report on total bone mineral gain or hip bone density in adolescent girls consuming caffeine but continues to be a subject of concern (Lloyd, Rollings, Kieselhorst, Eggli, & Mauger, 1998).

GREEN TEA

Green tea (Camellia sinensis) is promoted to assist in weight loss, to combat fatigue, aid digestion, and decrease headaches. This industry has made its mark. It is difficult not to see green tea sold in grocery stores, health food shops and the omnipresent coffee establishments. Green tea leaves are processed by steaming, differently than black tea leaves, thus enhancing the positive antioxidant effect of this tea.

The steaming method causes green tea leaves to combine with catechin and produce a milder form of tea. Active ingredients include caffeine, 2-amino-5-(N-ethylcarboxyamido)-pentanoic acid, catechins, and polyphenolic compounds. In vitro studies show green tea to be antibacterial, antimutagenic, and anticarcinogenic (Mukhtar, Wang, Katiyar, & Agarwal, 1992). Metabolic effects of green tea, increased metabolism and decreased appetite, may be due to the caffeine (one cup may contain 22–46 mg of caffeine) (Dulloo et al., 1999).

Side effects of green tea include those similar to caffeine and ephedra, including the symptoms of withdrawal. It is not recommend in those with cardiac arrhythmias, hypertension, gastrointestinal ulcers, or anxiety. Those taking stimulants and/or ami-nophylline need to also be warned of additive effects. A retrospective trial noted that microcytic anemia can occur in infants consuming daily green tea (Merhav, Amitai, Palti, & Godfrey, 1985).

GUARANA

Guaraná (Paullinia cupana) is a small shrub native to South America, and its fruit has a high stimulant content. The seeds from this fruit are touted to enhance athletic perfor-mance, suppress appetite, and act as an aphrodisiac.

Guaraná seeds contain a caffeine-like product along with xanthine derivatives. When a combination of Guaraná, Mate and Damiana was studied in overweight adults, gastric emptying was delayed, causing prolonged perceived gastric fullness. This small study also reported an associated weight loss over 45 days (Andersen & Fogh, 2001).

There are a number of energy drinks containing Guaraná. Teens should be coun-selled that the side effects of drinking these drinks are similar to those of ephedra and caffeine.

MATE

Yerba Mate (Ilex Paraguariensis), a member of the holly family, is a widely cultivated medium-sized evergreen tree native to South American countries. Yerba mate tea leaves are used as a diuretic, for weight loss, and for fatigue and depression. The primary active chemical constituents are caffeine (0.3–2.0%) and xanthine derivatives similar to the-ophylline. Like the other caffeine type herbals mentioned above, mate may cause insom-nia, gastric irritation, irritability, diuresis, and arrhythmias (Mate Monograph, Natural Medicines Comprehensive Database).

HOODIA

Hoodia gordonii is a plant which grows in the Kalahari Desert in southern Africa. Bushmen from this area have been using hoodia for centuries to help ward off hunger during long trips in the desert.

A steroidal glycoside termed P57AS3 (P57) has been isolated from Hoodia gordonii and may increase the content of ATP causing a decrease in hunger in rates (Tulp OL, 2001). Preliminary data suggests that overweight men who consume P57 have significantly lower calorie intake than those taking a placebo. Side effects have not been reported although liver function may be affected (Avula, Wang, Pawar, Shukla, Schaneberg, & Khan, 2006).

GINSENG

Ginseng (Panax Ginseng) has been purported to strengthen both mental and physical vitality. Ginseng may affect nitric oxide synthesis in endothelial tissue of lung, heart, and kidney. Stimulation of serotonin and dopamine pathways have also been implicated in the mechanism of action of this herb. Other effects may be related to activity on the hypothalamic-pituitary-adrenal system.

In a meta review, ginseng's effects on physical performance in young, active volunteers during cycle ergometer exercises have been reported. Four studies found no significant difference between ginseng and placebo, whereas three studies found a significant decrease in heart rate and increase in maximal oxygen uptake with ginseng (Vogler, Pittler, & Ernst, 1999).

Adverse effects may include nervousness, insomnia, hypoglycemia, altered platelet aggregation and GI disturbance associated with prolonged use. Due to the estrogen-like effect, ginseng has been reported to cause mastalgia and vaginal bleeding in women. Importantly, ginseng may interact with oral anticoagulants, antiplatelet agents, corticosteroids, and hypoglycemic agents (Ginseng). Natural Medicines Comprehensive Database.

ST. JOHN'S WORT

Based on historical writings, St. John's wort was used as a sedative and a treatment for malaria, as well as a balm for wounds, burns, insect bites, and mental disorders. St. John's wort is currently used for depression, anxiety, and sleep disorders.

Hypericin and hyperforin, two of at least ten active ingredients in St. John's wort, bind neuroreceptors and inhibit the reuptake of serotonin, norepinephrine, and dopamine. In mild depression, St. John's wort was superior to placebo (Gaster & Holroyd, 2000; Linde, Berner, Egger, & Mulrow, 2005). More recently, several studies comparing St. John's wort to selective serotonin reuptake inhibitors (SSRI) found comparable efficacy using high doses of St. John's wort and low doses of SSRIs (Shelton et al., 2001). This has not been confirmed in the treatment of more severe depression, although in the Hypericum Study there was also no difference between SSRI and placebo (Hypericum Depression Trial Study Group, 2002; National Center for Complementary and Alternative Medicine).

The incidence of side effects is low with St. John's wort. Noted are gastrointestinal (GI) symptoms, dizziness, phototoxicity, and confusion.

St. John's wort has been shown to induce the cytochrome P-450 metabolic pathway. Studies have shown a significant interaction with St. John's wort and cyclosporine, oral anticoagulants, oral contraceptives, and certain antiretroviral agents including indinavir. Serotonin syndrome may occur with concomitant use of St. John's wort and SSRI antidepressants.

KAVA

Kava is an important ceremonial drink in the South Pacific. Its calming and sedative effects are well established. The root of kava is used to formulate beverages, extracts, capsules, tablets, and topical solutions.

Kava may bind to GABA (γ-amino butyric acid) receptor complexes or it may work as a dopamine/norepinephrine antagonist. The opiate pathway is not utilized as naloxone does not reverse the effects of kava. A Cochrane Systematic Review found that kava does have an anti-anxiety effect compared with placebo (Pittler & Ernst, 2003).

Adverse effects include "kava dermopathy," a yellowing and flaking of the skin, associated with excessive use of kava, which resolves with discontinuation of the herb (Almeida & Grimsley, 1996). Reversible liver toxicity has been noted when kava is ingested (Clough, Bailie, & Currie, 2003). Reports from Germany, Switzerland, France, Canada, and the United Kingdom have linked kava use to at least 25 cases of liver toxicity, including hepatitis, cirrhosis, and liver failure. Although liver damage appears to be rare, the FDA believes consumers should be informed of this potential risk (Kava Linked to Liver Damage, NCCAM).

VALERIAN

Valerian has been used for centuries as a sedative agent and more recently as a sleep aid for those with insomnia and jet lag. It is also used for migraine headaches, fatigue, and intestinal cramps.

The sedative effects of valerian may be due to binding of GABA receptors. Several human trials confirm a mild sedative effect. From a Cochrane review, efficacy of valerian as a sedative or anxiolytic could not be determined (Miyasaka, Atallah, & Soares, 2006).

Side effects include headache, excitability, irritability, and cardiac disturbances. Valerian should not be taken when consuming sedatives and/or alcohol.

CHAMOMILE

Chamomile has been used for GI discomfort, peptic ulcer disease, infantile colic, and mild anxiety. Teas, liquid extracts, capsules, or tablets are produces from this lovely plant as well as ointments or creams. Chamomile contains chamazulene, acting like an anti-inflammatory agent, apigenin which binds to central benzodiazepine receptors and has a mild sedative effect (Viola et al., 1995), and bisapolol which has anti spasmodic properties in intestinal smooth muscle (Dombek, 1991).

No randomized or controlled trials have been reported to date in the adolescent population.

Chamomile is regarded as safe although cases of allergic reactions to chamomile have been reported. No significant side effects or herb drub interactions have been observed.

MELATONIN

Melatonin is a neurohormone that is primarily produced by the pineal gland, located behind the third ventricle in the brain. In the synthesis of melatonin, tryptophan is hydroxylated to 5-hydroxytryptophan, which in turn is decarboxylated to

5-hydroxytryptamine (serotonin). Melatonin may have a direct radical scavenging and antioxidant action.

It is unclear how melatonin works as a sleep aid, but three main hypotheses have been proposed. First, there may be a phase-shift of the endogenous circadian pacemaker; second, there is a reduction in core body temperature; and third, somogenic brain structures are directly affected (Melatonin Supplements, 2005).

It has been proposed, although not definitively proven, that in children and adolescent with learning disorders, those who are visually handicapped, and those with developmental delays and irregular sleep-wake patterns, melatonin can result in improvement in their sleep cycles (Gordon, 2000).

In a Cochrane review, melatonin, when taken close to destination bedtime, was tested for its ability to prevent jet lag, especially when five or more time zones were crossed. Its use has been recommended to adult travelers known to experience jet lag in an easterly direction, and especially if they have experienced jet lag on previous journeys (Melatonin for the Prevention and Treatment of Jet Lag, 2002).

In adolescents with delayed sleep-phase syndrome, one study reported that when treated with 3–5 mg/day of melatonin for an average of 6 months, the participants had quicker sleep onset, longer sleep duration and, interestingly, a decrease in school problems (Szeinberg, Borodkin, & Dagan, 2006).

In a meta review, sleep latency decreased significantly in adults with primary sleep disorders. There were no significant findings in adults with secondary sleep disorders (Buscemi et al., 2006).

Melatonin is considered relatively safe when used in the short term, over a period of days or weeks. The safety of long-term use in not known.

ECHINACEA

Echinacea (E. angustifola, E. pallida, and E. purpurea) is widely popular as a natural immune booster and has been traditionally used to prevent and treat colds and other infections. Elite figure skaters use Echinacea to boost the immune system prior to skating events (Ziegler, 2003).

Echinacea stimulates the alternate complement pathway and promotes nonspecific T-cell activation by binding to T-cells. Echinacea may increase interferon production, and the polysaccharides arabinogalactan and echinacin are felt to have immune-modulating effects on the body. Finally, Echinacea may also enhance natural killer cell activity.

Conflicting findings have been observed in studies of Echinacea. In a Cochrane review, Echinacea preparations were found to be better than placebo for the treatment of upper respiratory symptoms (Melchart, Linde, Fischer, & Kaesmayr, 1999). This was confirmed in a separate study (Fugh-Berman, 2003). In the pediatric population, Echinacea was not reported to prevent upper respiratory infections (URI) (Barrett et al., 2002; Taylor et al., 2003).

Side effects are usually mild and may include skin rash in those allergic to ragweed, GI upset, and diarrhea. A theoretic concern has been proposed cautioning those with progressive systemic diseases such as multiple sclerosis, tuberculosis, systemic lupus erythematosus, autoimmune diseases, and human immunodeficiency virus due to *Echinacea's* possible effects on the immune system.

FEVERFEW

Feverfew is well known for its use in the prevention and treatment of migraine headaches. Feverfew is thought to inhibit prostaglandin, thromboxane, and leukotriene synthesis. The mechanism of action for preventing migraine headaches is unknown. Two randomized trials have shown benefit of feverfew use for the prevention of migraines (Johnson, Kadam, Hylands, & Hylands, 1985). However, these studies did not address acute treatment of migraines.

Adverse effects include occasional mouth ulcerations, contact dermatitis, dizziness, diarrhea, and heartburn. Feverfew may interact with anticoagulants and antiplatelet agents due to its platelet aggregation inhibition.

GARLIC

Garlic is known as a natural cholesterol-lowering agent and has been touted as a topical antiseptic and an oral agent to increase physical strength.

Garlic causes a reduction in cholesterol synthesis by reducing the hepatic activity of beta-hydroxy-beta-methylglutaryl-CoA (HMG-CoA) reductase, an enzyme essential to cholesterol biosynthesis. A number of small studies have noted a modest reduction in the total cholesterol level when compared to placebo (Adoga, 1987). Other studies have found no reduction in cholesterol (Sorrentino, 1998).

Garlic may cause GI distress, including gas symptoms and skin irritation. Garlic may interfere with platelet aggregation therefore should not be used in patients on anticoagulant medication.

CREATINE

Creatine is a dietary supplement promoted for its ability to enhance muscle strength and physical endurance (Metzl, Small, Levine, & Gershel, 2001). Adolescent football players and "to be buff" enthusiasts have easy access to this supplement and frequently take it during the summer before a football season or return to a new year in high school. It may be helpful for enhancing muscle performance for high intensity repetitive burst exercise.

Interestingly, it is not officially banned by either the NCAA or the Olympic Committee, although many consider its use in competitive sport unethical and recommend caution in its use as it may be contaminated with other banned substances.

In humans, creatine is found primarily in muscle (i.e., 95%). This includes skeletal muscle, heart, and smooth muscle. The primary source of dietary creatine is meat

(1 g of creatine is found in 250 g of meat). In its phosphorylated intracellular form (creatine phosphate), creatine serves as an energy source for muscular work, providing the high-energy phosphate for adenosine triphosphate (Tjerung et al., 2000).

Creatine supplementation may increase skeletal muscle creatine stores by approximately 20%. Proposed theoretical mechanism of action is that creatine may lead to enhancement of exercise to uptake creatine and augment physiological adaptations to resistance training (Kraemer & Volek, 1999).

Creatine may be beneficial in some chronic illness, particularly when the clinical abnormalities are similar to the physiological and biochemical effects of creatine deficiency in the cell. Creatine supplementation may have a place in managing patients with muscular and neuromuscular disorders (e.g., inflammatory myopathy, mitochondrial cytopathy, or muscular dystrophy) (Tarnopolsky & Martin, 1999; Walter, 2000).

The most common method of loading with creatine involves the ingestion of 20–25 g per days (or 0.3 gm/kg per days in 4–5 doses throughout the day) for 5–7 days. The exact maintenance dose required to retain muscle creatine stores for various populations is not known; a daily dose of approximately 0.03 g/kg is recommended.

Adverse effects include diarrhea, nausea, vomiting, muscle cramping or pain and renal dysfunction (Koshy, Griswold, & Scheenberger, 1999; Prichard & Kaltra, 1998).

Important Note

As with all things concerning the health and wellbeing of adolescents, they need to be counselled repeatedly about their choices to use CAM treatments, especially herbal medicines and supplements. Information on contamination and herb/drug interaction is extremely to impart early and often (Halt, 1998; Saper et al., 2004). Adverse events associated herbal therapies should be reported as soon as possible to the FDA's MedWatch program by calling their toll-free number (1-800-332-1088) or through their Internet site (http://www.fda.gov/medwatch).

ACUPUNCTURE

Acupuncture originated as an ancient Chinese therapeutic treatment and is based on the theory that energy (*Qi*, Chi) flows along channels known as meridians, connected by acupuncture points (Kaptchuk, 1983; Stux & Pomeranz, 1998). Acupuncture needles manipulate the flow of *Qi*. European cultures have embraced acupuncture since the 1600s. Acupuncture has been practiced in the United States since the mid-twentieth century. Please see Chapter 6 on this subject.

Acupuncture may be beneficial in adolescent patients who have dental pain, postoperative nausea and vomiting, or chemotherapy nausea and vomiting (Tsao & Zeltzer, 2005). Other opportunities for use of acupuncture in the adolescent include those with migraine/tension headaches (Linde et al., 2005), dysmenorrhea (Helms, 1987; Pouresmail & Ibrahimzadeh, 2002), and substance abuse (Otto, 2003).

Complications include pneumothorax, angina, septic sacroilitis, epidural and temporomandibular abscess (Peuker, White, Ernst, Pera, & Filler, 1999).

MASSAGE

The effects of massage on sports performance in the adolescent goes without question, and research is needed to support this. Massage therapy is thought to decrease muscle tension, remove toxic metabolites, and facilitate oxygen transport to cells and tissues. There has been research on lactate clearance, delayed onset of muscle soreness, muscle fatigue, the psychological effect of massage, and injury prevention and treatment. Many research reports contain methodological limitations including inadequate therapist training, insufficient duration of treatment, and few subjects. Tissue healing and the psychological effects of massage are areas that merit further research (Morasaka, 2005).

Massage is an essential health intervention to consider for those with eating disorders. In a small placebo controlled study, massage was shown to decrease body dissatisfaction and anxiety in those with eating disorders (Field, Schanberg, et al., 1998; Hart et al., 2001). Massage was proposed to help those with eating disorders by decreasing levels of cortisol and increasing levels of serotonin and dopamine (Hart et al., 2001).

In a Cochrane review, massage was compared to an inert treatment (sham laser) in one study that showed that massage was superior, especially if given in combination with exercises and education. In the other seven studies, massage was compared to different active treatments. Massage was considered beneficial in patients with chronic low-back pain and continued at least one year after the cessation of treatment (Furlan, Brosseau, Imamura, & Irvin, 2006).

Massage may increase the attention span in adolescents with ADHD (Field et al., 1998), decrease pain in those with juvenile rheumatoid arthritis (Field, Hernandez-Reif, Seligmam, Krasnegor, & Sunshine, 1997), and can improve mood in teens with postpartum depression (Field et al., 1996). Massage augments lung function in those with cystic fibrosis (Hernandez-Reif et al., 1999) and improves overall control in those with asthma (Field, Henteleff, et al., 1998).

Side effects include temporary pain or discomfort, bruising, swelling, and breathing sensitivity or allergy to massage oils (http://www.abmp.com/home/index.html). Massage therapy is not recommended in patients with deep vein thrombosis, coagulopathy, fractures, or open/ healing wounds.

Homeopathic Medicine

Homeopathy aims to stimulate the body's own healing responses through the ingestion of extremely small doses of substances which can produce characteristic symptoms of illness when given in larger doses. This approach is called "like cures like."

Anecdotal support of the efficacy of homeopathy has been partially replaced with more scientific evidence. In a meta-analysis of 32 trials in adults, individualized homeopathy was significantly more effective than placebo in treating symptomatic seasonal allergies (Taylor, Reilly, Llewellyn-Jones, McSharry, & Aitchison, 2000). However, when the analysis was restricted to more methodologically sound trials, no significant effect was seen (Linde et al., 1997; Linde & Melchart, 1998). A second meta-analysis comparing trials of homeopathy and matched conventional medicine trials for respiratory tract infections, gynecological problems, musculoskeletal disorders demonstrated weak evidence for specific effects of homeopathic remedies (Berkowitz, 1994; De Lange deKlerk et al., 1994; Ernst & Kaptchuk, 1996; Shang et al., 2005).

Complications are rare and include aggravation of symptoms and a delay in seeking care.

Adolescent Case #4

Antoinette, 14, was recently diagnosed with systemic lupus erythematosis. Her family is devoutly Christian and would love to include a spiritual component to her interdisciplinary healing program. She is about to begin her pharmacological treatment which includes prednisone and immunosuppressants. She is panicking about the possibility of the side effects of acne and weight gain from the prednisone. Antoinette belongs to her youth group at church and has a daily spiritual practice of morning prayer and nightly Bible reading. How can you support her?

Adolescent Case #5

Tran is a 13-year-old with Type 1 Diabetes Mellitus which is poorly controlled. His parents feel that bringing in their monk would help with Tran's acceptance of his disease and involvement in his treatment. The monk wants to help but doesn't want to come in to the hospital, yet would like to talk with you, his provider, at the family's temple. Are you comfortable with this?

Adolescent Case #6

Simon, 15, has reflex neurodystrophy with chronic back pain. Multiple different regimens have failed including the use of pain medications, physical therapy, and psychotherapy. The family has searched the Internet and is open to yoga, chiropractic or Reiki as possible interventions. What can you tell him about these options?

Chiropractic

Chiropractic, founded by Daniel David Palmer (1845–1961), is based on the theory that all disease can be traced to malpositioned bones in the spinal column called "subluxations," which lead to the entrapment of spinal nerves. Subluxations produce symptoms of disease because optimal functioning of tissues and organs does not occur. Physical adjustment of the spine restores proper alignment of the spine by relieving nerve entrapments (Bronfort, 1999; Kaptchuk & Eisenberg, 1998; Meeker & Haldeman, 2002).

In an adult study comparing chiropractic spinal manipulation, sham manipulation, and a back education program, improvement was greater in the manipulation group than in other groups. Pain relief continued to the end of the 12-month evaluation period (Triano, Mc Gregor, Hondras, & Brennan, 1995). In separate studies, the results were not as encouraging and the researchers concluded that the effectiveness of chiropractic spinal manipulation for back pain was still a subject of debate (Cherkin, Deyo, Battie, Street, & Barlow, 1998; Ernst, 2003).

Complications include strokes, myelopathies, and radiculopathies after cervical manipulation (Stevinson, Honan, Cooke, & Ernst, 2001). Adverse outcomes are most likely to occur with a bleeding dyscrasia, when improper diagnosis is made, in the presence of a herniated disc, or when an improper manipulative method is utilized (Lee, Carlini, Mc Cormick, & Albers, 1995).

Mind-Body Therapies

What better place to begin talking about mind-body/ relaxation psychotherapies than in a chapter on the care of adolescents, especially those who may be having a tough time? Who better to start with—the teen or their parent? Meditative interventions have been used to decrease symptoms associated with stuttering, cancer treatment, sleep disorders, diabetic care, affective disorders, irritable bowel syndrome, and eating disorders.

Mindfulness meditation can be defined as a form of self-regulation that ebbs and flows as thoughts enter and leave the mind (Miller, Fletcher, & Kabat Zinn, 1995). The model of mindfulness meditation occurs when the patient looks at their thoughts and experiences from a detached perspective. Thoughts and experiences that come into awareness are acknowledged and then disappear from consciousness. This form of meditation has been used with the treatment of pain amplification disorders, depression, and other chronic conditions such as eating disorders.

Eating disorders can be, at times, an overwhelming problem that primarily affects adolescents. Standard treatments include frequent medical evaluations, nutritional interventions, and psychological treatments. CAM therapies integrated in the management of eating disorder often include meditation, yoga, and herbal remedies (Barabasz, 2007; Triassic, Tennankore, Vohra, & Katzman, 2004). In a study looking at CAM treatments in those with eating disorders, meditation was reported as a potential therapeutic alternative to psychotherapy where finances or geography decreased access to counseling (Garfinkel, 1997).

Spirituality

Adolescents and their families have incorporated spiritual exercises, including prayer, in their health practices for generations. Spirituality in the world of the adolescent takes many forms. It is fascinating to explore this with the teenager. They experience their faith in the synagogue or Sunday morning church; in the mosque; or in their temple.

They may experience their spirit guides on the soccer field, hiking in the mountains, or even when they text message their friend. Don't for a minute think that they haven't thought about this or that they have no beliefs or opinions on the subject. They do!

There are few pediatric/adolescent papers on this subject, yet religious practices are the most commonly used CAM therapy in the United States. In 2004, a comprehensive survey of more than 31,000 adults, 45 percent used prayer for health reasons, 43% prayed for their own health, approximately 25%had had others pray for them and 10% had participated in a group prayer (Barnes, Powell-Griner, Mc Fann, & Nahin, 2002).

Adolescent spiritual development may be as important to explore and follow as are the height and weight curves. Spirituality and religion may help mold a teenager's life by the enhancement of inner resources and can play an important role part in their moral development including socialization and world awareness of the sacred (Barnes, Plotnikoff, Fox, & Pendleton, 2000). There are many different views on how religion affects medical care both positively and negatively. The challenge is in the synthesis of the information and incorporation it into the basic health interview of the adolescent.

Adolescents with chronic diseases, along with their families, may understandably turn more frequently to spirituality and prayer than to other CAM interventions (Cotton et al., 2009). The focus of the discussion of spirituality should be on the fact that this intervention should be viewed as predominantly supportive rather than curative. This avoids the common trap pitting the biomedical against the spirituality, and recovery occurring only in the devout. No one should ever be left out of the discussion of mindful healing, no matter what their belief system.

Table 18-1. Seven Questions for Learning About Connections Families and Children Make Among Spirituality. Religion, Sickness, and Healing

1. How is ultimate health understood?

   (This question involves learning about how the ultimate purpose and possibility of human life is envisioned by the child and the family. It includes understandings of Ultimate Healing, such as salvation or enlightenment. It may also include what a child and/or family think happens after death. because in soma traditions, ultimate healing doesn't happen until then).

2. How are affliction and suffering explained?

   (This question addresses how the child and the family explain why affliction and suffering happen in more general terms. The child and family may have >1 explanation).

3. What are the different parts of a person?

   (Different spiritual/religious traditions think of a person as being, made up of different parte, such as body, mind, spirit, soul, or souls, vital forces, etc. Each tradition conceptualizes a human being differently. To know the parts is to know what can get sick, from the perspective of the child and the family. It also helps one understand a family's strong feelings with regard to some biomedical therapies).

4. How is the child's illness/sickness/disease understood and explained?

   (It is important to learn how family members describe and explain what has gone wrong for their child, and what the child thinks has happened. Causes in some spiritual/religious traditions may be seen as multiple, and may include variables like troubled relationships, divine will, punishment, or testing, the angry dead, demons, soul loss, or karmic influences).

Table 18-1. (Continued)

5. What intervention and/or care is seen as necessary?

(One can explore what the child and family see as necessary interventions for different conditions. Depending on how a family explains the child's condition, these interventions may include not only biomedical therapies but other approaches to healing such as a wide range of religious therapies. Frequently, families pursue >1 approach, although they may not discuss the nonbiomedical strategies they are using. The core issue is what a child and family think needs to be done for heeling to happen).

6. Who is seen as qualified to address the different parts that need healing?

(This question involves learning that different types of practitioner may be recognized as capable of treating different aspects of the illness. Pediatricians may be seen as the best qualified caregivers for certain dimensions and not for others. Families may seek help for their children from different kinds of practitioners, ranging from physicians to priests, acupuncturists, and shamans).

7. What do the child and family mean by efficacy, or healing?

(This question addresses what the family and the child mean when they say that something worked. They may or may not mean that the child's symptoms have gone away. One can also try to learn how children and their families explain it when an intervention does not appear to have worked, according to their understanding of efficacy. The key issue is what a child and a family mean by healing, The term may also have multiple meanings for them).

Source: From Barnes, L. L., Plotnikoff, G. A., Fox, K., & Pendleton S. (2000). Spirituality, religion, and pediatrics: Intersecting worlds of healing. *Pediatrics, 106*(4), S899–S908.

The important outcomes to be studied would be (quality of life) QOL/comfort with the treatment/the disease process itself and the ability to tolerate or even control the pain or discomfort associated with the diseases or the treatments.

Separate, but no less important, is the education of providers in incorporating a spiritual history into the health interview. Healthcare providers need to be aware that the overwhelming response to a question on spirituality/faith/ prayer will be affirmative. Should the spiritual interview stop at this point or should this be explored? What about the discomfort a provider may feel when the patient asks for guidance or even for their inclusion in prayer? See Table 18-1 for suggestions on how to talk about this with patients and their families. There are many unanswered questions on this subject that have still to be pondered, thoughtfully researched, and openly discussed (Armbruster, Chibnall, & Legett, 2003).

Reiki/Therapeutic Touch

Reiki is a traditional form of Japanese healing that was rediscovered by Dr. Mikai Usi in the late 1800s. Reiki, meaning "universal life energy," is based on the belief that when spiritual energy is channeled through a Reiki practitioner, the patient experiences balance and healing in mind, body, and spirit (Herron-Marx, Price-Knol, Burden, & Hicks, 2008).

Despite its popularity, there is a paucity of well-conducted research on theoretical mechanisms of action in Reiki, or on its efficacy.

Therapeutic touch also has a history steeped in tradition and has many potential uses. Therapeutic touch practitioners balance the flow of energy and may be helpful in reducing pain, improving wound healing, aiding relaxation, and in palliative care. As noted with Reiki, there are insufficient trials on mechanisms or efficacy yet research is highly recommended (Robinson, Biley, & Dolk, 2007).

Yoga

Yoga is taken from the Sanskrit word "yuga"; this has been translated to mean "to join" or "to yoke oneself;" to harness to a "discipline or a way of life" (Nayak & Shankar, 2004). Yoga includes meditation, relaxation, control of breathing, and various physical postures or asanas.

Yoga is an extremely important CAM therapy in the adolescent, and has been shown to be beneficial to those with chronic diseases such as cystic fibrosis, asthma, depression, and eating disorders. Yoga may be an effective intervention for the overweight adult. A meditation intervention for the treatment of binge eating disorders was studied, and results indicated that the number of binges dropped significantly over the course of treatment, with nine participants bingeing less than once a week and five participants bingeing less than once or twice a week post-treatment. Participants who spent time using eating mediation were subsequently able to change their bingeing behaviors with an increased sense of eating control, sense of mindfulness, and awareness of hunger cues and satiety cues (Kristeller & Hallett, 1999).

Yoga also may strengthen and increase muscle tone in the patient with an eating disorder. In a small, but thought-provoking, study examining the positive effects of yoga, eating disorder patients completed a yoga program in an observed setting. Eating disorder patients completed different exercise programs including one with yoga. Although the weights did not change in any groups, quality of life scales trended towards improvement (Thien, Thomas, Markin, & Birmingham, 2000). These results suggest preliminary positive uses for yoga and recommendations have included controlled longitudinal clinical trials.

The use of yoga to treat anxiety is based on anecdotal and empiric responses. The lack of controlled clinical trials and/or adequate statistical analysis makes it difficult to interpret the results of several articles which have attempted to examine the impact of yoga on anxiety or other affective states. In one study of patients with eating disorders, yoga was seen as a possible aid in reducing severe physical discomfort and feelings of guilt after eating (Giles, 1985). Recommendations from this chapter include scheduling yoga sessions before and after meals, to possibly helping to reduce many typical anxiety responses and in the alleviation of some of the problems of after-meal supervision.

Research on the physiological effects of yoga has also been sparse. In a study evaluating physiological and psychological effects of hatha-yoga in healthy women, there was a decline in heart rate during and after yoga practice with a return to normal baseline. Blood pressure showed no significant variation (Schell, Allolio, & Schonecke, 1993). The yoga group had significantly higher life satisfaction and positive temperament traits. In another study, yoga was noted to decrease food preoccupation in adolescents with eating disorders (Carei, 2007).

Yoga may help to develop strength and flexibility. Meditation, controlled breathing, and stretches may be an important adjunct treatment for sports performance, anxiety, hypertension, heart disease, depression, low-back pain, headaches, and cancer (Gupta, Khera, Vempati, Sharma, & Bijlani, 2006; Kirkwood, Rampes, Tuffrey, Richardson, & Pilkington, 2005).

Many different schools of yoga exist with varying curricula depend on the type of yoga being taught. Training may include techniques, anatomy and physiology, diet, philosophy, methodology, and personal practice. Although no license is required to teach yoga, attempts are being made to bring standardization to yoga instructors.

If a joint is stretched (flexed or extended) beyond its normal limit, an injury may occur. For example, hyperextension of the knee may aggravate a meniscal tear. Extreme poses should be avoided, despite their enthusiasm, in those youth with existing trauma or joint injuries.

Conclusion

Counselling adolescents about the variety of health options that are available to them and guiding them though a decision process is important and rewarding (American Academy of Pediatrics, 2001). As providers for this dynamic population we need to understand these choices, and support them if CAM use is safe and/or effective, thus reflecting respect for their healthcare preferences. Even with the best of intentions, some teens don't want to do anything about their health. Working closely with CAM providers can provide that edge that, through motivational interviewing, can help a teen navigate a chronic illness with the help of alternative adjunctive interventions. Improved communication can be addressed by following the recommendations in Table 18-2. Healthcare providers need to inquire regularly about CAM use and be nonjudgmental

Table 18-2. Talking with Your Patients about CAM

Be open-minded. Most patients are reluctant to share information about their use of CAM therapies because they are concerned their physicians will disapprove. By remaining open-minded, you can learn a lot about your patients' use of unconventional therapies. These strategies will help foster open communication.

Ask the question. I recommend asking every patient about his or her use of alternative therapies during routine history taking. One approach is simply to inquire, "Are you doing anything else for this condition?" It's an open-ended question that gives the patient the opportunity to tell you about his or her use of other healthcare providers or therapies. Another approach is to ask, "Are you taking any over-the-counter remedies such as vitamins or herbs?"

Avoid using the words "alternative therapy," at least initially. This will help you to avoid appearing judgmental or biased.

Don't dismiss any therapy as a placebo. If a patient tells you about a therapy that you are unaware of, make a note of it in the patient's record and schedule a follow-up visit after you have learned more—when you'll be in a better position to negotiate the patient's care. If you determine the therapy might be harmful, you'll have to ask the patient to stop using it. If it isn't harmful and the patient feels better using it, you may want to consider incorporating the therapy into your care plan.

Discuss providers as well as therapies. Another way to help your patients negotiate the maze of alternative therapies is by stressing that they see appropriately trained and licensed providers and knowing whom to refer to in your area. Encourage your patients to ask alternative providers about their background and training and the treatment modalities they use. By doing so, your patients will be better equipped to make educated decisions about their healthcare.

Discuss CAM therapies with your patients at every visit. Charting the details of their use will remind you to raise the issue. It may also help alert you to potential complications before they occur.

Source: Breuner, C. C. (2002). Complementary medicine in pediatrics: a review of acupuncture, homeopathy, massage, and chiropractic therapies. Current Problems in Pediatric and Adolescent Health Care, 32(10):353–384.

in their approach in order to help steer adolescents and their families towards a proper course to health (Kemper 2000).

Websites

General

AAP CHIM website

http://www.nccam.nih.gov National Center for Complementary and Alternative Medicine

http://www.amfoundation.org Alternative Medicine Foundation

Herbal Medicine

http://www.herbmed.org HerbMed database

http://www.herbs.org Herb Research Foundation

http://www.herbalgram.org American Botanical Council

http://www.naturaldatabase.com Natural Medicines Comprehensive Database

Mind-Body Medicine

http://www.umassmed.edu/cfm/clinical.cfm The Stress Reduction Clinic at the University of Massachusetts

http://www.holisticmedicine.org The American Holistic Medical Association

http://www.ahha.org The American Holistic Health Association

http://www.nicabm.com The National Institute for Clinical Applications of Behavioral

Medicine

http://www.cmbm.org The Center for Mind Body Medicine

Yoga

http://www.americanyogaassociation.org/

Acupuncture

http://www.aaom.org American Association of Oriental Medicine

http://www.acuall.org Acupuncture and Oriental Medical Alliance

http://www.medicalacupuncture.org American Academy of Medical Acupuncture

Chiropractic

http://www.amerchiro.org American Chiropractic Association

http://www.chiropractic.org International Chiropractors Association

Homeopathy

http://www.homeopathic.org National Center for Homeopathy

Massage

http://www.amtamassage.org American Massage Therapy Association

http://www.ncbtmb.com National Certification Board for Massage Therapy and Bodywork

REFERENCES

Adoga, G. I. (1987). The mechanism of the hypolipidemic effect of garlic oil extract in rats fed on high sucrose and alcohol diets. *Biochemical and Biophysical Research Communications, 142,* 1046.

Ahuja, J. (2001). Caffeine and theobromine intakes of children: Results from CSF II 1994–96, 1998. *Family Economics and Nutrition Review, 13*(2) 47–52. http://www.barc.usda.gov/bhnrc/foodsurvey/pdf/fenrv13n2p47.pdf.

Almeida, J. C., & Grimsley, E. W. (1996). Coma from the health food store: interaction between kava and alprazolam. *Annals of Internal Medicine, 125,* 940.

American Academy of Pediatrics. (2002). AAP Medical Home Initiatives for Children with Special Needs Project Advisory Committee: The medical home. *Pediatrics, 110*(1), 184–186.

American Academy of Pediatrics Division of Health Policy Research. (2001). Periodic Survey of Fellows #49: Complementary and Alternative Medicine (CAM) Therapies in Pediatric Practices. Retrieved April 8, 2007, from http://www.aap.org/research/periodicsurvey/ps49bexs.htm

Andersen, T., & Fogh, J. (2001). Weight loss and delayed gastric emptying following a South American herbal preparation in overweight patients. *Journal of Human Nutrition and Dietetics, 14*(3), 243–250.

Armbruster, C. A., Chibnall, J. T., & Legett, S. (2003). Pediatrician beliefs about spirituality and religion in medicine: Associations with clinical practice. *Pediatrics, 111*(3), e227–e235.

Avula, B., Wang, Y. H., Pawar, R. S., Shukla, Y. J., Schaneberg, B., & Khan, I. A. (2006). Determination of the appetite suppressant P57 in Hoodia gordonii plant extracts and dietary supplements by liquid chromatography/electrospray ionization mass spectrometry (LC-MSD-TOF) and LC-UV methods. *JAOAC Int, 89*(3), 606–611.

Barabasz, M. (2007). Efficacy of hypnotherapy in the treatment of eating disorders. *The International Journal of Clinical and Experimental Hypnosis, 55*(3), 318–335.

Barnes, L. L., Plotnikoff, G. A., Fox, K., & Pendleton, S. (2000). Spirituality, religion, and pediatrics: Intersecting worlds of healing. *Pediatrics, 106*(4), S899–S908.

Barnes, P. M., Powell-Griner, E., Mc Fann, K., & Nahin, R. L. (2002). Complementary and alternative medicine use among adults: United States, *CDC Advance Data Report #343*. 2004. Retrieved April 2, 2008, from nccam.nih.gov/news/report.pdf

Barrett, B. P., Brown, R. L., Locken, K., et al. (2002). Treatment of the common cold with unrefined Echinacea: A randomized, double-blind, placebo-controlled trial. *Annals of Internal Medicine, 137*(12), 939–946.

Berkowitz, C. D. (1994). Homeopathy: Keeping an open mind. *Lancet, 344*, 701.

Bernstein G. A. (1998). Caffeine withdrawal in normal school aged children. *Journal of American Academy of Adolescent and Child Psychiatry, 37*(8), 858–865.

Bielroy, L. (2004). Complementary and alternative interventions in asthma, allergy, and immunology. *Annals of Allergy, Asthma & Immunology, 93*(Suppl 1), S45–S54.

Braun, C. A., Bearinger, L. H., Halcón, L. L. & Pettingell, S. L. (2005). Adolescent use of complementary therapies. *Journal of Adolescent Health, 37*, 76.

Breuner, C. C. (2002). Complementary medicine in pediatrics: a review of acupuncture, homeopathy, massage, and chiropractic therapies. *Current Problems in Pediatric and Adolescent Health Care, 32*(10):353–384.

Breuner, C. C., Barry, P., & Kemper K. J. (1998). Alternative medicine use by homeless youth. *Archives of Pediatrics & Adolescent Medicine, 152*(11), 1071–1075.

Bronfort, G. (1999). Spinal manipulation: Current state of research and its indications. *Neurologic Clinics, 17*(1), 91–111.

Buscemi, N., Vandermeer, B., Hooton, N., Pandya, R., Tjosvold, L., Hartling, L., et al. (2006). Efficacy and safety of exogenous melatonin for secondary sleep disorders and sleep disorders accompanying sleep restriction: Meta-analysis. *BMJ, 332*(7538), 385–393.

Carei, T., Breuner, C. C., & Fyfe Johnson, A. (2007). The evaluation of yoga in the treatment of eating disorders. *Journal of Adolescent Health, 40*(2), S31–S32.

Cherkin, D. C., Deyo, R. A., Battie, M., Street, J. & Barlow, W. (1998). A comparison of physical therapy, chiropractic manipulation, and provision of an educational booklet for the treatment of patients with low back pain. *New England Journal of Medicine, 339*(15), 1021–1029.

Clough, A. R., Bailie, R. S., & Currie, B. (2003). Liver function test abnormalities in users of aqueous kava extracts. *Journal of Toxicology. Clinical Toxicology, 41*(6), 821–829.

Cohen, E., Mackenzie, R. G., & Yates, G. (1991). HEADSS: A psychosocial risk assessment instrument: implications for designing effective intervention programs for runaway youth. *Journal of Adolescent Health, 12*(7), 539–544.

Cotton, S., Kudel, I., Roberts, Y., Pallerla, H., Tsevat, J., Succop, P., & Yi, M. (2009). Spiritual Well-Being and Mental Health Outcomes in Adolescents With or Without Inflammatory Bowel Disease. *Journal of Adolescent Health, 44* (5), 485–492.

De Lange de Klerk, E. S. M., Blommers, J., et al. (1994). Effect of homeopathic remedies medicines on daily burdens of symptoms in children with recurrent upper respiratory infections. *British Medical Journal, 309*: 1329–1332.

Dombek, C. (Ed.). (1991). *Lawrence Review of Natural Products*. St Louis Facts and Comparisons.

Dulloo, A. G., Duret, C., Rohrer, D., Girardier, L., Mensi, N., Fathi, M., et al. (1999). Efficacy of a green tea extract rich in catechin polyphenols and caffeine in increasing 24-h energy expenditure and fat oxidation in humans. *The American Journal of Clinical Nutrition, 70*(6), 1040–1045.

Ellison, R. C. (1993). Caffeine intake and salivary levels in children. Paper presented at the 7th International Caffeine Workshop, Santorini, Greece.

Ernst, E. (2003). Chiropractic spinal manipulation for back pain. *British Journal of Sports Medicine, 37*(3), 195–196.

Ernst, E., & Kaptchuck, T. J. (1996). Homeopathy revisited. *Archives of Internal Medicine, 156,* 2162.

Faw, C., Ballentine, R., Ballentine, L., & van Eys. J. (1977). Unproved cancer remedies. A survey of use in pediatric outpatients. *JAMA, 238,* 1536–1538.

Field, T., et al. (1996). Massage and relaxation therapies' effects on depressed adolescent mothers. *Adolescence, 31*(124), 903.

Field, T., et al. (1998). Adolescents with attention deficit hyperactivity disorder benefit from massage therapy. *Adolescence, 333,* 103.

Field, T., Henteleff, T., Hernandez-Reif, M., Martinez, E., Mavunda, K., Kuhn, C., & Schanberg, S. (1998). Children with asthma have improved pulmonary functions after massage therapy. *Journal of Pediatrics, 132*(5), 854–858.

Field, T., Hernandez-Reif, M., Seligmam, S., Krasnegor, J., & Sunshine, W. (1997). Juvenile rheumatoid arthritis: Benefits from massage therapy. *Journal of Pediatric Psychology, 22*(5), 607–617.

Field, T., Schanberg, S., Kuhn., C., Field, T., Henteleff, T., Mueller, C., et al. (1998). Bulimic adolescents benefit from massage therapy. *Adolescence, 33,* 131.

Friedman, T., Slayton, W. B., Allen, L. S., Pollock, B. H., Dumont-Driscoll, M. & Mehta, P., et al. (1997). Use of alternative therapies for children with cancer. *Pediatrics, 100*(6), E1.

Fugh-Berman, A. (2003). Echinacea for the prevention and treatment of upper respiratory infections. *Seminars in Integrative Medicine, 1*(2), 106–111.

Furlan, A. D., Brosseau, L., Imamura M., & Irvin, E. (2006). Massage for low-back pain. *The Cochrane Library* (ISSN 1464–780X) (3).

Gardiner, P., & Kemper, K. J. (2000). Herbs in pediatric and adolescent medicine. *Pediatrics in Review, 21*(2), 44.

Garfinkel, P. E. (1997). Dorian BJ Factors that may influence future approaches to the eating disorders. *Eating and Weight Disorders, 2*(1), 1–16.

Gaster, B., & Holroyd, J. (2000). St John's wort for depression: A systematic review. *Archives of Internal Medicine, 160,* 152–156.

Giles, G. (1985). Anorexia nervosa and bulimia: An activity-oriented approach. *The American Journal of Occupational Therapy, 39*(8), 510–517.

Ginseng. Natural Medicines Comprehensive Database Website. Retrieved December 8, 2007, from www.naturaldatabase.com

Gordon, N. (2000). The therapeutics of melatonin. A pediatric perspective. *Brain & Development, 22*(4), 213–217.

Gupta, N., Khera, S., Vempati, R. P., Sharma, R., & Bijlani, R. L. (2006). Effect of yoga based lifestyle intervention on state and trait anxiety. *Indian Journal of Physiology and Pharmacology, 50*(1), 41–47.

Halt, M. (1998). Moulds and mycotoxins in herb tea and medicinal plants. *European Journal of Epidemiology, 14,* 269.

Hart, S., Field, T., Hernandez-Reif, M., Nearing, G., & Shaw, S. (2001). Anorexia nervosa symptoms are reduced by massage therapy. *Eating Disorders. The Journal of Treatment and Prevention, 9*(4), 289–299.

Helms, J. M. (1987). Acupuncture for the management of primary dysmenorrhea. *Obstetrics and Gynecology, 69,* 51–56.

Hernandez-Reif, M., Field, T., Krasnegor, J. Martinez, E., Schwartzman, M., & Mavunda, K. (1999). Children with cystic fibrosis benefit from massage therapy. *Journal of Pediatric Psychology, 24,* 176.

Herron-Marx, S., Price- Knol, F., Burden, B., & Hicks, C. (2008). A systematic review of the use of Reiki in healthcare. *Journal of Alternative and Complementary Medicine, 14*(1)37–42.

How Does Hoodia Gordonii work on Appetite Suppression. Retrieved September 3, 2008, from http://www.cellhealthmakeover.com/hoodia-p57.html

Huestis, R. D., Arnold, L. E., & Smeltzer, D. J. (1975). Caffeine versus methylphenidate and d-amphetamine in minimal brain dysfunction: A double-blind comparison. *The American Journal of Psychiatry, 132*(8), 868–870.

Hypericum Depression Trial Study Group. (2002). Effect of *Hypericum perforatum* (St. John's wort) in major depressive disorder: A randomized controlled trial. *Journal of the American Medical Association, 287*(14), 1807–1814.

Johnson, E. S., Kadam, N. P., Hylands, D. M., & Hylands, P. J. (1985). Efficacy of feverfew as prophylactic treatment of migraine. *British Medical Journal, 291*(6495), 569–573.

Kaptchuk, T. (1983). *The web that has no weaver.* New York: Congdon and Weed.

Kaptchuk, T. J., & Eisenberg, D. M. (1998). Chiropractic: Origins, controversies, and contributions. *Archives of Internal Medicine, 158*(20), 2215–2224.

Kava Linked to Liver Damage. Retrieved December 11, 2007, from http://nccam.nih.gov/health/alerts/kava/

Kemper, K. J. (2000). Holistic pediatrics = Good medicine. *Pediatrics, 105*(1 Pt 3), 214–218.

Kirkwood, G., Rampes, H., Tuffrey, V., Richardson, J., & Pilkington, K. (2005). Yoga for anxiety: A systematic review of the research evidence. *British Journal of Sports Medicine, 39*(12), 884–891; discussion 891.

Ko, J., Lee, J. I., Muñoz-Furlong, A., Li, X. M. & Sicherer, S. H. (2006). Use of complementary and alternative medicine by food-allergic patients. *Annals of Allergy, Asthma & Immunology, 97,* 365–369.

Koshy, K. M., Griswold, E., & Scheenberger, E. E. (1999). Interstitial nephritis in a patient taking creatine [letter]. *The New England Journal of Medicine, 340,* 814–815.

Kraemer, W. J., & Volek, J. S. (1999). Creatine supplementation. Its role in human performance. *Clinics in Sports Medicine, 8*(3), 651–666.

Kristeller, J. L., & Hallett, B. (1999). An exploratory study of a meditation-based intervention for binge eating disorder. *Journal of Health Psychology, 4*(3) 357–363.

Lee, A. C. C., & Kemper, K. J. (2000). Homeopathy and naturopathy. *Archives of Pediatrics & Adolescent Medicine, 154,* 78–80.

Lee, K. P., Carlini, W. G., Mc Cormick, G. F., & Albers, G. W. (1995). Neurologic complications following chiropractic manipulation: A survey of California neurologists. *Neurology, 45*(6), 1213–1215.

Linde, K., & Melchart, D. (1998). Randomized controlled trials of individualized homeopathy: A state-of-the-art review. *Journal of Alternative and Complementary Medicine, 4*(4), 371.

Linde, K., Berner, M., Egger, M., & Mulrow, C. (2005). St. John's wort for depression: Meta-analysis of randomized controlled trials. *British Journal of Psychiatry, 186,* 99–107.

Linde, K., Clausius, N., Ramirez, G., et al. (1997). Are the clinical effects of homeopathy placebo effects; a meta analysis of placebo-controlled trials. *Lancet, 350,* 834.

Linde, K., Streng, A., Jurgens, S., Hoppe, A., Brinkhaus, B. & Witt, C., et al. (2005). Acupuncture for patients with migraine. *JAMA, 293,* 2118–2125.

Lloyd, T., Rollings, N. J., Kieselhorst, K., Eggli, D. F., & Mauger E. (1998). Dietary caffeine intake is not correlated with adolescent bone gain. *Journal of the American College of Nutrition, 17*(5), 454–457.

Loman, D. G. (2003). The use of complementary and alternative healthcare practices among children. *Journal of Pediatrics and Healthcare, 17,* 58–63.

Mate Monograph, Natural Medicines Comprehensive Database. Retrieved December 2007, from www. naturaldatabase.com

Meeker, W. C., & Haldeman, S. (2002). Chiropractic: A profession at the crossroads of mainstream and alternative medicine. *Annals of Internal Medicine, 136*(3), 216–227.

Melatonin for the prevention and treatment of jet lag. (2002). *Cochrane Database of Systematic Reviews,* (2), CD001520.

Melatonin supplements, often taken for difficulty in sleeping, appear to be safe when used over short periods at high doses, according to a report by the Agency for Healthcare Research and Quality (2005). http://www.ahrq.gov/clinic/evrptpdfs.htm#melatonin.

Melchart, D., Linde, K., Fischer, P., & Kaesmayr, J. (1999). Echinacea for preventing and treating the common cold. *The Cochrane Database of Systematic Reviews,* (1), CD000530.

Merhav, H., Amitai, Y., Palti, H., & Godfrey, S. (1985). Tea drinking and microcytic anemia in infants. *American Journal of Clinical Nutrition, 41*(6), 1210–1213.

Metzl, J. D., Small, E., Levine, A. R., & Gershel, J. C. (2001). Creatine use among young athletes. *Pediatrics, 108*(2), 421–425.

Miller, J. J., Fletcher, K., & Kabat Zinn, J. (1995). Three year follow up and clinical implications of a mindfulness meditation based states reduction intervention in the treatment of anxiety disorders. *General Hospital Psychiatry, 17*(3); 192–200.

Mind-Body Medicine: An Overview (NCCAM). Retrieved April 3, 2008, from http://nccam.nih.gov/health/backgrounds/mindbody.htm#intro

Miyasaka, L. S., Atallah, A. N., & Soares, B. G. (2006). Valerian for anxiety disorders. *Cochrane Database of Systematic Reviews, 18*(4), CD004515.

Morasaka, A. (2005). Sports massage: A comprehensive review. *The Journal of Sports Medicine and Physical Fitness, 45*(3), 370–380.

Mukhtar, H., Wang, Z. Y., Katiyar, S. K., & Agarwal, R. (1992). Tea components: Antimutagenic and anticarcinogenic effects. *Preventive Medicine, 21,* 351–360.

National Center for Complementary and Alternative Medicine. *St. John's Wort and the Treatment of Depression.* National Center for Complementary and Alternative Medicine Web site. Retrived December 10, 2007, from http://nccam.nih.gov/

Nayak, N. N., & Shankar, K. (2004). Yoga: A therapeutic approach. *Physical Medicine and Rehabilitation Clinics of North America, 15*(4), 783–798.

Neuhouser, M. L., Patterson, R. E., Schwartz, S. M., Hedderson, M. M., Bowen, D. J., & Standish, L J. (2001). Use of alternative medicine by children with cancer in Washington State. *Preventive Medicine, 33*(5), 347–354.

Otto, K. C. (2003). Acupuncture and substance abuse: A synopsis, with indications for further research. *The American Journal on Addictions, 12*(1), 43–51.

Paramore, L. C. (1997). Use of alternative therapies: Estimates from the Robert Wood Johnson Foundation national access to care survey, US Cancer Pain Relief Committee. *Journal of Pain and Symptom Management, 13,* 83–89.

Peuker, E. T., White, A., Ernst, E., Pera, F., & Filler, T. (1999). Traumatic complications of acupuncture. *Archives of Family Medicine, 8,* 553–558.

Pittler, M. H., & Ernst, E. (2003). Kava extract for treating anxiety. *Cochrane Database of Systematic Reviews,* (1), CD003383.

Pouresmail, Z., & Ibrahimzadeh, R., (2002). Effects of acupressure and ibuprofen on the severity of primary dysmenorrhea. *Journal of Traditional Chinese Medicine, 22,* 205–210.

Prichard, N. R., & Kaltra, P. A. (1998). Renal dysfunction accompanying oral creatine supplements. *Lancet, 351,* 1252–1253.

Rapoport J. L. Berg, C. J., Ismond, D. R., Zahn, T. P., & Neims, A. (1984). Behavioral effects of caffeine in children. Relationship between dietary choice and effects of caffeine challenge. *Archives of General Psychiatry, 41*(11), 1073–1079.

Retrived January 9, 2009, from http://www.abmp.com/home/index.html

Reznick, M., et al. (2002). Use of complementary therapy by adolescents with asthma. *Archives of Pediatrics & Adolescent Medicine, 156*, 1042–1044.

Robinson, J., Biley, F. C., & Dolk, H. (2007). Therapeutic touch for anxiety disorders. *Cochrane Database of Systematic Reviews, (3)*, CD006240.

Sanders, H., Davis M. F., Duncan B., Meaney J. F., Haynes J., & Barton L. L. (2003). Use of complementary and alternative medical therapies among children with special healthcare needs in southern Arizona. *Pediatrics, 111*, 584–587.

Saper, R. B., Kales, S. N., Paquin, J., Burns, M.J., Eisenberg, D.M. & Davis, R.B., et al. (2004). Heavy metal content of ayurvedic medicine products. *JAMA, 292*, 2868–2873.

Sawni-Sikand, A., Schubiner, H., & Thomas, R. L. (2002). Use of complementary/alternative therapies among children in primary care pediatrics. *Ambulatory Pediatrics, 2*(2), 99–103.

Sawyer, M. G., Gannoni, A. F., Toogood, I. R., Antoniou, G., & Rice, M. (1994). The use of alternatives therapies by children with cancer. *The Medical Journal of Australia, 169*, 320–322.

Schell, E., Allolio, B., & Schonecke, W. (1993). Physiological and psychological effects of hatha-yoga exercise in healthy women. *International Journal of Eating Disorders, 41*, 46–52.

Shang, A., Huwiler- Muntener, K. H., Juni, P., Dörig, S., Sterne, J. A., et al. (2005). Are the clinical effects of homeopathy placebo effects? Comparative study of placebo controlled trials of homeopathy and allopathy. *Lancet, 366*, 726–732.

Shekelle, P. G., Hardy, M. L., Morton, S. C., Maglione, M., Mojica, W. A., Suttorp, M. J., et al. (2003). Efficacy and safety of ephedra and ephedrine for weight loss and athletic performance: A meta-analysis. *JAMA, 289*(12), 1537–1545.

Shelton, R. C., Keller, M. B., Greenberg, A., Dunner, D. L., Hirschfeld, R. & Thase, M. E., et al. (2001). Effectiveness of St. John's wort in major depression, a randomized control trial. *JAMA, 285*, 1807.

Smitherman, L. C., Janisse, J. & Mathur, A. (2005). The use of folk remedies among children in an urban black community: Remedies for fever, colic, and teething. *Pediatrics, 115*: e297–e304.

Sorrentino, M. (1998). Garlic: Is the "stinking rose" good for the cholesterol count? *Altern Med Alert, 1*(9), 97.

Southwood, T. R., Malleson, P. N., Roberts-Thomson, P. J., & Mahy, M. (1995). Unconventional remedies used by patients with juvenile arthritis. *Pediatrics, 85*, 150–154.

Spigelblatt, L., Laine-Ammara, G., Pless, I. B., & Guyver, A. (1994). The use of alternative medicine by children. *Pediatrics, 94*, 811–814.

Stein, M. A., Krasowski, M., Leventhal, B. L., Phillips, W., & Bender, B. G. (1996). Behavioral and cognitive effects of methylxanthines. A meta-analysis of theophylline and caffeine. *Archives of Pediatrics & Adolescent Medicine, 150*(3), 284–288.

Stem, R. C., Canda, E. R., & Doershuk, C. F. (1992). Use of non-medical treatment by cystic fibrosis patients. *The Journal of Adolescent Health, 13*, 612–615.

Stevinson, C., Honan, W., Cooke, B., & Ernst, E. (2001). Neurological complications of cervical spine manipulation. *Journal of the Royal Society of Medicine, 94*:107–110.

Stux, G., & Pomeranz, B. (1998). *Basics of acupuncture.* Germany: Springer Verlag.

Szeinberg, A., Borodkin, K., & Dagan, Y. (2006). Melatonin treatment in adolescents with delayed sleep phase syndrome. *Clinical Pediatrics (Phila), 45*(9), 809–818.

Tarnopolsky, M., & Martin, J. (1999). Creatine monohydrate increases strength in patients with neuromuscular disease. *Neurology, 52*(4), 854–857.

Taylor M. A., Reilly D, Llewellyn-Jones R. H., McSharry C., & Aitchison T. C, (2000). Randomized controlled trial of homoeopathy versus placebo in perennial allergic rhinitis with overview of four trial series. *British Medical Journal, 321*, 471–476.

Taylor, J. A., Weber, W., Standish, L., et al. (2003). Efficacy and safety of Echinacea in treating upper respiratory tract infections in children: A randomized controlled trial. *JAMA, 290*(21), 2824.

Thien, V., Thomas, A., Markin, D., & Birmingham, C. (2000). Pilot study of a graded exercise program for the treatment of anorexia nervosa. *International Journal of Eating Disorders, 28*(1), 101–106.

Tjerung, R. L., Clarkson, P., Eichner, E. R., et al. (2000). The physiological and health effects of oral creatine supplementation. *Medicine and Science in Sports and Exercise, 32,* 706–717.

Triano, J. J., Mc Gregor, M., Hondras, M. A., & Brennan, P. C. (1995). Manipulative therapy versus education programs in chronic low back pain. *Spine, 20*(8), 948–955.

Triassic, L., Tennankore, D., Vohra, S., & Katzman, D. K. (2004). The use of herbal remedies by adolescents with eating disorders. *The International Journal of Eating Disorders, 35*(2), 223.

Tsao, J. C., & Zeltzer, L. K. (2005). Complementary and alternative medicine approaches for pediatric pain: A review of the state-of-the-science. *eCAM, 2*(2), 149–159.

Tulp, O. L., Harbi, N. A., Mihalov, J., DerMarderosian, A. (2001). Effect of Hoodia plant on food intake and body weight in lean and obese. LA/Ntul//-cp rats. *FASEB J, 15*(4):A404.

Viola, H., Wasowski, C., Levi de Stein, M., Wolfman, C., Silveira, R., Dajas, F., et al. (1995). Apigenin, a component of Matricaria recutita flowers, is a central benzodiazepine receptors-ligand with anxiolytic effects. *Planta Medica, 61*(3), 213–216.

Vogler, B. K., Pittler, M. H., & Ernst, E. (1999). The efficacy of ginseng. A systematic review of randomized clinical trials. *European Journal of Clinical Pharmacology, 55*(8), 567–575.

Walter M. C. (2000) Creatine monohydrate in muscular dystrophies: A double-blind, placebo-controlled clinical study. *Neurology, 54*(9), 1848–1850.

Wilson, K. M., & Klein, J. D. (2002). Adolescents' use of complementary and alternative medicine. *Ambulatory Pediatrics, 2,* 104–110.

Yussman, S., Wilson, K., Graff, C., et al. (2002). Herbal products and their association with substance abuse in adolescents. *Journal of Adolescence Health, 30,* 122.

Ziegler, P. (2003). Dietary intake of elite figure skating dancers. *Nutrition Research, 21*(7), 983–992.

19

Integrative Developmental/Behavioral Pediatrics

SANFORD NEWMARK

KEY CONCEPTS

- Integrative therapies play an increasingly important role for children with common biobehavioral challenges such as ADHD, autism, and sleep disorders.
- The prevalence of the use of CAM therapies by families, both in ADHD and autism is extremely high.
- Autism is a genetically based neurodevelopmental disease whose expression is partly or completed influenced by environmental triggers. It is associated with significant gastrointestinal, metabolic, and autoimmune abnormalities
- The most common and effective non-conventional treatment of autism, often known as the biomedical approach, concentrates on direct treatment of these abnormalities, usually through dietary changes and nutritional supplements.
- There has been explosive increase in the prevalence of the diagnosis of ADHD and the concurrent use of prescription psychotropic medications; this necessitates a thorough evaluation and integrative approach for children with this diagnosis.
- Nutritional evaluation, including the possibility of food sensitivities, should be an essential part of the integrative approach to ADHD.
- Sleep problems are common in children and teens and respond well to integrative approaches.

■

Introduction

Neurodevelopmental disorders, especially ADHD and autism, have become an increasingly important and sometimes frustrating aspect of modern pediatric practice. Physicians and other practitioners are being asked to diagnose, treat, and monitor these conditions on an ever-more frequent basis, often without the necessary time and skills to feel comfortable in this role. To complicate matters further, in both of these conditions, many parents are unhappy with conventional medical treatment and have questions about diet, herbs, nutritional supplements, and other interventions that physicians do not know how to answer. The purpose of this chapter is to outline an integrative approach to these two neurodevelopmental issues and discuss the nature and research evidence for the main non-conventional treatments that are currently being used. In addition, pediatric sleep problems are discussed, with an emphasis on behavioral and other non-pharmacologic treatment.

Autism

Autism is a neurodevelopmental disorder characterized by deficits in social interaction, language development, and a restricted or stereotypical pattern of interests and activities. Formerly a rare condition unfamiliar to most professionals, autism is now a topic of widespread interest and coverage in both the media and professional journals. The prevalence of autism has increased at least tenfold in the last 20 years, from about 5 to 6 per 10,000 children to 67/10,000 in the most recent Center for Disease Control study (Center for Disease Control and Prevention, 2007). There is no scientific agreement as to the cause of this rapid increase in prevalence, often referred to as an "epidemic" in the media. It is likely some combination of increased awareness and case-finding, a loosening of the diagnostic criteria, and a true increase in the occurrence of the disorder.

Complicating matters still further, other diagnostic categories such as autistic spectrum disorder (ASD), pervasive developmental disorder, and Asperger's syndrome have been added to the mix, including children with some features of autism but who do not meet the full criteria. However, the Brick Township study separated out autism from ASD and Asperger's syndrome and still recorded a prevalence of 40/10,000 of autism itself (Bertrand et al., 2001).

REGRESSIVE AUTISM

Regressive autism refers to children who have normal development until the age of 1 to 2 years, after which there is a loss of language, social interaction, and other developmental milestones. It is this type of autism which has caused the widespread public concern over the influence of the MMR and mercury-containing vaccines on the development of autism. Available studies indicate that regressive autism accounts for only 20%–50% of autism, although there is surprisingly little good research available on this point (Tuchman, 2006). In a recent study by Ozonoff, almost half of those children who experienced true regression were not developing normally before the regression occurred, indicating a possibility for earlier intervention (Ozonoff, Williams, & Landa, 2005).

ETIOLOGY

Autism is though to be a genetically based disorder whose expression may be partially or completely based on environmental factors. There is a 62%–90% concordance rate in identical twins versus a 0%–10% concordance rate in fraternal twins (Muhle, Trentacoste, & Rapin, 2004). There have been many gene loci associated with autism, but no single gene or even group of genes has been definitively linked to this disorder (Shastry, 2003). There has been little scientific research concerning what environmental factors may trigger the expression of this disease. Although some patients and physicians interested in alternative treatment of autism are concerned about the role of mercury and immunizations in triggering the development of autism, there are many other possible environmental triggers, both natural and man-made.

In general, it has been felt that whatever the genetics and triggering factors, autism is a brain disorder that is hard-wired before birth, a type of "static encephalopathy." However some recent neuroanatomical research has shown ongoing neuroinflammation and brain growth abnormalities that are more indicative of a chronic disease process, perhaps of an autoimmune nature (Vargas, 2005). This suggests a pathophysiologic basis for some of the biomedical treatments which will be discussed below.

Recent research has shown ongoing neuroinflammation in autism, raising the possibility that autism is at least partially an ongoing chronic disease rather than a static encephalopathy.

CAM Therapies for Autism

CAM therapies are used with great frequency in the treatment of autism. A study in 2006 showed that 74% of families of children with autistic spectrum disorder were using some type of CAM therapy. Although these included the full spectrum of CAM therapies, the highest frequency of use, over 54% of families, involved what were termed biologically based therapies, including modified diets, vitamins and minerals, and other nutritional supplements (Hanson et al., 2007). Several other studies have demonstrated similarly high frequency of use, from 30% in a regional referral center to 92% in two primary care practices (Harrington, Rosen, Garnecho & Patrick, 2006; Levy, Mandell, Merhar, Ittenbach, & Pinto-Martin, 2003; Wong & Smith, 2006).

The widespread use of these biologically based therapies reflects the very high acceptance, among both families and many healthcare providers, of what is commonly referred to as a "biomedical" approach to autism. The basis of this approach is as follows: although autism is a genetically based syndrome triggered by certain fetal, neonatal, and early childhood stimuli, the syndrome is associated with a variety of nutritional, gastrointestinal, metabolic, and autoimmune abnormalities. Further, interventions resulting in full or partial correction of these abnormalities can lead to improvements in the core symptoms of autism. The following sections will examine the evidence for the existence of these biochemical abnormalities, and the evidence that interventions can have a positive effect on the autistic behavior.

Autism is associated with a variety of nutritional, gastrointestinal, metabolic, and autoimmune abnormalities. Interventions resulting in full or partial correction of these abnormalities may lead to improvements in the core symptoms of autism.

THE GASTROINTESTINAL SYSTEM

Children with autism have a wide variety of both gastrointestinal symptoms and clear gastrointestinal pathology. The incidence of GI problems in autism is generally in the range of 30 to 40% of children. Symptomatically, the most common reports are of chronic constipation or diarrhea, and chronic abdominal pain.

GI pathology is common and widespread. One study of children with autism and GI symptoms showed that 69.4% of subjects had reflux esophagitis, 42% had chronic gastritis, and 67% had chronic duodenitis (Horvath, Papadimitriou, Rabsztyn, Drachenberg, &Tildon, 1999). It should be noted that many of these children are nonverbal and cannot express GI discomfort. These children may react to pain by exhibiting behaviors not obviously referable to the GI system, such as self-stimulation or temper tantrums.

There have been several studies demonstrating definite pathology of the small and large bowels. Torrente performed biopsies of 25 children with autism, and found duodenitis in almost all of the children. He described increased lymphocytic proliferation in both the epithelium and lamina propria (Torrente et al., 2002). Horvath also documented significant dissacharridase deficiencies in a population of children with autism and gastrointestinal symptoms (Horvath et al., 1999).

Dysbiosis, or abnormalities of gastrointestinal microflora, is also thought to be a common problem. Rosseneu (2003) analyzed 80 children with autism and GI symptoms and found that 61% had growth of abnormal aerobic gram negative endotoxin producing bacteria. It should be remembered that these aerobic gram negative bacteria are producers of endotoxin, which could cause ongoing bowel damage. Fifty-five percent had overgrowth of *Staphylococcus aureus* and 95% had overgrowth of pathogenic *E. coli*. Of note, there were no abnormal amounts of yeast noted in this study. In a fascinating pilot study, 11 of these children were treated with a non-absorbable antibiotic and not only did the abnormal flora disappear, but both GI symptoms and autistic behaviors decreased significantly. This study did not have a control group, and unfortunately, after 2 months, the abnormal bacteria returned to pretreatment levels. In another study, Vancomycin treatment of children with regressive autism and diarrhea resulted in decreased autistic behaviors as measured by blinded observers (Sandler et al., 2000).

An overgrowth of yeast is widely felt to be part of dysbiosis and responsible for many gastrointestinal and behavioral symptoms of autism, and many children are treated with antifungal agents as part of their "bowel detoxification" protocol. The evidence for this yeast overgrowth is very limited. As aforementioned, Rosseneu's study failed to identify any yeast among the abnormal bacteria, and there have been no good controlled studies evaluating yeast overgrowth in autism. Some research as shown the presence of urine organic acids suggestive of yeast overgrowth in children with autism, but the significance of these byproducts is unclear. There is widespread use of such antifungals as nystatin, fluconazole, and ketoconazole, with much anecdotal evidence of positive results, but no controlled studies.

Another gastrointestinal abnormality commonly attributed to children with autism is called the "leaky gut" phenomena or increased intestinal permeability. In a study by D'Eufemia examination of 21 autistic children with no known intestinal disorders, there was confirmed increased intestinal permeability in 43%, as opposed to none of the control group (D'Eufemia et al., 1996). Horvath examined 25 children with autism and GI symptoms using Lactulose/Mannitol testing, and found 76% had altered intestinal permeability (Horvath & Perman, 2002).

Increased intestinal permeability or "leaky gut" syndrome is a very real problem in many children with autism. This may relate to an increased incidence of food sensitivities.

FOOD SENSITIVITIES/ALLERGIES

Food sensitivities or allergies are also thought to play an important role in the pathophysiology of autism. The evidence for this is indirect, but suggestive. In one study, 36 children with autism were compared to healthy controls, and had significantly higher levels of IgA, IgG, and IgM antigen-specific antibodies for such specific food proteins as lactoglobulin, casein, and beta-lactoglobulin than did the controls (Lucarelli et al., 1995). Also, a study by Jyonouchi, Sun, and Itokazu (2002) showed that children with autism had higher intestinal levels of inflammatory cytokines directed against specific dietary proteins than did controls.

AUTOIMMUNITY

There are a number of studies that suggest that autoimmune abnormalities are very common in children with autism. Some of these can be directly linked to the central nervous system. Connolly et al. (1999) examined the sera of children with autism for antibrain antibodies. IgG antibrain antibodies were present in the sera of 27% of children and only 2% of controls. IgM antibodies were present in 36% of the sera of autistic children and in 0% of controls. Singh, Warren, Averett, and Ghaziuddin (1997) evaluated the prevalence of antibodies to various brain structures in 68 autistic children and 30 controls and found that 49% of autistic children had serum antibodies to the caudate nucleus as opposed to 0% of controls. Most recently, Cabanlit, Wills, Goines, Ashwood, and Van de Water (2007) described a significantly increased incidence of brain-specific (thalamic and hypothalamic) autoantibodies in the plasma of children with autism compared to controls. It is not clear whether these antibodies represent ongoing autoimmune neurological insult or are an epiphenomena of earlier central nervous system damage caused by other factors. As mentioned earlier, neuroanatomical studies have shown signs of chronic inflammation in the autistic brain.

An autoimmune connection is also suggested by research showing a significantly higher incidence of autoimmune disease in families of children with autism (Sweeten, Bowyer, Posey, Halberstadt & McDougle, 2003). In fact, the prevalence of autoimmunity in families with an autistic child was actually higher than in those families with a child with autoimmune disease.

The issue of whether autistic children have functional deficiencies in their immune regulation, however, is not clear. Although some studies have shown abnormalities of T cell or NK cell function, the evidence is preliminary and inconclusive at this time.

METABOLIC DISORDERS

There have been a number of studies which have demonstrated some abnormalities in the metabolic functioning of children compared to controls. One study in the *American Journal of Clinical Nutrition* demonstrated that relative to the control children, the children with autism had significantly lower baseline plasma concentrations of methionine, SAM (*S*-adenosylmethionine), homocysteine, cystathionine, cysteine, and total glutathione. They also had significantly higher concentrations of SAH (*S*-adenosylhomocysteine), adenosine, and oxidized glutathione (James et al.,

2004). This metabolic profile is consistent with impaired capacity for methylation (significantly lower ratio of SAM to SAH) and increased oxidative stress. In another study, activities of erythrocyte superoxide dismutase and erythrocyte and plasma glutathione peroxidase in autistic children were significantly lower than normal (Yorbik, Sayal, Akay, Akbiyik, & Sohmen, 2002), indicating decreased activity of antioxidant enzyme systems.

An excellent review article by McGinnis (2006) documented a number of positive markers of oxidative stress in children with autism. Among other factors, he cites such indirect markers for greater oxidative stress as (1) lower endogenous antioxidant enzymes and glulathione; (2) lower antioxidant nutrients; (3) higher organic toxins and heavy metals; (4) higher xanthine oxidase and cytokines; and (5) higher production of nitric oxide (NO), a toxic free-radical.

Both autoimmune and metabolic abnormalities, including increased markers of oxidative stress, have a higher prevalence in autistic than control children.

HEAVY METAL TOXICITY

It is a widespread belief among many clinicians and families involved in the alternative treatment of autism that increased body levels of heavy metals, especially mercury, are an important part of the pathophysiology of autism. The evidence for this is minimal. However, one study in Texas did showed a direct correlation between the incidence of autism and the amount of mercury expelled from industrial pollution (Palmer, Blanchard, Stein, Mandell & Miller, 2006). In fact, for each 1000 pounds of environmentally released mercury, there was a 43% increase in the rate of special education services and a 61% increase in the rate of autism.

Although there is not room here for an in-depth discussion of the tremendous increase in the prevalence of autism and ADHD over the last 25 years, the role of environmental toxin exposure cannot be overlooked. Not only has lead been definitively shown to cause developmental problems, even at levels previously thought to be safe, but there is strong evidence that environmental mercury, polychlorinated biphenyls, and other environmental toxins may have significant developmental impact (Stein, Schettler, Wallinga, & Valenti, 2002). The concern about mercury is also linked to the assumption that the thimerosal contained in, and later withdrawn from, infant immunizations, is a major factor in the rise in autism prevalence. Since children with autism are likely not exposed to more mercury or other heavy metals than other children, it is postulated that these children have impaired abilities to detoxify or excrete mercury and other heavy metals. This is thought to be due to the various methylation, sulfation, and antioxidant deficiencies discussed previously.

What is the evidence that there is specifically an increased body burden of mercury and other heavy metals in children with autism? There is surprisingly little. One of the problems in discussing heavy metal toxicity is that there are no simple tests for determining body levels of heavy metals. Blood tests for mercury are not useful because mercury remains in the tissues and not the circulation. Hair analysis has been used, but it is not clear that these tests adequately reflect body burdens of mercury. In conventional toxicology, mercury toxicity is measured by giving a dose of a chelating agent, such as EDTA or DMSA, and then measuring urine mercury levels. There is no significant body of data using this procedure to compare autistic children and controls. One study compared blood and hair levels of autistic children with those of controls and found no significant differences. It should be noted that this did not examine urine levels after chelation (Ip, Wong, Ho, Lee, & Wong, 2004). A study by Adams did show that children with autism had significantly higher levels of mercury in their baby teeth than typically developing children (Adams, Romdalvik, Ramanujam, & Legator, 2007). Bradstreet et al. (2003) performed a retrospective analysis of 221 children and 18 controls that had been treated with 3 doses of DMSA. Heavy metal concentrations in the urine were then analyzed, showing urinary concentrations of mercury were significantly higher in the 221 autistic children than in the 18 controls. Limitations of this study were that it was a retrospective study with non-random selection of controls, and that the imbalance between the number of cases and the control group was very large. Selection bias is a concern for both the controls and autistic children.

In summary, although it is clear that mercury is a potent neurotoxin, especially in the developing brain, the idea that mercury exposure is a significant cause of autism is at this point largely unproven. There is need of a prospective study comparing post-chelation urinary heavy metal levels in autistic children as compared to controls. In addition, chelation therapy is widely recommended by biomedical practitioners for children with autism, based on the assumption that removing these metals will result in improvement in autistic symptoms. There is no scientific support for this contention at this point in time. It should be noted that there are possible electrolyte imbalances that could accompany chelation therapy, and if used at all, should be done carefully under the direction of an experienced practitioner.

Although it is possible that prenatal or postnatal exposure to mercury and other environmental toxins may play a role in the development of autism, there is no good evidence of the efficacy of chelation therapy.

Nutritional Deficiencies

It is a tenet of the biomedical approach that nutritional deficiencies are widespread and important in autism. It is thought that these are mainly linked to poor digestion and absorption of nutrients due to the aforementioned gastrointestinal problems, as well as abnormalities in the metabolic processing of nutrients. The evidence for these nutritional deficiencies however, is somewhat uneven and rarely complete. The most convincing area is that of omega-3 fatty acids.

OMEGA-3 FATTY ACID DEFICIENCY

Vancassel et al. (2001) evaluated levels of omega-3 fatty acids and other polyunsaturated fatty acids in the serum of children with autism compared to controls. Children with autism had 23% lower levels of plasma omega-3 fatty acids than did controls. Autistic children also had 20% lower levels of plasma polyunsaturated fatty acids compared with the controls. Bell found that children with autism had both increased signs of clinical fatty acid deficiencies and abnormalities of RBC membrane Omega-3 fatty acid levels (Bell et al., 2004).

The reason for this is unclear. Since there is no evidence that children with autism have different levels of omega-3 fat intake than control children, one would have to postulate a difference in digestion, absorption, or metabolism. As will be discussed below, children with ADHD have similar omega-3 abnormalities, as well as patients with other neurodevelopmental disorders.

There is good evidence that children with autism have a deficiency of omega-3 fatty acids.

Integrative Therapies for Autism

CONVENTIONAL BEHAVIORAL APPROACHES

Speech therapy is almost universally recommended to deal with the language deficits of children with autism. Anecdotally, it is felt to be effective by almost all parents and most professionals. However, there is surprisingly little solid research supporting the efficacy of speech therapy for autism. Although some studies have shown specific areas of language improvement, there are no good randomized and controlled studies.

Intensive behavioral therapy is also employed therapy for children with autism. In this type of therapy, direct behavioral intervention by trained facilitators occurs in home and school settings from 20 to 40 hours a week. There are a number of specific methods, such as Lovas, Floortime, and Applied Behavior Analysis. Intervention is directed at increasing appropriate social and language behavior while decreasing self-stimulatory activities. A 2003 review in the *Canadian Journal of Psychiatry* concluded that "delivering interventions for more than 20 hours weekly that are individualized, well planned, and target language development and other areas of skill development significantly increases children's developmental rates, especially in language, compared with no or minimal treatment" (Bryson, Rogers, & Fombonne, 2003).

ALTERNATIVE BEHAVIORAL APPROACHES

Another modality commonly employed with children with autism is sensory integration therapy. It is clear that children with autism have significant sensory issues. They often do not enjoy touching, can be upset by noisy environments, and exhibit other sensory difficulties. Sensory integration therapy is often recommended to reduce the intensity of these problems. This usually involves a variety of sensory stimuli administered under controlled conditions. As with the above therapies, there is only anecdotal evidence of effectiveness. There have been a number of small studies, but any evidence of efficacy is preliminary at best.

A second alternative behavioral modality is auditory integration therapy. This is based on the idea that abnormalities in auditory processing contribute significantly to the difficulties of autistic children. Essentially, auditory integration therapy attempts to reprogram and "integrate" the auditory system by sending specific randomized and filtered sound frequencies through earphones worn by the autistic child. This is usually done in 20 thirty-minute sessions over a period of 10 days or so. There are many anecdotal reports of efficacy, but studies so far are uncontrolled or are limited to very small numbers A systematic review of the few controlled studies showed equivocal results and found insufficient evidence to support its use (Sinha, Silove, Wheeler, & Williams, 2006).

Nutrition

DIETARY INTERVENTIONS

The gluten-free casein-free (GFCF) diet is the most common biomedical intervention employed in children with autism. The rationale for this approach is the belief that food sensitivities, especially to gluten and casein are common in autism. These sensitivities can then produce, not only gastrointestinal symptoms, but gut inflammation and increased intestinal permeability ("leaky gut"). The ensuing exposure to foreign proteins is believed to lead to many of the neurological and behavioral manifestations of autism. In general, for the GFCF diet, parents are advised to strictly avoid all foods containing gluten or casein for periods of 60 days or more.

The anecdotal evidence for the efficacy is abundant. In various support groups, listservs, and other situations bringing together parents of children with autism, the GFCF diet is often described as promoting significant positive changes in gastrointestinal symptoms, language, socialization, and other autistic behaviors.

The research evidence is limited. There are only two controlled studies of the gluten-free, casein-free diet in the treatment of autism, but both showed positive results. In the first study, by Knivsberg, ten matched pairs of children with autism were randomized to a GFCF diet or a placebo control for one full year (Knivsberg, Reichelt, Hoien, &

Nødland, 2002). Behaviors were then evaluated by blinded observers using the DIPAB, a Danish instrument for measuring autistic traits. Post-intervention, the diet group had a mean DIPAB rating of 5.60, significantly (p = 0.001) better than the control group rating of 11.20. Specifically, social contact increased in 10 of 15 of the treated children, while ritualistic behaviors in that group decreased in 8 of 11 children. In the second study, by Lucarelli, autistic children were found to have decreased behavioral symptoms after 8 weeks on a dairy elimination diet (Lucarelli et al., 1995).

It can be difficult to balance the enthusiasm for this diet with the limited evidence. One problem is that the GFCF diet is often started in conjunction with a number of nutritional supplements and other interventions, making it difficult to know if behavioral or other improvements can be clearly attributed to the diet. Although it is a difficult diet in terms of parental time and energy, there should little adverse effect if nutritional status, particularly weight and calcium intake, is monitored.

Although there is much anecdotal evidence of the efficacy of the GFCF diet for autism, research is limited. If recommended, it should be done when no other interventions are introduced.

SUPPLEMENTS

There are many nutritional supplements used in the treatment of autism, including omega-3 fatty acids, probiotics, zinc, vitamin B-6, and other multivitamin and mineral supplements.

OMEGA-3 FATTY ACIDS

Omega-3 fatty acids are widely used in the treatment of autism. The evidence for their use is not robust but is the results are encouraging. In a pilot study, 18 children were given an omega-3 fatty acid supplement (with 247 mg of omega-3s and 40 mg of omega-6s) for 3 months (Patrick & Salik, 2005). Their language skills were measured at baseline, and again after the three-month trial. There was a highly significant increase in language skills over a wide variety of measures. Next, a randomized double-blind placebo-controlled study evaluated the effects of 1.5 mg total omega-3 fatty acids on children with autistic disorders accompanied by severe tantrums, aggression, or self-injurious behavior (Amminger et al., 2007). This study, although small, did show significant advantages of omega-3s over placebos.

Another study of relevance concerned the use of omega-3 fatty acids in developmental coordination disorder (DCD) (Richardson & Montgomery, 2005). While not part of the autistic spectrum, DCD is relevant because children with this disorder present with some of the features of autism spectrum disorders. In this double-blind controlled trial,

117 children were given either an omega-3 fatty acid supplement or placebo for three months. Treated children made startling gains in reading, spelling, and mathematical skills compared to the placebo group. For example, the average reading scores in the treatment group advanced 9.5 months in 3 months, as opposed to an increase of 3.5 months in the placebo group.

It should be noted that there are no well-accepted guidelines for the dosage of omega-3 fatty acids or the optimal ratio of DHA and EPA. Given the relatively low cost and safety of this intervention, it seems a reasonable approach, although it is clear that much more research is needed.

> There is good evidence that children with autism have a deficiency of omega-3 fatty acids and suggestive evidence that omega-3 supplementation can be helpful in autism. Given the high safety profile, this seems a reasonable intervention.

PROBIOTICS

Probiotics are used frequently in the biomedical treatment of autism. As discussed previously, it is speculated that children with autism have abnormal gut flora, as well as increased intestinal permeability. Unfortunately, treatment with antibiotics for presumed bowel bacterial overgrowth seems to result in only temporary changes in bowel flora. Probiotics are recommended in the hopes of normalizing bowel flora as well as healing the inflamed intestinal lining. Again, despite widespread use and anecdotal reports of efficacy, there have been no well-designed studies concerning the impact of probiotics in the treatment of autism.

ZINC

Zinc is one of the most widely recommended single minerals for children with autism. Much of the rationale for its use is based on research by Dr. William Walsh of the Pfeiffer Institute in Chicago, who found that copper to zinc ratios were increased in over 85% of children with autism (Walsh, 2003). He also found that a dysfunction of metallothionein, a protein involved in the regulation of these and other metals, was present in 99% of 503 autistic children. Unfortunately, this research was published by the Pfeiffer Institute only and not in any peer-reviewed journals. There are, at this point, no controlled studies indicating the efficacy and safety of zinc supplementation in the treatment of autism.

METABOLIC INTERVENTIONS

There are a number of metabolic interventions that are intended to treat presumed defects in methylation, sulfation, and other metabolic processes. These include the use of methylcobolamin (methyl-B12), folic acid derivatives (folinic acid), and trimethylglycine (TMG) or dimethylglycine (DMG). While one study did demonstrate correction of abnormal laboratory values of metabolic factors in autistic children, there has been no published randomized controlled trial to date demonstrating safety and efficacy of these interventions. This is an area ripe for well-designed intervention trials, especially as there is some evidence that children with autism and their families may, in fact, have an increased frequency compared with the general population of single nucleotide polymorphisms in the methylenetetrahydrofolate reductase (MTHFR) and other methylation genes (James et al., 2006).

OTHER CAM THERAPIES

Complementary therapies such as homeopathy, craniosacral therapy and other manipulative therapies, Reiki and other energy medicine modalities, biofeedback, and traditional Chinese medicine have all been employed. There are scattered anecdotal reports of efficacy, but no research evidence exists to support their use in the treatment of autism.

ADHD

CONVENTIONAL APPROACH

ADHD is a developmental disorder consisting of difficulties with attention, distractibility and impulsivity. It is felt to be a disorder of executive dysfunction, with imaging studies showing abnormalities in the prefrontal cortex and other areas. Dopamine and norepinephrine are the main neurotransmitters suspected in the pathophysiology, and are the ones most affected by stimulant treatment. The most recent evidence is that ADHD is not a single disorder with a single dysfunction, but a multifaceted syndrome related to various genetic, biologic, environmental, and psychosocial factors. One recent study showed that cortical development in the prefrontal cortex in children with ADHD showed a 3-year delay compared with controls but normalized after that time, "suggesting that ADHD is characterized by delay rather than deviance in cortical maturation" (Shaw et al., 2007). Conventional treatment is classically based on a combination of behaviormanagement and pharmacotherapy, usually the long-term use of stimulants such as methylphenidate and dextroamphetamine and their derivatives. An estimated 2.5 million children currently are currently taking stimulants in the United States (Nissen, 2006). Many studies have shown these medications to be effective in reducing ADHD symptoms in the short term but there are few longer term studies. The MMTA study is the longest study to have followed children over time (Satterfield et al., 2007). Assigned to one of four groups, 579 children were evaluated for intensive multicomponent behavior therapy (Beh), intensive medication management (MedMgt), the combination (Comb), and routine community care (CC). At 14 months, the two medicated groups improved significantly compared to the other groups. At that time, the study became observational only. At 24 months there was still benefit, although much less robust. However, a recent update showed that at 3 years all groups showed improvement over time, but treatment groups did not differ significantly on any measure at 36 months.

Adverse effects of stimulants occur in up to 30% of children with ADHD, commonly including gastrointestinal symptoms, decreased appetite, headaches, tics, and sleep problems (Schachter, Pham, King, Langford, & Moher, 2001). Some parents also complain of more subtle side-effects such as "teariness," decreased joy or enthusiasm, irritability, or that their child "is just not himself or herself." These latter effects have not been formally researched. A recent FDA advisory panel recommended that a warning be issued for stimulants because of the substantial risk of hallucinations in children, which were estimated to be between 2% and 5% (New warning about ADHD drug, 2005).

Although stimulants are generally effective in the short term, there remain questions about long-term efficacy, and significant side effects are common.

The frequency of the use complementary or alternative medicine in children with ADHD is high. Although studies have varied, the most recent two studies have shown frequency of use of 64% and 67% respectively (Sinha & Efron, 2005; Siubberlield, Wray, & Parry, 1999). Modified diet, vitamin and nutritional supplements, and herbal therapies were the most common treatments used. Parental discomfort with children being on long-term stimulant medication and the fear of serious side-effects are among the most common reasons for seeking alternative care. Unfortunately, there are hundreds of products available over the Internet and elsewhere which purport to treat or even cure ADHD. Most of these have little or no research documenting their safety or efficacy. This emphasizes the need for health professionals to become familiar with both an integrative approach to ADHD and to the various CAM treatments available.

INTEGRATIVE APPROACH

An integrative approach to the problem of ADHD begins with a thorough assessment both of the child as an individual, and of his relationship to the family, school, and community. It is essential that a practitioner take the time to talk to the child and parents, alone and together, as well as teachers, counselors, and other relevant persons. Standardized evaluation forms such as the Conners or Vanderbilt are necessary but never sufficient to make the diagnosis. This type of assessment will avoid the common pitfall of misdiagnosing ADHD in children with such conditions as depression, anxiety, sleep apnea, a difficult temperament, learning disabilities, and giftedness. Sometimes, the problem can be as simple as a misfit between a child and his or her teacher or school. It should be remembered that such factors as parental depression, marital discord, or any abusive relationship could play a major role in both diagnosis and treatment options.

Given confirmation of the diagnosis of ADHD what would be involved in a truly integrative approach to the problem? Before considering the various nutritional and CAM therapies available, it is important to emphasize that the child is not just a patient with ADHD, but a person with a unique set of strengths and challenges, both of which are highly effected by his or her physical and emotional environment. An integrative treatment plan should aim as much at supporting the child's strengths and optimizing his family and social environment as it does at identifying and treating his individual weaknesses.

A thorough evaluation of the child in the context of his family school and community is essential to making the diagnosis of ADHD. Standardized questionnaires are only a small part of the assessment.

DIETARY MODIFICATIONS AND FOOD SENSITIVITIES

Nutritional interventions are the most common alternative to stimulants. They are generally based on the assumption that children may be allergic or sensitive to some food protein, sugar, or additive, and that this sensitivity causes changes in behavior. Most professionals and families do not feel that these nutritional issues are the sole cause of ADHD, but that they can have significant impact on the severity of symptoms.

The first important attempt at nutritional intervention in ADHD was the Feingold diet (Feingold, 1975). In 1973, Feingold published his study claiming that 50% of treated children improved after elimination of all food colorings and naturally occurring salicylates. This required the elimination of almost all processed foods and many fruits and vegetables. Despite its difficulty, this became an extremely popular diet. However, the results of subsequent research were mixed, failing to validate these findings in many cases. A thorough review of these by Wender reaches the conclusion that the Feingold diet is most likely effective for, at most, a small percentage of children with ADHD (Wender, 1986). The Feingold diet, now called the Feingold program, is still quite popular, but focuses mainly on the elimination of artificial colors, flavors, sweeteners, and certain preservatives with most natural salicylates eventually added back to the diet.

However other more focused studies on artificial colors, flavors, and preservatives demonstrate that these substances can definitely have an impact on ADHD or hyperactive behavior. Bateman, in 2004, studied 273 three-year-olds with hyperactivity. After an initial washout period, they were given a drink with either food coloring and sodium benzoate or placebo (Bateman et al., 2004). There was a statistically significant increase in hyperactivity in those given the active substance compared to placebo. McCann et al. (2007) completed a double-blind, placebo-controlled study examining effects of artificial food coloring and additives (AFCAs) on hyperactive behavior in 3- to 4-year-old and 8- to 9-year-old children from the general population. All children had AFCAs removed from their diet for the 6-week trial and then consumed either AFCA drinks or placebo. There was increased global hyperactivity in the 3- to 4-year-olds and the 8- to 9-year-olds after consuming the AFCAs.

Other investigators have examined the role of allergy or sensitivity to certain foods ADHD. Egger, Carter, Graham, Gumley, and Soothill (1985) placed 76 children on an oligoantigenic or "few foods" diet in an open label trial, and 62 of these children improved. In the second, double-blinded placebo-controlled phase of the study, those children who reacted demonstrated significantly increased ADHD symptoms when given the actual offending foods compared to placebo. Carter et al. (1993) performed a very similar study with 59 of 78 children improving during the open trial and a positive result in the double blind aspect of the trial. Boris and Mandel (1994) employed a similar research design and the results were again significant. Interestingly, in all cases, artificial colors and flavors were among the most common offenders.

There is good evidence that food sensitivities, especially to artificial colors and flavors, may play a role in the pathophysiology of ADHD.

The role of sugar is an area of controversy. Although many parents of children with and without ADHD notice adverse or hyperactive reactions to large amounts of sugar, research has not substantiated this connection. An excellent review of these studies by Scholl, Burshteyn, and Cea-Aravena (2003) addresses this issue and points out some methodological limitations that may be responsible for some negative studies.

For parents and practitioners attempting to determine if food sensitivities are provoking or worsening ADHD symptoms, there are many practical difficulties. The oligoantigenic diet described is very difficult and impractical for most families. Some practitioners use some type of modified elimination diet, eliminating the most common food allergens, (such as wheat, dairy, corn, soy, chocolate, nuts, and citrus) as well as artificial colors and flavors and preservatives, for some period of time. The foods are then reintroduced one by one. One can attempt to eliminate foods one at a time, but if there is more than one food sensitivity, the effect can be attenuated. The use of food allergy testing is common, but even the more reliable IgE tests may not be specific or sensitive enough to predict behavioral food reactions. IgG and other "alternative" food testing has minimal research to justify its use.

An interesting area is that of the relationship of the glycemic index to hyperactive behavior. Although no studies have examined this issue, it makes sense that children who eat foods high on the glycemic index may have volatile blood sugar levels which are reflected in their behavior. As Dr. David Ludwig of Boston's Children Hospital states, "A child eats a breakfast that has no fat, no protein, and a high glycemic index— let's say a bagel with fat-free cream cheese. His blood sugar goes up, but pretty soon it crashes, which triggers the release of stress hormones like adrenaline. What you're left with, at around 10 am, is a kid with low blood sugar and lots of adrenaline circulating in his bloodstream. He's jittery and fidgety and not paying attention. That's going to look an awful lot like ADHD to his teacher" (Scholastic Parent & Child, 2007). This is an area in need of significant research, given the dietary habits of many American children.

Nutritional supplements

OMEGA-3 FATTY ACIDS

Omega-3 fatty acids are the most used and well-researched nutritional supplements in the treatment of children with ADHD. These are essential fatty acids, so termed because the human body cannot synthesize them and thus they must be supplied in the diet. Omega-3 fatty acids, eicosapentaenoic acid (EPA) and docosahexaenoic acid (DHA), have a number of important functions, one of which is that they are essential to normal brain development and function. A growing body of research indicates that children with ADHD may have low levels of omega-3 fatty acids (Burgess, Stevens, Zhang, & Peck, 2000).

A number of studies have looked at the treatment of ADHD with omega-3 fatty acid supplementation. Overall, these results have been positive, as detailed in a review by Richardson in 2006. In one study (Richardson, 2006), children with ADHD and learning disabilities were given omega-3s or placebo for 12 weeks, and those in the active treatment group had impressive improvements compared to placebo in all areas of ADHD (Richardson & Puri Basant, 2002). In a 2007 study by Sinn, 132 children were given either omega 3s(with GLA), the same supplement with micronutrients, or placebo (Sinn, & Bryan, 2007). There were statistically significant improvements in the treatment groups versus the placebo, but no extra benefit of adding micronutrients. Given the relative safety of omega-3s, and the positive research findings, this would seem a very reasonable intervention. The total required dosage of omega-3 and the optimal ratio of DHA/EPA are not yet clearly delineated. Most studies use a combination of DHA and EPA, often up to 1000mg of total DHA and EPA.

As with autism, there is reasonable evidence that omega-3 fatty acid deficiency is common in ADHD and that supplementation may be effective.

ZINC AND FERRITIN

Although a number of individual vitamins and minerals are used empirically in the treatment of ADHD, there has been little research in this area for the role of zinc, which has shown promise in several studies. In one, Zinc reduced hyperactivity impulsivity and socialization in ADHD children, but did not reduce inattention (Bilici et al., 2004). In another, adding zinc to methylphenidate treatment showed a statistically significant improvement over methylphenidate alone (Akhondzadeh, Mohammadi, & Khademi, 2004). In a 2005 study, serum zinc levels correlated positively with inattention in a group of American children with ADHD (Arnold et al., 2005).

There have several studies about the role of iron in ADHD. Konofal showed that children who have ADHD had lower serum ferritin levels than children without ADHD and that the severity of symptoms correlated with low ferritin levels (Sever, Ashkenazi, Tyano, & Weizman, 1997). These children were not anemic. In an open-label study, iron supplementation was found to improve symptoms of ADHD in non-anemic children; however as of yet there are no controlled studies of iron treatment for ADHD (Lozoff & Georgieff, 2006). Lozoff and others have shown that there are negative cognitive and neurophysiologic correlates to iron-deficiency anemia in infancy, which may not resolve with later treatment (Lozoff & Georgieff, 2006). From a global perspective, Galler has shown a higher incidence of deficits in attention, as well as intelligence quotient, in children who had malnutrition as infants (Galler, Ramsey, Morley, Archer, & Salt, 1990).

There are no good studies confirming the effectiveness of any other vitamins or minerals in the treatment of ADHD.

Electroencephalographic Biofeedback

Electroencephalographic biofeedback is a fascinating area of research and treatment for ADHD. It is based on the principle that the EEG pattern of children with ADHD is quantitatively different than of children without ADHD, generally showing hypoarousal (with a decreased ratio of beta to theta waves) or sometimes hyperarousal. In one study, EEG analysis was over 85% sensitive and specific in distinguishing ADHD from non-ADHD children (Chabot, Merkin, Wood, Davenport, & Serfontein, 1996). EEG biofeedback or neurofeedback uses a series of sessions, usually 30 to 50, to teach patients to alter their quantitative EEG to a more normal pattern. This is usually done using positive reinforcement in a video game or other format.

There have been a number of controlled trials of EEG neurofeedback in ADHD, most reporting positive results (Butnik, 2005; Fuchs, Birbaumer, Lutzenberger, Gruzelier & Kaiser, 2003). However, other researchers point out significant methodological flaws to most of the studies, including small numbers, especially the lack of randomized assignment to treatment group and suitable control groups (Sandra & Russell, 2005). Since the children are receiving many hours of direct therapist time, wait-list controls or others not receiving similar attention may not be adequate. When neurofeedback is successful, it is unclear how well it generalizes to school and home situations and for how long. At this point, it would be fair to say that from a scientific standpoint, neurofeedback is a promising but not proven treatment for ADHD. From a practical point of view, the time commitment and financial cost is substantial. However, if successful, the benefits of long-term improvement without pharmaceutical treatment would be significant.

Homeopathy

There have been a number of studies of homeopathy for the treatment of ADHD, many of them showing positive results, but only three randomized, controlled trials in the literature. Strauss reported improvement in treated patients versus placebo in children both taking and not taking methylphenidate (Strauss, 2000). A limitation of this study is that there were only five children in each group. Frei did a larger randomized placebo-controlled crossover study with 62 children who had responded to an initial open trial of homeopathy, and found significant improvement in the treated versus placebo group (Frei et al., 2005). On the other hand, in another randomized trial, Jacobs found no difference between a placebo group and those treated with homeopathy (Jacobs, Williams, Girard, Njike, & Katz, 2005). The placebo children in this trial had a full homeopathic consult, the non-specific effect of which may have obscured the difference between groups.

Overall, given the relatively high safety and reasonable cost, homeopathic treatment is a reasonable alternative for those patients who are interested.

Traditional Chinese Medicine

Although no research trials of TCM appear in the usually reviewed medical journals, there have been a number of research studies concerning the treatment of ADHD with both acupuncture and Chinese herbal medicine. Several successful open trials were reported by Arnold in his 2001 review in the *Annals of the New York Academy of Sciences* (Arnold, 2001). In a Townsend Newsletter of 2003, Flaws describes six studies of TCM herbal treatment and acupuncture, some open and using methylphenidate treatment as a control group (Flaws, 2003). All of these showed effectiveness of the TCM modalities. These are not randomized studies and research protocols in China may not meet current western standards, but this information indicates the possibility that TCM may be an effective modality and should be investigated more thoroughly.

Botanicals

There are a number of botanical products that have been used in the treatment of ADHD, but there are only three for which there is at least some scientific research. One open label study of a combination of ginkgo biloba and panax quinquefolius showed improvements in ADHD symptoms after 4 weeks of treatment (Lyon, Cline, Totosy de Zepetnek, Shan Pang, & Benishin, 2001). Since both of these herbs are known to have nootropic effects to improve memory and learning, there is a biological justification to their use. However without any control group, one cannot draw conclusions about efficacy.

Pycnogenol, a standardized extract from the French Maritime pine tree (*Pinus pinaster*) is widely touted as an effective treatment for ADHD. After some positive case reports innon-randomized trials, Trebatická, in the *European Journal of Pediatrics* (2006) conducted a randomized, placebo-controlled and double-blind study of pycnogenol in 61 children with ADHD (Trebatická et al., 2006). After 4 weeks of treatment, the treatment group improved significantly compared to placebo. One month after treatment was discontinued, symptoms returned to baseline. The mechanism of action of pycnogenol is proposed to be increased production of nitric oxide, which regulates dopamine and norepinephrine release and uptake.

The third herbal product with research support is a combination of valerian and lemon-balm. Both of these herbs are widely known for their relaxant effects. In a study by Muller (2006), 918 children with hyperkinesis and dyssomnia were treated with for 4 weeks with "Euvagel" a combination of valerian and lemon balm. Seventy percent of children with hyperkinesis and 80% with insomnia improved significantly. There were no significant adverse effects. There was, however, no control group. Also, the children had some combination of hyperkinesis and dyssomnia, not ADHD. There was no assessment of any symptoms related to concentration or distractibility.

Other Interventions

One small controlled trial of yoga for children with ADHD showed improvements in some of the variables tested but not others (Jensen & Kenny, 2004). The study was probably underpowered and needs to be repeated with a larger group. In another adolescents were randomized to massage therapy or simply relaxation therapy (Khilnani, Field, Hernandez-Reif, & Schanberg 2003). Both groups improved, but there was no significant difference between the groups.

A recent book by Louv (2005) made the claim that lack of nature and green space is responsible for ADHD and other mental health disorders, coining the term "nature deficit disorder." This was based on anecdotal evidence only. However in a recent study by Kuo on this same topic, 450 parents completed a survey on the effects of "green" or non-green activities on the behavior of their children with ADHD (Kuo, & Taylor, 2004). There was a significant tendency for the green activities to result in decreased

ADHD symptoms. Although this study clearly has limitations, it suggests a possible role for nature or natural settings which should be tested by more rigorous research.

An Integrative Approach to Sleep Problems in Children

Sleep problems are quite common in children, with 20%–30% of children from infancy to adolescence having sleep disorders (Meltzer & Mindell, 2006; Mindell, Kuhn, Lewin, Meltzer, & Sadeh, 2006). Infants and younger children tend to have problems with bedtime or nighttime awakening, while in adolescence changes in circadian rhythms and increased societal stress often result in sleep-onset insomnia and inadequate total sleep. These sleep problems can have serious health-related consequences for both these children and their families. Children with disturbed sleep have been shown to have poorer school performance, poorer function on tests of neurobehavioral function (including attentional issues), abnormal mood regulation, more health-related problems, and decreased overall quality of life (Dahl & Lewin, 2002; Mindell et al., 2006). Parents of children with sleep problems have also shown to have higher incidences of depression and poorer family functioning.

Although pharmaceutical interventions can be effective for sleep, they have a number of drawbacks, including alterations of normal sleep architecture, residual effects on cognitive functioning, physiologic side-effects, and the development of tolerance. An integrative approach would examine the problem in the context of the child, family, and community, and use a range of behavioral and other non-pharmaceutical treatments with less potential for harm.

BEHAVIORAL METHODS

Most sleep problems in babies and young children are problems of bedtime difficulties, delayed sleep-onset, and nighttime awakenings (excluding obstructive sleep apnea, a non-behavioral sleep problem usually requiring surgical intervention). These are highly amenable to relatively simple behavioral interventions which, on the whole, are aimed at redefining the bedtime and sleep environment, especially as regards the parental regulation of and response to the child's sleep. These interventions, which include standardized bedtime routines, sleep hygiene, extinction, graduated extinction (i.e., the Ferber method) and others have been shown to have very high overall success. In fact, one review of 52 studies showed an across-the-board efficacy rate of 80% for behavioral treatment of sleep disorders of infants and young children (Tuchman, 2006). Therefore, in this age group, behavioral interventions should always be the first line of approach.

Adolescent sleep disorders tend to be those of an altered Circadian rhythm leading to later sleep onset and awakening. In itself, this would not be a problem, but the early awakening demanded by school schedules results in decreased sleep and overall sleep debt. This can have an impact on mood, attention, memory, behavior, and academic performance (Ozonoff et al., 2005). Behavioral intervention in adolescence would be based on regulation of sleep hygiene, and perhaps, on a community level, of changing school hours to account for these physiological differences. Most sleep problems, especially in younger children, will respond very well to relatively simple behavioral interventions.

MIND-BODY INTERVENTIONS

Mind-body interventions such as self-hypnosis, guided imagery, and relaxation are used by many practitioners with great effectiveness. There are a number of case reports, but no controlled studies addressing this issue in children. This is, however, an intervention with almost no risk of harm, reasonable cost, and the potential to solve sleep problems by allowing the child to draw upon his or her own resources. In my own practice and those of my colleagues, I have seen long-term sleep problems resolve with one teaching session accompanied by an audiotape sent home for practice.

Music therapy has long been used informally by parents, and formally by practitioners to treat sleep disorders. In one study, music therapy was compared to chloral hydrate for the purpose of inducing sleep in children about to have an EEG (Loewy, Hallan, Friedman, & Martinez, 2006). Ninety percent of the children were successfully sedated with music therapy without additional intervention, as opposed to only 50% of those treated with chloral hydrate.

BOTANICALS

There are many botanicals which have been used to treat sleep disorders. I will focus on those of well-established safety; valerian, lemon balm, and German chamomile. All of the above have been used for centuries for relaxation and insomnia, and all are on the US GRAS (Generally Recognized as Safe) list in the amounts usually found in foods. Short-term studies have shown safety in all of the above, but no long-term studies in children are available (Natural Medicines Comprehensive Data Base).

A number of studies have shown that valerian is effective for sleep disorders in both adults and children. In the previously cited study in the ADHD section, a valerian lemon-balm combination was shown to improve dyssomnia as well as hyperkinesis in children with both problems (Muller, 2006). In another small, placebo-controlled study in children with intellectual deficits, valerian reduced sleep latency, increased total sleep time, and improved total quality of sleep (Francis & Dempster, 2002). Numerous studies have demonstrated that valerian has no negative behavioral effects during waking hours. However, many practitioners do not appreciate that it usually takes 7 to 28 days for the full effect of valerian to occur, making it a more useful long-term than short-term treatment. Its rather unpleasant smell and taste can also be a limiting factor.

Chamomile has been used effectively for infants with colic in at least two studies, but it is unclear if this is related to a sedative or a gastrointestinal effect (Gardiner, 2007). There are no studies of chamomile as a treatment for insomnia in children.

Aromatherapy is often felt to be effective in the treatment of insomnia, lavender being one of the more commonly used oils. A single-blind randomized study in middle-aged adults showed good efficacy for mild insomnia, as did another study with college-age females, but there have been no studies in children (Lee & Lee, 2006; Lewith, Godfrey, & Prescott, 2005).

MELATONIN

Melatonin is commonly used in the treatment of sleep disorders in children. Several studies have shown it to be effective in both normal children and those with developmental disorders (Pillar et al., 2000; Ross, Davies & Whitehouse, 2002; Smits et al., 2003). Although only 0.1 to 0.3 mg of melatonin would replicate naturally occurring peak melatonin levels, most studies have used 1 to 5 mg/dose. Melatonin appears to be safe in children at these doses in the short term, however, there are no long-term safety studies. Melatonin has many non-sleep related functions, including a role in gonadal development and immunity, and it should not be assumed that there cannot be long-term safety issues. Melatonin appears to be a safe and effective treatment for pediatric sleep problems on a short-term basis. There is no safety data for long-term treatment.

Conclusion

For both autism and ADHD, here are a number of treatment modalities that can be part of an integrative approach. Although few of these have been definitively proven to be efficacious, many show promise and have very low potential for harm. Thus, while further research proceeds, it seems reasonable for physicians to become aware of these various approaches and be willing to discuss, recommend, or monitor them in those families who so desire. Sleep problems are predminent in our children and may have significant behavioral consequences. Behavioral interventions are often effective, and can be supplemented with several effective non-pharmacologic approaches.

Oxford Chapter Autism Case

David is a 3-year-old boy who comes to see you after being recently diagnosed with autism by a pediatric neurologist. His parents state that they were told that speech and occupational therapy were the only viable therapeutic options, along with a special preschool. His parents are distraught and wonder if there is anything else that can be done.

Pregnancy and delivery: He was the product of a normal pregnancy. Delivery was somewhat complicated by a tight nuccal cord and a difficult vacuum extraction, but Apgars were 6 and 8 and his neonatal course was benign.

Development:
—Never developed any language.
—No words, only occasional babbling. Seems to understand some language—No hx regression
—Gross fine motor WNL; mildly delayed fine motor.
—Minimal eye contact, frequent flapping and staring at lights.

PMH
—He was a very colicky infant who was treated early for gastroesophageal reflux. Several formula changes were attempted and he ended up on Nutramigen until 1 year old. However he seemed to be able to tolerate milk after that.
—David has had chronic loose to watery stools his entire life. Parents were assured these were normal for his age.
—Chronic nasal congestion with multiple ear infections treated with antibiotics.

Diet
—Very picky eater. Likes "white" foods, especially macaroni and cheese and bread.
—Rarely eats fruits and vegetables.

ROS
Nose—chronic congestion.
Abdomen—watery stools, sometimes appears to be experiencing abdominal pain.
Skin—dry, intermittent eczema.

Relevant PE
General—little eye contact, frequent flapping, no spontaneous language, some echolalia.
Eyes—prominent allergic shiners.
Nose—congested.
Skin-dry, with eczematous patches.

Neuro-Gross motor normal (nl), fine motor delayed, no focal findings.

Questions
1. What treatments would you recommend for this child?
2. Do you think some type of elimination diet would be helpful?
3. What supplements could be useful?
4. Besides a biomedical approach, are there other CAM therapies that might be worth trying?

REFERENCES

Adams, J. B., Romdalvik, J., Ramanujam, V. M., & Legator M. S. (2007). Mercury, lead, and zinc in baby teeth of children with autism versus controls. *Journal of Toxicology and Environmental Health A, 70*(12), 1046–1051.

Akhondzadeh, S., Mohammadi, M. R., & Khademi M. (2004). Zinc sulfate as an adjunct to methylphenidate for the treatment of attention deficit hyperactivity disorder in children: A double blind and randomized trial [ISRCTN64132371]. *BMC Psychiatry, 4*(1), 9.

Amminger, G. P., Berger, G. E., Schafer, M. R., Klier C., Friedrich M. H., & Feucht M. (2007). Omega-3 fatty acids supplementation in children with autism: A double-blind randomized, placebo-controlled pilot study. *Biol Psychiatry, 61*(4), 551–553.

Arnold, L. (2001). Alternative treatments for adults with attention-deficit hyperactivity disorder (ADHD). *Annals of the New York Academy of Sciences, 931*, 310–341.

Arnold, L. E., Bozzolo, H., Hollway, J., Cook, A., DiSilvestro, R. A., Bozzolo, D. R., et al. (2005). Serum zinc correlates with parent- and teacher-rated inattention in children with attention-deficit/hyperactivity disorder. *Journal of Child & Adolescent Psychopharmacology, 15*(4), 628–636.

Bateman, B., Warner J. O., Hutchinson E, Dean T, Rowlandson P, Gant C, et al. (2004). The effects of a double blind, placebo controlled, artificial food colorings and benzoate preservative challenge on hyperactivity in a general population sample of preschool children. *Archives of Disease in Childhood, 89*, 506–511.

Bell, J. G. MacKinlay E. E., Dick J. R., MacDonald D. J., Boyle R. M., & Glen A. C. (2004). Essential fatty acids and phospholipase A$_2$ in autistic spectrum disorders. *Prostaglandins, Leukotrienes and Essential Fatty Acids, 71*(4), 201–204.

Bertrand, J., Mars, A., Boyle, C., Bove, F., Yeargin-Allsopp, M., Decoufle, P., et al. (2001). Prevalence of autism in a United States population: The Brick Township, New Jersey, investigation. *Pediatrics, 108*(5), 1155–1161.

Bilici, M., Yildirim, F., Kandil, S., Bekaroglu M., Yildirmis S., Deger O., et al. (2004). Double-blind, placebo-controlled study of zinc sulfate in the treatment of attention deficit hyperactivity disorder. *Progress in Neuro-psychopharmacology & Biological psychiatry, 28*(1), 181–190.

Boris, M., & Mandel, F. S. (1994). Foods and additives are common causes of the attention deficit hyperactive disorder in children. *Annals of Allergy, 72*(5), 462–468.

Bradstreet, J., Geier, D., Kartzinel, J., et al. (2003). A case-control study of mercury burden in children with autistic spectrum disorders. *Journal of American Physicians and Surgeons, 8*(3), 76–79.

Bryson, S. E., Rogers, S. J., & Fombonne, E. (2003). Autism spectrum disorders: Early detection, intervention, education, and psychopharmacological management. *Canadian Journal of Psychiatry, 48*(8), 506–516.

Burgess, J. R., Stevens, L., Zhang, W., & Peck L. (2000). Long-chain polyunsaturated fatty acids in children with attention-deficit hyperactivity disorder. *The American Journal of Clinical Nutrition, 71*(1 Suppl), 327S–330S.

Butnik, S. M. (2005). Neurofeedback in adolescents and adults with attention deficit hyperactivity disorder. *Journal of Clinical Psychology, 61*(5), 621–625.

Cabanlit M, Wills, S., Goines, P., Ashwood P., & Van de Water J. (2007). Brain-specific autoantibodies in the plasma of subjects with autistic spectrum disorder. *Annals of the New York Academy of Sciences, 1107*, 92–103.

Carter, C. M., Urbanowicz, M., Hemsley, R., Mantilla, L., Strobel, S., Graham, P. J., et al. (1993). Effects of a few food diet in attention deficit disorder. *Archives of Disease in Childhood, 69*(5), 564–568.

Center for Disease Control and Prevention. (2007). Prevalence of the autism spectrum disorders in multiple areas of the United States surveillance years 2000 and 2002. National Center on Birth Defects and Developmental Disabilities; Retrieved September 17, 2007, from http://www.cdc.gov/ncbddd/dd/addmprevalence.htm

Chabot, R. J., Merkin, H., Wood, L. M., Davenport, T. L., & Serfontein, G. (1996). Sensitivity and specificity of QEEG in children with attention deficit or specific developmental learning disorders. *Clinical Electroencephalography, 27*(1), 26–34.

Connolly, A. M., Chez, M. G., Pestronk, A., Arnold S. T., Mehta S., & Deuel R. K. (1999). Serum autoantibodies to brain in Landau-Kleffner variant, autism, and other neurologic disorders. *The Journal of Pediatrics, 134*(5), 607–613.

D'Eufemia, P., Celli, M., Finocchiaro, R., Pacifico L., Viozzi L., Zaccagnini M., et al. (1996). Abnormal intestinal permeability in children with autism. *Acta Paediatrica, 85*(9), 1076–1079.

Dahl, R. E., & Lewin, D. S. (2002). Pathways to adolescent health sleep regulation and behavior. *The Journal of Adolescent Health, 31*, 175–184.

Egger, J., Carter, C. M., Graham, P. J., Gumley D., & Soothill J. F. (1985). Controlled trial of oligo-antigenic treatment in the hyperkinetic syndrome. *Lancet, 1*(8428), 540–545.

Feingold, B. (1975). *Why your child is hyperactive*. New York: Random House.

Flaws, B. (2003). Recent Chinese medical research on the treatment of ADHD—Chinese Medicine Update *Townsend Letter for Doctors and Patients*.

Francis, A. J., & Dempster, R. J. (2002). Effect of valerian, Valeriana edulis, on sleep difficulties in children with intellectual deficits: Randomized trial. *Phytomedicine, 9*, 273–279.

Frei, H., Everts R., von Ammon K., Kaufmann F., Walther D., Hsu-Schmitz S. F., et al. (2005). Homeopathic treatment of children with attention deficit hyperactivity disorder: A randomized, double blind, placebo controlled crossover trial. *European Journal of Pediatrics, 164*, 758–767.

Fuchs, T., Birbaumer, N., Lutzenberger, W., Gruzelier J. H., & Kaiser J. (2003). Neurofeedback treatment for attention-deficit/hyperactivity disorder in children: A comparison with methylphenidate. *Applied Psychophysiology and Biofeedback, 28*(1), 1–12.

Galler, J. R., Ramsey, F. C., Morley, D. S., Archer, E., & Salt P. (1990). The long-term effects of early kwashiorkor compared with marasmus. IV. Performance on the national high school entrance examination. *Pediatric Research, 28*(3), 235–239.

Gardiner, P. (2007). Complementary, holistic, and integrative medicine: Chamomile. *Pediatrics in Review, 28*(4), e16–e18.

Hanson, E., Kalish, L. A., Bunce, E., Curtis C., McDaniel, S., Ware, J., et al. (2007). Use of complementary and alternative medicine among children diagnosed with autism spectrum disorder. *Journal of Autism and Developmental Disorders, 37*(4), 628–636.

Harrington, J. W., Rosen, L., Garnecho A., & Patrick, P. A. (2006). Parental perceptions and use of complementary and alternative medicine practices for children with autistic spectrum disorders in private practice. *Journal of Developmental and Behavioral Pediatrics, 27*(2 Suppl), S156–161.

Horvath, K., & Perman, J. A. (2002). Autism and gastrointestinal symptoms. *Current Gastroenterology Reports, 4*(3), 251–258.

Horvath, K., Papadimitriou, J. C., Rabsztyn, A., Drachenberg, C., &Tildon, J. T. (1999). Gastrointestinal abnormalities in children with autistic disorder. *Journal of Pediatrics, 135*(5), 559–563.

Ip, P., Wong, V., Ho, M., Lee J., & Wong W. (2004). Mercury exposure in children with autistic spectrum disorder: A case-control study. *Journal of Child Neurology, 19*(6), 431–434.

Jacobs, J., Williams A. L., Girard C, Njike V. Y., & Katz D. (2005). Homeopathy for attention-deficit/hyperactivity disorder: A pilot randomized-controlled trial. *The Journal of Alternative and Complementary Medicine, 11*(5) 799–806.

James, S. J., Cutler, P., Melnyk, S., Jernigan S, Janak L, Gaylor D. W., et al. (2004). Metabolic biomarkers of increased oxidative stress and impaired methylation capacity in children with autism. *The American Journal of Clinical Nutrition, 80*(6), 1611–1617.

James, S. J., Melnyk, S., Jernigan, S., Cleves M. A., Halsted C. H., Wong D. H., et al. (2006). Metabolic endophenotype and related genotypes are associated with oxidative stress in children with autism. *American Journal of Medical Genetics. Part B, Neuropsychiatric genetics, 141*(8), 947–956.

Jensen, P. S., & Kenny, D. T. (2004). The effects of yoga on the attention and behavior of boys with attention-deficit/hyperactivity disorder (ADHD). *Journal of Attention Disorders, 7*(4), 205–216.

Jyonouchi, H., Sun, S., & Itokazu, N. (2002). Innate immunity associated with inflammatory responses and cytokine production against common dietary proteins in patients with autism spectrum disorder. *Neuropsychobiology, 46*(2), 76–84.

Khilnani, S., Field, T., Hernandez-Reif, M., & Schanberg S. (2003). Massage therapy improves mood and behavior of students with attention-deficit/hyperactivity disorder. *Adolescence, 38*(152), 623–638.

Knivsberg, A. M., Reichelt, K. L., Hoien, T., & Nødland M. (2002). A randomized, controlled study of dietary intervention in autistic syndromes. *Nutr Neurosci, 5*(4), 251–261.

Konofal, E., Lecendreux, M., Arnulf, I., & Mouren M. C. (2004). Iron deficiency in children with attention-deficit/hyperactivity disorder. *Archives of Pediatrics & Adolescent Medicine, 158*(12), 1113–1115.

Kuo, F. E., & Taylor, A. F. (2004). A potential natural treatment for attention-deficit/hyperactivity disorder: Evidence from a national study. *American Journal of Public Health, 94*(9), 1580.

Lee, I. S., & Lee, G. J. (2006). Effects of lavender aromatherapy on insomnia and depression in women college students. [Korean] *Daehan Ganho Haghoeji, 36*(1), 136–143.

Levy, S. E., Mandell, D. S., Merhar, S., Ittenbach, R. F., & Pinto-Martin, J. A. (2003). Use of complementary and alternative medicine among children recently diagnosed with autistic spectrum disorder. *Journal of Developmental and Behavioral Pediatrics, 24*(6), 418–423.

Lewith, G. T., Godfrey, A. D., & Prescott, P. (2005). A single-blinded, randomized pilot study evaluating the aroma of *Lavandula augustifolia* as a treatment for mild insomnia. *Journal of Alternative & Complementary Medicine, 11*(4), 631–637.

Loewy, J., Hallan, C., Friedman, E., & Martinez, C. (2006). Sleep/sedation in children undergoing EEG testing: A comparison of chloral hydrate and music therapy. *American Journal of Electroneurodiagnostic Technology, 46*(4), 343–355.

Louv, R. (2005) *Last child in the woods: Saving our children from nature-deficit disorder.* New York: Algonquin Books of Chapel Hill.

Lozoff, B., & Georgieff, M. (2006). Iron deficiency and brain development. *Seminars in Pediatric Neurology, 13*(3), 158–165.

Lucarelli, S., Frediani, T., Zingoni, A. M., Ferruzzi F., Giardini O., Quintieri F., et al. (1995). Food allergy and infantile autism. *Panminerva Medica, 37*(3), 137–141.

Lyon, M. R., Cline, J. C., Totosy de Zepetnek, J., Shan J. J., Pang P., & Benishin C. (2001). Effect of the herbal extract combination Panax quinquefolium and Ginkgo biloba on attention-deficit hyperactivity disorder: A pilot study. *J Psychiatry Neurosci, 26*(3), 221–228.

McCann, D., Barrett, A., Cooper, A., Crumpler D., Dalen L., Grimshaw K., et al. (2007). Food additives and hyperactive behavior in 3-year-old and 8/9-year-old children in the community: A randomized, double-blinded, placebo-controlled trial. *Lancet, 5,* 5.

McGinnis, W. R. (2004). Oxidative stress in autism. *Alternative Therapies in Health and Medicine, 10*(6), 22–36.

Meltzer, L. J., & Mindell, J. A. (2006). Sleep and sleep disorders in children and adolescents. *Psychiatric Clinics of North America, 29*(4), 1059–1076.

Mindell, J. A., Kuhn B., Lewin D. S., Meltzer L. J., & Sadeh A. (2006). Behavioral treatment of bedtime problems and night wakings in infants and young children. *Sleep, 10*(29), 1263–1276.

Muhle, R., Trentacoste, S. V., & Rapin, I. (2004). The genetics of autism. *Pediatrics 113*(5), E472–E486.

Muller, S. F. (2006). A combination of valerian and lemon balm is effective in the treatment of restlessness and dyssomnia in children. *Phytomedicine, 13*(6), 383–387.

Natural Medicines Comprehensive Data Base-Updated 3/28/08. http://www.naturaldatabase.com

New warning about ADHD drug. (2005). *FDA Consum, 39*(2), 3.

Nissen, S. E. (2006). ADHD drugs and cardiovascular risk. *The New England Journal of Medicine, 354*(14), 1445–1448.

Ozonoff, S, Williams, B. J., & Landa, R. (2005). Parental report of the early development of children with regressive autism. *Autism, 9*(5), 461–486.

Palmer, R. F., Blanchard, S., Stein, Z., Mandell D., & Miller C. (2006). Environmental mercury release, special education rates, and autism disorder: An ecological study of Texas. *Health Place, 12*(2), 203–209.

Patrick, L., & Salik, R. (2005). The effect of essential fatty acid supplementation on language development and learning skills in autism and asperger's syndrome. *Autism-Asperger's Digest*, 36–37

Pillar, G., Shahar, E., Peled, N., Ravid, S., Lavie, P., & Etzioni, A. (2000). Melatonin improves sleep-wake patterns in psychomotor retarded children. *Pediatric Neurology, 23*, 225–228.

Richardson, A. J. (2006). Omega-3 fatty acids in ADHD and related neurodevelopmental disorders. *International Review of Psychiatry, 18*(2), 155–172.

Richardson, A. J., & Montgomery, P. (2005). The Oxford-Durham study: A randomized, controlled trial of dietary supplementation with fatty acids in children with developmental coordination disorder. *Pediatrics,115*(5), 1360–1366.

Richardson, A. J., & Puri Basant, K. (2002). A randomized double-blind, placebo-controlled study of the effects of supplementation with highly unsaturated fatty acids on ADHD-related symptoms in children with specific learning difficulties. *Progress in Neuro-Psychopharmacology & Biological Psychiatry, 26*, 233–239.

Ross, C., Davies P., & Whitehouse W. (2002). Melatonin treatment for sleep disorders in children with neurodevelopmental disorders: An observational study. *Developmental Medicine & Child Neurology, 44*, 339–344.

Rosseneu, S. (October 3, 2003). *Aerobic gut flora in children with autism spectrum disorder and gastrointestinal symptoms.* Paper presented at the Defeat Autism Now Conference, San Diego, CA.

Sandler, R. H., Finegold, S. M., Bolte, E. R., Buchanan C. P., Maxwell A. P., Väisänen M., et al. (2000). Short-term benefit from oral vancomycin treatment of regressive-onset autism. *Journal of Child Neurology, 15*(7), 429–435.

Sandra, K. L., & Russell, A. (2005). Barkley clinical utility of EEG in attention deficit hyperactivity disorder. *Applied Neuropsychology, 12*(2), 64–76.

Satterfield, James, H., Faller, Katherine, J., Crinella, Francis, M., et al. (2007). A 30-year prospective follow-up study of hyperactive boys with conduct problems: Adult criminality. *Journal of the American Academy of Child and Adolescent Psychiatry, 46*(5), 60.

Schachter, H. M., Pham, B., King, J., Langford S, & Moher D. (2001). How efficacious and safe is short-acting methylphenidate for the treatment of attention-deficit disorder in children and adolescents? A meta-analysis. *CMAJ, 165*(11), 1475–1488.

Schnoll, R., Burshteyn, D., & Cea-Aravena, J. (2003). Nutrition in the treatment of attention-deficit hyperactivity disorder: A neglected but important aspect. *Applied Psychophysiology and Biofeedback, 28*(1), 63–75.

Scholastic Parent & Child. (2007). Turn off the TV to fight fat and ADHD: Television commercials can affect your child's diet, and in turn, his learning. Scholastic Inc. Retrieved September 5, 2007, from http://content.scholastic.com/browse/article.jsp?id¼1441

Sever, Y., Ashkenazi, A., Tyano, S., & Weizman A. (1997). Iron treatment in children with attention deficit hyperactivity disorder. A preliminary report. *Neuropsychobiology, 35*(4), 178–180.

Shastry, B. S. (2003). Molecular genetics of autism spectrum disorders. *Journal of Human Genetics, 48*(10), 495–501.

Shaw, P., Eckstrand, K., Sharp, W., Blumenthal, J., Lerch, J. P., Greenstein, D., et al. (2007). Rapoport attention-deficit/hyperactivity disorder is characterized by a delay in cortical maturation. *PNAS, 104*(49)19649–19654.

Singh, V. K., Warren, R., Averett, R., & Ghaziuddin M. (1997). Circulating autoantibodies to neuronal and glial filament proteins in autism. *Pediatric Neurology, 17*(1), 88–90.

Sinha, D., & Efron, D. (2005). Complementary and alternative medicine use in children with attention deficit hyperactivity disorder. *Journal of Pediatrics & Child Health, 41*(1–2), 23–26.

Sinha, Y., Silove, N., Wheeler, D., & Williams K (2006). Auditory integration training and other sound therapies for autism spectrum disorders: a systematic review. *Archives of Disease in Childhood, 91*(12), 1018–1022.

Sinn, N., & Bryan, J. (2007). Effect of supplementation with polyunsaturated fatty acids and micronutrients on learning and behavior problems associated with child ADHD. *Journal of Developmental and Behavioral Pediatrics, 28*(2), 82–91.

Siubberlield, T. G., Wray, T. A., & Parry, T. S. (1999) Utilization of alternative therapies in attention-deficit hyperactivity disorder. *Pediatr Child Health, 35*, 450–453.

Smits, M. G., van Stel H. F., van der Heijden K, Meijer A. M., Coenen A. M., & Kerkhof G. A. (2003). Melatonin improves health status and sleep in children with idiopathic chronic sleep-onset insomnia: A randomized placebo-controlled trial. *Journal of the American Academy of Child and Adolescent Psychiatry, 42*(11), 1286–1293.

Stein, J., Schettler, T., Wallinga, D., & Valenti, M. (2002). In harm's way: Toxic threats to child development. *Journal of Developmental & Behavioral Pediatrics, 23*(1 Suppl), S13–s22.

Strauss, L. C. (2000). The efficacy of a homeopathic preparation in the management of attention deficit hyperactivity disorder. *Journal of Biomedical Therapy, 18*(2) 197.

Sweeten, T. L., Bowyer S. L., Posey D. J., Halberstadt G. M., & McDougle C. J. (2003). Increased prevalence of familial autoimmunity in probands with pervasive developmental disorders. *Pediatrics, 112*(5), e420.

Torrente, F., Ashwood, P., Day, R., Machado, N, Furlano R. I., Anthony, A, et al. (2002). Small intestinal enteropathy with epithelial IgG and complement deposition in children with regressive autism. *Molecular Psychiatry, 7*(4), 375–382,

Trebaticka, J., Kopasova, S., Hradecna, Z., et al . (2006). Treatment of ADHD with French maritime pine bark extract, Pycnogenol. *European Child & Adolescent Psychiatry, 15*(6), 329–335.

Tuchman, R. (2006). Autism and epilepsy: What has regression got to do with it? *Epilepsy Currents, 6*(4), 107–111.

Vancassel, S., Durand, G., Barthelemy, C., Lejeune B., Martineau J., Guilloteau D., et al. (2001). Plasma fatty acid levels in autistic children. *Prostaglandins, Leukotrienes, and Essential Fatty Acids, 65*(1), 1–7.

Vargas, D. L. (2005). Neuroglial activation and neuroinflammation in the brain of patients with autism. *Ann Neurol, 57*(1), 67–81.

Walsh, W. (2003). Metallothionein and autism. Presented at Defeat Autism Now Conference. San Diego (CA), October 3, 2003.

Wender, E. H. (1986). The food additive-free diet in the treatment of behavior disorders: A review. *Journal of Developmental and Behavioral Pediatrics, 7*(1), 35–42.

Wong, H. H., & Smith, R. G. (2006). Patterns of complementary and alternative medical therapy use in children diagnosed with autism spectrum disorders. *Journal of Autism and Developmental Disorders, 36*(7), 901–909.

Yorbik, O., Sayal, A., Akay, C., Akbiyik D. I., & Sohmen T. (2002). Investigation of antioxidant enzymes in children with autistic disorder. *Prostaglandins, Leukotrienes, and Essential Fatty Acids, 67*(5), 341–343.

20

Integrative Pediatric Gastroenterology

GERARD A. BANEZ AND RITA STEFFEN

KEY CONCEPTS

- Pediatric functional gastrointestinal disorders (FGIDs) are increasingly conceptualized from a biopsychosocial perspective, which acknowledges the reciprocal influences of multiple physiological, psychological, and environmental factors and their interactions along the central nervous system/enteric nervous system or "brain-gut" axis.
- Despite the existing evidence base for conventional treatments of FGIDs, not all children benefit from these treatments and interest in complementary and alternative approaches has been growing.
- Biofeedback and self-hypnosis are mind-body therapies that have been found effective in treating childhood functional abdominal pain (FAP).
- Peppermint oil has been shown to reduce pain severity in adolescents with irritable bowel syndrome, one subtype of FAP.
- Literature on CAM therapies and constipation/encopresis suggests that self-hypnosis, massage, and reflexology have clinical potential and are safe complements to the more established treatments of dietary fiber, increased water consumption, and biofeedback.
- Existing literature on CAM approaches for pediatric FGIDs consists mostly of case series and single case reports, and more rigorous clinical research, including studies of the placebo response, will be critical for the growth of the field.

- Increased fiber with biofeedback-assisted low arousal was effective and efficient as a treatment modality for FAP (p. 429).
- Children who had 4-weekly sessions of guided imagery with progressive muscle relaxation were more likely than a comparison group to have 4 or less days of abdominal pain each month and no missed activities (p. 430).
- After 2 weeks, 75% of adolescents with IBS receiving peppermint oil had reduced severity of abdominal pain (p. 432).
- Abdominal massage is an easily learned technique that can encourage peristalsis, relieve flatulence, precipitate bowel opening, and retrain bowel function in children with constipation/encopresis (p. 440).
- Children undergoing six sessions of reflexology which replaced enemas had more frequent stools and less soiling accidents (p. 441).

Functional gastrointestinal (GI) disorders are characterized by "chronic or persistent (GI) symptoms occurring in the absence of biochemical or structural abnormalities, tissue damage, or inflammation" (Fleischer & Feldman, 1999). Functional abdominal pain (FAP) and constipation/encopresis are the most common functional GI disorders in children and adolescents. Consistent with other functional GI disorders, these disorders are increasingly conceptualized from a biopsychosocial perspective, which acknowledges the reciprocal influences of biological, psychological, and social contributing factors. Despite the existing evidence base for conventional treatments, interest in complementary and alternative medicine (CAM) approaches to these disorders has been growing. In this chapter, we will review the existing literature on CAM approaches for FAP and constipation/encopresis in children and adolescents. Our focus is on those approaches that have undergone formal evaluation. For that reason, certain potentially useful but, as of yet, unevaluated treatments will not be described. The National Center for Complementary and Alternative Medicine (NCCAM), grouping of CAM practices into five domains (Whole Medical Systems, Mind-Body Medicine, Biologically Based Practices, Manipulative and Body-Based Practices, and Energy Medicine), will be used.

Functional Abdominal Pain

Functional abdominal pain refers to abdominal pain that is not associated with a specific physical or organic cause. There is no serious, life-threatening illness underlying the pain. Historically, the term "recurrent abdominal pain" (Apley, 1975; Apley & Naish, 1958) was used to refer to FAP. More recently, the symptom-based classification of FAP by the Rome team has grown in popularity (Rasquin et al., 2006). Studies of the prevalence of FAP have found disparate results, with rates ranging from 9% to almost 25% (Apley & Naish, 1958; Oster, 1972). In general, population-based studies suggest that FAP is experienced by 10%–15% of school-age children (Apley, 1975; Apley & Naish, 1958) and almost 20% of middle school and high school students (Hyams, Burke, Davis, Rzepsaki, & Andrulonis, 1996). As children grow older, the incidence of FAP appears to decrease in boys but not girls (Apley & Naish, 1958; Stickler & Murphy, 1979) As noted, FAP is increasingly viewed from a biopsychosocial perspective (e.g., Drossman, 2000; Walker, 1999). This perspective acknowledges the reciprocal influences of multiple physiological, psychological, and environmental factors and their interactions along the central nervous system/enteric nervous system or "brain-gut" axis. For example, a child with abdominal pain but with no psychosocial problems as well as good coping skills and social support is predicted to have a better outcome than the child with pain as well as coexisting emotional difficulties. The child's clinical outcome (e.g., daily function and quality of life) is predicted, in turn, to affect the severity of the disorder.

Much of the interest in CAM approaches for pediatric FAP stems from the fact that not all children benefit from conventional treatments (reassurance and general advice, symptom-based pharmacological therapies, and psychological/behavioral treatments). Currently, the empirical support for CAM treatments lags behind the interest level but is growing. In our literature search, we identified papers on the following CAM intervention strategies: Chinese herbal medicine, biofeedback, self-hypnosis, yoga, acupuncture, various probiotics, peppermint oil, and other biologically based practices. Some of the studies included child as well as adult participants. These studies were not limited to children with pain of a functional nature, and some included children with organic pain as well. At present, case series and single case reports outnumber randomized controlled trials of CAM practices.

WHOLE MEDICAL SYSTEMS

Chinese Herbal Medicine

The use of herbs is a practice of traditional Chinese medicine, which is based on the concept that disease results from disruption in the flow of qi and imbalance in the forces of yin and yang. Two studies (Bensoussan et al., 1998; Leung et al., 2006) examined the treatment of irritable bowel syndrome (IBS), a subtype of FAP, with traditional Chinese herbal medicine, and reported conflicting results. In a randomized controlled trial of

116 (adult) patients who fulfilled Rome's criteria for a diagnosis of IBS, Bensoussan and colleagues (1998) found that Chinese herbal formulations offered improvement in symptoms for some patients with IBS. Patients were randomly assigned to 1 of 3 treatment groups: individualized Chinese herbal formulations ($n = 38$), a standard Chinese herbal formulation ($n = 43$), or placebo ($n = 35$). They received 5 capsules 3 times daily for 16 weeks and were evaluated regularly by a traditional Chinese herbalist and by a gastroenterologist. Compared with patients in the placebo group, patients in the active treatment groups (individualized and standard Chinese herbal medicine) had significant improvement in bowel symptom scores as rated by patients and by gastroenterologists and significant global improvement as rated by patients and by gastroenterologists. Patients reported that treatment significantly reduced the degree of interference with life caused by IBS symptoms. At the conclusion of 16 weeks of treatment, Chinese herbal formulations individually tailored to the patient proved no more effective than standard Chinese herbal medicine treatment. On follow-up 14 weeks after the completion of treatment, only the individualized Chinese herbal treatment group maintained improvement.

In contrast to this, Leung et al. (2006) found that the use of a standard preparation of traditional Chinese medicine extracts did not lead to global symptom improvement in 119 patients that fulfilled Rome criteria for diarrhea-predominant IBS. Patients were randomized to receive a standard preparation of traditional Chinese medicine extracts that contained 11 herbs ($n = 60$) or a placebo with similar appearance and taste ($n = 59$) for 8 weeks after a 2-week run-in period. There was no significant difference in the proportion of patients with global symptom improvement between the traditional Chinese medicine and placebo groups at week 8 and at week 16. Moreover, there was no difference between the two groups in individual symptom scores and quality-of-life assessment at all time points.

Together, these studies suggest that individualized Chinese herbal treatment, as compared to standard Chinese herbal medicine, shows more promise for offering sustained improvement in symptoms for some patients with IBS. In light of the conflicting results, however, more studies examining traditional Chinese herbal treatment are clearly needed. Studies examining (1) the relative therapeutic efficacy of individualized and standard Chinese herbal treatment, and (2) the use of these treatments specifically with children and adolescents will be necessary to characterize the role of traditional Chinese medicine in the management of IBS and other types of childhood FAP.

Mind-Body Medicine

BIOFEEDBACK Various types of biofeedback therapy have been used to treat FAP. Electrocardiogram (ECG) and pneumograph (PNG) biofeedback provide the patient and the practitioner with valuable information for effective treatment of FAP. ECG biofeedback devices have the capability to separate cardiac rhythms into separate spectral bands and are able to calculate the patient's vagal tone, an indicator of their autonomic nervous system's ability to achieve and maintain homeostasis. By watching the display of moment-to-moment psychological activity with the patient, the practitioner can coach the patient in resonant frequency training by instructing him or her to increase activity in the low-frequency range and decrease activity in the very low- and high-frequency ranges. This method of focusing on the "peak" of activity in the low frequency range is an efficient method of familiarizing the patient with his or her own unique physiological response. The practitioner and patient can also validate the intervention by monitoring session-to-session improvements and comparing them to changes in the patient's pain frequency or severity.

Pneumograph biofeedback monitors respiratory activity to facilitate training in abdominal breathing a particularly helpful treatment for FAP. With strain gauges around both the chest and abdomen, the patient learns to decrease chest movement and increase abdominal movement. The practitioner also explains the effects of shallow breathing and demonstrates with a capnometer, when available. With this guidance, the patient learns to breathe fully, slowly, and evenly, utilizing the diaphragm muscle.

Additionally, electrodermograph (EDG) biofeedback consisting of skin conductance/resistance can be used for training the patient to reduce worry and anxiety, thermal biofeedback measuring peripheral skin temperature can be used to vasodilate and enhance blood flow, and electromyography (EMG) can be used to train the patient in muscle relaxation, if indicated. Each of these types of biofeedback provides immediate feedback, which assists the learning process as well as the patient's sense of control and understanding of personal physiology.

In a study examining biofeedback as one component of a behavioral treatment protocol for FAP, Humphreys and Gervitz (2000) compared four different treatment protocols using a pre-test/post-test control group design. Participants in the research were 64 children and adolescents with FAP. They were randomly assigned into four groups: (1) fiber-only comparison group; (2) fiber and skin temperature biofeedback; (3) fiber, skin temperature biofeedback, and cognitive-behavioral procedures; and (4) fiber, skin temperature biofeedback, cognitive-behavioral procedures, and contingency management training for parents. The results revealed that all groups showed improvement in self-reported pain. The active treatment groups, however, showed significantly more improvement than the fiber-only comparison group. Because the addition of cognitive-behavioral parent support components did not seem to increase treatment effectiveness, the authors concluded that increased fiber with biofeedback-assisted low arousal was effective and efficient as a treatment modality for FAP.

SELF-HYPNOSIS Hypnosis is an altered state of awareness within which an individual experiences heightened suggestibility. Self-hypnosis refers to the use of hypnosis by an individual to achieve a personal goal. It is a simple, non-invasive self-regulation technique that has been used to treat various pediatric health conditions, including

FAP. Weydert and her colleagues (2006) evaluated the two primary components of pediatric hypnotherapy—relaxation and mental imagery—as treatment for FAP in a randomized controlled trial of 22 children, aged 5–18 years. Participants were randomized to learn either breathing exercises alone or guided imagery with progressive muscle relaxation. Both groups had 4-weekly sessions with a therapist. Children who learned imagery with relaxation had a significantly greater decrease in the number of days with pain than those who learned breathing exercises alone after 1 and 2 months. They also had a significantly greater decrease in days with missed activities after 1 and 2 months. During the 2 months of follow-up, more children who had learned relaxation and mental imagery met the threshold of ≤ 4 days of pain each month and no missed activities.

Additional evidence for the therapeutic efficacy of self-hypnosis is found in several case series reports. In four of five FAP patients, Anbar (2001) found that pain resolved within 3 weeks after a single session of self-hypnosis instruction. Sokel, Devane, and Bentovim (1991) reported that all six of their FAP patients were able to use self-hypnosis to reduce or remove pain so that they were able to resume normal activities within a mean period of 17.6 days. Browne (1997) reported that seven children with FAP were treated with brief hypnotherapy and subsequently rated at follow-up as improved. Finally, Ball, Shapiro, Monheim, and Weydert (2003) found that children with long-standing FAP that was refractory to conventional therapy had a decrease in their complaints of pain during and following relaxation and mental imagery.

YOGA In 2006, Kuttner and colleagues conducted a preliminary randomized study of yoga as a treatment for adolescents with IBS. Participants were 25 adolescents aged 11–18 years with IBS, who were randomly assigned to either a yoga or wait list control group. Before the intervention, both groups completed questionnaires assessing gastrointestinal symptoms, pain, functional disability, coping, anxiety, and depression. The yoga intervention consisted of a 1-hour instructional session, demonstration and practice, followed by 4 weeks of daily home practice guided by a video. After 4 weeks, adolescents repeated the baseline questionnaires. The wait-list control group then received the yoga intervention and 4 weeks later completed an additional set of questionnaires. Adolescents who completed the intervention reported lower levels of functional disability, less use of emotion-focused avoidance, and lower anxiety following the intervention than adolescents in the control group. When the pre- and post-intervention data for the two groups were combined, adolescents had significantly lower scores for gastrointestinal symptoms and emotion-focused avoidance following the yoga intervention. Adolescents found the yoga to be helpful and indicated they would continue to use it to manage their IBS. Additional research on the benefits of yoga will be important for establishing its clinical effectiveness for IBS and other subtypes of FAP.

COGNITIVE-BEHAVIORAL PROCEDURES Cognitive-behavioral procedures such as self-management training for children (e.g., distraction techniques, progressive muscle relaxation, coping statements) and contingency management training for parents (e.g., reinforcement of well-behavior, ignoring nonverbal, pain behaviors) have emerged as a probably efficacious treatment for childhood FAP (e.g., Sanders et al., 1989, 1994). These procedures were considered CAM in the past but have become mainstream treatments for FAP.

Energy Medicine

ACUPUNCTURE Acupuncture is practice of traditional Chinese medicine that seeks to aid healing by restoring the yin-yang balance and the flow of qi. A prospective, blinded, sham acupuncture-controlled trial of traditional Chinese acupuncture (Forbes et al., 2005) found that acupuncture was relatively ineffective in treating IBS. Participants in this research were 60 patients with well-established IBS. Patients in treated and sham groups improved significantly during the study. Several secondary outcome measures favored active treatment, but an improved symptom score occurred more often with sham therapy. For no criterion was statistical significance approached.

Two additional acupuncture studies were identified. Yanhua and Sumei (2000) reported on the treatment of 86 cases of epigastric and abdominal pain by scalp acupuncture. Significant improvement resulted from the insertion of just a few needles. Xiaoma (1988) described electroimpulse acupuncture treatment of 110 cases were clinically cured with disappearance of symptoms and signs. These studies had mixed age samples and, like the hypnotherapy studies, were not prospective controlled investigations. The latter study assessed children with presumably organic pain, and the extent to which its findings can be generalized to FAP is uncertain.

Biologically Based Practices

LACTOBACILLUS In a double-blind randomized controlled trial, Gawronska et al. (2007) found that *Lactobacillus rhamnosus GG* (LGG) appeared to moderately increase treatment success, particularly among children with IBS. One hundred and four children who fulfilled the Rome II criteria for functional dyspepsia (FD), IBS, or FAP were assigned to receive LGG ($n = 52$) or placebo ($n = 52$) for 4 weeks. For the overall study population, those in the LGG group were more likely to have treatment success (no pain) than those in the placebo group (25% versus 9.6%). For children with IBS ($n = 37$), those in the LGG group were more likely to have treatment success than those in the placebo group and reduced frequency of pain, but not pain severity. For the FD group and FAP group, no differences were found.

In contrast, another double-blind randomized control trial (Bausserman & Michail, 2005) found that LGG was not superior to placebo in the treatment of abdominal pain in children with IBS but may help with perceived abdominal distention. Fifty children fulfilling Rome II criteria for IBS were given LGG or placebo for 6 weeks. No difference in other gastrointestinal symptoms, except for perceived abdominal distention, was seen.

Niv, Naftali, Hallak, and Vaisman (2005) reported that IBS symptoms did not improve with probiotic treatment with Lactobacillus reuteri. Fifty-nine patients with IBS were randomized for treatment in a double-blind, placebo-controlled 6-month trial, and 39 concluded the study. Both groups (treatment and placebo) improved significantly in all the studied parameters with no significant differences between groups. The authors reported that a strong placebo effect and a lack of uniformity of the IBS population may have hindered a clearer demonstration of the effect.

BIFIDOBACTERIUM INFANTIS 35624 Whorwell et al. (2006) provided preliminary evidence that Bifidobacterium infantis 35624 may have utility in IBS. After a 2-week baseline, 362 primary care IBS patients, with any bowel habit subtype, were randomized to either placebo or freeze-dried, encapsulated B. infantis at a dose of 1×10^6, 1×10^8, or 1×10^{10}, cfu/mL for 4 weeks. *B. infantis* at a dosage level of 1×10^8 cfu was significantly superior to placebo and all other bifidobacterium doses for abdominal pain, a composite score for IBS symptoms and scores for bloating, bowel dysfunction, incomplete evacuation, straining, and the passage of gas.

PEPPERMINT OIL In a randomized, double-blind controlled study (Kline, Kline, DiPalma, & Barbero, 2001), 42 children with IBS were given pH-dependent, enteric-coated peppermint oil capsules or placebo. After 2 weeks, 75% of those receiving peppermint oil had reduced severity of pain associated with IBS.

ARTICHOKE LEAF EXTRACT In a double-blind, randomized controlled trial (Holtmann et al., 2003), 247 patients with FD were recruited and treated with either a commercial artichoke leaf extract (ALE) or a placebo. The overall symptom improvement over the 6 weeks of treatment was significantly greater with ALE than with the placebo. Patients treated with ALE showed significantly greater improvement in global quality-of-life scores.

FOLK REMEDIES (TEA) A study of folk remedies for a Hispanic population (Risser & Mazur, 1995) found that tea (chamomile, cinnamon, honey, and lemon) was commonly used to treat childhood abdominal pain. Participants were 51 Hispanic caregivers, mostly mothers, attending a primary care facility serving a primarily Hispanic population. The authors failed to specify whether the children's pain was functional or organically caused. No outcome data were reported.

CONSTIPATION/ENCOPRESIS

Constipation not only refers to infrequent stooling (<3 bowel movements/week) but also includes hard or large stools that may be accompanied by pain. Constipation is not a disease but a symptom that is common among children. Encopresis, a term coined in the 1920s (Potosky, 1925), refers to the involuntary loss of stool causing soiling accidents in the underwear. It is the appropriate medical term when the child is over 4 years old and the diagnosis has been deemed functional, that is, not secondary to other physical or organic causes. Constipation and encopresis are common in pediatric patients and may constitute up to 25% of referrals to pediatric gastroenterologists (Loening-Baucke, 1993).

The standard medical treatment for constipation and fecal soiling is a combination of stool softeners, enemas, and/or suppositories for disimpaction (clearing a large, hard fecal mass that has accumulated in the rectum) and maintaining frequent bowel movements. A combination of patient education, a bowel training program of timed toilet sitting after meals, and other behavioral techniques are frequently used. Though these strategies are often effective, there is a great deal of interest in CAM approaches to constipation/encopresis.

WHOLE MEDICAL SYSTEMS

Homeopathy

Homeopathy is a system of medical treatment that was developed in the 1800s. It is based on the law of dilutions—the more dilute the remedy, the more power it has to heal a patient's symptoms—and the law of similars—a remedy that causes a symptom is used to treat the same symptom in a sick person, or "like cures like." In an observational case series (Olsen, 2003), a homeopathic treatment with Sanicula aqua, a mineral water from Ottawa, Illinois, was used to treat constipation in children. Three children, ages 1 ½ to 3 years, were given this mineral water with good results 1 month to 1 year later. There was no evidence cited to suggest that Sanicula aqua has curative properties that are not in plain water.

In another case series (Hossain, 2006), a 7-year-old boy with severe constipation was successfully treated with the homeopathic remedy, Carcinosin. The text did not define Carcinosin or speculate as to why it worked. There were two adult patients in this case series, and both responded to the remedy as well. Because the report provided little specific information, Carcinosin cannot as of yet be recommended for treatment of childhood constipation.

A case report described homeopathic treatment in an 8-month-old boy with chronic constipation and Hirschsprung's disease (Higley, 1998). The extent of the bowel involvement with Hirschsprung's was not detailed. The boy was given a bowel nosode, Morgans Gaertners 200, which is made from bacteria growing in the bowel, and its remedy, lycopodium 30. Later, silica 500 and its bowel nosode, Gaertners Bach 200, were added. Sulfur 30 was given to treat eczema separately. No information was presented about the substances given nor was any follow-up evaluation done. Higley reported that "a few months later," the boy no longer needed laxatives and was given prune juice, a home remedy laxative. Since this 8-month-old boy was in an age range at risk for potentially fatal enterocolitis secondary to Hirschsprung's disease, this treatment cannot be recommended for this children this age.

Overall, published reports on homeopathic approaches for childhood constipation/encopresis have not been specific about the remedies given and their mechanisms of action. The infrequent case reports found on these practices underscore the limitations of this literature, including the lack of standardization and the possible dangers in some homeopathic therapies. Little rigorous clinical research on homeopathic approaches currently exists.

Chinese Herbal Medicine

Ohya and colleagues (2003) described the use of a traditional Chinese herbal medicine, Dai-kenchu-to (DKT), to treat children with obstructive bowel diseases. DKT is composed of ginseng root, zanthoxylum fruit (pepper), dried ginger rhizome, and maltose powder. Ohya et al. treated 46 pediatric patients over a 5 ½ year period, 21of whom had chronic constipation. Ages of the subjects ranged from 5 months to 15 years. Six children in this study had postoperative ileus, and 12 had constipation, some with obstructive symptoms after large abdominal surgeries (one with anorectal anomaly, three with Hirschsprung's disease, two with functional bowel obstructions, and one with SMA syndrome). DKT was mixed with 5–10 ml warm water and given two to three times daily. Bowel movements were evaluated 2 to 4 weeks later. Successful laxation was achieved in 18 of the 21 children with chronic constipation, and DKT was subsequently discontinued in 15 of the 18. Of the 46 total children and adolescents, 39 patients (85%) improved. There were no side effects or risks of DKT reported. Long term follow up data were not available.

This study was done by pediatric surgeons who were vigilant to rule out Hirschsprung's disease and ready to move to exploratory laparotomy in a timely manner if DKT failed to relieve the abdominal distention and open up the bowels. The study did not report objective data to support its findings, such as anorectal manometric values or clinical scoring, but the clinical results are encouraging.

Iwai and colleagues (2006) measured the effect of DKT on anorectal manometric parameters for 10 children (ages 6–13 years, mean 8.6 years) with severe chronic constipation and 5 children (ages 7–17 years, mean 11.5 years) with severe constipation after surgery for anorectal malformations. On the basis of their clinical scoring system, it appeared that rectal reservoir function, as measured with manometry, improved secondarily in response to normal bowel habits. Because of the small number of patients, the significance of this improvement could not be statistically analyzed.

Though these studies of DKT are encouraging, more rigorous research is clearly needed. Randomized controlled trials with larger samples will be important for better evaluating clinical efficacy. As with Ohya et al. (2003), special precautions may be necessary for certain patients who are medically at-risk .

Ayurveda

In India, Ayurveda is the most popular indigenous constipation medicine. Ayurveda, which literally means "the science of life," is a whole medical system that aims to integrate the body, mind, and spirit to prevent and treat disease. The principles and practices of Ayurveda were first recorded in Sanskrit in 400 BC, but the specific substances used and their proportions are often elusive.

Ramesh and colleagues (1998) used Misrakasneham, an Ayurvedic liquid which contains 21 herbs, castor oil, ghee, and milk, with cancer patients with opioid-induced constipation. Misrakasneham is a liquid purgative and has been in the Ayurvedic formulary for 13 centuries. Fifty patients participated in this study, one of which was 15 years old and the rest were adults. All had advanced cancer and were treated in a palliative care unit. The patients were randomly assigned to two groups, one receiving Misrakasneham and the other getting Sofsena, a stimulant laxative that contains Senna. The specific doses or proportions were not reported. The authors concluded that although there was no significant difference between the two groups, the results indicated that Misrakasneham was taken in smaller amounts and had a tolerable taste, acceptable side-effect profile, and lower cost. These factors, in the authors' opinion, made Misrakasneham a good choice for prophylaxis in opioid-induced constipation, albeit they acknowledged a need for more research on Ayurvedic medicines in palliative care. While positive, additional research on the use of Ayurvedic medicine with children and adolescents is needed before this approach can be recommended clinically.

BIOLOGICALLY BASED PRACTICES

Fiber

Loening-Baucke and her colleagues (2004) evaluated whether fiber supplementation with glucomannan (a fiber gel polysaccharide extract of the Japanese konjac root) was more beneficial than placebo in the treatment of children who had functional constipation with or without encopresis. In a double-blind, crossover study, fiber and placebo were given daily as 100 mg/kg body weight daily (maximal 5g/d) with 50 ml fluid/500 mg for 4 weeks each. Parents were asked to have children sit on the toilet four times daily after meals and to maintain a stool diary. Forty-six chronically constipated children were recruited, and 31 children completed the study. These 31 children (16 boys and 15 girls) were 4.5 to 11.7 years of age (mean age: 7 ± 2 years). All children had functional constipation, and 18 had encopresis when recruited for the study. The results found that children who had constipation alone were more likely to be treated successfully (69%) than those who had constipation and encopresis (28%). Overall, glucomannan was beneficial in the treatment of constipation with and without encopresis. Children who had encopresis and who were already being treated with laxatives also benefited from the additional fiber.

Herbs

The herbal laxatives, including psyllium seed, cascara sagrada, and senna, are approved by the Food and Drug Administration (FDA) for treatment of constipation and encopresis. Psyllium seed (*Plantago ovata*) is a soluble fiber that needs to be taken with adequate fluid as it absorbs water and expands in the gut (Gardiner et al., 2007). It is available without a prescription, but an allergic reaction is possible. It is contraindicated in intestinal obstruction, fecal impaction, and narrowing in the gastrointestinal tract. Cascara sagrada (*Rhamnus purshiana*) and senna (*Sennae folum*) stimulate the colon and are approved by the FDA for children over 2 years of age. There is a potential for dependence to develop if they are overused. Gardiner and colleagues (2007) reported that the American Academy of Pediatrics has judged senna and cascara to be safe in breast-feeding mothers (American Academy of Pediatrics, 2005).

Foods

Prunes (*Prunus domesticus*) also contain a colon stimulant (diphenylisation) and have antioxidant activity that helps to absorb oxygen-free radicals. Since prunes act as a stimulant, however, it is actually safer for a child to take stool softeners or bulk agents that act by attracting water into the intestine. Castor oil (*Ricinus communis*) is thought to increase fluid secretion but is not indicated for long-term use (Ladas et al., 2006). Because it is readily available over-the-counter, the potential for abuse exists.

A study investigating Fruitlax, a combination of raisins, currants, prunes, figs, and dates, was conducted with children with chronic neurologic conditions causing paralysis or limitation of motion, a risk factor for developing constipation because of inability to exercise (Day & Monsma, 1995). Seven of the 8 children (ages 3–9 years) showed improvement in specific factors related to bowel movements. The following factors were monitored: amount, frequency, color, and consistency of stool; effort in straining to stool, and number of laxatives, suppositories, and enemas used. The duration of treatment in the 7 children ranged from 24 to 77 days, with an average of 42.6. Results showed little or no effort required to pass stools. There was an increase in softer stools, but the number of hard stools increased in some children. There was a trend to requiring fewer enemas and stimulant laxatives . Unfortunately, while these results are positive, it is difficult to determine how much of the improvement was truly related to Fruitlax because other treatments were also being used at the same time.

BIOLOGICALLY BASED PRACTICES

Probiotics consisting of combinations of living microorganisms have been used to treat constipation and diarrhea. A probiotic is live bacteria that benefit the host through their effects on the gastrointestinal tract. Prebiotics are food substances that may also be given as useful substrates to stimulate the growth or activity of potentially health promoting bacteria. Together, they are called symbiotic therapy and are intended to improve survival and implantation of health-promoting, live bacteria which restore the balance of these favorable species. Several studies that have assessed the efficacy and safety of probiotics. Most of these focused on adult patients, but some included children and adolescents.

Lactobacillus

A randomized, double-blind, placebo-controlled trial comparing lactulose to Lactobacillus GG, a probiotic (Banaskiewicz et al., 2005), as a treatment for constipation in children showed the Lactobacillus GG to be ineffective. Eighty-four children (ages 2–16 years of age) were enrolled in a trial in which they received either lactulose 1 mg/kg/day plus Lactobacillus GG 10^9 colony forming units (n = 43) or a placebo (n = 41 subjects). The primary outcome measure of treatment success, ≥ 3 bowel movements per week and no fecal soiling, was similar in both groups at 12 weeks (28/41 [68%] versus 31/43 [72%] respectively; P = .70) and again at 24 weeks (27/41 [64%] vs 27/42 [65%]). The authors concluded that Lactobacillus GG, at least at the dose used, is not an effective adjunct to lactulose in managing constipation in patients 2 to 16 years of age.

In a prospective, double blind, placebo-controlled trial, Niv and colleagues (2005) studied another *Lactobacillus* species, reuteri ATCC 55730, for the treatment of IBS. The youngest patient in the series was 19 years old. The treatment was found to be ineffective for IBS, including the constipation-predominant IBS patients.

Amenta, Cascio, Fiori, and Venturini (2006) studied the oral supplement zir fos (bifidobacterium longum W11 + FOS actilight) in 297 patients (age range: 8–78 years) with constipation and obesity on a weight- loss diet. Improvement in constipation was associated with younger adults (35 ± 12 years) who were compliant or adherent to taking at least 17/20 daily doses of zir fos. There were no data on the number of pediatric patients in the study, but the results revealed that zir fos was not effective in children because the only group that improved was between ages 35 ± 12 years. The data reported does not segregate patients ≤18 years as a subgroup, thus the youngest patients may have worsened or remained unchanged.

Lactobacillus reuteri, a different bacterial species, was used to treat patients who fulfilled Rome II criteria for IBS. Ten of 54 patients (18.5%) in this study had constipation. The youngest patient was 19 years old, and the oldest was 70 years old. Their symptoms did not improve, and this finding was attributed to the strong placebo effect as well as a lack of uniformity of the IBS population.

MIND-BODY MEDICINE

Behavioral Therapies

Behavioral techniques have become standard adjuncts to medical therapies in the treatment of constipation and encopresis. Timed toilet sitting after meals is often recommended when stool softeners are prescribed. Specific exercises to accompany the toilet sitting are sometimes recommended (Brooks et al., 2000). Consultation with pediatric psychologists is also standard treatment for constipation and encopresis in children. Individual therapy includes combinations of relaxation training, positive and negative reinforcement, cognitive behavioral therapy, hypnosis and other techniques, including biofeedback.

Kisch and Pfeffer (1984) described inpatient psychiatric treatment of constipation and encopresis in a 12 year old boy with behavior problems. Their interventions included nutritional consultation, timed toilet sitting, individual and group therapy, and staff support and supervision. After 2 months of therapy, the boy passed a stool in the toilet, and he gradually improved. He was followed in outpatient therapy, but long term follow-up was not reported. This approach was considered a CAM practice at that time, but constipation/encopresis are now almost always treated on an outpatient basis.

Self-Hypnosis

A study of relaxation-mental imagery (RMI) (self-hypnosis) in the management of 505 pediatric behavioral encounters (Kohen et al., 1984) included a subset of children with encopresis. The children with encopresis practiced RMI, and, at the conclusion of 2 years of data collection, 12 demonstrated significant improvement. Four demonstrated initial improvement but did not practice their exercises, and three children did not improve. The authors concluded that self-hypnosis is a useful tool for managing a variety of pediatric problems (e.g., enuresis, generalized anxiety, anxiety about pelvic examinations, pain, obesity, habit problems, headaches, and asthma). They also noted that the use of self-hypnois was associated with shorter office visits, and there was often spillover of therapeutic success into other areas of the child's life.

A case report (Tilton, 1980) of an 8-year-old boy using trance (not fully described) achieved by a television screen technique, 15 minutes a week for 4 weeks, described success in treating his enuresis and encopresis. The follow-up was short—one call a month after completing this treatment—but revealed continued success. This patient also stopped sucking his thumb during treatment. A second case report (Linden, 2003) of therapeutic play and hypnosis used to treat a 4½-year-old boy with constipation and encopresis was also successful. There was no long-term follow-up reported.

Group Behavioral Treatment

A study of group behavioral treatment of children with encopresis who failed standard medical treatment (Stark et al., 1990) used group appointments with a total of 18 children ages 4–11 years. Six sessions of 3–5 families were completed. These sessions promoted enema clean-out, increased dietary fiber intake, and appropriate toileting techniques. Fiber consumption increased by 40%, appropriate toileting by 116%, and soiling accidents decreased by 83%. These changes were sustained at 6 months follow-up. Although the content of therapy is standard, the use of groups provides a cost-effective alternative to one-on therapy.

Health Visitor Teams

A variation on this approach, reported in New Zealand, is the use of health visitor teams composed of nurses (Smith et al., 2006). Results were compiled from a survey to identify types of care provided and to gather information on how to improve the service. A questionnaire was completed for each child seen during a 1-month period. A total of 34 children with constipation/encopresis were seen in the home, and the families were given educational information on fluid intake, diet, and stool softeners. The treatment emphasis was on dietary intervention as opposed to laxatives. No study results were reported. The authors found a need for improved information for parents, early intervention with escalating advice/treatment to remedy the constipation, and consistent guidelines to be provided by healthcare professionals.

Play Therapy

The use of play with clay (Feldman et al., 1993) was reported in an observational study of 6 consecutively recruited children, all boys, ages 4–12 years. All had intractable constipation and encopresis. Brown clay was used as a metaphor for fecal material, and the children played creatively with no interpretations made. Four children were cured of constipation after 2 months of therapy, and no relapse was reported during 1 year of follow-up. One child improved significantly, and the remaining child withdrew from treatment after three sessions. Modeling clay therapy was used before any biofeedback was used and deemed a cost-effective treatment modality. This report is limited by the small number of patients enrolled, and the modeling clay method has not been adopted in general practice since the time of this publication.

Biofeedback

Biofeedback has been used as adjunctive therapy for constipation and fecal incontinence since the 1970s. Biofeedback and behavior therapy, including timed toilet sitting and prescribed exercises, are no longer considered CAM practices. Along with laxatives and stool softeners, they have become a part of mainstream treatment.

MANIPULATIVE AND BODY-BASED PRACTICES

Chiropractic and massage therapy are the interventions found in this domain of CAM therapies. Chiropractors study the neurological learning or programming of the central nervous system (brain and spinal cord) with respect to locomotion, posture, sensory input, and body kinetics. Disturbances in the vertebral column are treated with corrective manipulations, and many ailments and diseases are treated in this manner. Like doctors of osteopathy (DOs), chiropractors believe that misalignment of the spine is a major source of morbidity, and spinal manipulation is their main therapeutic option.

In a case report (Quist & Duray, 2007), an 8-year-old boy unresponsive to allopathic treatment with laxatives, fluid, and fiber was found to have "sacral chiropractic subluxation complex." He was treated with manipulation of the sacral area using diversified adjusting procedures in addition to external massage of the abdomen. Massage began in the right lower quadrant and followed the course of the colon in a clockwise direction. He received 2 treatments per week for 4 weeks, and was having normal bowel movements after treatment. Follow-up 13 years later revealed continuing normal bowel function.

A case report of a 5-year-old girl with severe chronic constipation (Eriksen ,1994) showed a dramatic change in bowel function following chiropractic upper cervical spine correction by manual manipulation. Follow-up 2 months later revealed continuing regular bowel movements. The author referred to the occipito-attlantoaxial subluxation (or a misalignment of the bones of the base of the skull with the uppermost bones of the spinal column) complex having an effect on the lumbo-pelvic region.

Constipation is among the many problems in children that have been attributed to vertebral subluxation and related pelvic dysfunction. Ressel and Rudy (2004) attempted to describe 650 children with a wide variety of somatic, visceral, and immune complaints. They felt that the effects of their newly reported subluxation were responsible directly or indirectly for "a number of neurological patterns and kinesiopathological reflexes that can propagate a myriad of conditions" and maintained that correction would restore the body to homeostasis. Unfortunately, the heterogeneous nature of the sample and the multiple outcome measures used do not allow for a clear understanding of the relation between subluxation and constipation/encopresis. As with some of the other CAM practices reviewed, more rigorous controlled research on chiropractic therapies is needed.

Massage

An observational study (Richards, 1998) reported on the use of abdominal massage in 10 patients, 4 of whom were children, ages 4–11 years. Laxatives were available if needed, and a diary of bowel movements and laxative use was maintained over a 4–6 week period. The massage technique used a tennis ball which was pressed into the right lower quadrant and along the colon in its distribution down to the suprapubic area. Massage resulted in increased frequency of stooling and decreased use of laxatives. The authors stated that abdominal massage encourages peristalsis, relieves flatulence and can precipitate bowel opening, be used to retrain bowel function, and it can be learned easily by a caregiver and used for someone with chronic disabilities. It is safe, non-invasive, and can be self-administered, although it is contraindicated in patients who have hernias, recent surgery, or scarring.

ENERGY MEDICINE

Acupuncture

Broide and colleagues (2001) treated 17 children who had chronic constipation with 5 weekly placebo acupuncture sessions followed by 10 weekly true acupuncture sessions.

Frequency of bowel movements improved from 1.4 per week at baseline to 5.6 per week in female subjects after the 10 true acupuncture sessions were completed. Basal panopioid levels were measured and were noted to be lower at baseline in constipated children but gradually increased to control levels after 10 true acupuncture sessions.

A study using acupuncture with traditional Chinese medicine to treat rectal prolapse in 38 patients (Jingfang et al., 2003) included 12 children ages 6–10 years as well as several adolescents and adults aged 50–70 years. Some of this diverse group of participants had "habitual constipation," while others had diarrhea. The authors reported 35 cases (93%) cured and 3 patients (7%) improved with this treatment. Because acupuncture and traditional Chinese medicine were combined, it is difficult to establish the extent to which improvement was related to acupuncture alone.

Reflexology

Reflexology is a complementary form of treatment that has origins in several ancient cultures (Coates, 2002). Reflexology posits that surface areas of the feet have nerve or other direct pathways from the soles of the feet to organs. The underlying theory behind reflexology is that applying pressure with the fingers to certain areas on the soles of the feet restores the energy flow to certain parts of the body.

The largest study of reflexology was an observational study (Bishop, 2003) treating 50 children between three and 14 years of age who suffered from chronic constipation and encopresis. Six sessions of clinical reflexology were completed for 48 of the 50 children enrolled. Reflexology was used to replace enema administration in this cohort. The results demonstrated increased frequency of stooling and decreased incidence of soiling. The manuscript does not address follow-up to assess maintenance of this positive treatment.

Summary and Recommendations

The existing literature on CAM approaches for FAP and constipation/encopresis in children and adolescents consists of more case series and single case reports than randomized controlled trials. Many of these reports are observational in nature. Heterogeneous samples (e.g., combined child and adult participants, multiple presenting problems), combinations of treatments, and variable outcome measures are not uncommon. Despite this, several CAM approaches emerge as promising treatments. For FAP, in addition to cognitive-behavioral procedures, biofeedback, self-hypnosis, and peppermint oil appear to be the most promising, while yoga, artichoke leaf extract, and *Bifidobacterium infantis* 35624 also have some empirical support. The literature on CAM therapies and constipation/encopresis suggests that self-hypnosis, massage, and reflexology have clinical potential and are safe complements to more established treatments of dietary fiber, increased water consumption, and biofeedback.

In light of the increasing interest in CAM practices and the promise suggested in early reports, more rigorous clinical research will be critical for the growth of this field.

Of particular importance will be randomized controlled trials with larger samples of pediatric patients with functional GI disorders, standard outcome measures, and longer term follow-up. More detail about the nature of CAM practices, their rationale, and safety is essential. Because some positive outcomes may be associated with a placebo effect, the placebo effect and the intention/expectation of the patient to be healed regardless of the type of therapy is also a critical and under-researched topic.

An integrative and holistic approach to FAP and constipation/encopresis encourages blending of CAM approaches with empirically supported conventional approaches. CAM approaches that have some evidence base and are safe, affordable, and acceptable to the child and family can be used in conjunction with established treatment strategies. As more is learned about the efficacy and safety of certain CAM practices for these functional GI disorders, we anticipate that the integration of these approaches and conventional treatments will become increasingly standard and best practice.

REFERENCES

Amenta, M., Cascio, M. T., Di Fiori, P., & Venturini, T. (2006). Diet and chronic constipation: benefits of symbiotic zir fos (bifidobacterium longum W11 + FOS actilight. *Acta Bio-medica: Atenei Parmensis, 77*(3), 157–162.

Anbar, R. D. (2001). Self-hypnosis for the treatment of functional abdominal pain in childhood. *Clinical Pediatrics, 40*, 447–451.

Apley, J. (1975). *The child with abdominal pains* (2nd ed.). London: Blackwell.

Apley, J., & Naish, N. (1958). Recurrent abdominal pain: A field survey of 1,000 school children. *Archives of Diseases of Childhood, 7*, 7–9.

Ball, T. M., Shapiro, D. E., Monheim, C. J., & Weydert, J. A. (2003). A pilot study of the use of guided imagery for the treatment of recurrent abdominal pain in children. *Clinical Pediatrics, 42*(6); 527–532.

Baker, S., Liptak, G., & Colletti, R. (1999). Constipation in infants and children: evaluation and treatment: A medical position statement of the North American Society for Pediatric Gastroenterology and Nutrition. *Journal of Pediatric Gastroenterology and Nutrition, 29,* 612–626.

Banaszkiewicz, A., & Szajewska, H. (2005). Ineffectiveness of Lactobacillus GG as an adjunct to lactulose for the treatment of constipation in children: A double-blind, placebo-controlled trial. *Journal of Pediatrics, 146*, 364–369.

Bausserman, M., & Michail, S. (2005). The use of Lactobacillus GG in irritable bowel syndrome in children: A double-blind randomized control trial. *Journal of Pediatrics, 147*(2), 197–201.

Bensoussan, A., Talley, N., Hing, M., et al. (1998). Treatment of irritable bowel syndrome with Chinese herbal medicine: A randomized trial. *Journal of the American Medical Association, 280*(18), 1585–1589.

Bishop, E., McKinnon, E., Weir, E., & Brown, D. W. (2003). Reflexology in the management of encopresis and chronic constipation. *Paediatr Nursing, 15*(3), 20–21.

Broide, E., Pintov, S., Portnoy, S., Barg, J., Klinowski, E., & Scapa, E. (2001). Effectiveness of acupuncture for treatment of childhood constipation. *Digestive Diseases and Sciences, 46*(6), 1270–1275.

Brooks, R. C., Copen, R. M., Cox, D. J., Morris, J., Borowitz, S., & Setphen, J. (2000). Review of the treatment literature for treatment of childhood constipation. *Annals of Behavioral Medicine, 22,* 260–267.

Browne, S. E. (1997). Brief hypnotherapy with passive children. *Contemporary Hypnosis, 14,* 59–62.

Castillejo, G., Bullo, M., Anguera, A., Escribano, J., & Salas-Salvado, J. (2006). A controlled, randomized double-blind trial to evaluate the effect of a supplement of cocoa husk that is rich in dietary fiber on colonic transit in constipated pediatric patients. *Pediatrics, 118,* e641–e648.

Chase, J., Robertson, V. J., Southwell, B., Hutson, J., & Gibb, S. (2005). Pilot study using transcutaneous electrical stimulation (interferential current) to treat chronic treatment-resistant constipation and soiling in children. *Journal of Gastroenterology and Hepatology, 20*(7), 1054–1061.

Coates, E. (2002). Clinical reflexology. *Practical Nursing, 23*(9), 32.

Day, R. A., & Monsma, M. (1995). Fruitlax: Management of constipation in children with disabilities. *Clinical Nursing Research, 4*(3), 306–322.

Di Lorenzo, C. (2000). Childhood constipation: Finally some hard data about hard stools. *Journal of Pediatrics, 136,* 4–7.

Drossman, D. A. The functional gastrointestinal disorders and the Rome II process. In D. A. Drossman, N. J. Corazziari, & N. J. Talley, et al. (Eds.), *Rome II: The functional gastrointestinal disorders* (pp. 1–29). Lawrence, KS: Allen Press.

Eisenberg, D. M., Kessler, R. C., Foster, C., Norlock, F. E., Calkins, D. R., & Delbanco, T. L. (1993). Unconventional medicine in the United States. Prevalence, costs, and patterns of use. *New England Journal of Medicine, 328,* 246–252.

Eriksen, K. (1994). Effects of upper cervical correction on chronic constipation. *Chiropractic Research Journal, 3*(1), 19–22.

Feldman, P. C., Villanueva, S., Lanne, V., & Devroede, G. (1993). Use of play with clay to treat children with intractable encopresis. *Journal of Pediatrics, 122*(3), 483–488.

Fleischer, D., & Feldman, E. J. (1999). The biopsychosocial model of clinical practice in functional gastrointestinal disorders. In P. Hyman (Ed.), *Pediatric functional gastrointestinal disorders.* New York, NY: Academy Professional Information Services.

Forbes, A., Jackson, S., Walter, C., et al. (2005). Acupuncture for irritable bowel syndrome: A blinded placebo controlled trial. *World Journal of Gastroenterology, 11*(26), 4040–4044.

Gardiner, P., & Kemper, K. J. (2005). For GI complaints: Which herbs and supplements spell relief?

Gawronska, A., Dziechciarz, P., Horvath, A., & Szajewska, H. (2007). A randomized double-blind placebo-controlled trial of Lactobacillus GG for abdominal pain disorders in children. *Alimentary Pharmacology & Therapeutics, 25*(2), 177–184.

Higley, P. (1998). Continence with nature's help. *Nursing Times, 94*(32), 79–80.

Holtmann, G., Adam, B., Haag, S., Collet, W., Grünewald, E., & Windeck, T. (2003). Efficacy of artichoke leaf extract in the treatment of patients with functional dyspepsia: A six-week placebo-controlled, double-blind, multicentre trial. *Alimentary Pharmacology & Therapeutics, 18* (11–12), 1099–1105.

Hossain, M. A. (2006). The management of constipation. *National Journal of Homeopathy, 8*(2), 118–122.

Humphreys, P. A., & Gervitz, R. N. (2000). Treatment of recurrent abdominal pain: Components analysis of four treatment protocols. *Journal of Pediatric Gastroenterology and Nutrition, 31,* 47–51.

Hyams, J., Burke, G., & Davis, P. M., et al. (1996). Abdominal pain and irritable bowel syndrome in adolescents: A community-based study. *Journal of Pediatrics, 129,* 220–226.

Iwai, N., Kume, Y., Kimura, O., Ono, S., Aoi, S., & Tsuda, T. (2007). Effects of herbal medicine dai-kenchu-to on anorectal function in children with severe constipation. *European Journal of Pediatric Surgery, 17*(2), 115–118.

Jingfang, G. (2003). Treatment of prolapse of rectum with acupuncture combined with TCM drugs in 38 cases. *Journal of Traditional Chinese Medicine, 23*(2), 121.

Kemper, K. J. (1996). Seven herbs every pediatrician should know. *Contemporary Pediatrics, 13,* 79.

Kisch, E. H., & Pfeffer, C. R. (1984). Functional encopresis: Psychiatric inpatient treatment. *American Journal of Psychotherapy, 38*(2), 264–271.

Kline, R. M., Kline, J. J., Di Palma, J., & Barbero, G. J. (2001). Enteric-coated, pH-dependent peppermint oil capsules for the treatment of irritable bowel syndrome in children. *Journal of Pediatrics, 138,* 125–128.

Kohen, D. P., Olness, K. N., Colwell, S. O., & Heimel, A. (1984). The use of relaxation-mental imagery (self-hypnosis) in the management of 505 pediatric behavioral encounter. *Journal of Developmental and Behavioral Pediatrics, 5*(1), 21–25.

Kuttner, L., Chambers, C. T., & Hardial, J., et al. (2006). A randomized trial of yoga for adolescents with irritable bowel syndrome. *Pain Research and Management, 11*(4), 217–23.

Leung, W. K., Wu, J. C., & Liang, S. M., et al. (2006). Treatment of diarrhea-predominant irritable bowel syndrome with traditional Chinese herbal medicine: A randomized placebo-controlled trial. *American Journal of Gastroenterology, 101*(7); 1574–1580.

Linden, J. H. (2003). Playful metaphors. *The American Journal of Clinical Hypnosis, 45*(3), 245–250.

Loening-Baucke, V. (1993). Chronic constipation in children. *Gastroenterology, 105*(5), 1557–1564.

Loening-Baucke, V., Miele, E., & Staiano, A. (2004). Fiber (Glucomannan) is beneficial in the treatment of childhood constipation. *Pediatrics, 113,* e259–e264.

McGuire, J. K., Kulkarni, M. S., & Baden, H. P. (2000). Fatal hypermagnesemia in a child treated with megavitamin/megamineral therapy. *Pediatrics, 105*(2), E18.

Morais, M. B., Vitolo, M. R., Aguirre, A. N., & Fagundes-Neto, U. (1999). Measurement of low dietary fiber intake as a risk factor for chronic constipation in children. *Journal of Pediatric Gastroenterology and Nutrition, 29*(2), 132–135.

Niv, E., Naftali, T., Hallak, R., & Vaisman, N. (2005). The efficacy of *Lactobacillus reuteri* ATCC 55730 in the treatment of irritable bowel syndrome—a double blind, placebo-controlled, randomized study. *Clinical Nutrition, 24*(6), 925–931.

Ohya, T., Usui, Y., Arii, S., & Iwai, T. (2003). Effect of dai-kenchu-to on obstructive bowel disease in children. *American Journal of Chinese Medicine, 31*(1), 129–135.

Olsen, S. (2003). Sanicula aqua. Water as medicine. *American Journal of Homeopathic Medicine, 96*(3), 211–224.

Oster, J. (1972). Recurrent abdominal pain, headache and limb pains in children and adolescents. *Pediatrics, 50,* 429–436.

Quist, D. M., & Duray, S. M. (2007). Resolution of symptoms of chronic constipation in an 8-year-old male after chiropractic treatment. *Journal of Manipulative and Physiological Therapeutics, 30*(1), 65–68.

Ramesh, P. R., Kumar, K. S., Rajagopal, M. R., Balachandran, P., & Warrier, P. K. (1998). Managing morphine-induced constipation: A controlled comparison of an ayurvedic formulation and senna. *Journal of Pain and Symptom Management, 16*(4), 240–244.

Rasquin, A., Di Lorenzo, C., Forbes, D., Guiraldes, E., Hyams, J. S., Staiano, A., & Walker, L. S. (2006). Childhood functional gastrointestinal disorders: Child/adolescent. *Gastroenterology, 130,* 1527–1537.

Ressel, O., & Rudy, R. (2004). Vertebral subluxation correlated with somatic, visceral and immune complaints: An analysis of 650 children under chiropractic care. *Journal of Vertebral Subluxation Research (JVSR)*, 23.

Richards, A. (1998). Continence. hands on help…therapeutic massage. *Nursing Times, 94*(32), 69.

Risser, A. L., & Mazur, L. J. (1993). Use of folk remedies in a Hispanic population. *Archives of Pediatric and Adolescent Medicine, 149*, 978–981.

Roma, E., Adamidis, D., Nikolara, R., Constantopoulos, A., & Messaritakis, J. (1999). Diet and chronic constipation in children: The role of fiber. *Journal of Pediatric Gastroenterology and Nutrition, 28*, 169–174.

Sanders, M. R., Rebgetz, M., & Morrison, M. M., et al. (1989). Cognitive-behavioral treatment of recurrent nonspecific abdominal pain in children: An analysis of generalization, and maintenance side effects. *Journal of Consulting and Clinical Psychology, 57*, 294–300.

Sanders, M. R., Shepherd, R. W., Cleghorn, G., & Woolford, H. (1994). The treatment of recurrent abdominal pain in children: A controlled comparison of cognitive-behavioral family intervention and standard pediatric care. *Journal of Consulting and Clinical Psychology, 62*, 306–314.

Smith, D., & Derrett, S. (2006). Constipation services for children: The role of health visitor teams. *British Journal of Nursing (Mark Allen Publishing), 15*(4), 193–195.

Sokel, B., Devane, S., & Bentovim, A. (1991). Getting better with honor: Individualized relaxation/self-hypnosis techniques for control of recalcitrant abdominal pain in children. *Family Systems Medicine, 9*, 83–91.

Stark, L. J., Owens-Stively, J., Lewis, A., & Guevremont, D. (1990). Group behavioral treatment of retentive encopresis. *Journal of Pediatric Psychology, 15*(5), 659–671.

Stickler, G. B., & Murphy, D. B. (1979). Recurrent abdominal pain. *American Journal of Diseases in Childhood, 133*, 486–489.

Stockton, C. A. (2005). Natural Medicine Comprehensive Database [database online]. Natural Medicine Comprehensive Database 1995, Updated: February 27, 2006. American Academy of Pediatrics: The Transfer of Drugs and Other Chemicals into Human Milk.

Tilton, P. (1980). Hypnotic treatment of a child with thumb-sucking, enuresis and encopresis. *The American Journal of Clinical Hypnosis, 22*(4), 238–240.

Tokuda, Y., Takahashi, O., Ohde, S., Shakudo, M., Yanai, H., & Shimbo, T. (2007). Gastrointestinal symptoms in a japanese population: A health diary study. *World Journal of Gastroenterology, 13*(4), 572–578.

Walker, L. S. (1999). The evolution of research on recurrent abdominal pain: history, assumptions, and a conceptual model. In P. J. McGrath & G. A. Finley (Eds.), *Chronic and recurrent pain in children and adolescents* (pp. 141–172). Seattle, WA: International Association for the Study of Pain.

Wang, X. M. (1988). Electroimpulse acupuncture treatment of 110 cases of abdominal pain as a sequela of abdominal surgery. *Journal of Traditional Chinese Medicine, 8*, 269–270.

Weydert, J. A., Shapiro, D. E., Acra, S. A., et al. (2006). Evaluation of guided imagery as treatment for recurrent abdominal pain in children: A randomized controlled trial. *BMC Pediatrics, 6*, 29.

Whorwell, P. J., Altringer, L., Morel, J., et al. (2007). Efficacy of an encapsulated probiotic *Bifidobacterium infantis* 35624 in women with irritable bowel syndrome. *American Journal of Gastroenterology, 132*(2), 813–816.

Yanhua, S., & Sumei, Y. (2000). The treatment of 86 cases of epigastric and abdominal pain by scalp acupuncture. *Journal of Chinese Medicine, 62*, 27–29.

21

Integrative Pediatric Intensive Care

DAVID M. STEINHORN AND SHEILA WANG

KEY CONCEPTS

- Care on pediatric intensive care units (PICU) has evolved based upon two overarching principles: (i) the best care is provided by a multidisciplinary team incorporating the expertise of many allied medical arts in an open and mutually respectful manner and (ii) the focus of care is the patient (child) and his/her family with the assumption that the family will be the child's greatest source of strength and support.
- It is a challenge for medical teams in pediatric intensive care units to attend to the psycho-social-spiritual needs of their patient.
- PICU's as currently designed do not reflect optimal healing features. One of the most problematic aspects of intensive care is the constant presence of activity, lights, and noise from patients, staff, machines, and bedside monitors. The environment is often perceived as stressful for staff, patients, and their families.
- When the stress is reduced, the patient can shift toward a restorative or healing state. Integrative interventions such as massage or energy healing in the PICU can serve as adjuncts in grounding the patient and reducing stress.
- The most commonly utilized integrative modalities in the PICU setting are massage, energy healing techniques, music therapy, aromatherapy, pet therapy, relaxation imagery, and hypnosis. Acupuncture is provided in some PICUs as an adjunct in pain and symptom management.
- Education of all PICU medical team members about integrative approaches is important and must be included routinely in PICU staff programs if these approaches are to succeed.

Introduction

The care provided to children requiring intensive care services is both physically and emotionally challenging for patients, their families and the medical staff who work there. Very young children may be extremely fragile when struggling with life-threatening illness or extensive surgical interventions. They frequently benefit from an environment which is maximally nurturing and supportive to insure optimal recovery. Integrative medicine practitioners who have the opportunity to work in the intensive care environment will benefit from an understanding of the complexity and timeliness of much of the activity surrounding patient care. This information will allow those not familiar with the PICU environment to integrate their service with the other demands of patient care.

The journey of intensive care for children has moved from triumph to triumph. However, in the process the public has perceived that although medicine has succeeded on the technical level, it has lost much of it human touch, becoming more impersonal and forbidding.

—*I. David Todres, 2006*

Background

With these sobering words, one of the fathers of contemporary pediatric critical care summarized his observation of hospital-based care for children with life-threatening illness. The technical advances and increased understanding of disease are astounding from a historical perspective. These advances have led to the ability to correct and treat or palliate previously fatal conditions in children and to save many extremely premature infants who would have died or suffered profound disability as recently as 10–15 years ago. Our successes have also created a new group of patients who live with chronic disability or who may yet succumb to their primary disease at a much later time.

Pediatric critical care has evolved over the last three decades into an internationally recognized subspecialty with a training and certification process overseen by the American College of Graduate Medical Education. While often confused in the public's mind with neonatology (the care of premature and newborn infants up to 28 days of age) or pulmonary medicine, pediatric critical care specialists care for children from the newborn period up to older teenager. In some circumstances, many young adults are cared for in pediatric intensive care units who have survived childhood conditions such as congenital heart disease or other chronic, complex childhood conditions. By their nature, pediatric intensive care units are commonly multidisciplinary and provide specialized medical and nursing care for children with diseases of any vital organ system.

The mission of critical care and the tacit contract with the patient/family are always to return children to as long and meaningful a life as is possible while minimizing unnecessary burden and suffering. Unfortunately, meaningful survival is not always possible. In such circumstances, the death of a child represents a specialized aspect of intensive care. It requires a close partnership between intensive care and the specialists caring for the child as well as the team of specialists who will subsequently work with the family and surviving siblings.

Family-centered Care in Pediatric Intensive Care

Over the last decade, care on pediatric intensive care units has evolved based upon two overarching principles: (1) the best care is provided by a multidisciplinary team incorporating the expertise of many allied medical arts in an open and mutually respectful manner and (2) the focus of care is the patient (child) and his/her family with the assumption that the family will be the child's greatest source of strength and support (Ridling, Hofmann, & Deshler, 2006). The underlying tenets of family-centered care are familiar to most integrative medicine practitioners. They demand (1) that people are treated with dignity and respect; (2) that information is provided completely and in an unbiased manner to affirm and support the parents' right to make critical decisions; (3) that a patient's and family's strengths be enlisted to enhance self control and autonomy; and (4) that institutional policy and program development involve patients, families, and professionals (Care, I.f.F.-C). Such care reflects the respect of the healthcare providers for choices made by the patient and family based upon their own cultural, religious and personal beliefs of what is proper and best for their child. It implies a partnership between families and medical team in striving to achieve the best possible outcome for the pediatric patient. However, providing comprehensive family-centered care in the PICU setting is challenging for bedside nurses who must contend with dozens of tasks every hour such as the administration of scheduled medications, observation of monitors, charting vital signs and patient data, and dealing with the plethora of machines and their attendant alarms, all the while not forgetting the small patient in the big bed in front of them. It continues to be a challenge for the medical team to attend to the human needs of their patient (Alliex & Irurita, 2004; Kelleher, 2006; Wilkin & Slevin, 2004).

Daily Routines on the PICU

The majority of PICUs have adopted a predictable routine of "rounding" as a multidisciplinary team early in the morning and once again as a smaller group late in the afternoon. Large PICUs are typically staffed with physicians and nurse practitioners and operate "24/7" to respond immediately to changes in a patient's condition. In many units, an additional set of rounds takes place around 10 pm with the on-call team. The purpose of rounds is to cover every aspect of the patient's care that may impact the health status or be relevant for recovery including physical, emotional and social concerns of the team members. The schedule of rounding reflects the dynamic nature of treatment in the critical care setting and the constant need for patient oversight and adjustment of support. In many patients, support is adjusted on an hourly or even minute-to-minute basis as the status changes. Short-lived alterations in blood pressure or oxygen level can produce significant secondary consequences and may have a profound long-term impact on outcomes, if not corrected immediately. Thus, finding a calm time for interventions by integrative medicine practitioners may be difficult. In our institution, it is not uncommon to have interventions interrupted by urgent diagnostic procedures, respiratory therapy interventions or visits by medical consultants. Rather than feeling demeaned, the integrative medicine practitioners must realize that the PICU team's first priority will always be achieving physiologic stability in the patient. To be successful and welcome in the PICU setting, a practitioner must be flexible above all else and leave ego at the door (even if the physicians don't!).

A WORD ABOUT STRESS: THE PICU IS STRESSFUL, BUT SOME STRESS IS UNAVOIDABLE...

One of the most noticeable aspects of intensive care is the constant presence of activity, lights, and noise (Smith, Hefley, & Anand, 2007) from patients, staff, machines, and bedside monitors. The environment is often perceived as stressful both for staff, patients, and their families. One must recognize that stress is a term which is used loosely by many disciplines and has come to have a generally pejorative connotation. From a psychological point of view, stress reflects psychic tension resulting from forces that offset a state of psychic equilibrium. From a physiologic perspective, a state of stress is one which perturbs the normal balance of activity within the body. Both psychological and physical stress commonly elicits the so-called fight or flight response. This response is associated with increased output of hormones such as cortisol, catecholamines, glucagon, and growth hormone, as well as changes in the autonomic nervous system's balance characterized by reduced vagal tone compared to sympathetic activity (Porges, 2007). Such stress responses are vital to the survival of patients with acute life-threatening disease. On the other hand, prolonged and sustained stress can adversely affect wound healing, immune function and psychological state (Cohen, Daj, & Smith, 1991; Kiecolt-Glaser, Glaser, Cacioppo, & Malarkey 1998; Kiecolt-Glaser, Marucha, Malarkey, Mercado, & Glaser, 1995; Rahe, 1964). For the alert young child admitted to the PICU, painful procedures (e.g., blood drawing and IV placement) as well as the presence of the PICU team (e.g., strangers and lack of parental protection) are frequently perceived as additional threats very much like a small animal being overwhelmed by a larger predator. While it might be counterproductive to attempt to reduce normal physiologic stress responses in acutely ill or newly admitted PICU patients, we believe that efforts to alleviate unnecessary stress and to create a healing environment at the bedside of critically ill patients are potentially very useful. While it is clear in certain specialized circumstances, for example, very premature infants, that excessive environmental and tactile stimulation has adverse effects on recovery, it has been more difficult

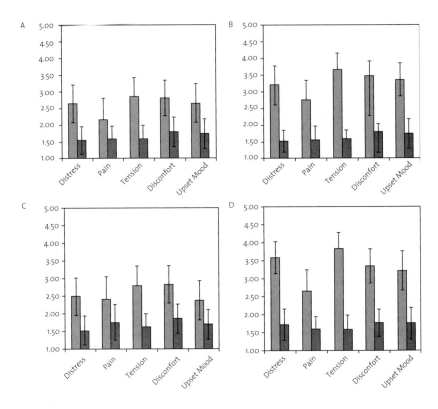

FIGURE 21-1. Panels A and C: Parent ratings of their child's level of Distress, Pain, Tension, Discomfort and Upset Mood Before and After Receiving (A) Touch Healing ($n = 378$) and (C) Massage ($n = 233$), respectively. Panels B and D: Parent ratings of their own level of Distress, Pain, Tension, Discomfort and Upset Mood Before and After Receiving (B) Touch Healing and (D) Massage. Data represent mean±SD. responses on a 1–5 scale. Mean + SD). For all results, $p<0.0001$ for pre- (light bars) / post-(dark bars) comparisons

to demonstrate this point for older children and adults. To reduce psychological and physical stress when appropriate, integrative medicine interventions can often enhance a patient's sense of well-being as demonstrated in Figure 21-1 even when potent drugs may not be effective.

Conceptually, trauma or illness throws a child into a state of stress or threat (Figure 21-2). Persistent, unrelieved stress may lead to progressive organ system failure and even death unless means to mitigate the stress are applied, for example, antibiotics for bacterial infections, surgery to remove dead tissue or restore function, or an integrative approach to reduce anxiety, fear, and depression. When the stress and inflammatory responses are reduced, the patient can shift towards a restorative or healing state. In our experience working with patients in the PICU, interventions such as massage or energy healing can serve as adjuncts in grounding the patient and replacing harsh

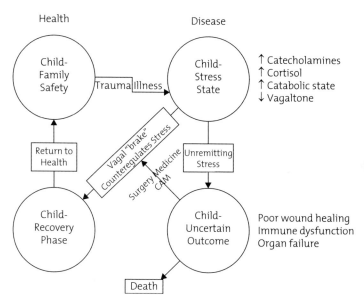

FIGURE 21-2. Conceptual framework depicting the impact of life-threatening illness on a child and the necessary mitigation of the stress response to enter a recovery phase.

tactile stimuli with periods of comfort and nurturing. We have seen numerous patients with delirium in the ICU, so-called ICU syndrome (Baker, 2004), who have dramatically calmed, relaxed and often fallen asleep during energy healing treatments, avoiding the need for higher doses of sedative medications. Often, the integrative medicine intervention is seen by the parents and nurses as an important turning point in the patient's recovery. While many other restorative processes are clearly underway in such patients, it is hard to ignore the temporal association with the intervention. While investigations of integrative medicine interventions in the PICU are limited, such observations must serve as stimuli for further prospective and, ideally, controlled investigations of PICU patients' responses to complementary interventions.

Finding Opportunities for Integrative Medicine Interventions

In the ideal PICU world, all interactions with patients would communicate our intention to promote safety, healing, and wellbeing; however, it is clear that that is often not the case in the hospital setting. In a recent discussion of care for children alone in the hospital, Zengerle-Levy (2006) points out several attitudes of nursing staff which are important for the care of a hospitalized child: (a) being a parent-minded nurse; (b) sustaining human connections; (c) receiving the patient as a child; and (d) renewing the spirit of the child. One can see that many of these attitudes resonate closely with integrative medicine practitioners' own feelings of compassion and the desire to promote

Table 21-1. Examples of Situations in the PICU Potentially Benefiting
from CAM Interventions

- Delirium and agitation
  - Due to head trauma, stroke or drowning
  - Due in newborns to in utero drug exposure
  - Patient confusion due to multiple psychoactive medications
- To relieve air hunger
- As an adjunct in pain management
- In fearful or emotionally distraught patients
- In situations of feeling hopeless
- In terminally ill patients as an aid in end-of-life transition

healing. From such a perspective, a wide range of clinical circumstances could be suitable for the application integrative healing modalities to augment and complement the conventional therapy being provided. Table 21-1 includes a sampling of possible situations for which such interventions are applied in our program and elsewhere.

In addition to treating the child/patient, parents benefit from both massage and energy healing methods as depicted in Figure 21-1. Treating parents not only benefits them but also allows them to be a more supportive presence for their child. Because the parents are the greatest source of security and comfort for most children, more fully supporting parents fulfills a fundamental principle of family-centered care (Care, I.f.F.-C; Ridling et al., 2006; Tomlinson, Thomlinson, Peden-McAlpine, & Kirschbaum, 2002).

SPECIFIC MODALITIES APPLIED IN THE PICU

The availability of randomized, controlled studies in the PICU is very limited. Critical readers of the complementary medicine literature will quickly realize that well controlled studies are often difficult in this field due to the difficulty of finding suitable cohorts to study, the small number of patients available at any single center, and general disagreement even among experts as to what a suitable control group is for various complementary interventions. Another issue that has been persistently vexing in carrying out studies in hospitalized children is the high background noise in the data set caused by interruptions in protocolized treatments or, in the PICU setting, the underlying physiologic instability of our patients. Thus, much of our approach to the use of integrative modalities in the PICU is based upon our experience with them in other hospital-based settings.

One of the most universally voiced requests of parents of critically ill children is for the PICU medical team to do anything that might help their child. It goes without saying that in our society, any child admitted to the PICU will receive *all* medical therapies and services that the physician leaders feel might benefit the patient. Contrary to the public's perception, in pediatric medicine, there is rarely a consideration for a family's financial or socioeconomic status in making clinical decisions. The only exceptions to this statement may pertain to organ transplantation for which the parents' ability to understand and follow through on critical post-transplant medications and care are vital to the success of the procedure.

The most commonly utilized integrative modalities in the PICU setting are massage (Bartolome, Cid, & Freddi, 2007; Beider, Mahrer, & Gold, 2007; Gasalberti, 2006; Vickers et al., 2007), energy healing techniques (Eschiti, 2007), music therapy (Kemper & Danhauer, 2005; Lee, Chung, Chan, & Chan, 2005; Sahler, Hunter, & Liesveld, 2003; Southby, 2006; Standley, 2002; Stouffer, Shirk, & Polomano, 2007; Twiss, Seaver, & McCaffrey, 2006), aromatherapy (Fitzgerald et al., 2007; McDowell, & McDowell, 2005), pet therapy (Gasalberti, 2006; McDowell, 2005), relaxation imagery (Bartolome et al., 2007; Lassetter, 2006; Sahler et al., 2003), and hypnosis (Butler, Symons, Henderson, Shortliffe, & Spiegel, 2005). In addition, acupuncture (NIH Consensus Conference, 1998), is provided in some institutions as an adjunct in pain and symptom management (Kemper et al., 2000; Rusy, Hoffman, & Weisman, 2002; Zeltzer et al., 2002) although it is generally not offered for young infants (Golianu, Krane, Seybold, Almgren, &Anand, 2007). In some ethnic communities, the input of traditional healers, shamans and other practitioners is given significant weight by families in making medical decisions. In light of the profound role that faith and cultural belief systems play in patient and family expectations, it behooves the PICU team to support and encourage such beliefs even if they are at odds with the clinician's own belief systems. Whether such responses are through the skill of indigenous healers or the placebo effect, the benefit to patients and families is undeniable.

Our program has provided over 800 interventions utilizing massage or energy healing interventions. All of these procedures were carried out in the PICU or hospital setting with careful attention to universal precautions for patient contact and adherence to conventional isolation measures when indicated. The data from many of these interventions which were carried out under the auspices of the Institutional Review Board are summarized in Figure 21-1. The safety record for these interventions is pristine with only one episode of mild dizziness reported in a pain clinic patient who was being seen for dizziness in the first place. Therefore, it is fair to say that the provision of this service to hospitalized children appears to be safe and well tolerated without evidence for displacement of necessary medical hardware, that is, intravenous catheters or arterial lines, or known transmission of infections.

THE ABSENCE OF HARM DOES NOT PROVE THE PRESENCE OF A BENEFIT...

While the safety record of most integrative medicine interventions is far better than many conventional therapies, the absence of harm should not necessarily be an open invitation to provide such interventions. Outside of the hospital, parents are entitled to seek out most integrative therapies for their children without any limitations by legal bodies. In the hospital setting, on the other hand, the concept of evidence for each medical decision has been elevated to an almost godlike level. All decisions regarding patient care within the hospital must conform to a basic assessment of risk vs. anticipated benefit. Integrative interventions should similarly be chosen based upon the anticipated benefit to the patient. Unfortunately, the role of complementary interventions is not generally agreed upon by western clinicians making judgment the most valuable tool in selecting appropriate interventions. In general, we try to accede to parents' requests for integrative treatments when (1) we can identify a qualified individual to provide the treatment in the PICU; (2) there is no strong theoretical contraindication to the requested treatment (e.g., bleeding risk from acupuncture in a patient with a bleeding disorder); and (3) it does not pose a risk to other therapies underway with the patient.

THE INTEGRATIVE PRACTITIONER IN THE PICU: LIKE A NIGHTINGALE FLYING THROUGH A HURRICANE...

When planning for integrative treatment of patients in the PICU, a practitioner should become familiar with the diagnosis and general condition of the patient. The practitioner should become familiar with the organization of the medical record and should develop rapport and face recognition with the PICU nurses and physicians to permit open communication about patients. As in most aspects of hospital-based healthcare, well-established hierarchies and routines exist. Most integrative medicine practitioners have extensive experience and training with adults in clinic or private practice settings; however, the world of the PICU will be very different from anything they have previously experienced. To successfully integrate into the PICU setting, it is incumbent upon *the practitioner* to develop an open and understanding relationship with the PICU staff. While many of the nurses may welcome the practitioners' presence, most practitioners find that they must earn the respect of the team to be heard and to be effective advocates for the patient. This can best be accomplished by demonstrating the benefit of what they have to offer on a case-by-case basis. Building trust takes months or years and cannot be hurried.

It is important to consider the topic of communication between conventional PICU providers and integrative medicine practitioners. All integrative medicine disciplines have developed their own unique jargon for assessing a patient's condition as well as explaining what they do for the patient. Traditional Chinese medicine (TCM), for example, uses terminology such as "heat," "cold," "dampness," "wind," "summer heat," "dryness," etc. which sound quaint although foreign to western clinicians, but which have very specific meaning to the TCM practitioner. While the National Center on Complementary and Alternative Medicine classifies integrative practices based upon the presumed mechanism of action (http://nccam.nih.gov/health/whatiscam/), even practitioners of similar *mechanistic* modalities, for example, Reiki, touch healing, energy healing, acupuncture, may use similar terms in very different ways. We have witnessed integrative practitioners attempting to explain a patient's condition to allopathic physicians using terminology from their own tradition only to have the physician shake his/her head in disbelief at the incomprehensible explanation just offered. Because our goal is to help the patient first and foremost, we must strive for clarity and simplicity in communicating about patients. Our desire to change western medicine's attitudes towards integrative medicine must wait for a more suitable opportunity. Once trust and rapport have been established, the integrative practitioner can begin to share the deeper aspects of their healing art.

Summary

As stated at the beginning of this chapter, the PICU represents a remarkable environment for both patients and healthcare providers. Extraordinary capacity exists to sustain life in the most fragile of patients, although the ability to restore health and function is often elusive. The PICU environment, therefore, offers an opportunity to create a window of time during which a patient can begin to recover. When recovery is not possible or death is inevitable, the PICU can offer an important point of transition during which patients and families can be prepared for the closure of life and the transition to whatever may come next for the patient and the surviving family. It is our feeling that integrative medicine can offer many patients important and meaningful help for any of the eventual outcomes. For those who have the potential to recover, integrative medicine can help to ground, comfort and support the ill child as they heal and to maintain an emotional, energetic bond between parent and child. For those patients who will not survive, integrative approaches may assist in easing suffering and pain and may provide as easy a transition as possible. In both contexts in the PICU setting, integrative medicine interventions express the clinician's desire to help the patient and their family in ways that drugs and machines cannot.

REFERENCES

Alliex, S., & Irurita, V. (2004). Caring in a technological environment: How is this possible? *Contemporary Nurse, 17*, 32–43.

Baker, C. (2004). Preventing ICU syndrome in children (Cover story). *Pediatric Nursing, 16*(10), 32–35.

Bartolome, S., Cid, J., & Freddi, N. (2007) Analgesia and sedation in children: Practical approach for the most frequent situations. *Jornal de Pediatria, 83*, S71–82.

Beider, S., Mahrer, M. & Gold, J. (2007). Pediatric massage Therapy: An overview for clinicians. *Pediatric Clinics of North America, 54*(6), 1025–1041.

Butler, L. D., Symons, B. K., Henderson, S. L., Shortliffe, L. D., & Spiegel, D. (2005). Hypnosis reduces distress and duration of an invasive medical procedure for children.*Pediatrics, 115*(1), e77–85.

Care, I.f.F.-C.: Bethesda, MD.

Cohen, S., Daj, T., & Smith, A. (1991). Psychological stress and susceptibility to the common cold. *The New England Journal of Medicine, 325*, 606–612.

Eschiti, V. S. (2007). Healing touch. *Dimensions of Critical Care Nursing, 26*(1), 9–14.

Fitzgerald, M., Culbert, T., Finkelstein, M., Green, M., Johnson, A., & Chen, S. (2007). The effect of gender and ethnicity on children's attitudes and preferences for essential oils: A pilot study. *Explore, 3,* 378–385.

Gasalberti, D. (2006) Alternative therapies for children and youth with special health care needs. *Journal of Pediatric Health Care, 20*(2), 133–136.

Golianu, B., Krane, E., Seybold, J., Almgren, C., Anand, K. J. (2007). Non-pharmacological techniques for pain management in neonates. *Seminars in Perinatology, 31*(5), 318–322.

Kelleher, S. (2006). Providing patient-centered care in an intensive care unit. *Nursing Standard, 21,* 35–40.

Kemper, K. J., & Danhauer, S. C. (2005). Music as therapy. *Southern Medical Journal, 98*(3), 282–288.

Kemper, K. J., Sarah, R., Silver-Highfield, E., Xiarhos, E., Barnes, L., & Berde, C. (2000). On pins and needles? Pediatric pain patients' experience with acupuncture. *Pediatrics, 105,* 941–947.

Kiecolt-Glaser, J., Glaser, R., Cacioppo, J. T., & Malarkey W. B. (1998). Marital stress: Immunological, neuroendocrine, and autonomic correlates. *Annals of the New York Academy of Sciences, 840,* 656–663.

Kiecolt-Glaser, J. K., Marucha, P. T., Malarkey, W. B., Mercado, A. M., & *Glaser,* R. (1995). Slowing of wound healing by psychological stress. *Lancet, 346,* 1194–1196.

Lassetter, J. H. (2006). *The Effectiveness of Complementary Therapies on the Pain Experience of Hospitalized Children.* 196–208.

Lee, O., Chung, Y., Chan, M., & Chan, W. 2005. Music and its effect on the physiological responses and anxiety levels of patients receiving mechanical ventilation: A pilot study. *Journal of Clinical Nursing,* 14(5):609-620.

McDowell, B. M. (2005). *Ask the Expert. Nontraditional Therapies for the PICU - Part 2.* 81–85.

McDowell, B. M., & McDowell, B. M. (2005). *Ask the Expert. Nontraditional Therapies for the PICU — Part 1.* 29–32.

NIH Consensus Conference. (1998). Acupuncture. *The Journal of the American Medical Association, 280,* 1518B4.

Porges, S. W. (2007). The polyvagal perspective. *Biological Psychology, 74*(2), 116–143.

Rahe, R. (1964). Social stress and illness onset. *Journal of Psychosomatic Research, 8,* 35–44.

Ridling, D., Hofmann, K., & Deshler, J. (2006). *Family-centered care in the pediatric intensive care unit.* In B. Fuhrman & J. Zimmerman (Eds.), *Pediatric critical care* (pp. 106–116). Philadelphia: Mosby-Elsevier.

Rusy, L., Hoffman, G., & Weisman, S. (2002). Electroacupuncture prophylaxis of postoperative nausea and vomiting following pediatric tonsillectomy with or without adenoidectomy. *Anesthiology, 96,* 300–305.

Sahler, O., Hunter, B., & Liesveld, J. (2003). The effect of using music therapy with relocation imagery in the management of patients undergoing bone marrow transplantation: A pilot feasibilitiy study. *Alternative Therapies in Health and Medicine, 9,* 70–74.

Smith, A., Hefley, G., & Anand, K. J. S. (2007). Parent bed spaces in the PICU: Effect on parental stress. *Pediatric Nursing, 33,* 215–221.

Southby, H. V. (2006). A personal reflection. *Dimensions of Critical Care Nursing, 25*(4), 172–174.

Standley, J. M. (2002). A meta-analysis of the efficacy of music therapy for premature infants. *Journal of Pediatric Nursing, 17*(2), 107–113.

Stouffer, J. W., Shirk, B. J., & Polomano, R. C. (2007). Practice guidelines for music interventions with hospitalized pediatric patients. *Journal of Pediatric Nursing, 22*(6), 448–456.

Todres, I. D. (2006). *History of pediatric critical care.* In B. Fuhrman & J. Zimmerman (Eds.), *Pediatric critical care* (pp. 7–14). Philadelphia: Mosby-Elsevier.

Tomlinson, P. S., Thomlinson, E., Peden-McAlpine, C., & Kirschbaum, M. (2002). Clinical innovation for promoting family care in pediatric intensive care: Demonstration, role modeling and reflective practice. *Journal of Advanced Nursing, 38*(2), 161–170.

Twiss, E., Seaver, J., & McCaffrey, R. (2006). The effect of music listening on older adults undergoing cardiovascular surgery. *Nurs Crit Care, 11*(5), 224–231.

Vickers, A., et al. (2007). Massage for promoting growth and development of preterm and/or low birth-weight infants (Review). In *The Cochrane Library*, Wiley.

Wilkin, K., & Slevin, E. (2004). The meaning of caring to nurses: An investigation into the nature of caring work in an intensive care unit. *Journal of Clinical Nursing, 13*, 50–59.

Zeltzer, L. K., Tsao, J. C., Stelling, C., Powers, M., Levy, S., & Waterhouse, M. (2002). A phase I study on the feasibility and acceptability of an acupuncture/hypnosis intervention for chronic pediatric pain. *J Pain Symptom Management, 24*, 437–446.

Zengerle-Levy, K. (2006). Nursing the child who is alone in the hospital nursing the child who is alone in the hospital. *Pediatric Nursing, 32*(3), 226–237.

22

Integrative Pediatric Mental Health (Assessment and Treatment Using an Ecological Perspective)

SCOTT M. SHANNON

KEY CONCEPTS

- Children are complex, constantly changing and have plastic brains of enormous potential. Remember that change and growth are the cornerstones of development.
- In all ecological models, any attempt to isolate and label individual pathology is less valuable then understanding the interdependent relationships that enhance or diminish the individual's ability to sustain the well point of true health.
- Clinicians must be trained in and aware of systems concepts as family dynamics are often playing a significant role in a child's emotional/behavioral struggles yet are often hidden, and difficult to fully appreciate.
- The current DSM-based diagnostic system is flawed and elicits grave concerns about the reliability and validity of these diagnoses as applied to children and teens, as well as concerns about the potential negative consequences of labeling when based on this system.
- Reviews of current pediatric psychopharmacology practice suggest we are prescribing well beyond our existing science. To some extent, this is being driven by desperation: the perception of inadequate alternative treatment options for children with emotional and behavioral challenges, in the face of escalating clinical needs and healthcare access limitations.
- Treatment must be strength-based.
- The process of mindful assessment and artful choices in integrative mental health treatment carry tremendous importance;

the mere substitution of alternative modalities for conventional medications is a tiny part of this process. Multi-modal treatments that respect the ecological nature of the child are most likely to be helpful in the long run.

■

Children's Mental Health

This chapter presents an overview of children's mental health from the integrative perspective. The author provides an integrative perspective for the evaluation and care of children that present with common mental health issues. The focus of this chapter is on depressive disorders, anxiety disorder, and bipolar disorder. The treatment of problem behaviors and attention disorders are explored more thoroughly in Chapter 19. This chapter highlights the process of evaluating the whole child and selecting appropriate interventions. For a more in-depth review of the current evidence base for various interventions many other excellent resources are available (Kaplan & Shannon, 2007; Kemper & Shannon, 2007; Lake, 2007; Lake & Spiegel, 2007).

What Is Mental Health?

Mental health and mental illness are complex abstractions with little firm ground. In psychiatry we do not have clear guidance from cellular pathology, biochemical tests, or neuro-imaging. The human nervous system remains far too complex and variable for scientists to provide clinically useful precise biological explanations for mental health or illness.

Currently the pre-eminent model for understanding the etiology of mental illness is the stress-diathesis model. In this framework, we presume a baseline state of mental health unless compromised by the interaction of genetics and environmental stressors. Thus, the individual with their unique genetic predisposition (diathesis) encounters the unique environment found in that person's life. These environmental stressors trigger (presumably via genomics) the expression of underlying predispositions inherited in the genetic code. Sadly, this model has not demonstrated much useful clinical utility. It has yet to be structured in a manner that is that can be proved or disproved. To quote one recent integrative textbook, "Western psychiatry can be understood as an eclectic worldview that incorporates diverse psychological, social, and biological explanatory modes, none of which is verifiable and many of which are not even testable using existing empirical models" (Lake, 2007).

The Integrative model postulates that mental and emotional health is but one aspect in the continuum of health of mind-body-spirit. In this viewpoint the range of human experiences (both in health and illness) can be thought of as a reflection of physical, mental, emotional, social, environmental, and spiritual hierarchies that are interdependent and interconnected. The essence of this model is ecological in that multiple nesting levels of levels of organization co-exist within each individual. The description of healthcare can also be explained using the ecological model. Health becomes the homeostatic point in which all of these nesting hierarchies are in a dynamic state of balance. Biological science is rapidly moving towards descriptive models of self-correcting systems and self-organization. These models also create our first demonstrable progress in outlining models of life itself. We know for example that ecosystems are self-correcting. The core foundation of all living organisms is the ability to resist entropy and move to more and more complex states. In this model, good health can be seen as the sustained ability to achieve an equilibrium that is stable within a narrow range.

Illness becomes any sustained deviation from this core state of balance whether biological, psychological, or spiritual. In this perspective, the delineation of endocrine versus GI versus neurological versus psychiatric, etc. is also rather arbitrary and often creates gaps in our understanding of the whole process. Processes that dysregulate often dysregulate more than one level of these linked human systems. Symptoms often cross these false boundaries as well.

Also, as the triggers for dysregulation can occur in any body system and be expressed on the neurological/psychological level. For example, many triggers can lead to the expression of ADHD symptoms of hyperactivity, impulsivity, and inattention in children. These include lead toxicity, closed head injury, food sensitivity, thyroid dysfunction, zinc deficiency, early malnutrition, iron deficiency, early sexual trauma, and Fragile X Syndrome. Many of our psychiatric illnesses can be best viewed as a final common pathway expressing dysregulation in the child's ecosystem. Using this model, the illness label holds less value than identifying (if possible) the triggers and supporting the systems return to a healthy state of balance.

Our Current Situation

Children bear a significant burden of psychiatric illness. There is mounting evidence that many if not most, lifetime psychiatric disorders will first appear in childhood or adolescence. Estimates of prevalence and incidence vary from site to site and study to study but the median prevalence of functionally impairing child and adolescent psychiatric disorders in 12% (Costello, Egger, et al., 2005).

Since 1991, 12-month rates of attempted suicide have remained constant at 8%, cigarette use has fallen steadily, use of marijuana rose through 1997 and since fallen while cocaine use doubled through 1999 and has held steady. Anxiety disorders have the highest prevalence at 8%, disruptive disorders at 7% and major depression at 4% (Costello, Egger et al., 2005).

The range in these studies can be enormous. For example, the prevalence rates of ADHD ranged from 1% to 13% with a median of 3%. With Bipolar Disorder, the current situation is much less clear. Case definition and diagnostic criteria remain in flux. However, one recent study found a 40-fold rise in the number of children diagnosed with bipolar illness in an outpatient setting from 1994 to 2003 (Moreno, Laje, et al., 2007).

Worldwide psychiatric issues constitute a massive problem. Using disability as a measure of the burden of illness rather than mortality, psychiatric illnesses account for over 50% of DALY (Disability Adjusted Life Years). According to a recent WHO survey, American adolescents have the highest rates of depression, substance abuse, psycho-somatic symptoms (headache, abdominal pain) and psychiatric medication use in the developed countries that were surveyed (Currie et al., 2004). The US consumes 80% of the world's stimulant medication.

Treatment in the United States remains problematic. Only 20% of children under 18 with significant psychiatric issues ever receive treatment. Children make up about one quarter of the population in the United States, but only one ninth of our mental health/ substance abuse dollars go to this population in spite of a similar burden of illness and a vastly greater potential for real prevention (Costello, Egger, et al., 2005).

Unique Issues with Children's Mental Health

Children's mental health presents significant challenges for the primary care practi-tioner. Clinical manifestations vary according to the developmental stage of each child. The variety, complexity and variability of symptoms make children's mental health assessments more difficult than those of adults.

The first level of challenge can be found inherent in the complexity of the growing child. Children learn, adapt and change quickly. The 5-year-old child's brain has twice the neurons of the adult brain and is extremely dynamic and responsive to the child's environment. In fact, extreme plasticity may be the single greatest defining character-istic of the child's brain. This ability to adapt and respond to the varied environmental influences may be both the greatest strength and the greatest liability in the child's psy-chological/behavioral adjustment.

If the environment is positive, caring, supportive, sensitive, engaged, and appro-priately stimulating the brain will respond with enhanced dendritic interconnections, cerebral blood vessels, self-regulation, cognitive depth and emotional reserve. On the other hand, if the environment is negative, conflictive, insensitive, disengaged, abu-sive, or inappropriately stimulating (excessive screen time, overt sexuality, and graphic violence) the brain will hardwire patterns of aggression, dysphoria, dysregulation, and learning problems that may become life long patterns. While theses extremes represent the extremes of early environments, the situations that practitioners encounter may be unique combinations of both positive and negative influences. Children vary enor-mously in their reactivity to these environmental influences and in their resiliency.

Trauma, particularly chronic physical abuse or sexual abuse can profoundly derail a child's future. Bruce Perry, MD, PhD and others have demonstrated that these insults in the first 5 years will profoundly alter neurological development. Perry has also demonstrated similar patterns with neglect; at times resulting in the loss of 30% of the neocortex (Perry & Pollard, 1998). These extreme cases often become chronic psychiatric patients because of their neurological adaptation to trauma and neglect. However, the real challenges for the primary care practitioners are the subtler, milder cases. For example, the mildly depressed mom who is often emotionally unavailable for her infant, or the alcoholic father that only binges once a month and then becomes loud, hostile, and threatening What about the immature parents that rent violent and sexual movies to watch at home in the presence of their 5 year old? What about the overwhelmed single mom who repeatedly sets her 3-year-old in front of a 4-hour stream of "appropriate" children's movies robbing him of emotional interaction? What about the violent and aggressive 6-year-old from "the good family" where the father is actually a tyrannical monster behind closed doors? These types of cases are all too common in practice and often fly under the radar of recognition.

All too often mild cases of trauma, abuse, and neglect go unrecognized. Hidden abuse, neglect, and trauma make it easy to blame the child and label it as psychiatric illness when it is, in reality, the marvel of neurological plasticity that presents our challenge.

It is crucial that we understand the plasticity of the child's brain and hold awareness about the power of environmental factors such as nutrition, screen time, media content, parental mental health, social pressures, and trauma to alter the path of development. We need to move beyond blaming the brain, faulty genetics, and neurochemistry in cases of child psychiatric disorders. We must see that both parents and practitioners have the power to alter this early environment and significantly redirect the path of neurological and emotional development.

One of the most complex issues in children's mental health rarely gets discussed. This relates to the parent's mental health. Every parent brings his/her own individual issues into the marriage and into the family dynamics. These issues can be massive (such as alcoholism, severe depression, and recurring pattern of abuse, etc.) or they can be subtle. This section concerns the more subtle issues. The parents' needs can drive some features of parenting and clearly color the concerns that bring the child into treatment. Parents become the agents of the child and they frame the treatment concerns. Sadly, sometimes the parents' needs are so great they remain unaware of the child's internalized suffering (anxiety, depression, Post-traumatic stress disorder [PTSD], etc.) Sometimes it is the fit between the child and the parent's personality that is the real source of the problem. As practitioners, we must realize that the parent's own issues affect their perspective and their expectations for their child. Often this dims the actual presentation. If we spend a few moments to assess this issue it may help us to intervene and understand the child's needs more completely.

As we grow and mature, all individuals have a variety of unmet emotional needs. We all carry unfulfillable dreams: we really wanted to make a career move, we really wanted to go to college, we really wanted to travel more, etc. Carl Jung MD said that there is no greater power in the psyche of an individual than their parent's unfulfilled dreams. These and other more subtle issues mix together in the marriage and affect how the child is raised. These expectations, hopes, wishes, and frustrations are different for every child. Often, most of these issues remain unconscious and outside the parent's awareness. Yet, it can have a profound influence on the growing child. Do parents (or parent) "need" this learning disabled child to be a superior student to get to law school (that dad never reached)? Do the parent(s) "need" this low motor skills child to be a competitive athlete? Do the parent(s) need this reactive and somewhat volatile child to be less like their own abusive parent? If we as practitioners can hold awareness of these parental dynamics in our awareness it will allow us to assess and treat the child more effectively.

Concerns: Conventional Care

The conventional approach to children's mental health presents some grave concerns for the integrative practitioner. These concerns cover both the diagnostic and treatment systems of modern day child psychiatry. This section will review a few significant concerns in each arena.

The diagnostic system for children's mental health is based on the criteria outlined in the *Diagnostic and Statistical Manual—4th Edition* (*DSM-IV*). Psychiatry is the only specialty that does not base its diagnostic system on verifiable tissue pathology. There are no blood tests, brain scans, or other methods to verify psychiatric diagnosis. It is based on personal report, history from parents, interview, and personal judgment. Most of the psychiatric illnesses diagnosed in childhood are based on adult illness criteria that are extrapolated to children. A recent review article confirms a common perception that the reliability of clinical diagnosis remains poor in adult clinical practice (Aboraya, 2006). In child psychiatry the extrapolation of adult diagnostic criteria, the shifting cognitive depth of children, the high rates of co-morbidity (typically three axis I diagnoses per symptomatic child), and the presence of multiple developmental lines create a moving playing field that results in even lower rates of reliability. It should be noted that reliability is fair using structured clinical interviews that are not practical in clinical practice. Experts on DSM agree that the childhood portion of DSM is problematic and in need of significant revision (due in 2012).

The psychiatric label brings some benefits for the child: insurance reimbursement, proper treatment and prognostic guidelines (if diagnosis is correct). However, the diagnostic label also carries a number of negative consequences. These include the all too common concern when the diagnosis is incorrect. Children often outgrow problems quickly, one of the joys of pediatric practice. However, labels can endure and create inappropriate expectation or prognostic pessimism. For example, about one third of kids with Obsessive–compulsive disorder will remit naturally within 2 years. A label (even when correct) can overly narrow treatment when multiple issues exist and only one is identified. The label often creates damage to the child's self-esteem and carries unfortunate stigma. Labels may all too often lead to a pharmacology-oriented approach that disempowers patient/parents and further narrows our treatment approach. Finally, in one of the bitter ironies of our dysfunctional system, a child may require one of a biological "parity" diagnosis to qualify for the highest level of insurance reimbursement. Yet, later this same label may be the source of insurance denial for any future coverage.

While most experts agree that diagnostic reliability in clinical practice of child psychiatry remains inadequate, the concerns over validity triggers even more debate. DSM has no theoretical basis and contains many different explanatory paradigms (psychodynamic, behavioral, biological, etc.). It is based on an outdated reductionistic model that moves us further from the much-needed broader integrative/holistic perspective for the whole child.

Concerns: Treatment System

The conventional treatment system for children's mental health turns to one of three common avenues of care: behavioral/parenting, psychotherapies, or pharmacological interventions. Recently we have seen a trend towards the increasing use of psychiatric medication in children and a relative reduction in other treatment options. Previously, federal monies provided the majority of financial support for psychiatric research, now the vast majority comes from the pharmaceutical industry. In a recent *New York Times* article, psychiatry was the specialty that had the highest level of financial support to doctors directly from the pharmaceutical industry (www.nytimes.com/2007/05/10/health/10psyche.html). These and a number of other complex factors have come together creating a strong push to medicalize and medicate behavioral issues in pediatric populations (For an excellent discussion of these topics see Diller, 1998, 2006).

In the last 15 years the use of psychiatric medications in children has more than tripled (Zito, Safer, et al., 2003). The use of anti-psychotic medications has risen five-fold from 1993 to 2002 and over 80% of the application of these medications is towards non psychotic indications. (Olfson, Blanco, et al., 2006) The use of psychiatric medications in a preschool (age 2–4 years) population are rising rapidly (Zito, Safer, et al. 2007). If these trends continue unabated, within 25 years over half of all American children will be on psychiatric medication. In the modern clinical practice of children's mental health we have witnessed a dramatic escalation of pharmacological interventions and a narrowing of other treatment options. This narrowing of treatment and thought in conventional child psychiatry flies in the face of a neuroscience that acknowledges the responsiveness of the child's brain (plasticity) and the ability of many external influences to alter the child's gene expression (genomics).

Finally, the evidence base in child psychiatry fails to document either adequate efficacy or long-term safety from early and prolonged medications. This is a grave concern. Of all the categories of psychiatric medication in kids, only the stimulant category has adequate documentation of efficacy and safety in children. Some of the other categories, especially anti-psychotics have inadequate testing in children in every aspect: long-term efficacy, short-term efficacy, short-term safety, and long-term safety. Some categories like SSRI anti-depressants have a mediocre efficacy record (only 1 of 15 anti-depressants have achieved an FDA indication for childhood depression) and a deteriorating safety record (black box warning for suicidality, persistent pulmonary hypertension in exposed neonates, etc.).

Another grave concern comes from the area of polypharmacy. This is one of the most notable trends in pediatric psychopharmacology. As of November 2006, we had 1.6 million pediatric patients on two or more psychiatric medications and rapidly climbing. (New York Times November, 2006 www.nytimes.com/2006/11/23/health/23kids.html) There is no science to support or encourage this trend.

An Ecological Perspective

Lead by the developments in modern physics, the clear movement in modern science has been away from narrow reductionistic and mechanistic models towards systems oriented, interactive representations. For example, we have moved from a simple mechanistic view of genetics to the much more interconnected and responsive systems perspective of genomics. In biological science we have learned that the more complex the system, the less helpful that reductionist analysis becomes. Theoretical physicist Frijof Capra (1996) said, "The great shock of twentieth century science is that systems can't be understood by analysis. The properties of the parts can only be understood from the whole.". The child's brain is the most complex system in the known universe. A model that focuses on narrow biochemical pathology in the child's brain and responds with reflectively narrow biochemical interventions represents an outdated perspective. A more accurate and modern perspective would embrace the interconnected and adaptive value of context in the child's life. Ecological science is the epitome of this type of model.

Ecology arrived as an outgrowth of the holistic reaction to the extremes of biological reductionism in the early twentieth century. An ecological perspective provides the most useful and current scientific model for understanding the complex nature of childhood behavior, emotional health, and brain function. We must learn to assess the context of the child's life if we are to understand the responses of his/her central nervous system.

In an ecological approach, the outdated emphasis on pathology is replaced by a focus on neuroplasticity, adaptability, and reactivity. Children are magnificently responsive to the context in which they develop and function. Often, this environmental responsiveness may be the source of the "illness" that we identify. For example, excessive screen time that occurs early in development of neurological controls of attention, focus, and executive function may result in attentional adaptation towards narrowly focused, high-paced, electronic delivery (TV, video games, etc.) and away from the slower, but more complex, nature of typical human environment (classroom activities, story time, family life). This excessive early stimulation will make these children proficient at video games but ineffective in classroom and prone to disorganization. Preliminary data supports this perspective (Christakis, Zimmerman, et al., 2004). PTSD is another possible example of disorder created by neurological and biochemical reaction to the environment. The trauma experienced by the child creates alternations in the neuro-hormonal milieu (i.e., increased cortisol), which, in turn, has neurotoxic effects in the hippocampus and other areas of the child's developing brain. This is why PTSD looks quite different when it develops in childhood as compared to PTSD that occurs in adults with a fully developed CNS.

Ecological Assessment

The key to understanding the child's unique ecosystem lies in the creation of a comprehensive model for assessment. The history of psychiatry moved forward notch by notch with the expansion of perspective (Freud's model of id, ego, superego, and the unconscious; the power model of Adler; the family systems model of Bowen; the bio-psycho-social model of Engel; the modern model of neurochemistry; etc.) The ecological model must be progressively comprehensive and inclusive. One such model would assess environmental, physical, mental, emotional, social, and spiritual realms, as key components of the child's ecosystem.

The environment would include a wide range of issues including such things as environmental toxins including mercury, lead, air pollution, and pesticides. It would also encompass the amount of sunlight and time in nature that the child experiences. The physical and emotional environments in the home are also other factors. Is the house cluttered, stressful, and noisy, or is it ordered, pleasing, and calm?

In the physical realm we would consider the biological family history of illness as this gives the best overall insight about genetic predisposition. The diet and ongoing nutrition of the child offers a crucial component. Both micronutrient and macronutrient patterns create the biochemical foundation for proper brain development. The personal history of illness offers critical understanding of physiological predispositions. The amount of sleep, exercise habits, relative fitness, and body habitus create the basis for proper stress management. Under this category we would also consider temperament and constitution, which are often underappreciated as significant physiological factors. Laboratory tests and issues related to chronic illness are considered here also.

The mental realm includes many factors commonly considered in the psychology of resilience. These would include the mental traits of positive mental attitude, engagement, and perseverance. Issues related to learning style (auditory, visual, kinesthetic, etc.) are also important. We must understand the learning preferences and challenges for every child. General consideration of cognitive capacity and formal learning disorders would also be included here. Stage of cognitive development, educational background, resources, and general level of intellectual stimulation all merit consideration. Finally, the level of perceptiveness, self-awareness, sensitivity, memory, and processing speed also factor into the mental realm. Once we grasp the learning style and characteristics of the child we must assess the goodness of fit with their school. A misfit with school may lead a child to failure, despair, and psychiatric symptoms.

The emotional realm generally includes the level of emotional reactivity, emotional tone, and self-control. Prior trauma or losses will be crucial features to assess in this realm of the child's life. A chronic abuse or neglect history will create considerable liability for any child in the emotional realm. Every child has a different pattern of ambient mood and affect. How expressive is the child at a healthy baseline? Also of concern here is the emotional tone between the parents and the general emotional tone, supportiveness and acceptance found in the household(s). If divorced, are the parents supportive of each other or still at war?

In the social realm, the history, nature, quality, and depth of the parent–child bonds create a crucial foundation for the child's physical, emotional, mental, social, and spiritual health. The Harvard Mastery of Stress Study, which followed Harvard students from the 1950s into the 1990s, provided evidence for this. No other factor (smoking, blood-pressure, weight, etc.) offered better predictive quality for mid-life physical health than a self-perceived rating of parent–child closeness offered at the beginning of the study (Russek & Schwartz, 1997).

Beyond this, the nature, quality, variety, and stability of peer relationships are a crucial barometer of social health. An often-overlooked factor is the important role that adults other than parents play in children's lives: neighbors, family-friends, coaches, teachers, and pastors, for example. In an era when extended family plays less of a role in children's lives, these other adults can make a major difference to children. Various studies of resilient children have confirmed the powerful ability of one outside adult to turn a child's life around (Stewart & Sun, 2004).

Fit is another parent–child factor that carries significant weight in our assessment of the child. Every child is different. Parents with many children are aware that their connection, comfort, and ease of interaction vary from child to child. Most parents are more drawn to one child than another and this is perfectly normal. Fit becomes a practical concern only when there is a conflict in the fit between parent and child. We can call this bad chemistry or a personality clash, but when this occurs it stresses both parent and child significantly. Unless it is addressed well, the child will be much more likely to become labeled and pathologized. When the number of positive outside adult relationships is limited, more pressure is placed on the parent–child relationship, and there may be more problems when there is an issue of fit (personality/temperament clash). Factors of interpersonal awareness (sensitivity and empathy) should be assessed here as well. Traits such as introversion/extroversion provide more helpful information about how the child connects with others and her social world.

Modern medicine and psychiatry ignored the importance of spirituality for far too long. Only in the last 20 years has medicine begun to appreciate the power of faith, religion, and spiritual community. Families with an intact belief system are healthier, happier, and more prone to stay intact. The specifics of the belief system do not seem to matter; rather the crucial factor seems to be regular attendance and active participation/practice for the family. Children seem to benefit in a wide variety of ways from the presence of an intact belief system and ongoing religious/spiritual practice.

The Treatment Plan

The treatment plan will flow naturally from the assessment. A broad and comprehensive assessment is crucial in understanding the child's ecosystem. Only then can we appreciate more of the contextual influences upon the child's plastic and responsive nervous system. True ecological understanding requires that we also appreciate the specific qualities of the child that drive the contextual responses. This is an area that is difficult to fully describe, as it is so specific for each child. Perhaps the best way in which to summarize the ecological assessment would involve a list of relative strengths and challenges for each child over the six realms. Thus, a hypothetical list might look something like for a 9-year-old boy presenting with attentional problems:

Environmental
- Strengths: lots of time in nature
- Challenges: chaotic, over-stimulated home

Physical
- Strengths: physically fit, constitutionally strong, athletic, negative family history
- Challenges: inadequate sleep, poor nutrition-excessive sweets in diet and inadequate protein

Mental
- Strengths: above average verbal skills, reading comprehension
- Challenges: slow in math, poor-fit with school

Emotional
- Strengths: strongly positive, joyful mood; positive supportive parental marriage
- Challenges: lack of emotional self-control, awareness

Social
- Strengths: broad range of friendships, close with both parents
- Challenges: tendency to be aggressive or impulsive with friends

Spiritual
- Strengths: generous and compassionate nature
- Challenges: lack of family spiritual practice

The treatment plan will flow from the information. Treatment in conventional child psychiatry has narrowed and is now mostly focused on symptomatic treatment of the presenting chief complaint. An integrative treatment model will consider the ecological assessment above and address as many of these issues as is practical. The treatment plan must be comprehensive and reflect content.

The challenges must be supported and acknowledged. For example, with this boy an integrative treatment plan would attempt to calm the home environment, increase his sleep, improve his diet, consider his school fit, build emotional self-awareness, and improve self-control. The treatment must address crucial challenges or triggers. His strengths can function as crucial tools to help him navigate his current struggles: build on his athletic prowess for more success experiences; emphasize his strengths in verbal skills and reading in the classroom; leverage his friendships to support the needed changes in self-control and awareness; focus positive one on one parent time to coach and support homework and needed behavioral changes.

There can be no cookbook recipe here for different diagnoses. The ecological assessment is an inquiry in individuality and the integrative treatment plan must reflect that uniqueness and must be tailored to the child's own ecosystem.

The treatment plan must be prioritized. Obviously, we can't address every challenge and strength. Rather, we must focus on these issues that are the most relevant to the current concerns. For the boy in the example, his current spiritual challenge is a background issue. His presentation comes from the mental (school/learning) realm, so that will predominate. Physical (i.e., diet and sleep) and environmental issues typically act as a foundation (for positive or negative) of functioning and can be quite relevant to most issues. For this boy, emotional, and social issues are secondary. His treatment plan would prioritize environmental, physical, and mental interventions.

The treatment plan must also reflect the child/family belief system. For example, if a family has a strong belief in medications they would be prioritized. Conversely, if the child/family has s strong preference for a natural approach that avoids psychiatric medications, the practitioner should make every effort to respect those wishes in creating a personalized treatment plan.

Clearly, the child's ecosystem and central nervous system are rapidly changing and never static. We must recognize that diagnosis and presentation change rapidly. We should make every treatment plan as fluid and dynamic as the child is, and should reevaluate frequently.

Ecosystems are defined by complexity of inter-relationships. Thus, narrow, "silver-bullet" interventions rarely last. Multi-faceted interventions that reflect the complex relationships in the child's ecosystem are more likely to bring positive adaptation. Powerful, narrow interventions may carry many hidden long-range repercussions that we can't anticipate. For example, the developmental and neuro-endocrine effects of long-term use of psychiatric medications are mostly unknown. All care for children should embody the precautionary principle: employ extreme caution where the effects and risks are not established.

Finally, the treatment plan must honor the self-healing capacity of every child. Scientists now recognize that self-correction is a central quality of ecosystems. The stronger and more diverse the ecosystem the greater the capacity there is for self-correction. In individual organisms we can describe this trait as homeostasis: the ability to maintain and self-correct an internal milieu.

The conventional model in child psychiatry places far stronger emphasis on models of pathology than on models of health. The ecological model is posited on the inherent self-correcting capacity of the ecosystem. Growing from the work of Nobel Prize winning chemist Ilya Prigogine (Prigogine & Geheniau, 1986), we now have chemical models of self-organizing systems. This ability to self-organize and self-correct is the basis of life and a crucial foundation for our approach to mental and emotional problems in children.

In summary, an integrative treatment plan should have the following characteristics:

1. Be comprehensive
2. Be contextual
3. Address challenges and triggers
4. Be strength-based
5. Be individualized
6. Be prioritized
7. Be dynamic
8. Be multi-faceted
9. Honor self-healing capacity
10. Respect the belief system of the child/family

The treatment plan can be integrative as well. This can mean a combination of ecological care and allopathic care. Allopathic treatment models (against illness) are typically symptom focused and narrow. The integrative model allows us to judiciously combine broader ecological interventions with allopathic approaches. Interestingly, many of the common complementary and alternative (CAM) approaches are actually allopathic in nature. For example, St. John's Wort (SJW) is a symptom-based herbal intervention for depression that treats the signs and symptoms of this mood disorder. SJW does not address the ecological nature of depression or correct fundamental deficiencies in the same way that B vitamins or essential fatty acids do. Furthermore, there has been no randomized controlled trial of SJW in young children. Thus, SJW can be considered an herbal form of allopathic (against illness) intervention. In the integrative model, allopathic interventions are not negative, merely narrow in scope.

The Issue of Diagnosis

In an ecological model the tendency to find isolated distinct pathology in the child is greatly diminished. Rather, the pathology becomes the negative context and forces that elicit the current response. Obviously, the child and the environmental influences interact to create a specific response. Although we can characterize the response of the child with a psychiatric label, it is more helpful to understand the child and their context (nutrition, family dynamics, learning style, social connections, etc.) if we are to move towards anything more than simple symptomatic control. A much deeper level of treatment flows from the ecological model that begins to appreciate the triggers for symptom expression. Once addressed, these triggers will diminish and symptoms will then abate reflecting the self-correcting nature of the human brain. For example, a child with a conflictual fit with one parent and a poor fit in his school will often become depressed. Rather than move to treatment with a serotonin reuptake inhibitor such as fluoxetine, address the issues of fit and the depression will improve on its own accord without pharmacological support. Simple pharmacotherapy alone may simply mask the reasonable response to the unreasonable context in which the child is immersed.

Given the malleable and plastic responsiveness of the child's brain, simple generic labels that identify the broad type of symptomatic presentation that the child presents with (i.e., mood, anxiety, disruptive, or attentional) may be the most accurate. We should move to a more specific label with a child only when it designates a specific, safe, and well-proven treatment. OCD is one example (exposure and response prevention). In psychiatry, we have a large number of diagnostic categories and very few specific treatments. For example, SSRIs are used in mood disorders, anxiety disorders, eating disorders, and sexual dysfunction. Anticonvulsants are used in epilepsy, mood disorders, and aggressive dyscontrol. Antipsychotics are used in schizophrenia, mood disorders, and disruptive disorders.

Facets of Integrative Treatment

By its very nature, the integrative treatment of pediatric mental health issues is broad, diverse, and creative. The number and variety of treatment options are vast. This section will provide a brief overview of the major categories and a few of the specific treatments approaches within each category.

Lifestyle interventions include interventions that improve the quality and duration of sleep (such as proper sleep hygiene and focused cognitive behavior therapy, CBT). Exercise and activity that improve fitness can range from recreational soccer to kick boxing classes to local swim teams. High levels of screen time have been shown to relate to high levels of levels of obesity (Crooks, 2000). A family hike or bike ride each weekend benefits children in a number of ways. Finally, something called social rhythms therapy has been proved to benefit bipolar illness by enhancing stability and predictability of basic routines in the individual's life (Frank, Kupfer, et al., 2005). Simply having set and predictable wake time, bedtime, meal times, and bath time improves emotional stability in bipolar patients. In a German study, intensive lifestyle therapy improved depression as well as counseling and medications (Hamre, Witt, et al., 2006).

Personality factors can play a huge role in how resilient or resistant to stress children are. If parents can role model positive mental attitude and engaged problem solving in their own lives this will have a beneficial effect for their children. Furthermore, parents can encourage their children to take reasonable risks and be prepared to watch them fail occasionally. In this circumstance, step back and focus on problem solving and re-engagement. Emphasize the process itself.

The child's diet and nutrition creates the foundation for structure and function in the developing CNS. Diet has a pronounced and pervasive influence on both the developmental and treatment of psychiatric symptoms. Examples include the corrective power of B vitamins, minerals, essential fatty acids, and combinations formulas on mood (Kaplan & Shannon, 2007) as well as the effects of food additives on attention (McCann, Barrett, et al., 2007). There are many examples of a nutritional deficiency model in which the patient's illness can be viewed as in-born errors of metabolism secondary to genetic idiosyncrasies or single nucleotide polymorphisms (SNPs) (Kaplan, Crawford, et al., 2007). These enzymatic inefficiencies make some children much more prone to symptomatic expression with a typical American diet. The treatment options either dramatically enhancing the available metabolic endpoint to overcome these metabolic inefficiencies or to supply the needed endpoint products themselves. For example, imagine that young Johnny has a strong family history of mood disorders that revolve around a SNP inefficiency of omega-3 EFA metabolism. Treatment could involve either a diet high in flaxseed (omega-3 precursor) or merely supplying the omega-3 metabolites (EPA and DHA) directly for CNS function.

Key: Improvement of diet alone is typically not enough for most symptomatic patients and supplementation is required for effective correction of these in born errors of metabolism.

Some children will have food sensitivities or food allergies that cause alterations in mood or behavior (Bischoff, 2007; Teufel, Biedermann, et al., 2007). About 6%–10% of children have either allergies or sensitivities to food and about 1% cannot tolerate gluten (Bangash, 2005). The most common sensitivities are dairy, wheat, corn, soy, eggs, citrus, tree nuts, peanuts, and shellfish. Some indicators of food related problems include family history of allergy, history of eczema or colic, chronic abdominal pain, long bone pain, bad breath, bad foot odor, insomnia, chronic headaches, or rhinorrhea. If a patient has two or more positives, consider an elimination diet or referral to a nutritional specialist.

Multivitamin combination formulas have demonstrated significant value in a wide range of problems including bipolar disorder, behavior disorders, and cognitive functioning (Jiang, 2006; Kaplan, Crawford, et al., 2007). Five studies documented here represent RCTs. Geseh (2002) gave juvenile offenders a vitamin, mineral and EFA combination and found significant reductions in violent acts and rule infractions. Four peer-reviewed studies in psychiatric journals have indicated significant benefit from the use of a proprietary vitamin mineral supplement called EM Power in bipolar disorder (Kaplan, Crawford, et al., 2007).

The number of studies exploring the value of essential fatty acids (EFAs) has mushroomed in the last 5 years. The current database provides strong evidence that EFAs play a crucial role in cognitive and emotional functioning (Freeman, Hibbeln, et al., 2006; Peet & Stokes, 2005). Eicosapentanoic acid (EPA) appears to play a pre-dominant role in the mood disorders while docasahexanoic acid (DHA) plays a more pronounced role in cognitive development and learning disorders. These Omega-3 EFAs form the foundation of neuronal development in the young child's brain. They are crucial for both the structure and function of all neurons secondary to their role in phospholipids and the second messenger system.

Recent studies indicate that children's diets are not balanced and only 1% meet food pyramid guidelines. A JAMA review article (Fletcher & Fairfield, 2002) found that suboptimal intake of micronutrients was a risk factor for chronic illness and data supported the use of vitamin supplementation as a tool to reduce chronic illness in adults. Given the dramatically elevated nutrient demands in the pediatric population the conclusion seems clear: all children, particularly those with mental health issues should take nutritional supplementation as a core facet of their care and treatment.

The family arena plays a central and crucial role in the child's emotional development. This includes a variety of family issues including parenting skills, parent–child fit, marriage, and support/acceptance. The modern shift towards biochemistry has unfortunately diminished our appreciation for the fundamental power that family interventions carry for symptomatic children.

Parenting skills often reflect the ability to be firm, consistent, and positive in limit setting and boundaries. These issues are most pronounced for disruptive and explosive children who are out of control. Often a depressed primary care giver feels overwhelmed. A number of recent studies document the increased risks for psychological diagnosis in children who live with a depressed mother (Hammen & Brennan, 2003). The risks include not just mood disorders but behavioral and attentional disorders as well, further documenting the ecological nature of children's mental health. These studies also document that a substantial portion of children lose their label if mom improves (Weissman, Pilowsky, et al., 2006).

Parent–child fit involves the comfortable blending or clashing of personalities, temperaments, and styles of a parent with a child. Most often it is not an issue. However, when present it can drive many psychiatric problems. Fit can often be labeled as psychiatric illness and may at times represent a scapegoating of the child.

The quality and emotional tone of the marriage creates a pervasive and forceful influence for every child. A positive, loving, supportive and understanding marriage radiates innumerable benefits to the child. Conversely, a high conflict divorce with custody battles may be the most emotionally damning family experience possible. Our work lies between these poles. Do not lose sight of the value of marital therapy for pediatric mental health issues, as it is not easy to appreciate the style and tone of a marriage from the vantage point of an office visit with a younger child.

In some ways, all of these family issues come back to the parents. They may be ignorant of specific skills, or their individual emotional development may be compromised in some way. This, in turn, may have adverse effects on the marriage and on their children. Parenting challenges our own emotional health and offers deep rewards if we meet these challenges with real awareness. When addressed with awareness parenting can burn away our own narcissism and selfishness, open our heart and can tear at our emotional scars. The book *Parenting from the Inside Out* (Seigel & Hartzell, 2003) explores this complex topic well.

The primary job of every school-aged child is that of student. Children who find school easy and fun have less emotional and behavioral concerns. Personality factors, cognitive factors, and specific learning styles play a key role in this process. The two crucial personality traits are introversion/extroversion and approach/avoidance. The introverted, avoidant or anxious younger child may struggle with school. He or she may do better with smaller schools and need more help with transitions. The Small Schools Project (smallschoolsproject.com) has documented that children attending small schools do better in performance, attendance and graduation rates (Cleary & English, 2005).

Parents and professionals should keep a watchful eye on the fit of this child with the schooling process. The cognitive issues often encompass general measures of intelligence and specific learning disorders. The child that has subnormal or gifted intelligence will require special support and consideration in school selection.

Finally, the specific learning style of each child will determine what type of school and curriculum path will be most optimal. Learning styles vary from child to child. A child may be a visual/verbal, visual/nonverbal, auditory, or kinesthetic learner. Experts also now recognize many types of basic human intelligences (Gardner, 1983, 2004). These include logical, linguistic, musical, kinesthetic, spatial, interpersonal, intrapersonal, and naturalistic. We will tend to find a child's gifts, and joys strongly connected to their innate preferences in this arena. The combination of intelligence type and learning style will determine the best school fit for the child. Poor school fit (a child with musical and physical gifts who is a kinesthetic leaner placed in a rigorous narrow "college prep" school) will create an increased likelihood of psychiatric symptoms. Parents should be encouraged to understand the power of intelligence type, learning style and school fit, and follow the child's passions and gifts.

Environmental Issues

Environmental issues are increasing threats to the health of children in the twenty-first century. As considered here, the environment includes the chemical environment (pesticides, herbicides, heavy metals, chemicals like bis-phenol A, etc.), psychological environment (television, print, internet, etc.) and the sociocultural environment (poverty, materialism, sexuality, commercialism, violence, sexism, etc.). Increasingly, all those caring for children must actively advocate for the identification and removal of toxins in whatever form they take. It is clear that the pervasive reach of these toxins exact a massive toll on our children's mental health.

Children vary widely in their exposure to these issues and their susceptibility to the burden imposed. We must be creative, educational, and persistent in our role as advocates for health. We often fail to make the connection between these environmental toxins and psychiatric symptoms. We have evidence that lead toxicity debilitates attentional skills all the way down to our lowest measurable threshold (Banerjee, Middleton, et al., 2007; McMichael, Baghurst, et al., 1994). We have strong evidence that exposure to violence is associated with violent behaviors. Some of the issues here are controversial (the neurological effects of EMF) while others are very difficult to measure (the pervasive sexualization of our culture). The best direction here is to individually assess each child's environment, assess the symptom pattern and forcefully advocate and intervene for the child as indicated.

Psychotherapy

In the treatment of mental health issues in children we have a wide array of therapeutic tools. Psychotherapy has a long-standing traditional role. The psychotherapeutic modalities vary by age, level of parental involvement, and philosophy. In general, the younger the age of the child the greater the level of parental involvement indicated. For example, when addressing a behavioral attachment issue with a 4 year old, the vast majority of the work should be with the parents. However, if dealing with existential depression in a 17 year old, the majority of the work will be with the teen.

Children vary widely in the ability and inclination to participate in verbally based psychotherapy. Many boys don't fare well with this modality. Play therapy has a role with young children. If behavior problems are part of the presentation, it is important to also teach parenting skills. In general, the more behavioral issues, the more parental involvement required. Often, this will require family therapy for the preteen and teen. Marital therapy is a must if the level of tension and hostility is high or sense of connection is low in the marriage. Family therapy is an underutilized modality. Group therapy, an extremely powerful tool for teens, is also significantly underutilized.

Recently, we have witnessed the emergence of a variety of approaches based on the principles of mindfulness. Dialetical behavior therapy (DBT) is the most prominent. This evidence based technique combines aspects of CBT and mindfulness. The majority of the early research involved adult patients with Borderline personality disorder (Linehan, Armstrong, et al., 1991). However, it has shown great promise in mood disorders and suicidality. A variety of pilot studies in pediatric populations echo the nine positive RCTs for adults. Recent studies have documented improvements in the pediatric age range for a variety of problems based in mood, affect, or behavioral regulation. Often run in groups, DBT is really a training course in the enhancement of self-awareness and self-regulation (Rathus & Miller, 2002). This modality is highly recommended. In many ways DBT is closer to psycho-education than to psychotherapy.

In general the key issues in psychotherapy involve the proper fit of personal chemistry, parental involvement, therapeutic style, and specific skill set with the child's issues. For OCD the therapist should be skilled in exposure response prevention (ERP) as this is a proven and specific skill set (Bolton & Perrin, 2007). The therapist must monitor responses and be quite willing to recommend change for lack of fit or progress. Three-month blocks are adequate for periodic reassessment. Psychotherapy is not useful for every child but if trauma, anxiety, or depression are present than a trial is usually warranted.

Eye movement desensitization and reprocessing (EMDR) is a relatively new psychtherapeutic technique that involves the use of eye movements across the midline with some verbal or internal processing. The evidence base is strongest in the trauma and PTSD but appears to have value for anxiety disorders and perhaps mood disorders as well (van der Kolk, Spinazzola, et al., 2007).

NON-TRADITIONAL THERAPIES

Art, music, and dance therapies are non-traditional therapies that may have a role in the treatment of children. The evidence base is currently small but promising (Whitehead-Pleaux, Zebrowski, et al., 2007). Many children do not process auditory information very well and these modalities offer excellent alternatives. Also, if the child has an artistic, musical, or kinesthetic gift/interest, than these referrals may be extremely useful on many levels.

Another underappreciated tool is the therapeutic use of the outdoors and adventure. Experiential therapy, adventure therapy, or outdoor education can be another amazing tool in the positive transformation of a child. These experiences can help alter the perspective and mindset of a depressed or substance abusing teen. They can also function as a positive anchor for a teen growing up in a highly dysfunctional family. The down side is that they are often expensive and time limited. So after-care and continuity are crucial. The most successful treatment recommendations are often creative and intuitive, based upon the unique make up of the identified patient.

Mind-Body Therapies

Practitioners have a wide range of mind-body tools to choose from. The specific techniques range from the ancient (Tai Chi and meditation) to the modern (biofeedback and guided imagery). Hypnosis and relaxation skills can help children deal with a variety of issues including pain and anxiety. Meditation and mindfulness skills have been well researched and appear to improve nearly every measured mediator of autonomic balance and psychological health (Grossman, Niemann, et al., 2004). Mindfulness skills can even be adapted for use with prepubertal patients (Ott, 2002). Tai Chi and mindfulness have been successfully demonstrated in a Boston Public Middle School (Wall,

2005). A variety of mind-body techniques significantly reduced the symptom load of students in war torn Kosovo (Gordon, Staples, et al., 2004). Relaxation therapy proved to be as effective as CBT in a RCT of 30 depressed adolescents (Reynolds & Coats, 1986). Given that most mental health problems are associated with increased levels of stress, mind-body skills can be a useful adjunct for many symptomatic children.

Biochemical Therapies

Psychiatric medications and herbal preparations constitute the bulk of biochemical therapies. Compounds found naturally in food are considered nutritional supplementation for this discussion. Psychiatric medications do play a role in the integrative treatment of pediatric mental health issues. The optimum approach may be a three-tiered treatment plan. The first tier prioritizes safe educational, environmental, lifestyle, family, diet changes, and nutritional approaches. The second tier can be other therapies including mind-body, herbal remedies, psychotherapies, and other CAM modalities. Psychiatric medications fall into the third tier because of the elevated levels of risk and power. An exception may be made for families that have a belief system favoring prescription medication or rejecting CAM approaches. In these cases the first tier of care should remain the same.

An integrative approach to the use of psychiatric medications in pediatric population involves seven basic principles:

1. Use low doses. Engage the power of the placebo to the benefit of all. Use the power of suggestion.
2. Advance doses slowly. Allow the body and nervous system time to adjust.
3. Drug holidays. Once or twice a year assess the child's symptom level by slowly tapering the dose and monitoring symptoms.
4. Multi-modal care. Never make psychiatric medications the sole approach.
5. Use targeted nutritional adjuvants. For example, B vitamins and folate should always be given with anti-depressants in order to enhance response and reduce the doses required.
6. Avoid poly-pharmacy whenever possible. We simply have no science to guide us.
7. Employ physiological supports. For example, use Omega-3 oils with neuroleptics (black box warning for weight gain and Type II diabetes) to reduce the risks of hyperlipidemia.

Herbal remedies contain both new and time-honored interventions for mental health. Saint John's Wort has a substantial and growing evidence base for use in depressive disorders (Linde & Knuppel, 2005) including three open trials. Kava-Kava has found a rather recent appreciation for its benefit in anxiety disorders. Whenever possible use the same preparations that have been involved in the key studies for a particular herb.

For example, when possible employ the same SJW formulation used in many of the prominent controlled trials. Finally, realize that quality varies widely for herbal preparations. Choose brands known to emphasize quality control, periodic assays, and product monitoring. This may often result in narrow brand recommendations and higher price range. Random retail surveys of herbal preparations demonstrate a disturbing range of product quality (ConsumerLab.com). Caveat Emptor.

Energy

A wide range of energy-based modalities can be applied to benefit mental health concerns. These approaches include the use of light, electricity, and human energy (Chi, prana, etc.). Light therapy has a proven role in treating mood disorders (with or without a seasonal rhythm). A recent meta-analysis of randomized controlled trials of light therapy found bright light treatment for non-seasonal depression is effective, the effect size being quite similar to that for anti-depressant trials (Golden, Gaynes, et al., 2005). Cranial electrical stimulation (CES) involves the use of low voltage, low amperage current from one ear lobe to the other. Previously called electro-sleep, this little used therapy has good evidence that is can reduce anxiety and improve mood (Passini, Watson, et al., 1976). Qi Gong is an ancient Chinese martial art that develops skills and awareness in the internal manipulation of the body's own energy (Chi). Qi Gong has wide ranging evidence supporting its value for a range of mental health issues (Shannon, 2002). Therapeutic Touch is a gentle physical technique often practiced by nurses in health care settings. There are no RCTs with children for these therapeutic modalities. Daylighting, the enhanced natural sunlight in classrooms has been found to improve school performance, reduce illness, and improve attendance (Manuel, 2003).

Biomechanical Modalities

Only a few of the available biomechanical therapies have been evaluated in psychiatric illness. Therapeutic massage promotes positive changes in a wide variety of physiological measures: blood flow, muscular relaxation, autonomic balance, and lymphatic drainage. In one study of massage in depressed patients it decreased cortisol levels and improved the levels of serotonin and dopamine (Field, Hernandez-Reif, et al., 2005). Massage reduced aggression is adolescent inpatients (Diego, Field, et al., 2002). A brief daily back rub reduced anxiety and improved cooperation in child and adolescent psychiatric inpatients (Field, Morrow, et al., 1992). The infants of depressed mothers derived significant benefit from maternal massage with higher scores on a variety of measures in the Brazelton scale (Field, Hernandez-Reif, et al., 2006). Given the persistent and significant negative effects of maternal depression (Weissman, Pilowsky, et al., 2006), this approach can support the infant's well-being into the future. In massage, the specific technique appears to be less important than the gentle, caring touch of a concerned attentive adult. Parents can be easily taught to touch and soothe their children. A prior history of physical or sexual abuse makes the application of "good touch" both more important and challenging. Osteopathic cranial manipulation may offer considerable benefit to children with a history of birth trauma, chronic headaches or severe learning disabilities.

Traditional Modalities

Acupuncture, homeopathy, and ayurvedic medicine form three of the most important time honored approaches to healing. Acupuncture has a growing research base with evidence building for its effectiveness with both depression and anxiety. A systematic review of randomized controlled trials of acupuncture of depressed adults suggested significant benefits equal to those of anti-depressant medications (Leo & Ligot, 2007). Another meta-analysis (Mukaino, Park, et al., 2005) found that electro-acupuncture was as effective as anti-depressant medications. Kemper (Kemper, Sarah, et al., 2000) demonstrated that acupuncture was well-received in a pediatric population. Other studies have found reduction in anxiety following acupuncture (Karst, Winterhalter, et al., 2007).

Symptom-Oriented Treatment

In an ecological perspective the treatment of mental health issues moves from a diagnostically based treatment model to a symptom-based model. In this way the treatment becomes more dynamic, more personalized and less rigid. This approach also tends to reduce our use of psychopharmacology. As previously mentioned, the treatment plan must be comprehensive and prioritized, emphasizing the realms in the child's life that have the most distress. Given all of this, each treatment plan will be quite unique and individualized. This section will present treatment plans for broad symptoms emphasizing commonly employed approaches with an evidence base. These lists are meant to be a general guide to be customized for the individual child or teen.

Symptom-oriented treatment

1. Depressed mood (flat, slowed, apathetic)
    a. Environments: sunlight, light therapy (30–60 minute 10,000 lux, in am), pets, atmosphere of joy and support in home. Reduced screen time.
    b. Physical: aerobic exercise (20 minutes, 3–4 times a week). More physical activity, B vitamins (B-complex 50 mg with 1 mg of folate), Omega-3 oils (1–2 g of EPA), chromium picolinate (400 mcg BID—atypical depression, hypersomnia/hyperphagia). SAMe (200–600 mg BID on empty stomach). Vitamin C (1000 mg in AM). Dietary improvements (enough protein and reduce sugar). Acupuncture trial (teens).
    c. Mental:psychotherapy (CBT), proper fit in school with learning style and support of specific intelligence, gifts, talents, etc.
    d. Emotional: expressive therapies: dance, art, music, family therapy, group therapy

    e. Social: recreation, sports, church groups, social skills groups (younger kids), after school clubs.

    f. Spiritual: forgiveness, gratitude journal, proper religious attendance, volunteer work.

2. Depressed mood (agitated, irritable)

    a. Environmental: sunlight, light therapy (30–60 minutes in AM; 10,000 Lux), time in nature, pets, atmosphere of peace and harmony in home. Reduction of screen time.

    b. Physical: physical activity (walking, hiking, etc.) aerobic exercise (20 minutes 3–4 times per week), dietary improvements (reduce sugar, eliminate caffeine), B-complex (50 mg with 1 mg of folate). St. John's Wort (900 mg per day of quality product divided BID). Inositol (2–4 g BID or TID), EFA (1–2 g of EPA), Vitamin C (1000 mg in AM), 5-HTP (50–200 mg BID). Acupuncture trial (teens), massage therapy. Support of proper sleep hygiene.

    c. Mental: psychotherapy (DBT, CBT, or Hakomi), relaxation therapy or mindfulness practice or Tai Chi, proper fit in school for learning style. Support of specific intelligence(s), gifts, talents.

    d. Emotional: expressive therapies: dance, art, or music. Family therapy. Group therapy

    e. Social: recreation, sports, church group. Social skills group (younger kids), after school groups.

    f. Spiritual: forgiveness, gratitude journal. Prayer. Religious services. Volunteer work.

3. Mood dysregulation (rage, lability, aggression)

    a. Environmental: social rhythms therapy (enhanced predictability of sleep, meals, and other routines), sense of peace and harmony in home. Reduction of screen time. Pets and time in nature. Elimination of violence (TV, video games, DVD, etc.).

    b. Physical: physical activity. Aerobic exercise (20 minutes 3–4 times per week), dietary improvements (reduction of sugar, eliminate caffeine, more complex carbohydrates) EFAs (2–4 g of EPA per day). EM Power Plus [proprietary vitamin mineral product tested in bipolar disorder] (5 capsules three times daily). Massage therapy. Inositol (2–4 g TID).

    c. Mental: psychotherapy (DBT), relaxation therapy, mindfulness practice, martial arts, proper fit in school for learning style. Support of specific intelligence(s), gifts, talents.

    d. Emotional: experiential therapies: dance, art, music. Family therapy. Group therapy.

    e. Social: recreation, sports, church groups, social skills group (younger kids), after school clubs.

    d. Spiritual: gratitude journal, prayer, religious services, and volunteer work.

4. Anxiety
   a. Environmental: strive for a calm, peaceful, predictable home life. Parents should role model peace, calm, and practice relaxation skills themselves, Pets, Avoid media violence, emphasize positive and relaxing entertainment, time in nature
   b. Physical: enhanced physical activity: swimming, walking or biking. Dietary improvements: reduce sugar, eliminate caffeine, and adequate protein. Vitamin C (1000 mg), B-complex (50 mg), Inositol (2–4 g two or three times daily). L-Theanine (100–200 mg) twice daily. Consider 50 to 150 mg 5-HTP twice daily. Massage therapy. Consider Acupuncture if acceptable.
   c. Mental: relaxation training or Tai Chi or Mindfulness meditation. Psychoeducational formats (books, DVDs, etc.) to enhance knowledge of anxiety and coping techniques. Adjust school size and style as needed, prevent bully issues. Psychotherapy with connected and reassuring therapist. Exposure and Response Prevention (ERP) if OCD features. Higher doses of 5-HTP (300–400 mg) if OCD features.
   d. Emotional: consider arts, crafts or other relaxing hobbies. Journaling.
   e. Social: may need to support one on one time with gentle peers.
   f. Spiritual: support spiritual path. Prayer and ritual may provide solace (Kaplan & Shannon, 2007; Kemper & Shannon, 2007; Lake, 2007; Lake & Spiegel, 2007; Shannon, 2002).

Safety Issues

Psychiatric medications have rather significant health and safety risks in adults. In a child with a growing nervous system most of these concerns are unexplored. By comparison, the integrative modalities discussed in this chapter appear to carry risks that are orders of magnitude safer. For example, over 100,000 Americans die each year from the correct use of prescription medications (Lazarou, Pomeranz, et al., 1998) and it is the sixth leading cause of death in the United States. Outside of the banned supplement ephedra (abused as a weight loss stimulant), only a handful of Americans die each year from herbal supplements in spite of enormous unsupervised use (Mills, 2007). A few notable safety concerns do stand out and merit discussion.

Kava Kava has been documented to reduce anxiety. However, there have been a number of deaths from liver failure associated with it (Ernst, 2007). These appear to be related to a manufacturing issue using non-rhizome components. Until this issue is clarified a ban on clinical use is warranted. Any of the stimulant or anti-depressant products (ginkgo, sun exposure, SJW, 5-HTP) can trigger manic cycling in predisposed patients (Fahmi, Huang, et al., 2002). Any patient with a bipolar presentation or family history must be approached with real caution. Acupuncture with pre-pubertal children is challenging. Acupuncture treatment itself can cause bruising, trigger premature labor or, rarely, cause a pneumothorax. St. John's Wort can cause sun sensitization. SAMe can elicit nausea, headaches or insomnia. Meditation must be recommended cautiously in any patient with a history of psychosis. All of the vitamins being discussed here (including EM Power) fall in the safe range and are not associated with known toxicity. Many categories discussed here; lifestyle changes (exercise, sleep, etc.), learning environment adjustments, home environment adjustments, parenting support, relaxation, and coping skills, for example, are safe, practical, and support the child's health in a number of ways.

Case Study

Jennifer is a 12-year-old girl who comes to you with her mother, Gloria, with a chief complaint of depression. Jennifer has felt bad for 6 months, she tried cutting on herself and took six Tylenol once but never told anyone. A teacher told the school counselor and they now seek your help. Father is a workaholic and under-available. Mom is mildly depressed and grew up with an alcoholic father. Jennifer is slightly overweight, inactive, craves carbohydrates and spends 2–4 hours a day on her computer on a social networking site.

As you explore her ecosystem you find that the home environment is stressful and chaotic. Jennifer stays up late on the computer and only gets 7 1/2 hours of sleep each evening. Her diet is low in protein and high in processed foods. She thinks poorly of herself and hates her body.

Your intervention revolves around improving the environmental supports for Jennifer. You spend time educating mom and Jennifer about the need for more sleep, a better diet, and more activity. You explain the need to limit screen time to allow time for these other priorities. Screen time gets earned when these are accomplished. You outline reasonable nutrition and get both of them to pledge a diet with more protein, whole grains, daily breakfast, and no caffeine or soda. You outline basic supplementation that includes 1000 mg of vitamin C, 50 mg of B complex, and 1 g of EPA fish oil.

You spend time with mom emphasizing the need to address her depression and marital stress, as this is a factor in Jennifer's mood and environment. You support a yoga class for Jennifer and her dad and emphasize the need for him to be more involved in her life. Both Jennifer and her mom feel worse in winter so you prescribe a light box with 30 minutes each morning while eating breakfast. Jennifer has a nice connection with her youth minister, so you suggest regular visits with him until Jennifer feels much better. You recommend Jennifer take 200 mg of SAMe each morning and afternoon on an empty stomach, increasing to 400 mg twice daily in 1 week. Finally, you recommend Jennifer spend 10 minutes each night before bed filling in a gratitude journal. The parents are very pleased that they can avoid prescription medication at this point and understand that is could be a part of the plan if Jennifer fails to respond. You will see them back in 2 weeks to coach and suggest these changes.

Summary

The child's brain is the most complex eco-system in the known universe. We must strive to assess this ecosystem as comprehensively as possible. A thorough assessment will include an understanding of environmental, physical, mental, emotional, social, and spiritual concerns. The unique characteristics of each child provide a map of strengths, gifts, challenges, and style. The treatment flows from this map.

The treatment will be much more likely to be successful if it is plays on strengths and addresses stressed areas of the child's life. A multi-modal treatment model also will be more effective in the long run. Work with the belief system of the family and of the child. Re-assess your assessment and treatment response on a regular basis. Remember, children represent a moving target. If the child does not respond positively to the treatment approach, reassess your diagnosis and your treatment within 6 weeks. Do not lose the momentum for change.

Embrace the awesome vitality and healing capacity of this child. You should radiate acceptance, optimism and engagement. As a practitioner, your own personal mental, emotional, and spiritual health becomes either an effective tool or serious roadblock to every child's recovery. You must walk the talk. Finally, the greatest joy in this work comes from knowing the whole child well and witnessing their beauty as they rebalance and blossom.

REFERENCES

Aboraya, A. (2006). The reliability of psychiatric diagnosis revisited. *Psychiatry 2006, 3*(1), 41–50.

Banerjee, T. D., Middleton, F., & Farone, S. (2007). Environmental risk factors for attention-deficit hyperactivity disorder. *Acta Paediatrica, 96*(9), 1269–1274.

Bischoff, S. C. (2007). Food allergies. *Current Treatment Options in Gastroenterology, 10*(1), 34–43.

Bolton, D., & Perrin, S. (2007). Evaluation of exposure with response-prevention for obsessive compulsive disorder in childhood and adolescence. *Journal of Behavior Therapy and Experimental Psychiatry.*

Capra, F. (1996). *The web of life: A new scientific understanding of living systems.* New York: Anchor Books.

Christakis, D. A., Zimmerman, F. J., DiGiuseppi, D. A., & McCarty, C. A. (2004). Early television exposure and subsequent attentional problems in children. *Pediatrics, 113*(4), 708–713.

Cleary, M., & English, G. (2005). The small schools movement: Implications for health education. *The Journal of School Health, 75*(7), 243–247.

Costello, E. J., Egger, H., & Angold, A. (2005). 10-year research update review: The epidemiology of child and adolescent psychiatric disorders: I. Methods and public health burden. *Journal of the American Academy of Child and Adolescent Psychiatry, 44*(10), 972–986.

Crooks, D. L. (2000). Food consumption, activity, and overweight among elementary school children in an Appalachian Kentucky community. *American Journal of Physical Anthropology, 112*(2), 159–170.

Currie, C., Robert, C., Morgan, A., Smith, R., Settertobulte, W., Samdal, O., & Fantol, B. (2004). Young People's Health in Context, Health Behaviour in School-aged Children study: International Report from the 2001/2002 Survey. *Health Policy for Children and Adolescents No.4*. Copenhagen, Denmark. World Health Organization.

Diego, M. A., Field, T., & Kuhn, C. (2002). Aggressive adolescents benefit from massage therapy. *Adolescence, 37*(147), 597–607.

Diller, L. (1998). *Running on ritalin: A physician reflects on children, society and performance in a pill*. New York: Bantam Books.

Diller, L. H. (2006). *The last normal child*. Westport, CN: Praeger.

Ernst, E. (2007). A re-evaluation of kava (Piper methysticum). *British Journal of Clinical Pharmacology, 64*(4), 415–417.

Fahmi, M., Huang, C., & Smith, C. (2002). A case of mania induced by hypericum. *The World Journal of Biological Psychiatry, 3*(1), 58–59.

Field, T., Hernandez-Reif, M., Diego, M., Schanberg, S., & Kuhn, C. (2005). Cortisol decreases and serotonin and dopamine increase following massage therapy. *The International Journal of Neuroscience, 115*(10), 1397–1413.

Field, T., Hernandez-Reif, M., & Diego, M. (2006). Newborns of depressed mothers who received moderate versus light pressure massage during pregnancy. *Infant Behavior & Development, 29*(1), 54–58.

Field, T., Morrow, C., & Diego, M. (1992). Massage reduces anxiety in child and adolescent psychiatric patients. *Journal of the American Academy of Child and Adolescent Psychiatry, 31*(1), 125–131.

Fletcher, R. H., & Fairfield, K. M. (2002). Vitamins for chronic disease prevention in adults: Clinical applications. *The Journal of the American Medical Association, 287*(23), 3127–3129.

Frank, E., Kupfer, D. J., Thase, M. E., Mallinger, A. G., Schartz, J. R., Fagolini, A. M., et al. (2005). Two-year outcomes for interpersonal and social rhythm therapy in individuals with bipolar I disorder. *Archives of General Psychiatry, 62*(9), 996–1004.

Freeman, M. P., Hibbeln, J. R., Wisner, K., Davis, J. M., Mischoulon, D., Peet, M., et al. (2006). Omega-3 fatty acids: Evidence basis for treatment and future research in psychiatry. *The Journal of Clinical Psychiatry, 67*(12), 1954–1967.

Gardner, H. (1983). *Frames of mind: The theory of multiple intelligences*. New York: Basic Books.

Gardner, H. (2004). *The unschooled mind: How children think and how schools should teach*. New York: Basic Books.

Golden, R. N., Gaynes, B. N., Ekstrom, R., Hamer, R., Jacobsen, F., & Suppes, T. (2005). The efficacy of light therapy in the treatment of mood disorders: A review and meta-analysis of the evidence. *Acta Paediatrica, 162*(4), 656–662.

Gordon, J. S., Staples, J. K., & Santos, R. (2004). Treatment of posttraumatic stress disorder in postwar Kosovo high school students using mind-body skills groups: A pilot study. *Journal of Traumatic Stress, 17*(2), 143–147.

Grossman, P., Niemann, L., & Shultz, M. (2004). Mindfulness-based stress reduction and health benefits. A meta-analysis. *Journal of Psychosomatic Research, 57*(1), 35–43.

Hammen, C., & Brennan, P. A. (2003). Severity, chronicity, and timing of maternal depression and risk for adolescent offspring diagnoses in a community sample. *Archives of General Psychiatry, 60*(3), 253–258.

Hamre, H. J., Witt, C. M., & Link, D. (2006). Anthroposophic therapy for chronic depression: A four-year prospective cohort study. *BMC Psychiatry, 6*, 57.

Jiang, Y. Y. (2006). Effect of B vitamins-fortified foods on primary school children in Beijing. *Asia-Pacific Journal of Public Health, 18*(2), 21–25.

Kaplan, B. J., Crawford, S. G., Field, C., & Simpson, S. (2007). Vitamins, minerals, and mood. *Psychological Bulletin, 133*(5), 747–760.

Kaplan, B. J., & Shannon, S. (2007). Nutritional aspects of child and adolescent psychopharmacology. *Pediatric Annals, 36*(9), 600–609.

Karst, M., Winterhalter, M., & Drappen, G. (2007). Auricular acupuncture for dental anxiety: A randomized controlled trial. *Anesthesia and Analgesia, 104*(2), 295–300.

Kemper, K., & Shannon, S. (2007). Complementary and alternative treatment of pediatric mood disorders. *Pediatric Clinics of North America, 54*(6).

Kemper, K. J., Sarah, R., Silver-Highfield, E., Xiarhos, E., Barnes, L., & Berde, C. (2000). On pins and needles? Pediatric pain patients' experience with acupuncture. *Pediatrics, 105*(4 Pt 2), 941–947.

Lake, J. (2007). *Textbook of integrative mental health care.* New York: Thieme.

Lake, J., & Spiegel, D. (2007). *Complementary and alternative treatments in mental health care.* Arlington, VA: American Psychiatric Press Inc.

Lazarou, J., Pomeranz, B. H., & Walton, F. (1998). Incidence of adverse drug reactions in hospitalized patients: A meta-analysis of prospective studies. *JAMA, 279*(15), 1200–1205.

Leo, R. J., & Ligot, J. S. Jr. (2007). A systematic review of randomized controlled trials of acupuncture in the treatment of depression. *Journal of Affective Disorders, 97*(1–3), 13–22.

Linde, K., & Knuppel, L. (2005). Large-scale observational studies of hypericum extracts in patients with depressive disorders—a systematic review. *Phytomedicine, 12*(1–2), 148–157.

Linehan, M. M., Armstrong, H. E., & Smith, T. (1991). Cognitive-behavioral treatment of chronically parasuicidal borderline patients. *Archives of General Psychiatry, 48*(12), 1060–1064.

Manuel, J. S. (2003). Solar flair. *Environmental Health Perspectives, 111*(2), A104–A107.

McCann, D., Barrett, A., Cooper, A., Crumpler, D., Dalen, L., Grimshaw, K., et al. (2007). Food additives and hyperactive behaviour in 3-year-old and 8/9-year-old children in the community: A randomized, double-blinded, placebo-controlled trial. *Lancet: 370* (9598):1560–1567.

McMichael, A. J., Baghurst, P. A., & Almondorf, S. (1994). Tooth lead levels and IQ in school-age children: The Port Pirie Cohort Study. *American Journal of Epidemiology, 140*(6), 489–499.

Mills, S. (2007). Monitoring herbal safety: Current debate and resources Symposium report: Pharmacovigilance of herbal medicines: Current state and future direction, London, 24-26 April 2006. *Phytomedicine.*

Moreno, C., & Laje, G. (2007). National trends in the outpatient diagnosis and treatment of bipolar disorder in youth. *Archives of General Psychiatry, 64*(9), 1032–1039.

Mukaino, Y., Park, J., et al. (2005). The effectiveness of acupuncture for depression—a systematic review of randomized controlled trials. *Acupuncture in Medicine, 23*(2), 70–76.

Olfson, M., Blanco, C., et al. (2006). National trends in the outpatient treatment of children and adolescents with antipsychotic drugs. *Archives of General Psychiatry, 63*(6), 679–685.

Ott, M. J. (2002). Mindfulness meditation in pediatric clinical practice. *Pediatric Nursing, 28*(5), 487–490.

Passini, F. G., Watson, C. G., & Franklin, D. J. (1976). The effects of cerebral electric therapy (electrosleep) on anxiety, depression, and hostility in psychiatric patients. *The Journal of Nervous and Mental Disease, 163*(4), 263–266.

Peet, M., & Stokes, C. (2005). Omega-3 fatty acids in the treatment of psychiatric disorders. *Drugs, 65*(8), 1051–1059.

Perry, B. D., & Pollard, R. (1998). Homeostasis, stress, trauma, and adaptation. A neurodevelopmental view of childhood trauma. *Child and Adolescent Psychiatric Clinics of North America, 7*(1), 33–51, viii.

Prigogine, I., & Geheniau, J. (1986). Entropy, matter, and cosmology. *Proceedings of the National Academy of Sciences of the United States of America, 83*(17), 6245–6249.

Rathus, J. H., & Miller, A. L. (2002). Dialectical behavior therapy adapted for suicidal adolescents. *Suicide & Life-Threatening Behavior, 32*(2), 146–157.

Reynolds, W. M., & Coats, K. I. (1986). A comparison of cognitive-behavioral therapy and relaxation training for the treatment of depression in adolescents. *Journal of Consulting and Clinical Psychology, 54*(5), 653–660.

Russek, L. G., & Schwartz, G. E. (1997). Perceptions of parental caring predict health status in midlife: A 35-year follow-up of the Harvard Mastery of Stress Study. *Psychosomatic Medicine, 59*(2), 144–149.

Shannon, S. E. (2002). *Handbook of complementary and alternative therapies in mental health.* San Diego, CA: Academic Press.

Stewart, D., & Sun, J. (2004). How can we build resilience in primary school aged children? The importance of social support from adults and peers in family, school and community settings. *Asia-Pacific Journal of Public Health, 16*(Suppl), S37–S41.

Teufel, M., Biedermann, T., & Hannace, M. (2007). Psychological burden of food allergy. *World Journal of Gastroenterology, 13*(25), 3456–3465.

van der Kolk, B. A., Spinazzola, J., & Fox, C. (2007). A randomized clinical trial of eye movement desensitization and reprocessing (EMDR), fluoxetine, and pill placebo in the treatment of posttraumatic stress disorder: Treatment effects and long-term maintenance. *The Journal of Clinical Psychiatry, 68*(1), 37–46.

Wall, R. B. (2005). Tai Chi and mindfulness-based stress reduction in a Boston Public Middle School. *Journal of Pediatric Health Care, 19*(4), 230–237.

Weissman, M. M., Pilowsky, D. J., Wickramaratne, P. J., Talati, A., Wiseniewki, S. R., & Fava, M. (2006). Remissions in maternal depression and child psychopathology: A STAR*D-child report. *The journal of the American Medical Association, 295*(12), 1389–1398.

Whitehead-Pleaux, A. M., Zebrowski, N., Santos, F., & Eaton, F. (2007). Exploring the effects of music therapy on pediatric pain: Phase 1. *Journal of Music Therapy, 44*(3), 217–241.

Zito, J. M., Safer, D. J., DosReis, S., Gardner, J. F., Magder, L., & Soeker, K. (2003). Psychotropic practice patterns for youth: A 10-year perspective. *Archives of Pediatrics & Adolescent Medicine, 157*(1), 17–25.

Zito, J. M., Safer, D. J., Valluri, S., Gardner, J. F., Korelitz, J. J., & Mattison, D. R. (2007). Psychotherapeutic medication prevalence in Medicaid-insured preschoolers. *Journal of Child and Adolescent Psychopharmacology, 17*(2), 195–203.

23

Integrative Pediatric Oncology

SUSAN F. SENCER

KEY CONCEPTS

- More than half of the children being treated for cancer in the United States use some form of integrative medicine (IM), primarily to treat symptoms rather than to cure the cancer directly.
- Greater than 75% of childhood cancer is currently curable with conventional chemotherapy, radiation therapy and/or surgery; pediatric oncologists are concerned that widespread use of IM may compromise the improvements made in survival.
- "Integrative oncology" implies an evolving evidence-based specialty that uses complementary therapies in concert with medical treatment to enhance efficacy, improve symptom control, alleviate patient distress, and reduce suffering.
- The majority of IM used by cancer patients is parent/patient selected rather than provider prescribed.
- The integrative oncologist's role is one of maintaining currency with the available research as well as providing information on safe, compatible IM adjuvants.
- Interactions of herbal or other supplements with chemotherapy and/or radiation therapy is a real concern.
- The best care for cancer for children and young adults is at a pediatric cancer center affiliated with the Children's Oncology Group (COG).
- Pediatric specific research is essential to guide the addition of IM therapies into the array of therapies open to children with cancer to improve side effects and augment cancer therapy.

Background

Approximately 10,000 children in the United States under the age of 20 will be diagnosed with cancer annually (Ries et al., 1999). Acute lymphoblastic leukemia (ALL) is the largest group of pediatric cancers, accounting for 25% of all cases. Brain tumors constitute the next largest group; brain tumors and ALL, together with acute myelogenous leukemia (AML) account for almost half of children's cancer. Neuroblastoma and Wilms' tumor are the next most frequently diagnosed tumors in children. There is debate as to whether children's cancer incidence rates are increasing; clearly, between 1975 to 1979 and 1995 to 1997, overall pediatric cancer rates did increase by 11.5% (Ries et al., 1999). These increases were primarily from increases in the incidence of CNS tumors and ALL (Ries et al., 1999Smith, Freidlin, Ries, & Simon, 1998). Non-Hodgkin's lymphoma, hepatoblastoma, osteosarcoma, and germ cell tumors rates were also increased slightly (Devesa, & Fears, 1992; Groves, Linet, Travis, & Devesa, 2000; Ries et al., 1999; Smith et al., 1998). The timing of these increases coincides with rapid changes in diagnostic imaging for CNS tumors and therefore the rise in incidence of brain tumors may be reflective of improvements either in diagnosis or reporting rather than true increases (Smith et al., 1998). Cancer incidence rates appear to have leveled off over the last 20 years, but further data are needed (Ries, 1996; Ries et al., 1999).

The success over the last 50 years in treating children with cancer is one of the great medical "miracles" of the latter half of the twentieth century. Currently, more than 75% of children with cancer will be cured (Ries, 1996; Ries et al., 1999). In 1960 a child diagnosed with ALL had a four percent chance of 5 year event free survival (EFS) (Ries, 1996; Ries et al., 1999); the current EFS is close to 80% for ALL, with certain subgroups enjoying even higher rates of cure (Ries, 1996; Ries et al., 1999). Improvements in survival, although less dramatic, exist for most other pediatric cancers. These successes are due, in no small part, to the continued commitment of pediatric oncologists to treating all patients, whenever possible, on large scale, national or international clinical trials, which compare newer therapies with the previously rigorously trialed standard therapy.

Pediatric oncologists recognized early that, given the relatively small number of children's cancer cases, few pediatric institutions would be able to run clinical trials with enough patients to produce meaningful results. The National Wilms Tumor Study Group, the Intergroup Rhabdomyosarcoma Study Group, and the larger Pediatric Oncology Group and Children's Cancer Study Group were all formed to design and implement large scale clinical trials. In 2000, these four groups combined to create the Children's Oncology Group (COG). The best care for cancer for children and young adults is at a pediatric cancer center affiliated with COG. Importantly for the purposes of this chapter, COG from its inception has had a commitment to studying IM, through its IM subcommittee, in children with cancer. The premise behind the support is that

IM for children's cancers deserves the same scrutiny that has been given to combination chemotherapy and radiation regimens.

IM use has grown exponentially over the last several decades. A pioneer survey in the field in the 1970s showed that less than 10% of pediatric cancer patients were using IM (Faw, Ballentine, Ballentine, & vanEys, 1977). Paralleling the explosion in IM use in the adult population, more contemporary surveys have indicated use in the 70%–80% range for children with cancer, especially if prayer is included (Friedman et al., 1997; Kelly, 2004; Kelly et al., 2000). Most parents surveyed chose to use IM for their children to combat side effects of the cancer or the cancer therapy; rarely is IM used as the primary means to treat the cancer. The most common modalities used are prayer and spiritual healing, nutritional supplements, vitamins, massage and mind-body therapies (Fernandez, Stutzer, MacWilliam, & Fryer, 1998; Friedman et al., 1997; Kelly et al., 2000; McCurdy, Spangler, Wofford, Chauvenet, & McLean, 2003; Post-White, Sencer, & Fitzgerald, 2000). The inclusion of prayer in IM surveys is controversial and is felt by some researchers to unfairly inflate estimates of IM use. Factors associated with increased IM use are poor prognosis, prior IM use by the parent, higher parental education, older age of parents and religiosity (Kelly et al., 2000; McCurdy, Spangler, Wofford, Chauvenet, & McLean, 2003; Post-White et al., 2000).

Surveys such as these, while helping to identify areas for further research, also underscore the need by oncologists to more fully explore the IM "phenomenon." The current emphasis of pediatric oncology IM researchers is to move away from descriptive studies and toward interventional studies. Of great concern to pediatric oncologists is the fact that only half of patients surveyed, fearing disapproval, disclosed their use of IM to their providers (Friedman et al., 1997; Kelly et al., 2000; McCurdy et al., 2003), and that many children enrolled on cooperative group trials were also using IM, adding yet another potentially confounding layer to already complicated trial designs (Kelly et al., 2000). The majority of studies to date investigating IM in children with cancer have focused on IM as supportive care agents and have been limited institution projects, with hopes to move promising agents or modalities to group-wide trials.

THE ROLE OF THE INTEGRATIVE ONCOLOGIST

The National Center for Complementary and Alternative medicine has defined integrative medicine as the combination of "mainstream medical therapies and complementary and alternative therapies for which there is some high-quality scientific evidence of safety and effectiveness" (National Institutes of Health National Center for Complementary and Alternative Medicine, 2002). Integrative oncology combines the "high tech" world of oncology with "high touch" IM therapies. The pediatric integrative oncologist finds that the majority of parental queries about IM and cancer fall into four categories: (1) causation, (2) nutrition (3) supportive care options, and (4) direct anticancer therapeutic options. To this must be added the oncologist's concern about possible adverse events and interactions.

Causation

When a child is diagnosed with cancer, parental guilt is an almost universal response. The parents are concerned that they may have contributed to their child's disease, either genetically or through lifestyle and environmental choices. It is true that the majority of adult cancers can be linked to tobacco, obesity, dietary, or other lifestyle choices (Danaei, Vander Hoorn, Lopez, Murray, & Ezzati, 2005). That sort of environmental causation is tempting to posit for pediatric cancers as well, as we become more aware of the increasing environmental burden on the planet, resulting in global warming and shrinking water supplies. Nonetheless, scant evidence currently exists linking childhood cancer with pesticides, solvents, or other pollutants (Zahm & Devesa, 1995). Other than ionizing radiation and a few medications, there is no convincing evidence of environmental causation (Kimmel, 2005). We do know that there are critical periods for environmental exposures in the developing child, which include prior to conception, during pregnancy and after birth (Grigg, 2004). While certain environmental toxins have been linked to embryologic abnormalities and hormonal changes in children, we cannot currently say that there is overwhelming evidence linking them to the development of cancer in children. At this point, providers can reasonably assure parents that the cause of their child's cancer is unlikely to be due to anything they ate, smoked, drank, or where they lived. In particular, electromagnetic fields (EMF) have been extensively studied; there is weak, but not convincing evidence that EMFs are associated with the development of childhood cancer (Belson, Kingsley, & Homes, 2007). C3: Causes of Childhood Cancer Newsletter, produced monthly by the University of Minnesota's Epidemiology Research Program, is an excellent source of cutting edge information (www.cancer.umn.edu/c3).

Some children's cancers have a genetic basis, such as many cases of retinoblastoma, and some Wilms tumors (Robison, Buckley, & Bunin, 1995). Individuals with underlying chromosomal abnormalities, such as Down syndrome, have higher rates of cancer, as do children with chromosomal breakage syndromes (e.g., Bloom, Fanconi) (Hasle, Clemmensen, & Mikkelsen, 2000; Hirsch et al., 2004). Many children with these syndromes do not develop cancer, however, or develop cancer at later ages. This suggests that at least two chromosomal "hits" are required for cancer initiation (Knudson, 1986). This theory was brought to the forefront in the landmark work by Alfred Knudson in a clearly genetic disease—retinoblastoma (RB). He theorized that if the child had the RB gene, a second "hit" would still be required for the cancer to start (Knudson, 1986). Environmental exposures could thus constitute the second, or third, etc., "hit."

The majority of childhood cancers are not obviously genetically linked. Because most American families have one or more family members with cancer, however, they may presume that their family is more at risk. Most true "cancer families" are relatively easy to identify, because they have multiple family members who develop cancer during childhood or young adulthood. Li-Fraumeni syndrome families, for instance, have a germline mutation in the p53 tumor suppressor gene, which leads to brain tumors, leukemias, sarcoma, and breast cancers, among others (Li et al., 1988). Thankfully, these germline mutations are relatively rare.

As we understand more about the human genome and cancer predisposition we will hopefully be able to more effectively counsel families and individuals about possible preventive measures to reduce their risk.

Nutrition

All parents of children with cancer ask about which foods to feed their children, or foods to avoid. More and more children in America start their cancer journey already obese. Obesity can predispose to hyperglycemia (Cowey & Hardy, 2006), which can become especially problematic if steroids are added to the treatment regimen. We recognize now that hyperglycemia is a proinflammatant, and that both hyperglycemia and obesity contribute to worsened side effects and poorer outcomes (Butturini et al., 2007; Weiser et al., 2004). However, changes in diet can be difficult to accomplish at such a stressful time, and a balance must be sought in keeping the child and family unit's quality of life as positive as possible. Certainly, moving families toward an organic, hormone free diet can be a positive step. It may be easier, however, to effect dietary change with the off-therapy patient than the patient undergoing active therapy.

Epidemiological data have found an increased risk of certain adult cancers associated with decreased intake of specific foods in the adult population (Adami, Day, Trichopoulos, & Willett, 2001). While there has not been a convincing connection made with diet and development of children's cancers, it is the responsibility of the oncologist to help their patients prevent second, adult cancers. A recent survey found that 79% of survivors of childhood cancer did not meet the guidelines for fruit and vegetable consumption and only 48% were meeting recommended exercise guidelines (Demark-Wahnefried et al., 2005). The problem is compounded because many survivors of childhood cancer have significant metabolic syndrome (Oeffinger et al., 2003), which includes dyslipidemia, glucose intolerance, insulin resistance, obesity and hypertension, and which may in turn contribute to the formation of adult cancers (Cowey & Hardy, 2006). Physicians should encourage patients and families to consult with a registered dietician for a complete nutritional assessment and recommendations; family-based nutrition counseling, rather than individual, has been found to be more effective over the long-term in pediatric populations (Ammerman, Lindquist, Lohr, & Hersey, 2002).

Unfortunately, nutritional supplements are now increasingly sold through multi-level marketing schemes, which generate huge profits, often without reliable evidence.

Parents are pressured into buying multiple products, many with similar constituents, but fancier names. Clinicians should stress the importance of fresh, whole foods over supplements whenever possible; it is hard to overdose on a food, but quite easy with a supplement.

Supportive Care

Children with cancer experience a range of symptoms resulting from the cancer and its treatment. Conventional treatments are not always effective at relieving symptoms or reducing side effects. Children with cancer commonly use complementary/alternative medicine (IM) to cope with the side-effects of cancer therapy (Kelly et al., 2000; Post-White et al., 2000; Sawyer, Gannoni, Toogood, Antoniou, & Rice, 1994).

Integrative oncology, or the use of IM in conjunction with standard medical treatment, seeks to improve the supportive care available to patients and to determine through scientific clinical trials which adjuvant IM therapies are medically sound, effective, and compatible with standard chemotherapy and radiation. Over the last decade, scientific inquiry of IM therapies has shown that some of the agents previously considered on the fringe of medicine are sufficiently studied as to become part of the mainstream (Ladas, & Post-White, 2006). Some therapies have more evidence for effectiveness (e.g., hypnosis and acupuncture) than others (e.g., herbal therapies and homeopathy), and clinical trials in children lag behind IM trials in adults. Oncology especially is a very data driven field, relying upon the results of legions of researchers in preclinical and clinical trials to further drive developments. The backbone of these trials involves treating individuals with similar diseases in similar manners. Many IM therapies, on the other hand, have traditionally been studied or practiced within completely different frameworks. For instance, Traditional Chinese Medicine or Ayurvedic medicine practitioners are more apt to see an individual and his or her symptoms as reflective of an imbalance, and each individual may require an individual treatment plan, rather than standardized treatment plans. (Interestingly, as we learn more about genetic polymorphisms, which help explain why individuals with similar diseases act in dissimilar ways, we may perhaps begin to develop more individualized treatment plans, more in keeping with other frameworks.) Nonetheless, until biomechanistic explanations for the activities of IM therapies are discovered, they are unlikely to see widespread support among oncologists.

One framework which potentially explains the possible effectiveness of some IM interventions for managing symptoms in cancer is a psychoneuroimmune (PNI) model, which identifies the complex interactions among behavior, neural, endocrine and immune function and thus how the patient adapts to stressors (Ader, Felten, & Cohen, 2001). Understanding how stress can effect physiologic and immune responses provides a framework for understanding the role of mind-body and touch interventions. Interventions aimed at reducing stress help manage symptoms by reducing physiologic tension through relaxation and facilitating the use of coping strategies to manage or control the stressors (Post-White & Bauer, 2006). IM interventions can help children (and adults) modify their responses to stress of various sorts. This in turn leads to a better sense of comfort, participation in care, and control of their responses.

Helping families decide on whether, or which, IM modalities to consider requires an understanding of a family's belief system, as well as patient characteristics and preferences. Consideration should always be given toward the patient's developmental stages, in addition to the level of evidence available in the literature. Determining the level of evidence, however, can be problematic for the individual practitioner without the time or resources to fully investigate a particular supplement or modality. Many institutions and organizations, including the National Cancer Institute (NCI) have developed rating systems which compile and evaluate evidence. The Oncology Nursing Society has an excellent website which provides ranked information on evidence-based interventions for supportive care in a highly accessible format (http://www.ons.org/outcomes/pep.shtml).

Relief of cancer-related symptoms is the backbone of the supportive care of cancer patients. Complementary therapies can help reduce symptoms when conventional treatment does not bring satisfactory relief or causes undesirable side effects. Existing research demonstrates beneficial roles for some IM therapies. Mind-body medicine and biofield therapies may be particularly useful, especially for the management of symptoms for which conventional therapy is often ineffective. Hypnosis and imagery reduced anticipatory nausea and vomiting and pain in children with cancer (Jacknow, Tschann, Link, & Boyce, 1994; Kazak, Penati, Brophy, & Himelstein, 1998; Olness, 1981; Zeltzer, LeBaron, & Zeltzer, 1984). Music therapy may affect a child's emotional state (Barrera, Rykov, & Doyle, 2002) as well as immune function (Marwick, 1996). Body-based therapies such as massage are associated with improvements in mood and anxiety (Field et al., 1997). What follows is an overview of the most distressing symptoms of cancer therapy in children and some integrative approaches to their treatment. It should be recognized that some of these approaches have more evidence for their support than others, and much of the evidence is extrapolated from research with adults with cancer. The increased use of IM in children necessitates responsible investigation of these therapies to determine their safety and efficacy among children receiving treatment for cancer.

NAUSEA AND VOMITING

Nausea and vomiting related to chemotherapy (CINV) is one of the most distressing side effects of cancer therapy. The addition of 5HT3 antagonists to the armamentarium has changed the face of chemotherapy delivery, but nausea and vomiting nonetheless remain the primary complaint of cancer patients. IM offers a number of primary or adjuvant options to alleviate the discomfort and consequences of CINV including acupuncture, acustimulation, acupressure, aromatherapy, and the use of herbal remedies, such a ginger.

Acupuncture has a large body of data supporting its efficacy in the prevention and treatment of chemotherapy-induced nausea and vomiting (NIH Consensus Conference, 1998), including feasibility and acceptability in children with cancer (Reindl et al., 2006). One of the first IM clinical trials in COG was investigating the efficacy of electroacupuncture treatment, versus sham placebo, to reduce delayed CINV in pediatric and young adult patients with pediatric solid tumors; this study is currently still on-going.

For children averse to needles, acupressure wrist bands over the P6 point (in combination with modern antiemetics) have demonstrated effectiveness in decreasing the severity of acute nausea, although they were not as effective in controlling actual vomiting or delayed nausea (Ezzo et al., 2005; Roscoe et al., 2003; Treish et al., 2003). In a meta-analysis of 11 studies, acupressure was less effective in reducing nausea and vomiting than acupuncture, but could extend the duration of benefit of acupuncture (Ezzo et al., 2005).

Herbs are commonly used for cancer treatment symptom management in adults. Ginger (*Zingiber officinale*) has been shown to be effective for nausea and vomiting due to causes other than chemotherapy, with few side effects (Betz, Kranke, Geldner, Wulf, & Eberhart, 2005; Lien et al., 2003; Pongrojpaw & Chiamchanya, 2003). Further research is needed on the use of ginger as an adjunctive therapy for pediatrics, and theoretically should be avoided in patients with a bleeding diathesis.

Aromatherapy is the inhaled use of essential oils for therapeutic or medical purposes. Ginger, spearmint (*Mentha spicata*), and peppermint (*Mentha piperita*) are recommended for antiemetic and antispasmodic effects on the gastric lining and colon. Several studies show peppermint's efficacy in reducing CINV (Buckle, 2003). Aromatherapy massage was found to have a mild transient anxiolytic effect, which may be useful for the treatment of anticipatory nausea and vomiting (Cooke & Ernst, 2000). A limitation of these studies is the small sample sizes and lack of testing in a pediatric population. No significant side effects of aromatherapy have been reported in large reviews. One potential concern that has not been well studied is the case reports of children developing pubertal changes believed to be due to synthetic fragrances in detergents and air fresheners, as well as a case report of boys developing gynecomastia when exposed to lavender and tea tree oil (Henley, Lipson, Korach, & Bloch, 2007). Clearly, further work is needed to elucidate both safety and efficacy of aromatherapy in children, and only high-grade essential oils should be used for therapeutic purposes.

Hypnosis is especially effective in children for a variety of symptoms. One of the earliest works in the field of pediatric hypnosis showed its value in the pediatric oncology population (Olness, 1981). In more recent studies of children with cancer, Zeltzer and colleagues found hypnosis more effective than cognitive distraction/relaxation or placebo in reducing anticipatory and post-chemotherapy nausea and vomiting (Zeltzer, Dolgin, LeBaron, & LeBaron, 1991; Zeltzer et al., 1984).

MALNUTRITION

Chemotherapy and radiation therapy can lead to profound loss of appetite and weight loss, which can affect a child's quality of life. Having a nutritionist on staff is essential in helping educate parents about how to help their child to eat healthy foods; however, nutrition counseling on its own has not been found to be effective in improving the caloric content of patient's diets and preventing weight loss.

The wasting syndrome of cachexia has long been one of the hallmarks of cancer therapy. The use of appetite stimulants may be prescribed for severe weight loss but these have side effects and may be contraindicated in certain pediatric oncology populations (Meacham, Mazewski, & Krawiecki, 2003). In some cases, total parenteral nutrition is used. Enteral nutrition, either through eating or the use of nasogastrostomy or gastrostomy tubes, is preferred.

Clinical trials on Essential Fatty Acids (EFA) and cachexia provide encouraging support for the role of EFA as mediators of cytokine production and nutrition status, but show mixed results in treating cachexia per se (Falconer, Fear on, Ross, & Carter, 1994; Wigmore et al., 1996). Omega-3 Fatty Acid is the most well studied EFA; in general, Omega-3's have been found to have some small benefit to health, but results in treating patients with cancer are mixed (Hooper et al., 2006). No significant side effects have been attributed to Omega-3's, except perhaps for the mercury found in fish.

Immunocal, an un-denatured whey-protein derivative that provides precursors of glutathione has been used to supplement patients with HIV/AIDS and adolescents with cystic fibrosis. Immunocal was well-tolerated with no reports of adverse events (Grey, Mohammed, Smountas, Bahlool, & Lands, 2003; Micke, Beeh, & Buhl, 2002; Micke, Beeh, Schlaak, & Buhl, 2001), and children had weight gain and improved immune function and quality of life. A small pilot study in children with cancer also found improvements in weight gain and increased levels of reduced glutathione (Melnick et al., 2005).

CONSTIPATION

Constipation is frequently a problem in children being treated for cancer, particularly those patients receiving vincristine as part of their chemotherapy regimen. Adolescents and young adults are often most affected by vincristine-induced constipation that is not always responsive to conventional agents. There are no trials investigating the effectiveness of IM therapies as a treatment for constipation in children with cancer, but several studies have investigated the effectiveness of biofeedback in children with chronic constipation with encouraging results (Heymen, Jones, Scarlett, & Whitehead, 2003; Palsson, Heymen, & Whitehead, 2004). Yoga and abdominal massage have also been found to be helpful. Inactivity is a major contributor to constipation. Encouraging physical activity is essential, preferably through sports and activities the child has previously played. More and more programs are recognizing that physical activity plays a key role in maintaining a child's functioning throughout therapy. Not just constipation, but neuropathy, depression and fatigue are all positively affected by increasing exercise. In addition to dietary fiber, there are many herbs that are used as laxatives, but these may be contraindicated in some patients. Some of the most common herbal laxatives are senna, psyllium, aloe vera, and rhubarb.

DIARRHEA

Most of the published research investigating IM remedies for the treatment of diarrhea in pediatrics has been in newborns, malnourished children, or children with HIV/AIDS. As most of these populations have compromised immune systems and are challenged with similar side effects due to conventional treatment, it is plausible that these remedies may be applicable to children undergoing treatment for cancer.

Colostrum is the milk secreted by mammals within the first few days after giving birth; it contains high concentrations of antibodies (IgG, IgM, and IgA) as well as a broad array of cytokines (Kelly, 2003). Colostrum, either from cows or humans, has shown efficacy as a treatment for infection-induced diarrhea (Mitra et al., 1995; Sarker et al., 1998). One case series found colostrum reduced the duration of severe GVHD in children after an allogeneic bone marrow transplant (Inoue, Okamura, Sawada, & Kawa, 1998).

Probiotics have been investigated in children with viral or antibiotic-induced diarrhea. Use of lactobacillus gg in children with viral-induced diarrhea has shown encouraging results (Szajewska & Mrukowicz, 2001). Although no studies have been published in children with cancer, probiotics have been prescribed to newborns, another immunologically fragile population, with no reports of adverse events (Bin-Nun et al., 2005; Euler, Mitchell, Kline, & Pickering, 2005). Because probiotics contain live active organisms, there has been hesitation in prescribing their use among patients with compromised immune systems. Lactobacillus bacteremia and sepsis have been reported in immunocompromised patients and in infants. Although most of these products have been used safely for years, careful analysis of scientific research should be conducted before routinely recommending these products to immunosuppressed children (Salminen et al., 2004; Wolf, Wheeler, Ataya, & Garleb, 1998).

MUCOSITIS

Mucositis is a frequent side effect from cancer therapy and affects a large proportion of children undergoing treatment for cancer at some point in their therapy. In children undergoing bone marrow transplantation, mucositis can be especially debilitating and severely painful. The breakdown in the mucosal barrier is also a portal of entry for infection. Many times mucositis necessitates long-term administration of total parental nutrition due to the child's inability to swallow.

Once considered an alternative therapy, glutamine is a nutrition supplement that is routinely used for the prevention of mucositis among children with cancer.

Administration of glutamine was found to be effective in preventing the duration and severity of mucositis in children undergoing bone marrow transplantation (Anderson et al., 1998; Anderson, Schroeder, & Skubitz, 1998).

TRAUMEEL S is a homeopathic remedy that was found to be effective in reducing mucositis in children undergoing bone marrow transplantation in a small pilot study (Oberbaum et al., 2001). These findings were the basis for the first large scale IM clinical trial among children with cancer through COG. Results of this clinical trial did not confirm the earlierpilot study findings; Traumeel S was not effective in preventing or treating mucositis in pediatric bone marrow transplant patients (unpublished data).

NEUROPATHY

Neuropathies, particularly peripheral neuropathies, are a significant problem for children, especially those treated with vincristine or cisplatin. Neuropathy may exist and persist in children even after treatment for cancer. Children with ALL demonstrate decreased balance control 1 year after finishing therapy when compared to age matched controls (Wright, Galea, & Barr, 2005) and persistent fine motor coordination deficits are found in children with ALL during therapy (Hockenberry et al., 2007). Gross and fine motor deficits have been noted 5 years after completing therapy (Lehtinen et al., 2003). Persistent loss of somatosensation and strength may have a long-term impact on the child in terms of functional limitations, available choices of physical activities, and quality of life. In adult survivors of childhood ALL, it has been shown that survivors are less likely to report leisure-time physical activity as compared to controls (Florin et al., 2007). In children, these losses can be potentially even more devastating if they lead to changes in age appropriate development of motor and social skills.

Children who are treated for cancer are at risk for decreased physical function both during and after their treatment. Impaired physical function may lead to decreased overall activity levels and an increased risk of obesity, decreased bone mineral density, and eventual cardiovascular disease (Oeffinger et al., 2003). Increased emphasis on identifying neuropathic deficits and intervening, either with physical therapy, increased activity or supplementation will hopefully lead to improved physical function, increased physical activity, improved quality of life, and increased overall health during cancer treatment and survivorship.

Glutamine and Vitamin E are two supplements that have reported encouraging results for neuropathies in adults with cancer. Glutamine was found in breast cancer patients to decrease the incidence of motor weakness and abnormalities in gait (Vahdat et al., 2001). This use is currently being investigated in children with cancer (Ladas et al., 2006). Vitamin E decreased the incidence of neuropathy in the treatment group compared to the placebo group in adults with cancer (Argyriou et al., 2005); these encouraging results of Vitamin E's neuroprotective properties need to be followed up in the pediatric population.

FATIGUE

Fatigue is prevalent in persons with cancer at any age and is associated with malaise, lethargy, asthenia, and decreased mental attention and energy. Fatigue is a complex condition with many contributing mechanisms. One of the more promising avenues for decreasing fatigue is by increasing physical exercise. Health professionals often counsel cancer patients experiencing fatigue to rest and decrease their daily activities in order to conserve energy; this advice can cause paradoxical results (Dimeo et al., 2003). When muscles become inactive, they lose their power and force and become more fatigable (Al-Majid & McCarthy, 2001). As fatigue increases, the person with cancer becomes more sedentary which triggers a further downward spiral of physical capability and a continued increase in fatigue (Lucia, Earnest, & Perez, 2003). Multiple meta-analysis and systemic reviews have found exercise to be a safe and effective intervention for treating fatigue in adults undergoing cancer chemotherapy and bone marrow transplant (Knols, Aaronson, Uebelhar, Fransen, & Aufdemkampe, 2005; Mitchell et al., 2006; NCCN National Comprehensive Cancer Network, 2008).

Several isolated IM studies suggest potential efficacy for acupuncture, Healing Touch, and massage as a treatment for fatigue in adult cancer patients. Massage had no effect on fatigue in pediatric cancer patients receiving weekly massage for 4 weeks (Post-White, Fitzgerald, & Sencer, 2005), but mothers had less fatigue and greater vigor when they received massage while their children were in the hospital for cancer treatment (Iwasaki, 2005).

L-Carnitine is a supplement that has been used as a cardioprotectant for anthracy-cline therapy, as well as in individuals with inborn carnitine deficiency. In preliminary clinical studies, carnitine deficiency was found in the majority of adult cancer patients (Cruciani et al., 2004) and pediatric patients with AIDS and chronic illness presenting with fatigue (Esteban-Cruciani, 2001, 2002). Carnitine is required to carry fatty acids across the inner mitochondrial membrane where fat oxidation and adenysine triphosphate (ATP) synthesis take place (Winter et al., 1995). Several chemotherapy agents have been found to interfere with this network (Peluso et al., 2000), resulting in alterations in energy utilization and balance, which can contribute to skeletal muscle fatigue and cardiac muscle inefficiency. In a preliminary report of a randomized Phase II clinical trial, 1 week of carnitine supplementation reduced fatigue and improved functional status and mean free carnitine levels in adult hospice patients. Importantly, no adverse events were reported (Cruciani et al., 2004).

PAIN

The causes of cancer pain are myriad and include tumor infiltration into bone, muscle or bone marrow or other direct tumor effects. Painful complications of chemotherapy and radiation such as mucositis, infections, skin irritations and neuropathies, as well as procedural pain, also commonly afflict pediatric cancer patients. Visceral pain is particularly difficult to treat using conventional means, as narcotics are not always effective.

In addition, many parents are wary of narcotics, fearing addiction or dependency. It is important to debunk the myths surrounding narcotic use. Stressing that pain can blunt normal immune responses is often a successful way to help parents accept appropriate pain management techniques. Pediatric trained staff is needed to assess pain in children, as children are often unable to localize or vocalize pain. An integrated approach to pain management is necessary and needs to include state of the art pharmacologic and non-pharmacologic treatments. Access to pediatric pain specialists well versed in integrative approaches is ideal.

Mind-body therapies have gained acceptance for supportive care of children and adults with cancer, and several randomized control trials support the efficacy of relaxation, imagery, and hypnosis in alleviating cancer pain (Weiger et al., 2002). In children, most pain related hypnosis studies address procedural related pain (Hawkins, Liossi, & Ewart, 1998; Hilgard, & LeBaron, 1982; Smith, Barabasz, & Barabasz, 1996; Wild, & Espie, 2004; Zeltzer, & LeBaron, 1982). A large recent study of pediatric cancer patients undergoing lumbar puncture showed that therapist guided hypnosis is effective in reducing pain and anxiety (Liossi, & Hatira, 2003).

Acupuncture, once felt to be unproven and for which the mechanism of action is still not completely understood, is now practiced in pain clinics across North America and has been shown in multiple controlled clinical trials to reduce pain. It is also useful in managing many of the side effects of chemotherapy and radiation therapy, including nausea and vomiting, postchemotherapy fatigue, mucositis, and possibly insomnia and anxiety (Deng, Cassileth, & Yeung, 2004; Lu, 2005). Acupuncture has the added benefit of treating multiple patient complaints with one modality and does not require ingestion of a supplement to assure its efficacy. Acupuncture has been found to be safe and effective in children, and is acceptable to this population when presented in a positive light (Kemper et al., 2000; Reindl et al., 2006; Zeltzer et al., 2002).

Several small studies found massage effective in reducing short term pain in adults with cancer, but long term effects require further study (Weiger et al., 2002). Two small pediatric studies demonstrate reduced pain with juvenile rheumatoid arthritis (Field et al., 1997) and burn cares (Hernandez-Reif et al., 2001). Gaps in research remain, and efficacy studies with larger samples are needed to test effectiveness for chronic pain, long-term effects, and pediatric populations.

ANXIETY-INSOMNIA

Among persons with cancer, insomnia, fatigue, and anxiety are highly intercorrelated (Redeker, Lev, & Ruggiero, 2000). Several botanicals, including (*Valeriana officinalis)*, passionflower, and kava (*Piper methysticum*), have demonstrated some efficacy as "natural sedatives" based on both clinical and preclinical studies (Block, Gyllenhaal, & Mead, 2004), but have not been extensively used or studied in children with cancer. Although St. John's Wort has been shown to be effective for mild to moderate depression, it is a potent cytochrome P450 inducer and should not be used concomitantly with chemotherapy (Schrader, 2000). Kava kava was found more effective than placebo for reducing anxiety, stress, and insomnia and may be a viable nonpharmacologic remedy (Gurley et al., 2005), but reports of hepatotoxicity related deaths have been reported. German chamomile demonstrates anxiolytic activity in animals; however, there are few clinical trials testing efficacy and some indications that chamomile may interfere with anthracycline chemotherapy (Block et al., 2004).

Valerian appears to have a wide margin of safety and is not metabolized via the cytochrome enzymes, so therefore has less risk of interaction with chemotherapy agents (Gurley et al., 2005). In children, a small pilot study found Valerian more effective than placebo at reducing sleep latency and time awake at night, and increasing sleep time and quality of sleep (Francis & Dempster, 2002). Valerian can potentiate effects of sedatives, hypnotics, and anesthetics, and should be avoided prior to scheduled surgery (Block et al., 2004). There are no known studies determining long-range safety and efficacy or issues of tolerance and dependency. Melatonin is also widely used as a sleep aid and has an excellent safety profile; interesting preliminary research indicates it may also have some direct anti-cancer properties (Mills, Wu, Seely, & Guyatt, 2005).

Aromatherapy with inhaled lavender (*Lavendula angustifolia*) has been shown to have sedative effects (increased sleep time and greater drowsiness and relaxation) (Hardy, Kirk-Smith, & Stretch, 1995; Lis-Balchin & Hart, 1999; Masago et al., 2000; Schultz, Hubner, & Ploch, 1997; Schulz, Stolz, & Muller, 1994). Progressive muscle relaxation has been extensively studied and shown to be effective for improving sleep in persons with insomnia (Richards, Nagel, Markie, Elwell, & Barone, 2003). Several studies support potential efficacy for massage in reducing anxiety. In children, hypnosis is particularly effective in reducing anxiety and distress. Several studies by Zeltzer and colleagues found hypnosis more effective than cognitive distraction/relaxation or placebo in reducing anxiety in children with cancer (Francis & Dempster, 2002; Zeltzer, & LeBaron, 1982). Although Healing Touch and therapeutic touch are widely used in pediatric hospitals to reduce stress and anxiety, no studies were found in pediatrics (Kemper & Kelly, 2004). Again, exercise and physical activity in general lead to decreased fatigue and better sleep.

Childhood Cancer Survivors

As conventional medicine becomes increasingly effective at treating children with childhood cancer, the challenges of survivorship have become more apparent. Studies have estimated that 60%–70% of children will have at least one disability as a result of cancer therapy. Survivors are challenged with issues related to energy balance, fatigue, bone density, pain syndromes, and anxiety, and are at increased risk for heart disease, osteoporosis, infertility, and second malignancies (Oeffinger & Hudson, 2004).

Surveys in survivors of adult cancers have found that the use of IM extends into survivorship (Boon et al., 2003; Hann, Baker, Denniston, & Entrekin, 2005). This trend has also been observed in survivors of childhood cancer, who report they use IM to reduce risk of relapse, cope with late-effects from cancer therapy, or reduce their risk of developing a late-effect (Mertens et al., 2008). They did not significantly use IM more than the sibling or friend control, however (Mertens et al., 2008). One of the most frequent forms of IM used by survivors is biologic therapy in the form of nutritional or herbal supplements. Although the risk of interaction with a conventional agent is less of a concern in the survivor population than those on therapy, biologic therapies are not devoid of possible adverse effects. The chemistry and mechanism of action of many nutrition and herbal remedies are not well understood. Some biologic therapies have been found to stimulate cancer growth, particularly hormone-sensitive malignancies (Montbriand, 2004a, 2004b, 2004c, 2004d). Many supplements also stimulate the immune system (Goldrosen & Straus, 2004; Yang, 1996). It is unknown if biologic therapies that exert an effect on the immune system are safe for patients who have undergone bone marrow transplants as immune-enhancing remedies may increase a transplant recipient's risk of graft vs. host disease. Healthcare providers counseling survivors on IM should advise patients to be cautious in beginning treatment with certain classes of biologic therapies because of the theoretic increased risk for significant side effects or second malignancies.

Although more clinical data are needed, a number of IM remedies that have already been discussed may be useful to survivors of pediatric cancer. Dietary modifications, exercise interventions, yoga, tai chi, massage, acupuncture, and mind-body interventions all may be of benefit to the patient and have little risk of side effects. Lifestyle modification programs have been effective in decreasing the incidence of diabetes in children at risk for diabetes, preventing excess weight gain in healthy children, and reducing risk factors for cardiovascular disease (Campbell, Waters, O'Meara, Kelly, & Summerbell, 2002; Dietz, & Gortmaker, 2001; Hayman & Reineke, 2003; Mobley, 2004; Summerbell et al., 2003), and hence may benefit survivors of childhood cancer.

Childhood obesity is an emerging national health crisis among healthy children. This is compounded for survivors of childhood cancer, particularly for survivors of ALL, who are at increased risk for metabolic syndrome (Oeffinger et al., 2003). Reviews of intervention trials among healthy children have found no single intervention effective at treating or preventing obesity (Campbell et al., 2002; Summerbell et al., 2003). A multidisciplinary approach including IM therapies may help provide support for making lifestyle changes.

Palliative Care

IM therapies help to improve quality of life and improve symptoms across the continuum of treatment for childhood cancer, including care at the end of life. Integration of IM modalities into palliative care is a natural extension of "holistic" care. IM interventions, which are family centered and child-focused, can easily be delivered in the home, which is where most terminally ill children choose to be. The aim of the interventions is to minimize pain and suffering and to provide practical, emotional and physical support. The interdisciplinary nature of palliative care, including a team of doctors, nurses, social workers, child life specialists and other healthcare professionals, has set the stage for the integration of IM modalities into the care of the child suffering from unresponsive cancer.

Conventional therapy alone has not eliminated pain and suffering at the end of a child's life. Families report that the symptoms of anorexia, nausea, vomiting, constipation and diarrhea are not always adequately treated (Wolfe et al., 2000). Many oncologists find it easier to support use of more alternative modalities in the setting of a terminally ill child, as the risk benefit ratio changes significantly.

Palliative care should also include interventions offered to parents and siblings, as well as other caregivers, who can suffer both psychological and physical distress during the child's illness and after his or her death (Anghelescu, Oakes, & Hinds, 2006). These symptoms may include fatigue, depression, insomnia, and pain (headaches and musculoskeletal pain). IM interventions can ease the burden of this suffering.

Direct Anti-Cancer Effects

Most parents are also interested in the potential anti-cancer properties of herbs and other supplements. To understand how any biological agent can be effective against cancer, we need to recognize that the development of cancer cells in the body is a multistep process. Any of these steps may potentially be utilized as targets for therapy. The biological properties of malignant tumor cells can be summarized as follows (Hannahan & Weinber, 2000):

- Unchecked cellular growth due to acquisition of self-sufficiency in <u>growth signals</u>
- Unchecked cellular growth due to loss of sensitivity to anti-growth signals
- Loss of capacity for <u>apoptosis</u> which allows growth despite genetic errors and external anti-growth signals
- Loss of capacity for senescence, leading to cellular immortality
- Sustained <u>angiogenesis</u>, allowing the tumor to develop its own blood supply, thereby outgrowing the limitations of passive nutrient diffusion
- Invasion of neighboring tissues
- Distant <u>metastases</u>

Various IM therapies which have evidence for anti-cancer properties generally work to combat one or more of these mechanisms. Additionally, the environment surrounding the cancer cell has implications for tumor growth. An inflammatory state, for instance, is felt to be cancer promoting (Coussens & Werb, 2002). Natural whole products have the added theoretic advantage of being able to exert anticancer effects at multiple levels. Traditional chemotherapy works primarily by inhibiting the cancer cell's ability to replicate.

Many mushroom species have been found to have constituents that exhibit anticancer activity in vitro. Two proteoglycans from *coriolus versicolor*—PSK and PSP—show promise in adult clinical trials. They appear to boost immune function and enhance tumor infiltration by dendritic and cytotoxic T cells (Kidd, 2000). Miatake-D fractions and Shiitake components are other mushroom proteoglycans which have immuno-modulating effects and may induce apoptosis in cancer cells (Fullerton et al., 2000).

The rhizome turmeric contains two important classes of compounds, curcuminoids (including curcumin or diferuloylmethane) and turmerones that exert anticancer effects through a number of mechanisms including inhibition of NF-kB, STAT3, and COX-2. Curcumin has also been shown to be a substrate for p-glycoprotein (MDR protein) thus playing an important role in the amelioration of drug resistance of cancer cells. While various constituents of turmeric have clearly demonstrated direct and adjuvant anti-cancer activity, some studies including animal models of breast cancer show turmeric may inhibit chemotherapy-induced apoptosis. Therefore, a greater understanding of the interactions of turmeric with different types of chemotherapy is important before it is considered for concomitant use during chemotherapy (Kawamori et al., 1999; Mehta, Pantazis, McQueen, & Aggarwal, 1997; Somasundaram et al., 2002).

The active polyphenol constituent of green tea, epigallacatechin gallate (EGCG) is thought to induce apoptosis and tumor antiangiogenesis (Tosett, Ferrari, & De Flora, 2002). It may also inhibit enzymes involved in cellular communication (Yang, Prabhu, & Landau, 2001). While population studies have suggested a chemopreventive effective of green tea, the Food and Drug Administration (FDA) has concluded that it does not significantly reduce the risk of most cancers (Letter from FDA, 2005). The caffeine in tea has a stimulatory effect which may cause sleep disturbances or dysphoria in children. Theoretically, large doses of green tea can prolong coagulation studies.

Emerging data on Vitamin D reveal that low levels of 25(OH) D are associated with increased risks of certain cancers as well as higher mortality from these cancers (Lappe, Travers-Gustafson, Davies, Recker, & Heaney, 2007). Much of the population is deficient in Vitamin D, and certain chemotherapies have been found to contribute to deficiency as well. Finally, $1,25(OH)_2 D_3$ may have antitumor activity (Masuda & Jones, 2006). Supplementation with Vitamin D is safe and recommended for pediatric cancer patients.

Memorial Sloan Kettering Cancer Center (http://www.mskcc.org/mskcc/html/11570.cfm), M.D. Anderson (http://www.mdanderson.org/departments/CIMER/), and the National Cancer Institute (http://www.cancer.gov/cancertopics/pdq/cam/) all have evi-dence ranking systems for herbs and supplements commonly used by cancer patients.

Adverse Effects

Counseling patients on the safety and efficacy of IM is a challenge to healthcare pro-viders because of the dearth of well-designed research trials. Although non-biolog-ically based therapies are generally considered safe and the risk of interference with conventional therapies is low, some rare adverse events have been reported with chi-ropractic manipulations and acupuncture (Ernst, 2003; Vohra, Johnston, Cramer, &

Humphreys, 2007). Adverse events reported with the use of biologically based therapies include case reports of direct toxicity or contamination of herbs with heavy metals, prescription pharmaceuticals or microbes, particularly with herbs imported from developing countries (Ernst, 2002; Sencer & Kelly, 2007). Contamination with these compounds can have a detrimental impact on the growth and development of the pediatric patient, especially those who are immunocompromised.

Few studies have been carried out to assess herb/supplement-drug interactions; potential interactions are listed in Table 23-1 (Labriola & Livingston, 1999; Fugh-Berman, 2000). Although reports have documented that St. John's Wort, taken concomitantly with irinotecan, results in low levels of irinotecan through induction of cytochrome P450 CYP3A4 (Mathijssen, Verweij, de Bruijn, Loos, & Sparreboom, 2002), there are

Table 23-1. Common Supplements Which May Interfere with Drugs Used in Pediatric Oncology Practice

Bleeding diathesis (thrombocytopenia, anticoagulation therapy, etc)	Bleeding tendency may be increased by: Angelica root, Anise, Arnica flower, Black Cohosh, Asa foetida, Capsicum, Celery, Chamomiles, Clove, Denshen, Devils claw, Dong Quai, Evening primrose, Fenugreek, Feverfew, Garlic, Ginkgo biloba, Guarana, Horse chestnut, Licorice, Onion, Papain, Parsley, Passion flower, Quassia, Quinine, Red clover, Sweet clover, Sunflower seeds (Vitamin E)
	Effectiveness of anticoagulation leading to increased risk of bleeding may be increased by: Ginseng, Green tea, Plantain, Saint John's Wort, Turmeric, Alfalfa (Vitamin K), inositol hexaphosphate (IP-6)
Corticosteroids, Cyclosporine (Immunosuppressive agents)	Immunosuppression may be blocked by: Alfalfa sprouts, Echinacea, Licorice, Saint John's Wort, Vitamin E, Zinc
	Grapefruit juice may increase cyclosporine levels
	Immunosuppression may be reduced by: Cordyceps (with prednisolone); country mallow, ephedra, marshmallow (with dexamethasone)
Methotrexate	Agents that may increase hepatotoxicity: Echinacea, Black Cohosh, salicylate-containing herbs such as bilberry, cramp bark, meadowsweet, poplars, red clover, uva ursi, white willow, wintergreen. Gerimandu, Comfrey, Chaparral and Konbacha may also cause cumulative hepatotoxicity
Tamoxifen	Effectiveness may be decreased by Black Cohosh, Soy
Cisplatin	Toxicity may be increased by Selenium
Intraconazole	Effectiveness may be decreased by Grapefruit juice
Penicillin's	Effectiveness may be decreased by Khat
Etoposide	Toxicity may be increased by Saint John's Wort

only rare reports of clinically significant adverse interactions. Again, because clinical studies of most biologically based modalities are lacking, the safest time to add these therapies may be after chemo- and radiotherapy have been completed, when drug interactions are no longer a risk.

Patients with cancer are often encouraged by IM providers to take antioxidants to lessen the side effects of chemotherapy and radiation therapy. The use of antioxidants during conventional cancer therapy is controversial, however. Theoretically, antioxidants may affect chemo-/radio-therapeutic agents that generate free radicals, thus decreasing their effectiveness (Kelly, 2004). The use of antioxidants may nonetheless reduce side effects of cancer treatment, thus allowing for higher doses of chemotherapy to be administered (Conklin, 2000). Preclinical studies also support a potential role for antioxidants having a direct anticancer effect through pro-oxidant effects at certain concentrations.

Immunostimulants are another category of supplements widely used by cancer patients. Besides the Asian mushrooms already discussed, mistletoe (Ernst, Schmidt, & Steuer-Vogt, 2003) and other herbals (Block, & Mead, 2003) are felt to alter the immune system. Certainly many agents may increase absolute numbers of cytotoxic T lymphocytes or natural killer cells, or increase endogenous production of cytokines (Block, & Mead, 2003), but the effects of these quantitative changes on disease states are not well understood. Whether these actions have *in vivo* efficacy to fight cancer is not well defined at the current time, but must be further studied. No definitive answer has been found to these vexing questions, and therefore children on therapy should be discouraged from combining chemotherapy and radiation with high doses of antioxidants, and those with leukemia or lymphoma or following stem cell transplant should be discouraged from taking immunomodulators.

It is important to assess and document the child's use of IM, critically evaluate the evidence or lack of evidence, balance the potential risks with possible benefits, and assist the family in their choices and decisions regarding use of IM for their child with cancer. Healthcare providers should initiate open, non-judgmental discussions with patients and parents regarding IM use. Unexpected toxicities or responses to treatment may be a result of an interaction between IM remedies and will warrant close observation. Guidelines for monitoring patients combining IM with conventional therapy have been previously published (Weiger et al., 2002).

Challenges of Pediatric Oncology IM Research

Although IM therapies often have been criticized for being used despite a lack of evidence, hundreds of systematic reviews have evaluated specific therapies (Sampson, Campbell, Ajiferuke, & Moher, 2003). IM intervention trials have, however, historically lacked the control and rigor of randomized controlled medical trials. Research into IM therapies is complicated, however. Complex therapeutic systems such as traditional Chinese medicine are difficult to standardize, as many of the therapies are individualized to a certain patient instead of a particular disease, in contrast to the approach used in most clinical trials of conventional therapies. Recruitment to clinical trials of IM therapies may be hampered by emotional biases either for or against a particular therapy. To date, there is no critical mass of quality IM investigators. Some IM practitioners may also have little incentive to conduct trials of IM therapies since the therapies are already available in the mainstream. Large-scale clinical trials within the context of the cooperative group setting have been the hallmark of pediatric oncology research, and the large advances in survival have been the direct result of these endeavors. IM research should have the same rigorous examination.

This is not without its difficulties. Several barriers to mounting large-scale research studies of complementary therapies through COG have been identified (Sencer, Reaman, & Kelly, 2007). There are many different types of IM therapies in use by children with cancer but, again, few have been evaluated for safety and efficacy, much less other important variables such as dosage, provider effectiveness or cost. Research priorities are difficult to determine. In addition, firmly held preconceptions by physicians, patients and IM practitioners about individual therapies have made the design and execution of studies difficult. Institutional review boards (IRBs) at individual institutions have been reluctant to "take on" potentially controversial complementary modalities. As IM has become more accepted throughout the medical community, these issues have become less problematic. Many academic institutions, for instance, now have departments of integrative medicine.

Practicing Integrative Oncology

The integration of IM therapies with conventional treatment for childhood cancer within the setting of a children's hospital or large medical center offers several opportunities, especially the ability to provide multidisciplinary care and enhance research capabilities. However, there are some basic business challenges to providing integrative medicine services within the larger medical center. Systems for billing and collections for services provided by IM providers are not well established. Few insurance plans cover these services, and therefore most IM programs need to rely on philanthropic support. Ultimately, the provision of integrative medicine becomes a low priority for resource stressed institutions.

Administratively, IM offerings in medical settings require relevant policies and procedures, such as the proper credentialing of practitioners (Eisenberg et al., 2002). The licensing of IM providers varies state by state. The oversight of practitioners providing herbal counseling is not regulated by a governing body; in some states this therapy is provided by licensed naturopathic physicians, whereas in others, this service falls under the domain of registered dieticians who may have minimal training or interest in this area. Oncologists can help address their own potential malpractice liability issues when considering IM treatments by evaluating the level of clinical risk, documenting patient decision-making in the medical record, continuing to monitor conventionally, and being prepared to intervene conventionally when medically required. When referring to an IM practitioner, they should be aware of the professional licensure regulations, the scope of practice, and malpractice concerns of their own state (Cohen, 2006). Minimum requirements to be considered in evaluating a practitioner include verification of education, licensure, certification, continuing medical education credits, evidence of malpractice insurance, and review of malpractice liability history or misconduct charges. Pediatric institutions have the added burden of ensuring that practitioners who work with children are aware of the unique developmental, emotional and ethical needs of children and adolescents. In addition, the concept of informed consent (and ethical practice) mandates that our patients/parents be educated about their disease and the various treatment modalities available.

Conclusions

Whatever the term, integrative or holist, a good pediatric oncologist has always paid attention to the whole patient, within the micro- and macrocosm of his or her life. This includes, family, school, friends and the larger social structure. This also means preserving future function as much as possible, whether cognitive, physical, reproductive, or emotional.

Many IM therapies have the potential of improving quality of life. IM therapies may be considered in the management of symptoms of cancer and conventional treatment and for psychological support associated with the diagnosis of cancer. IM therapies may also be useful for end of life care. Some IM therapies may eventually be shown to have positive, direct anti-tumor action upon the cancer itself, although at this point no alternative therapies have been shown in any scientific study to effectively treat cancer in humans on a large scale.

The oncologist is no longer the sole, or perhaps even primary, source of information for most cancer patients and their families about their disease and its treatment. The Internet, in particular, has become a powerful tool allowing individuals to exchange information about therapies, both conventional and alternative. This rapid flow of information has contributed to the increased use of unproven therapies, since anecdotal tributes and commercial websites are often more readily accessible and understandable to the Internet user than are results of scientific studies.

Pediatric oncologists can point to the tremendous successes over the last 30 years in treating children with cancer and are understandably reluctant to diverge from this path. This hesitancy to consider less proven therapies has often created animosity or tension between provider and patients and their parents. The appeal of alternative cures arises from the daunting risks, costs, and potential side effects of many conventional treatments, or in the limited prospect for cure.

Nonetheless, caution should be employed in recommending biologically active agents. Enormous strides have been made in the care of children with cancer; we should not allow potentially life-saving therapies to be shortchanged in an effort to provide more "natural" therapies.

Until the evidence for or against a IM modality is more conclusive, the providers' role is to assess and document the child's use of IM, critically evaluate the evidence or lack of evidence, balance the potential risks with possible benefits, and assist the family in their choices and decisions regarding use of IM for their child with cancer.

Acknowledgments

The author would like to thank Kara Kelly, M.D., Janice Post-White, RN, PhD, FAAN, and Elena Ladas, MS, RD, for their work in the field and their words in the previous articles we have written together on this topic. She would also like to thank Mary Langevin, FNP, Casey Hooke, RN, PhD, CPON, Laura Gilchrist, PhD, Steven Melnik, M.D., Brooks Puchner, Cynthia Ford and Kelly Finstrom for their help in the preparation of this manuscript.

REFERENCES

Adami, H. O., Day, N. E., Trichopoulos, D., & Willett, W. C. (2001). Primary and secondary prevention in the reduction of cancer morbidity and mortality. *European Journal of Cancer,* 37(Suppl 8), S118–S127.

Ader, R., Felten, D., & Cohen, N. (2001). *Psychoneuroimmunology,* (3rd ed.). San Diego: Academic Press.

Al-Majid, S., & McCarthy, D. O. (2001). Cancer-inducted fatigue and skeletal muscle wasting: The role of exercise. *Biological Research for Nursing, 2,* 186–197.

Ammerman, A., Lindquist, C., Lohr, K. N., & Hersey, J. (2002). The efficacy of behavioral interventions to modify dietary fat and fruit and vegetable intake: A review of the evidence. *Preventative Medicine, 35,* 25–41.

Anderson, P. M., Ramsay, N. K., Shu, X. O., Rydholm, N., Rogosheske, J., Nicklow, R., et al. (1998). Effect of low-dose oral glutamine on painful stomatitis during bone marrow transplantation. *Bone Marrow Transplant, 22,* 339–344

Anderson, P. M., Schroeder, G., & Skubitz, K. M. (1998). Oral glutamine reduces the duration and severity of stomatitis after cytotoxic cancer chemotherapy. *Cancer, 83,* 1433–1439.

Anghelescu, D. L., Oakes, L., & Hinds, P. S. (2006). Palliative care and pediatrics. *Anesthesiology Clinics of North America, 24,* 145–161.

Argyriou, A. A., Chroni, E., Koutras, A., Ellul, J., Papapetropoulos, S., Katsoulas, G., et al. (2005). Vitamin E for prophylaxis against chemotherapy-induced neuropathy: A randomized controlled trial. *Neurology, 64,* 26–31.

Barrera, M. E., Rykov, M. H., & Doyle, S. L. (2002). The effects of interactive music therapy on hospitalized children with cancer: A pilot study. *Psychooncology, 11*(5), 379–88.

Belson, M., Kingsley, B., & Homes, A. (2007). Risk factors for acute leukemia in children: A review. *Environmental Health Perspectives, 115*(1), 138–145.

Betz, O., Kranke, P., Geldner, G., Wulf, H. & Eberhart, L. H. (2005). [Is ginger a clinically relevant antiemetic? A systematic review of randomized controlled trials]. *Forschende Komplementärmedizin und klassische Naturheilkunde, 12,* 14–23.

Bin-Nun, A., Bromiker, R., Wilschanski, M., Kaplan, M., Rudensky, B., Caplan, M., et al. (2005). Oral probiotics prevent necrotizing enterocolitis in very low birth weight neonates. *The Journal of Pediatrics, 147,* 192–196.

Block, K. I., Burns, B., Cohen, A. J., Dobs, A. S., Hess, S. M., & Vickers, A. (2004). Point-counterpoint: Using clinical trials for the evaluation of integrative cancer therapies. *Integrative Cancer Therapies, 3*, 66–81

Block, K. I., Gyllenhaal, C., & Mead, M. N. (2004). Safety and efficacy of herbal sedatives in cancer care. *Integrative Cancer Therapies, 3*, 128–148.

Block, K. L., & Mead, M. N. (2003). Immune system effects of Echinacea, ginseng, and astragalus: A review. *Integrative Cancer Therapies, 2*, 247–267.

Boon, H., Westlake, K., Stewart, M., Gray, R., Fleshner, N., Gavin, A., et al. (2003). Use of complementary/alternative medicine by men diagnosed with prostate cancer: Prevalence and characteristics. *Urology, 62*, 849–853.

Buckle, J. (2003). *Nausea and vomiting clinical aromatherapy: Essential oils in practice*, (2nd ed.) Arnold, UK: Churchill Livingstone.

Butturini, A., Dorey, F., Lange, B., Henry, D., Gaynon, P, Fu, C., et al. (2007). Obesity and outcome in Pediatric Acute Lymphoblastic Leukemia. *Journal of Clinical Orthodontics, 25*, 2063–2069.

Campbell, K., Waters, E., O'Meara, S., Kelly, S., & Summerbell, C. (2002). Interventions for preventing obesity in children. *Cochrane Database of Systematic Reviews*, CD001871.

Cohen, M. H. (2006). Legal and ethical issues relating to use of complementary therapies in pediatric hematology/oncology. *Journal of Pediatric Hematology/Oncology, 28*, 190–193.

Conklin, K. A. (2000). Dietary antioxidants during cancer chemotherapy: Impact on chemotherapeutic effectiveness and development of side effects. *Nutrition and Cancer, 37*, 1–18.

Connor, K. M., Davidson, J. R., & Churchill, L. E. (2001). Adverse-effect profile of kava. *CNS Spectrums, 6*, 848, 850–848, 853.

Cooke, B., & Ernst, E. (2000). Aromatherapy: A systematic review. *The British Journal of General Practice, 50*, 493–96.

Coussens, L., & Werb, Z. (2002). Inflammation and cancer. *Nature, 420*, 860–867.

Cowey, S., & Hardy, R. (2006). The metabolic syndrome: A high-risk state for cancer. *The American Journal of Pathology, 169*, 1505–1522.

Cruciani, R. A., Dvorkin, E., Homel, P., Culliney, B., Malamud, S., Shaiova, L., et al. (2004). L-carnitine supplementation for the treatment of fatigue and depressed mood in cancer patients with carnitine deficiency: A preliminary analysis. *Annals of the New York Academy of Sciences, 1033*, 168–176.

Danaei, G., Vander Hoorn, S., Lopez, A. D., Murray, C. J., & Ezzati, M. (2005). Causes of cancer in the world: Comparative risk assessment of nine behavioural and environmental risk factors. *Lancet, 366*(9499), 1784–1793.

Demark-Wahnefried, W., Werner, C., Clipp, E. C., Guill, A. B., Bonner, M., Jones, L. W., et al. (2005). Survivors of childhood cancer and their guardians. *Cancer, 103*, 2171–2180.

Deng, G., Cassileth, B. R., & Yeung, K. S. (2004). Complementary therapies for cancer-related symptoms. *The Journal of Supportive Oncology, 2*, 419–426.

Devesa, S. S., & Fears, T. (1992). Non-Hodgkins's lymphoma time trends: United States and international data. *Cancer Research, 52*(Suppl), S5432–S5440.

Dietz, W. H., & Gortmaker, S. L. (2001). Preventing obesity in children and adolescents. *Annual Review of Public Health, 22*, 337–353.

Dimeo, F., Schwarz, S., Fietz, T., Wanjura, T., Boning, D., & Theil, E. (2003). Effects of endurance training on the physical performance of patients with hematological malignancies during chemotherapy. *Supportive Care in Cancer, 11*, 623–628.

Eisenberg, D. M., Cohen, M. H., Hrbek, A., Grayzel, J, Van Rompay, M. I., & Cooper, R. A. (2002). Credentialing complementary and alternative medical providers. *Annals of Internal Medicine, 137*, 965–973.

Ernst, E. (2002). Heavy metals in traditional Indian remedies. *European Journal of Clinical Pharmacology, 57*, 891–896. (act #5)

Ernst, E. (2003). Serious adverse effects of unconventional therapies for children and adolescents: A systematic review of recent evidence. *European Journal of Pediatrics, 162*(2), 72–80.

Ernst, E., Schmidt, K., & Steuer-Vogt, M. K. (2003). Mistletoe for cancer? A systematic review of randomized clinical trials. *International Journal of Cancer, 107*(2), 262–267.

Esteban-Cruciani, N. V. (2001). Severe carnitine deficiency in children with AIDS: Improved functional activity status after supplementation. *Pediatric Research, 49.*

Esteban-Cruciani, N. V. (2002). High prevalence of carnitine deficiency in children with chronic illness. *Pediatric Research, 51.*

Euler, A. R., Mitchell, D. K., Kline, R., & Pickering, L. K. (2005). Probiotic effect of fructo-oligosaccharide supplemented term infant formula at two concentrations compared with unsupplemented formula and human milk. *Journal of Pediatric Gastroenterology and Nutrition, 40*, 157–164.

Ezzo, J., Vickers, A., Richardson, M. A., Allen, C., Dibble, S. L., Issell, B., et al. (2005). Acupuncture-point stimulation for chemotherapy-induced nausea and vomiting. *Journal of Clinical Oncology, 23*, 7188–7198.

Falconer, J. S., Fearon, K. C., Ross, J. A., & Carter, D.C. (1994). Polyunsaturated fatty acids in the treatment of weight-losing patients with pancreatic cancer. *World Review of Nutrition and Dietetics, 76*, 74–76.

Faw, C., Ballentine, R., Ballentine, L., & vanEys, J. (1977). Unproved cancer remedies. A survey of use in pediatric outpatients. *The Journal of the American Medical Association, 238*, 1536–1538.

Fernandez, C. V., Stutzer, C. A., MacWilliam, L., & Fryer, C. (1998). Alternative and complementary therapy use in pediatric oncology patients in British Columbia: Prevalence and reasons for use and nonuse. *Journal of Clinical Oncology, 16*(4), 1279–1286.

Field, T., Hernandez-Reif, M., Seligman, S., Krasnegor, J., Sunshine, W., Rivas-Chacon, R., et al. (1997). Juvenile rheumatoid arthritis: Benefits from massage therapy. *Journal of Pediatric Psychology, 22*(5), 607–617.

Florin, T. A., Fryer, G. E., Miyoshi, T., Weitzman, M., Mertens, A. C., Hudson, M. M., et al. (2007). Physical inactivity in adult survivors of childhood acute lymphoblastic leukemia: A report from the childhood cancer survivor study. *Cancer Epidemiology, Biomarkers & Prevention, 16*(7), 1356–1363.

Francis, A. J., & Dempster, R. J. (2002). Effect of valerian, Valeriana edulis, on sleep difficulties in children with intellectual deficits: Randomized trial. *Phytomedicine, 9*, 273–279.

Friedman, T., Slayton, W. B., Allen, L. S., Pollock, B. H., Dumont-Driscoll, M., Mehta, P., et al. (1997). Use of alternative therapies for children with cancer. *Pediatrics, 100*(6), E1–6.

Fugh-Berman, A. (2000). Herb-drug interactions. *Lancet, 355*, 134–138.

Fullerton, S. A., Samadi, A. A., Tortorelis, D. G., Choudhury, M. S., Mallouh, C., Tazaki, H., et al. (2000). Induction of apoptosis in human prostatic cancer cells with beta-glucan (Maitake mushroom polysaccharide). *Molecular Urology, 4*(1), 7–13.

Glade-Bender, J. A., Ladas, E. J, Sands, S., Kelly, K. M., Vahdat, L., Essmertny, O., Einer, M. A., et al. (2006). Pilot Study Investigating the Effects of Glutamine and Vincristine-induced Neuropathy in Pediatric Patients with Cancer. SIO abstracts, 2006.

Goldrosen, M. H., & Straus, S. E. (2004). Complementary and alternative medicine: Assessing the evidence for immunological benefits. *Nature Reviews. Immunology, 4*, 912–921.

Grey, V., Mohammed, S. R., Smountas, A. A., Bahlool, R., & Lands, L. C. (2003). Improved glutathione status in young adult patients with cystic fibrosis supplemented with whey protein. *Journal of Cystic Fibrosis, 2*, 195–98.

Grigg, J. (2004). Environmental toxins; their impact on children's heath. *BMJ, 89*(3), 244–250.

Groves, F. D., Linet, M. S., Travis, L. B., & Devesa, S. S. (2000). Cancer surveillance series: Non-Hodgkin's lymphoma incidence by histologic subtype in the United States from 1978 through 1995. *Journal of the National Cancer Institute, 92,* 1240–1251.

Gurley, B. J., Gardner, S. F., Hubbard, M. A., Williams, D. K., Gentry, W. B., Khan, I. A., et al. (2005). In vivo effects of goldenseal, kava kava, black cohosh, and valerian on human cytochrome P450 1A2, 2D6, 2E1, and 3A4/5 phenotypes. *Clinical Pharmacology and Therapeutics, 77,* 415–426.

Hann, D., Baker, F., Denniston, M., & Entrekin, N. (2005). Long-term breast cancer survivors' use of complementary therapies: Perceived impact on recovery and prevention of recurrence. *Integrative Cancer Therapies, 4,* 14–20.

Hannahan, D., & Weinber, R. A. (2000). The hallmarks of cancer. *Cell, 100*(1), 57–70.

Hardy, M., Kirk-Smith, M. D., & Stretch, D. D. (1995). Replacement of drug treatment for insomnia by ambient odor. *Lancet, 346,* 701.

Hasle, H., Clemmensen, I., & Mikkelsen, M. (2000). Risks of leukemia and solid tumors in individuals with Down's syndrome. *Lancet, 335*(9199), 165–169.

Hawkins, P. J., Liossi, C., & Ewart, B. (1998). Hypnosis in the alleviation of procedure related pain and distress in pediatric oncology patients. *Contemporary Hypnosis, 15,* 199–207.

Hayman, L. L., & Reineke, P. R. (2003). Preventing coronary heart disease: The implementation of healthy lifestyle strategies for children and adolescents. *The Journal of Cardiovascular Nursing, 18,* 294–301.

Henley, D. V., Lipson, N., Korach, K. S., & Bloch, C. A. (2007). Prepubertal gynecomastia linked to lavender and tea tree oils. *The New England Journal of Medicine, 356*(5), 479–485.

Hernandez-Reif, M., Field, T., Largie, S., Hart, S., Redzepi, M., Nierenberg, B., et al. (2001). Childrens' distress during burn treatment is reduced by massage therapy. *The Journal of Burn Care & Rehabilitation, 22,* 191–195.

Heymen, S., Jones, K. R., Scarlett, Y., & Whitehead, W. E. (2003). Biofeedback treatment of constipation: A critical review. *Diseases of the Colon and Rectum, 46,* 1208–1217.

Hilgard, J. R., & LeBaron, S. (1982). Relief of anxiety and pain in children and adolescents with cancer: Quantitative measures and clinical observations. *The International Journal of Clinical and Experimental Hypnosis, 30,* 417–442.

Hirsch, B., Shimamura, A., Moreau, L., Baldinger, S., Hag-alshiekh M, Bostrom, B., et al. (2004). Association of biallelic BRCA2/FANCD1 mutations with spontaneous chromosomal instability and solid tumors of childhood. *Blood, 103,* 2554–2559.

Hockenberry, M., Krull, K., Moore, K., Gregurich, M. A., Casey, M. E., & Kaemingk, K. (2007). Longitudinal evaluation of fine motor skills in children with leukemia. *Journal of Pediatric Hematology/Oncology, 29*(8), 535–539.

Hooper, L., Thompson, R., Summerbell, C., Ne, A., Moore, H., Worthinton, H., et al. (2006). Risks and benefits of omega-3 fats for mortality, cardiovascular disease, and cancer; systematic review. *BMJ, 332*(7544), 752–760.

Inoue, M., Okamura, T., Sawada, A., & Kawa, K. (1998). Colostrum and severe gut GVHD. *Bone Marrow Transplant, 22,* 402–03.

Iwasaki, M. (2005). Interventional study on fatigue relief in mothers caring for hospitalized children—effect of massage incorporating techniques from oriental medicine. *The Kurume Medical Journal, 52,* 19–27.

Jacknow, D., Tschann, J., Link, M., & Boyce, W. T. (1994). Hypnosis in the prevention of chemotherapy-related nausea and vomiting: A prospective study. *Journal of Developmental and Behavioral Pediatrics, 15,* 258–264.

Kawamori, T., Lubet R., Steele V. E., Kelloff G. J., Kaskey R. B., Rao C. V., et al. (1999). Chemopreventive effect of curcumin, a naturally occurring anti-inflammatory agent, during the promotion/progression stages of colon cancer. *Cancer Research, 59*, 597–601.

Kazak, A. E., Penati, B., Brophy, P., & Himelstein, B. (1998). Pharmacologic and psychologic interventions for procedural pain. *Pediatrics, 102*, 59–66.

Kelly, G. S. (2003). Bovine colostrums: A review of clinical uses. *Alternative Medicine Review, 8*, 378–394.

Kelly, K. M. (2004). Complementary and alternative medical therapies for children with cancer. *European Journal of Cancer, 40*(14), 2041–2046.

Kelly, K. M., Jacobson, J. S., Kennedy, D. D., Braudt, S. M., Mallick, M., & Weiner, M. A. (2000). Use of unconventional therapies by children with cancer at an urban medical center. *Journal of Pediatric Hematology/Oncology, 22*(5), 412–416

Kemper, K. J., & Kelly, E. A. (2004). Treating children with therapeutic and healing touch. *Pediatric Annals, 33*, 248–252.

Kemper, K. J., Sarah, R., Silver-Highfield, E., Xiarhos, E., Barnes, L., & Berde, C. (2000). On pins and needles? Pediatric pain patients' experience with acupuncture. *Pediatrics, 105*, 941–947.

Kidd, P. (2000). The use of mushroom glucans and proteoglycans in cancer treatment. *Alternative Medicine Review, 5*, 4–27.(1).

Kimmel, G. (2005). An overview of children as a special population—Relevance to predictive biomarkers. *Toxicology and Applied Pharmacology, 206*(2), 215–218.

Knols, R., Aaronson, N. K., Uebelhar, D., Fransen, J., & Aufdemkampe, G. (2005). Physical exercise in cancer patients during and after medical treatment: A systematic review of randomized and controlled trials. *Journal of Clinical Oncology, 23*(16), 3830–3842.

Knudson, A. G. (1986). Genetics of human cancer. *Annual Review of Genetics, 20*, 231–251.

Labriola, D., & Livingston, R. (1999). Possible interactions between dietary antioxidants and chemotherapy. *Oncology (Huntingt), 13*, 1003–1008.

Ladas, E., & Post-White, J. (2006). Complementary and alternative medicine in pediatric oncology. In B. Carroll, J. Finlay (Eds.). *Cancer in Children.* submission.

Lappe, J. M., Travers-Gustafson, D., Davies, K. M., Recker, R. R., & Heaney, R. P. (2007). Vitamin D and calcium supplementation reduces cancer risk: Results of a randomized trial. *Clinical Nutrition, 85*(6), 1586–1591.

Lehtinen, S. S., Huuskonen, U. E., Harila-Saari, A.H., Tolonen, U., Vainionpaa, L. K., & Lanning, B. M. (2003). Motor nervous system impairment persists in long-term survivors of childhood acute lymphoblastic leukemia. *Cancer, 94*, 2466–2473.

Letter from FDA. Green Tea and Reduced Risk of cancer Health Claim. June 30, 2005.

Li, F. P., Fraumeni, J. F., Jr, Mulvihill, J. J., Blattner, W. A., Dreyfus, M. G., Tucker, M. A., et al. (1988). A cancer family syndrome in twenty-four kindreds. *Cancer Research, 48*, 5358–5362.

Lien, H. C., Sun, W. M., Chen, Y. H., Kim, H., Hasler, W., & Owyang, C. (2003). Effects of ginger on motion sickness and gastric slow-wave dysrhythmias induced by circular vection. *American Journal of Physiology. Gastrointestinal and Liver Physiology, 284*, G481–G489.

Liossi, C., & Hatira, P. (2003). Clinical hypnosis in the alleviation of procedure-related pain in pediatric oncology patients. *The International Journal of Clinical and Experimental Hypnosis, 51*, 4–28.

Lis-Balchin, M., & Hart, S. (1999). Studies on the mode of action of the essential oil of lavender (*Lavandula angustifolia* P. Miller). *Phytotherapy Research, 13*, 540–542.

Lu, W. (2005). Acupuncture for side effects of chemoradiation therapy in cancer patients. *Semin Oncol Nurs, 21*, 190–195.

Lucia, A., Earnest, C., & Perez, M. (2003). Cancer-related fatigue: Can exercise physiology assist oncologists? *The Lancet Oncology, 4,* 616–625.

Marwick, C. (1996). Leaving concert hall for clinic, therapists now test music's charms. *The Journal of the American Medical Association, 275,* 267–268.

Masago, R., Matsuda, T., Kikuchi, Y., Miyazaki, Y., Iwanaga, K., Harada, H., et al. (2000). Effects of inhalation of essential oils on EEG activity and sensory evaluation. *Journal of Physiological Anthropology and Applied Human Science, 19,* 35–42.

Masuda, S., & Jones, G. (2006). Promise of vitamin D analogues in the treatment of hyperproliferative conditions. *Molecular Cancer Therapeutics,* 5797–5808.

Mathijssen, R. H., Verweij, J., de Bruijn, P., Loos, W. J. & Sparreboom, A. (2002). Effects of St. John's Wort on irinotecan metabolism. *Journal of the National Cancer Institute, 94,* 1247–1249.

McCurdy, E. A., Spangler, J. G., Wofford, M. M., Chauvenet, A. R., & McLean, T. W. (2003). Religiosity is associated with the use of complementary medical therapies by pediatric oncology patients. *Journal of Pediatric Hematology/Oncology, 25*(2), 125–129.

Meacham, L. R., Mazewski, C., & Krawiecki, N. (2003). Mechanism of transient adrenal insufficiency with megestrol acetate treatment of cachexia in children with cancer. *Journal of Pediatric Hematology/Oncology, 25,* 414–417.

Mehta, K., Pantazis, P., McQueen, T., & Aggarwal B. B. (1997). Antiproliferative effect of curcumin (diferuloylmethane) against human breast tumor cell lines. *Anticancer Drugs, 8,* 470–481.

Melnick, S. J., Rogers, P., Sacks, N., Kwyer, T. A., Halton, J., Ramachandran, C., et al. (2005). A Pilot Limited Institutional Study to Evaluate the Safety and Tolerability of Immunocal®, a Nutraceutical Cysteine Delivery Agent in the Management of Wasting in High-Risk Childhood Cancer Patients. 1st Annual Chicago Supportive Oncology Conference.

Mertens, A. C., Sencer, S., Myers, C. D., Recklitis, C., Kadan-Lottick, N., Whitton, J., et al. (2008). Complementary and alternative therapy use in adult survivors of childhood cancer: A report from the Childhood Cancer Survivor Study. *Pediatr Blood Cancer,* 501(1), 90–97.

Micke, P., Beeh, K. M., & Buhl, R. (2002). Effects of long-term supplementation with whey proteins on plasma glutathione levels of HIV-infected patients. *European Journal of Nutrition, 41,* 12–18.

Micke, P., Beeh, K. M., Schlaak, J. F., & Buhl, R. (2001). Oral supplementation with whey proteins increases plasma glutathione levels of HIV-infected patients. *European Journal of Clinical Investigation, 31,* 171–78.

Mills, E., Wu, P., Seely, D., & Guyatt, G. (2005). Melatonin in the treatment of cancer: A systematic review of randomized controlled trials and meta-analysis. *Journal of Pineal Research, 39*(4) 360–366.

Mitchell, Mitchell, S., Beck, S., Hood, L., Moore, K., & Tanner, E. (2006). *Putting evidence into practice: Fatigue interventions.* Pittsburg, PA: Oncology Nursing Society.

Mitra, A. K., Mahalanabis, D., Ashraf, H., Unicomb, L., Eeckels, R., & Tzipori, S. (1995). Hyperimmune cow colostrum reduces diarrhoea due to rotavirus: A double-blind, controlled clinical trial. *Acta Paediatrica, 84,* 996–1001.

Mobley, C. C. (2004). Lifestyle interventions for "diabesity": The state of the science. *The Compendium of Continuing Education in Dentistry, 25,* 207–202, 214.

Montbriand, M. J. (2004a). Herbs or natural products that decrease cancer growth. Part one of a four-part series. *Oncology Nursing Forum, 31,* E75–E90.

Montbriand, M. J. (2004b). Herbs or natural products that increase cancer growth or recurrence. Part two of a four-part series. *Oncology Nursing Forum, 31,* E99–E115.

Montbriand, M. J. (2004c). Herbs or natural products that protect against cancer growth. Part three of a four-part series. *Oncology Nursing Forum, 31,* E127–E146.

Montbriand, M. J. (2005). Herbs or natural products that may cause cancer and harm. Part four of a four-part series. *Oncology Nursing Forum, 32*, E20–E29.

National Institutes of Health National Center for Complementary and Alternative Medicine. (2002, May). Classification of complementary and alternative medical practices. NCCAM Publication No. D156.

NCCN (National Comprehensive Cancer Network) (2008). Cancer related fatigue. Clinical Practice Guidelines in Oncology - v1.2008. Retrieved April 10, 2008, from http://www.nccn.org/professionals/physician_gls?PDFfatigue.pdf

NIH Consensus Conference. (1998). Acupuncture. *The Journal of the American Medical Association, 280*, 1518–1524.

Oberbaum, M., Yaniv, I., Ben-Gal, Y., Stein, J., Ben-Zvi, N., Freedman, L. S., et al. (2001). A randomized, controlled clinical trial of the homeopathic medication TRAUMEEL S in the treatment of chemotherapy-induced stomatitis in children undergoing stem cell transplantation. *Cancer, 92*(3), 684–690.

Oeffinger, K. C., & Hudson, M. M. (2004). Long-term complications following childhood and adolescent cancer: Foundations for providing risk-based healthcare for survivors. *CA: A Cancer Journal for Clinicians, 54*, 208–236.

Oeffinger, K. C., Mertens, A., Sklar, C., Yasui, Y., Fears, T., Stovall, M., Vik, T., et al. (2003). Obesity in adult survivors of childhood acute lymphoblastic leukemia: A report from the childhood cancer survivor study. *Journal of Clinical Orthodontics, 21*(7) 1359–1365.

Olness, K. (1981). Imagery (self-hypnosis) as adjunct therapy in childhood cancer: Clinical experience with 25 patients. *The American Journal of Pediatric Hematology/Oncology, 3*(3), 313–321.

Palsson, O. S., Heymen, S., & Whitehead, W. E. (2004). Biofeedback treatment for functional anorectal disorders: A comprehensive efficacy review. *Applied Psychophysiology and Biofeedback, 29*, 153–174.

Peluso, G., Nicolai, R., Reda, E., Benatti, P., Barbarisi, A., & Calvani, M. (2000). Cancer and anticancer therapy-induced modifications on metabolism mediated by carnitine system. *Journal of Cellular Physiology, 182*, 339–350.

Pongrojpaw, D., & Chiamchanya, C. (2003). The efficacy of ginger in prevention of post-operative nausea and vomiting after outpatient gynecological laparoscopy. *Journal of the Medical Association of Thailand, 86*, 244–250.

Post-White, J., & Bauer, S. (2006). Psychoneuroimmunology: The mind-body connection. In R. Carroll-Johnson, L. Gorman, & N. Bush (Eds.), *Psychosocial nursing care along the cancer continuum,* 2nd ed., pp. 465–485). Pittsburg: Oncology Nursing Society.

Post-White, J., Fitzgerald, M., & Sencer, S. (2005). Massage therapy in childhood cancer. Highlighting Massage Therapy in CAM Research.

Post-White, J., Sencer, S., & Fitzgerald, M. (2000). Complementary therapy use in pediatric cancer. *Oncology Nursing Forum, 27*(2), 342–343.

Redeker, N. S., Lev, E. L., & Ruggiero, J. (2000). Insomnia, fatigue, anxiety, depression, and quality of life of cancer patients undergoing chemotherapy. *Scholarly Inquiry for Nursing Practice, 14*, 275–290.

Reindl, T. K., Geilen, W., Hartmann, R., Wiebelitz, K. R., Kan, G., Wilhelm, I. (2006). Acupuncture against chemotherapy-induced nausea and vomiting in pediatric oncology Interim results of a multicenter crossover study. *Supportive Care in Cancer, 14*, 172–176.

Richards, K., Nagel, C., Markie, M., Elwell, J., & Barone, C. (2003). Use of complementary and alternative therapies to promote sleep in critically ill patients. *Critical Care Nursing Clinics of North America, 15*, 329–340.

Ries, L. A. (1996). In A. Harras, B. K. Edwards, W. J. Blot, et al. (Eds.), *Cancer: Rates and risks.* Bethesda, MD: National Cancer Institute, 9–54.

Ries, L. A. G., Smith, M. A., Gurney, J. G., Linet, M., Tamra, T., Young, J. L., et al. (Eds). (1999). Cancer incidence and survival among children and adolescents: United States SEER Program 1975–1995, National Cancer Institute, SEER, Program. NIH Pub. No. 99–4649. Bethesda, MD.

Robison, L., Buckley, J., & Bunin, G. (1995). Assessment of environmental and genetic factors in the etiology of childhood cancers: The Children's Cancer Group Epidemiology Program. *Environmental Health Perspectives, 1103*(Suppl 6), 111–116.

Roscoe, J. A., Morrow, G. R., Hickok, J. T., Bushunow, P., Pierce, H. I., Flynn, P. J., et al. (2003). The efficacy of acupressure and acustimulation wrist bands for the relief of chemotherapy-induced nausea and vomiting. A University of Rochester Cancer Center Community Clinical Oncology Program multicenter study. *Journal of Pain and Symptom Management, 26,* 731–742.

Salminen, M. K., Tynkkynen, S., Rautelin, H., Poussa, T., Saxelin, M., Ristola, M., et al. (2004). The efficacy and safety of probiotic Lactobacillus rhamnosus GG on prolonged, noninfectious diarrhea in HIV Patients on antiretroviral therapy: A randomized, placebo-controlled, cross-over study. *HIV Clinical Trials, 5,* 183–191.

Sampson, M., Campbell, K., Ajiferuke, I., & Moher, D. (2003). Randomized controlled trials in pediatric complementary and alternative medicine: Where can they be found? *BMC Pediatrics, 3,* 1.

Sarker, S. A., Casswall, T. H., Mahalanabis, D., Alam, N. H., Albert, M. J., Brüssow, H., et al. (1998). Successful treatment of rotavirus diarrhea in children with immunoglobulin from immunized bovine colostrum. *The Pediatric Infectious Disease Journal, 17,* 1149–54.

Sawyer, M. G., Gannoni, A. F., Toogood, I. R., Antoniou, G., & Rice, M. (1994). The use of alternative therapies by children with cancer. *The Medical Journal of Australia, 160*(6), 320–322.

Schrader, E. (2000). Equivalence of St John's Wort extract (Ze 117) and fluoxetine: A randomized, controlled study in mild-moderate depression. *International Clinical Psychopharmacology, 15,* 61–68.

Schultz, V., Hubner, W., & Ploch, M. (1997). Clinical trials with phyto-psychopharmacological agents. *Phytomedicine, 4,* 379–387.

Schulz, H., Stolz, C., & Muller, J. (1994). The effect of valerian extract on sleep polygraphy in poor sleepers: A pilot study. *Pharmacopsychiatry, 27,* 147–151.

Sencer, S. F., Reaman, G. H., & Kelly, K. M. (2007). Complementary and alternative medicine utilization in childhood cancer, Truth or consequences. *American Society of Clinical Oncology,* 617–621.

Sencer, S., & Kelly, K. (2007). Complementary and alternative therapies in pediatric oncology. *Pediatric Clinics of North America, 54* 1043–1060.

Smith, J. T., Barabasz, A., & Barabasz, M. (1996). Comparison of hypnosis and distraction in severely ill children undergoing painful medical procedures. *Journal of Counseling Psychology, 43,* 187–195.

Smith, M., Freidlin, B., Ries, L., & Simon, R. (1998). Trends in reported incidence of primary malignant brain tumors in children in the United States. *Journal of the National Cancer Institute, 90,* 1269–1277.

Somasundaram, S., Edmund, N. A., Moore, D. T., Small, G. W., Shi, Y. Y., Orlowski, R. Z. (2002). Dietary curcumin inhibits chemotherapy incuded apoptosis in models of human breast cancer. *Cancer Research, 62,* 3868–3875.

Summerbell, C. D., Ashton, V., Campbell, K. J., Edmunds, L., Kelly, S., & Waters, E. (2003). Interventions for treating obesity in children. *Cochrane Database of Systematic Reviews,* CD001872.

Szajewska, H., & Mrukowicz, J. Z. (2001). Probiotics in the treatment and prevention of acute infectious diarrhea in infants and children: A systematic review of published randomized, double-blind, placebo-controlled trials. *Journal of Pediatric Gastroenterology and Nutrition, 33*(Suppl 2), S17–S25.

Tosett, F., Ferrari, N., & De Flora, S. (2002). Angioprevention: Angiogenesis is common and key target for cancer chemopreventive agents. *The FASEB Journal, 16,* 2–14.

Treish, I., Shord, S., Valgus, J., Harvey, D., Nagy, J., Stegal, J., et al. (2003). Randomized double-blind study of the Reliefband as an adjunct to standard antiemetics in patients receiving moderately-high to highly emetogenic chemotherapy. *Supportive Care in Cancer, 11,* 516–21.

Vahdat, L., Papadopoulos, K., Lange, D., Leuin, S., Kaufman, E., Donovan, D., et al. (2001). Reduction of paclitaxel-induced peripheral neuropathy with glutamine. *Clinical Cancer Research, 7,* 1192–1197.

Vohra, S., Johnston, B. C., Cramer, K., & Humphreys, K. (2007). Adverse events associated with pediatric spinal manipulation: A systematic review. *Pediatrics, 119*(1), e275–e283.

Weiger, W. A., Smith, M., Boon, H., Richardson, M. A., Kaptchuk, T. J., & Eisenberg, D. M. (2002). Advising patients who seek complementary and alternative medical therapies for cancer. *Annals of Internal Medicine, 137,* 889–903.

Weiser, M., Cabanillas, M., Konopleva, M., Thomas, D., Pierce, Escalante, C., et al. (2004). Relation between the duration of remission and hyperglycemia during induction chemotherapy for acute lymphocytic leukemia with a hyperfractionated cyclophosphamide, vincristine, doxorubicin, and dexamethasone/methotrexate-cytarabine regimen. *Cancer, 100*(6) 1179–1185.

Wigmore, S. J., Ross, J. A., Falconer, J. S., Plester, C. E., Tisdale, M. J., Carter, D. C., et al. (1996). The effect of polyunsaturated fatty acids on the progress of cachexia in patients with pancreatic cancer. *Nutrition, 12,* S27–S30.

Wild, M. R., & Espie, C. A. (2004). The efficacy of hypnosis in the reduction of procedural pain and distress in pediatric oncology: A systematic review. *Journal of Developmental and Behavioral Pediatrics, 25,* 207–213.

Winter, S., Jue, K., Prochazka, J., Francis, P., Hamilton, W., Linn, L., et al. (1995). The role of L-carnitine in pediatric cardiomyopathy. *Journal of child neurology, 10*(Suppl 2), 2S45–2S51.

Wolf, B. W., Wheeler, K. B., Ataya, D. G., & Garleb, K. A. (1998). Safety and tolerance of *Lactobacillus reuteri* supplementation to a population infected with the human immunodeficiency virus. *Food and Chemical Toxicology, 36,* 1085–1094.

Wolfe, J., Grier, H. E., Klar, N., Levin, S. B., Ellenbogen, J. M., Salem-Schatz, S., et al. (2000). Symptoms and suffering at the end of life in children with cancer. *The New England Journal of Medicine, 342,* 326–333.

Wright, M., Galea, V., & Barr, R. (2005). Proficiency of balance in children and youth who have had acute lymphoblastic leukemia. *Physical Therapy, 85*(8) 782–790.

Yang, C. S., Prabhu, S., & Landau, J. (2001). Prevention of carcinogenesis by tea polyphenols. *Drug Metabolism Reviews, 33,* 237–253.

Yang, G. (1996). Immunologic effect of traditional Chinese drugs. *Chinese Medical Journal, 109,* 59–60.

Zahm, S. H., & Devesa, S. (1995). Childhood cancer: Overview of trends and environmental carcinogens. *Environmental Health Perspectives, 103*(Suppl 6), 177–184.

Zeltzer, L. K., Dolgin, M. J., LeBaron, S., & LeBaron, C. (1991). A randomized, controlled study of behavioral intervention for chemotherapy distress in children with cancer. *Pediatrics, 88,* 34–42.

Zeltzer, L. K., Tsao, J. C., Stelling, C., Powers, M., Levy, S., & Waterhouse, M. (2002). A phase I study on the feasibility and acceptability of an acupuncture/hypnosis intervention for chronic pediatric pain. *Journal of Pain and Symptom Management, 24,* 437–446.

Zeltzer, L., & LeBaron, S. (1982). Hypnosis and nonhypnotic techniques for reduction of pain and anxiety during painful procedures in children and adolescents with cancer. *The Journal of Pediatrics, 101,* 1032–1035.

Zeltzer, L., LeBaron, S., & Zeltzer, P. M. (1984). The effectiveness of behavioral intervention for reduction of nausea and vomiting in children and adolescents receiving chemotherapy. *Journal of Clinical Oncology, 2*(6), 683–90.

24

Integrative Pediatric Pain Management

JOY A. WEYDERT AND MARK CONNELLY

KEY CONCEPTS

- We have a better understanding of pain as a multidimensional idiosyncratic experience influenced by many factors beyond just nociceptive input.
- As compared to nociceptive pain caused by chemical, mechanical, or thermal stimulation to receptors in the periphery signaling tissue injury, neuropathic pain is produced by changes in the central nervous system which cause enduring changes in the processing of sensory information.
- Mind-body interventions in the context of a child's pain are used to modify how the child understands the situation, focuses his/her attention, and perceives control. These interventions can thereby transform how pain gets encoded and expressed.
- Biologically based therapies helpful for children who suffer pain include, but are not limited to botanicals, animal-derived extracts, vitamins, minerals, fatty acids, amino acids, proteins, prebiotics and probiotics, whole diets, and functional foods.
- Manipulation therapies, massage and alternative therapies such as acupuncture and homeopathy are also helpful for acute and chronic pain in children.
- It has been demonstrated that children with chronic pain problems such as juvenile migraine, complex regional pain syndrome, and juvenile idiopathic arthritis can benefit from complementary and alternative treatments.

■

Integrative Approach to Acute and Chronic Pain

OVERVIEW

The understanding of pain has markedly evolved over the past several decades, though steadfast throughout history has been the recognition that unrelieved pain can interfere with all aspects of life (Payne, 2007). Pain that is suboptimally treated has deleterious effects on the immune system, wound healing, tumor growth, and gastrointestinal functioning due to neurochemicals and cortisol produced by stress. Beyond these physiological effects, however, pain impacts many aspects of both the individual and his or her family through its influence on physical functioning, mood, sleep, interpersonal relationships, social activities, and ability to work or attend school. For these reasons, healthcare providers must both assess pain characteristics *and* the impact of pain on the whole person so as not to exclusively treat pain from a biomedical perspective.

The most commonly cited definition of pain was established by The International Association for the Study of Pain (IASP) more than a decade ago. This definition states that pain is "an unpleasant sensory and emotional experience associated with actual or potential tissue damage, or describe in terms of such damage" (Merskey, 1994). This definition has helped move the understanding of pain beyond prior more reductionist views by incorporating sensory, emotional, and cognitive phenomenon and acknowledging that observable physical pathology need not be present for one to experience pain. Increasingly we are recognizing why and how an individual's perception of pain is influenced by prior experience, cognitive development, cultural background, personal expectations and beliefs, and social context. Recognizing these domains as integral to the pain experience is fundamental in both effectively assessing and addressing pain from an integrative perspective.

Complementary and alternative methods for pain management are increasingly being used by both adult and pediatric patients. In the general population, chronic pain is in fact among the primary reasons for which complementary and alternative methods are used (Astin, 1998; Bausell, 2001; Eisenberg, 1998). In the sections that follow, we present information on the basic pathophysiology of pain and the general approach to a holistic assessment of pain in children. Subsequently, we give an overview of how specific complementary and alternative modalities have been applied to pain problems encountered in pediatric practice, with particular attention to issues of safety and empirical support.

PATHOPHYSIOLOGY

Nociceptive Pain

The first stage of the nociceptive pain pathway is typically referred to as transduction, or the conversion of chemical information into an electrical signal at the sensory neurons located peripherally in skin, muscles, joints, and viscera. These nociceptors, which are fully present at birth, become activated by chemically mediated changes induced by noxious mechanical, inflammatory, or thermal stimuli. The peripheral nociceptors convert the chemical information into an electrical impulse following depolarization of the cell membrane. Depolarization itself depends on many factors, including the functioning and stability of ion channels and the exchange of sodium (Na^+), potassium (K^+), chloride (Cl^-), calcium (Ca^{++}), and magnesium (Mg^{++}).

In the second stage of the pain pathway, or transmission, the depolarizing electrical signal travels along the primary afferent fibers and enters the dorsal horn of the spinal cord. This area of the dorsal horn may be activated by somatic stimuli (from skin, muscles, bones, etc.) or by visceral afferents (from internal organs) which, if they cross-fire, cause somato-visceral pain or "referred pain." Following synapses in the dorsal horn, the electrical impulses cross the midline to form the contra-lateral spinothalamic tracts that travel up through the brainstem to the thalamus, hypothalamus, amygdala, cingulate cortex, and higher brain centers, causing limbic and autonomic activation. Projections from the thalamus ultimately send information regarding the location, quality and intensity of pain to the primary sensory cortex, where all inputs are generally thought to culminate in pain perception (Chen H, 2004).

An integral but only relatively recently studied feature of the pain processing system is the ability to modulate pain signals to influence pain perception. Inhibitory pathways originating in the higher brain centers have the capacity to entirely transform nociceptive signals. These descending pathways are immature at birth likely from delayed maturation of inhibitory interneurons and low levels of serotonin and norepinephrine (Fitzgerald, 2003). In older infants, children, and adolescents, however, inhibition greatly improves and is mediated by the release of endogenous opioids, norepinephrine, and serotonin in the dorsal horn and through the release of the major inhibitory neurotransmitter, gamma-amino butyric acid (GABA), from the interneurons.

The "gate control" theory of pain modulation offered by Melzack and Wall in 1965 (and now updated as the "neuromatrix" theory of pain) first introduced the idea that the central inhibitory control processes of the brain include psychological factors such as emotional states (Melzack, 1965, 1999). Specialized networks of neurons in the brain forged between the thalamus, cortex, and limbic system regulate the autonomic, immune, and endogenous opioid systems. These connections allow for the promotion and modulation of the sensory, cognitive, and affective dimensions of the subjective pain experience (Melzack, 2007). Recent theories increasingly have focused on pain from the perspective of homeostasis (Craig, 2003; Gatchel, 2007), with chronic pain thought to represent unsuccessful attempts to restore homeostatic balance vis-à-vis what is perceived as an ongoing threat to the organism. This idea of balance in physiological systems is in fact largely consistent with some of the complementary and alternative approaches to pain and thus may offer a "mainstream" theoretical foundation to bridge previously disconnected conceptualizations of pain and stimulate novel studies.

Recognizing the psychological and social influences on pain processing has brought about a better understanding of pain as a multidimensional idiosyncratic experience influenced by many factors beyond just nociceptive input. Appropriate treatment, therefore, is best practiced with an integrated interdisciplinary approach that comprehensively addresses all of the dimensions of pain. Inadequate pain control often leads unnecessarily to greater disability, isolation, anxiety, fear, depression, and suffering. Further, persons with chronic pain are at risk for developing other concerning co-morbidities such as depression and sleep disorders which further aggravate the pain experience.

Neuropathic Pain and Pain Amplification

As opposed to nociceptive pain caused by chemical, mechanical, or thermal stimulation to receptors in the periphery signaling tissue injury, neuropathic pain is produced by neuroanatomical, neurochemical, and neurophysiological changes in the nerves of the peripheral and central nervous systems, leading to enduring changes in the processing of sensory information (Pediatric Chronic Pain Task Force, 2007). In the affected dorsal horn, nerve sensitization develops and leads to spontaneous (unprovoked) nerve activity through the release of excitatory neurotransmitters (aspartate and glutamate), a lowering of the activation threshold, and an increased responsiveness to a given stimulus. Some of these nerve fibers may develop new adrenergic receptors or ectopic neuronal pacemaker cells along the length of the nerve which have abnormal or dysfunctional sodium channels and increased adrenergic sensitivity (England, 1991). Still other neurons may develop abnormal electrical connections between adjacent demyelenated fibers or between sympathetic and sensory fibers (Macres, 1998).

The repetitive release of inflammatory neuropeptides [e.g., substance P, prostaglandins (PGE 2), nitric oxide, arachadonic acid, protein kinase C, glutamate, aspartate, and cyclo-oxygenase] all contribute to activating and promoting an ongoing pain cycle that is typically out of proportion with physical findings. As the cycle continues, repetitive stimulation of the neurons further results in prolonged discharges in the dorsal horn cells, spinothalamic tracts, thalamus, and/or cerebral cortex causing central sensitization and the up-regulation of excitatory receptors such as the N-methyl-D-aspartate (NMDA) receptor (Chen H, 2004). This persistent activation may also lead to the death of the inhibitory interneurons that produce serotonin, nor-epinephrine, or endogenous opioids. Treatment for this type of pain aims to restore the endogenous inhibitory systems and balance to the nervous system.

INTEGRATIVE ASSESSMENT OF PAIN

An integrative pain evaluation needs to include the biological, psychological, social, and spiritual factors in context with the child's developmental level (Bursch, 1998). At many pain clinics, multiple disciplines (e.g., physician, psychologist, social worker, nurse, physical therapist) work in concert to obtain this information.

The assessment typically begins with a thorough history of the current problem, including any significant events leading up to the initiation of the problems (e.g., trauma, illness, stressors, etc.). Subsequently, obtaining a thorough description of pain characteristics is critical as a guide to understanding the type of pain the child may be having (e.g., nociceptive versus neuropathic). For example, words such as sharp, dull, achy, pressure, tightness, stabbing, throbbing, tender, or nagging typically indicate somatic origin of pain and may be fairly localized. Words such as deep, achy, squeezing, cramping, or gnawing may indicate visceral pain, which is typically vaguer in nature. Words such as burning, tingling, numbness, "pins and needles," or shocking likely indicate neuropathic pain.

Obtaining a rating of average, best, and worst pain intensity also gives important information on pain variability, however, there has been a great deal of debate on the best method for obtaining these ratings in children. For preverbal children or children with mild to severe cognitive impairments, observational tools are generally required in conjunction with the parent's report of the child's baseline ("pre-pain") behavior if appropriate. The FLACC is a relatively well validated tool for this purpose and assesses the child's facial expression, leg position, activity level, cry, and consolability. The Non-Communicating Children's Pain Checklist also can be used in this population of children (Breau, 2002). For verbal children 3 years and older, or with children with a language barrier, a scale containing faces portraying varying pain intensity that the child can simply point to is recommended (Bieri, 1990; Hicks, 2001). For children aged 8 and above and who understand the concept, a visual analog scale (i.e., a 100 mm line typically with anchors "no pain" and "worst pain") or a numerical rating scale (i.e., requiring choosing a number between 0 and 10) can be used. Figure 24-1 provides examples of these pain scales.

It is especially important when assessing children with chronic pain to gather information about how pain is affecting academic, social, physical, and emotional functioning. Information on the extent of school and social activities missed gives insight into how well the child and family are coping with pain and may suggest the need for psychological interventions to assist with this. It also can be interesting to ask what the child and family would be doing or what would be different for them if the child no longer had pain. For some patients whose pain has become associated with escape or avoidance of unpleasant situations or ongoing reinforcement by family attention, they cannot imagine life to be any different without pain.

In addition to the typical pediatric history of past illnesses, surgeries, family history and social history, it is important to obtain a complete review of systems to assess for other constitutional symptoms that may be related to the current pain complaints. These symptoms may include shortness of breath (with no asthma history), dizziness or lightheadedness with standing, chronic constipation, or cold hands or feet which may indicate a dysregulated autonomic nervous system that needs to be addressed. Assessing the child's psychological status (sadness or flat affect, irritability, behavioral conduct, social involvement, emotional maturity, and current stressors) also is important. Ideally

Categories	Scoring		
	0	**1**	**2**
Face	No particular expression or smile disinterested	occasional grimace or frown, withdrawn	Frequent to constant frown, clenched jaw, quivering chin
Legs	Normal position or relaxed	Uneasy, restless, tense	kicking, rigid, or jerking
Activity	Lying quietly, normal position, moves easily	Squirming, shifting back and forth, tense	Arched, rigid, or jerking
Cry	No cry (awake or asleep)	Moans or whimpers, occasional complaint	Crying steadily, screams or sobs, frequent complaints
Consolability	Content, relaxed	Reassured by occasional touching, hugging, or talking to Distractable	Difficult to console or comfort

Each of the five categories (F) Face; (L) Legs; (A) Activity; (C) Cry; (C) Consolability is scored from 0-2, which results in a total score between zero and ten.

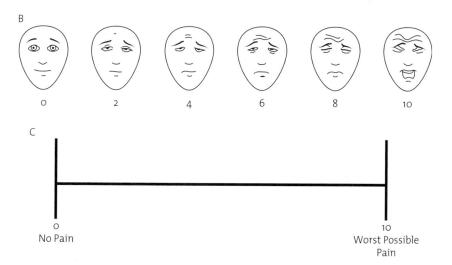

B

0   2   4   6   8   10

C

0
No Pain

10
Worst Possible
Pain

FIGURE 24-1. Example scales for pain assessment (FLACC, FPS-R, and Visual Analog Scale)

with a multidisciplinary approach to children with chronic pain, a full evaluation by a clinical psychologist would be done in conjunction with the medical interview. If this is not possible, be aware of the cues to depression and anxiety and make a referral for a full psychological evaluation if indicated.

Sleep is often disrupted in patients with acute or chronic pain, but so too, poor sleep can contribute to the pain experience. Studies have revealed relationships between the experience of recurrent or chronic pain and sleep disturbance in adolescents and these are often related to mood disturbances, decreased level of functioning and poorer overall quality of life (Palermo, 2005). Improving sleep along with addressing mood disturbances is important for effective treatment of pain.

As learned from osteopathic colleagues, it is helpful to obtain a full "accident and injury" history to assess for past traumas. This would include any birth trauma (forceps, vacuum extraction, difficult delivery, fetal distress) or falls during childhood (down stairs, off furniture, jungle gyms, trampolines, bikes, trees, etc.). This history would also include sports injuries, motor vehicle accidents, head injuries, or any injuries involving getting "the wind knocked out of them" or causing a loss of consciousness. Any of these traumas, even if seemingly minor, is an assault on the central nervous system which can lead to chronic stimulation and dysregulation of nerves to cause pain. These traumas may be cumulative over time so even remote trauma may contribute to current pain.

Observation of the child's general appearance, level of activity, pain behaviors, posture, gait, affect, and speech patterns need to be assessed throughout the entire visit and changes or consistency should be noted. If possible, observing these variables when the child is in the presence of parents as well as when the child is alone can be informative about the level of social influence on the pain presentation. A thorough physical examination needs to include comprehensive neurological and musculoskeletal evaluations.

CONVENTIONAL APPROACH TO PAIN MANAGEMENT

In general, conventional pain management is based on an acute pain model and often can be quite effectively applied in this context, although increasingly complementary and alternative methods are being used in concert with conventional pain treatment in acute pain situations as well. Acute pain may be related to procedures (IV starts, lumbar punctures, and sutures), trauma, surgery, or a symptom of a disease process (i.e., septic hip). In most of these cases, pain is self-limiting and treatment typically is for symptom management. For these types of pain, use of pharmacologic analgesics is indicated and effective. A good pediatric drug reference book can offer guidance on medication usage, dosages and side effects (Taketomo, 2007).

Various topical analgesics are available and should be used prior to the start of invasive procedures to reduce the pain experience. For acute pain of mild to moderate intensity, oral or intravenous non-opioid medications and non-steroidal anti-inflammatory drugs (NSAIDS) such as acetaminophen or ibuprofen are the conventional treatments of choice (Berde, 2002). For pain of moderate to severe intensity, typically IV or oral opioid medications are used. With rare exception, opioid analgesics are safe for the treatment of high levels of pain in children despite the continued prevalence of myths about addiction. Side effects such as reduced GI motility and pruritis do frequently occur on opioid medications but are easily managed with proper monitoring, medications, dosage reduction, or opioid rotation.

INTEGRATIVE APPROACH TO PAIN MANAGEMENT

An integrative approach to medicine is particularly applicable for pain management as it seeks to have a full understanding of the problem and all that contributes to it, engages in partnership with the patient and/or family to work on the solution, and offers a broader palate of therapeutic modalities that work synergistically to stimulate healing, recover balance and support the body's own resilience.

The National Center for Complementary and Alternative Medicine (NCCAM), a division of the National Institutes of Health (NIH) recognizes five domains that broadly characterize the "complementary and alternative" healing modalities. Listed below are these domains with a general overview of how they have been applied to pain problems in children and adolescents.

Mind-Body Therapies

The most widely used and empirically studied complementary and alternative treatments for both acute and chronic pain in children fall within the category of mind-body interventions. A main premise underlying the rationale for applying mind-body interventions to pain is that mental activities (e.g., perceptions, beliefs, memories, expectations, images, and intentions) have been demonstrated to be capable of directly (via neurobiological processes) and indirectly (via behavior) contributing to the expression of pain problems (McGrath, 1989, 1993, 2003, 2004; Watson, 2003). There are an increasing amount of fascinating studies using sophisticated neuroimaging and electroencephalogram techniques showing in real-time how mental activities directed in certain ways can transform pain processing both for better or worse (Borsook, 2006; deCharms, 2005; Goffaux, 2007; Koyama, 2005; Petrovic, 2001; Rainville, 2002).

Mind-body interventions in the context of a child's pain are used to modify how the child understands the situation, focuses his/her attention, and perceives control. These interventions can thereby transform how pain gets encoded and expressed. Much of children's understanding about pain and its significance comes directly from parents, and thus mind-body interventions for children's pain typically incorporate parents or caregivers in some fashion (e.g., as coaches, models, and active participants). In addition, given that pain may be associated with a number of other somatic symptoms as well as emotional distress and functional disability, often mind-body interventions for pain target multiple interrelated areas and not just pain intensity per se. In fact, particularly in the context of chronic pain in children, functional improvement (e.g., increased school attendance, improvements in mobility and physical activity, and increased social involvement) is often a primary target for mind-body therapies rather than exclusively pain reduction.

To our knowledge, there has been no published data on safety issues associated with mind-body therapies as applied to pediatric pain, which is part of their appeal for practitioners and families alike. However, there may be certain instances in which mind-body therapies (or their suggestion) can produce adverse effects and should be adapted or avoided. For example, depending on how the recommendation of cognitive-behavioral therapy (CBT) for chronic pain is made, the mere suggestion of "therapy" may be sufficient for some families to abandon care with the physician or team altogether. Also, in some cases mind-body therapies that involve focusing on and monitoring body responses may serve to escalate anxiety in some children that are already highly body-focused or that have body image disturbances.

With some notable exceptions, most mind-body interventions designed for children with pain complaints can be implemented by a variety of disciplines with relatively minimal formal training. Further, many mind-body pain interventions can be done by the child him or herself without needing a provider per se, or once the skill is learned from a provider "coach," the child can enact the strategy without necessarily requiring ongoing frequent contact. This requires a commitment on the part of the child and family, which clinicians need to assess and assist with if appropriate prior to making recommendations for these types of therapies.

Mind-body interventions used for pain are quite numerous. Some interventions that are used for pain management are reviewed below.

SELF-HYPNOSIS The use of self-hypnosis for the management of pediatric pain, particularly acute pediatric pain, is an increasingly common practice in both inpatient and outpatient pediatric settings. Coaching a child in self-hypnosis in the context of pain prevention or management typically involves helping the child to focus attention in a way that produces body responses incompatible with pain processing. Frequently this is done by invoking a child's natural ability to use his or her imagination while offering verbal suggestions that can transform the noxious sensation or its meaning to the child. Images often used during self-hypnosis (e.g., of "changing the channel" in the mind to a favorite place in which the child can get immersed, of finding a "pain volume switch" and turning it down, or of imagining immersing one's hand in a bucket of fluffy snow until it becomes numb) engage the child's sense of control over the situation and are capable of reducing sympathetic drive that can otherwise intensify any given pain experience (Lee, 1996). There is reasonable research supporting the efficacy of self-hypnosis on pain and anxiety associated with medical procedures (e.g., needle pain, dressing changes, lumbar puncture, intubation, voiding cystoure-throgram). Self-hypnosis has been less well studied in chronic pain conditions, but this technique does have demonstrated efficacy through randomized trials at least in children with chronic headaches (Hammond, 2007) and in recurrent abdominal pain (Weydert, 2006).

COGNITIVE-BEHAVIORAL THERAPY Conversely to self-hypnosis, formal CBT (including both behavioral and cognitive methods for managing pain and related disability) has been most widely used and studied in children with *chronic* pain disorders.

CBT by an appropriately trained practitioner is particularly recommended in a minority of cases for which beliefs and expectations about pain have become entrenched and are significant in maintaining the pain and/or disability for the child (Gauntlett-Gilbert, 2007; Konijnenberg, 2005; Palermo, 2005; Zeltzer, 2006). CBT typically involves 6 or more weekly sessions with a psychologist or other mental health professional. During these sessions, the child is taught a variety of pain coping skills that include relaxation training and methods for monitoring, identifying, and transforming thoughts that contribute to the emotions and behaviors thought to be maintaining pain and disability. Parents are often an integral part of this form of treatment and learn to change responses to their child's pain in a way that better empowers and supports their child's own adaptive coping efforts (Palermo, 2005). CBT has been supported through randomized studies to reduce pain and related emotional and academic disability associated with juvenile primary fibromyalgia (Degotardi, 2006; Kashikar-Zuck, 2005), sickle cell disease (Chen E, 2004), juvenile idiopathic arthritis (Walco, 1992), chronic headaches (Holden, 1999), chronic abdominal pain (Janicke, 1999), and Complex Regional Pain Syndrome Type I (Lee BH, 2002).

MEDITATION AND ACCEPTANCE-BASED THERAPY In principle, training in and regular implementation of meditative practices can influence the processing of pain by virtue of inducing an incompatible response (e.g., deep relaxation). Although there have been some adult studies evaluating the efficacy of mindfulness and transcendental meditation practices on pain and associated outcomes (Astin, 2003; Kingston, 2007; Morone, 2008), at the time of this writing we were unable to locate any published studies evaluating the application of meditation to pain conditions in children. However, given that there are limited if any safety issues associated with these approaches, the practice of meditation may be clinically recommended as an adjunctive pain management modality for children with idiopathic or disease-related chronic pain whose pain appears significantly influenced by stress and tension.

Recently, some tenets adapted from mindfulness meditation have begun being implemented in what is called "acceptance-based therapy" for adolescents with chronic pain disorders (Wicksell, 2005). Acceptance-based therapy for pain is based on the idea that the persistent attempt to "fight" pain can in fact itself produce disability. Instead, learning to live a valued life in the context of pain and accepting pain as a sensation that may or may not diminish is the central principle of the acceptance-based approach. This is an intriguing approach to the management of chronic pain and will likely generate many more studies in the upcoming years.

BIOFEEDBACK-ASSISTED RELAXATION TRAINING The processing of and response to pain signals inherently involve aspects of the autonomic nervous system that are not normally under much conscious control. Feedback on these autonomic nervous system parameters via auditory information and/or visual displays is capable of equipping children with insight into how components of the autonomic nervous system may be initiating and maintaining their pain. Pairing this feedback with training in relaxation techniques uniquely permits children the opportunity to observe how relaxation skills can positively influence some of the "automatic" internal processes of their body.

The clinical application of biofeedback for pediatric pain has thus far been primarily limited to certain chronic pain disorders. This approach has been studied adequately to recommend its use at least for recurrent tension-type and migraine headache in children (Eccleston, 2002, 2003; Holden, 1999), but there are several other potential pediatric pain applications of this approach that have yet to be studied. The ability to receive feedback on activity in areas of the brain that process and modulate pain signals has recently been exploited with some success in adult chronic pain patients (deCharms, 2005) and may begin to be used with children in the future. It should be noted, however, that there remains an active debate about whether any form of biofeedback has incremental efficacy on pain outcomes beyond training in relaxation approaches alone (NIH Technology Assessment Panel, 1996). This is a clinically relevant debate, given that biofeedback equipment and appropriately trained technicians can be quite prohibitive for pediatric centers with limited funds.

CREATIVE THERAPIES Music and other creative therapy interventions have been primarily used clinically in pediatric settings for the goal of reducing distress associated with pending medical or dental procedures or as a method of distraction during the procedure itself. There have been some case studies and small clinical trials on the use of music for reducing pain and distress in neonates and young children (up to age 7) and one recent trial of music therapy for pediatric headache, but no studies on other creative therapies for pediatric pain conditions. Data from the few pediatric studies conducted to date are somewhat conflicting, with some studies finding positive effects on reducing procedural distress or pain (Fowler-Kerry, 1987; Malone, 1996; Megel, 1999; Oelkers-Ax, 2007) and others finding no significant effects (Aitken, 2002; Arts, 1994; Marchette, 1991). Children generally enjoy these types of therapies and for some the results are clinically beneficial, especially in young or nonverbal children who may not be able to implement other mind-body approaches that require higher cognitive development.

VIRTUAL REALITY THERAPY Although not typically included in a list of mind-body therapies, virtual reality (VR) therapy has been increasingly applied to certain pediatric pain conditions with some success. One of the primary applications has been in children with acute pain from burn injuries. A randomized trial and multiple case studies have supported the use of VR for burn pain in children (Das, 2005; Hoffman, 2000; Steele,

2003). Other applications supported through small trials and case studies include using VR to reduce pain and distress associated with port access, venipuncture, and dental treatments (Gershon, 2004; Gold, 2006; Hoffman, 2001). Similar to self-hypnosis, this approach seems to work by helping to facilitate distraction and transforming how the noxious sensation gets perceived by the child.

Biologically Based Therapies

Biologically-based therapies include, but are not limited to botanicals, animal-derived extracts, vitamins, minerals, fatty acids, amino acids, proteins, prebiotics and probiotics, whole diets, and functional foods (NCCAM). The use of herbs or supplements helps support the many systems of the body with the goal of protecting and enhancing their function. Herbs contain combinations of many naturally occurring, biologically active compounds that work individually or synergistically, therefore they act in a wider, more general and less specific way than most single ingredient pharmaceutical drugs.

As with pharmaceutical agents, there is a paucity of studies on the use of botanicals or other biologically based therapies in children with pain. Despite this lack of evidence, many of these supplements are generally regarded as safe (GRAS) and can be used if monitored closely for their effectiveness (Cohen MH, 2005).

MAGNESIUM   Magnesium (Mg^{++}) is regarded as a natural muscle relaxant and pain reliever as it has depressant effects on nerve transmission and muscle contractility by antagonizing calcium-mediated channels. It also acts as an NMDA receptor antagonist so has potential pain relieving effects in migraine, tension headaches, neuropathic pain, fibromyalgia and other pain disorders (Cohen JS, 2002; Crosby, 2000). Even Epsom salts, which is 100% magnesium sulfate, is a known treatment either as a soak or a compress to relieve muscle pain from over-use or strains. Studies done specifically on the use of magnesium for pain have supported the efficacy of magnesium in reducing the frequency and severity of migraines in both adults (Demirkaya, 2000) and children (Wang, 2003). It has also been helpful in reducing pain and tenderness in adult fibromyalgia patients when taken orally as magnesium hydroxide with malic acid (Russell, 1995).

Lethal effects have been reported when excessive amounts (2400 mg daily for several days in an infant, ingestion of 2 boxes of Epsom salts in an adult) (Birrer, 2002; McGuire, 2000) were taken orally. Certain preparations of magnesium may cause diarrhea due to the unabsorbed salts in the intestine which is not necessarily dose related. Changing to a different preparation (i.e., magnesium glycinate, gluconate, aspartate, etc.) usually alleviates this problem. The recommended dose for chronic pain management in children is 9 mg/kg given 3 times daily.

GINGER   Ginger is used to relieve pain in inflammatory conditions through its inhibitory affects of cyclo-oxygenase (COX) and lipoxygenase pathways by one of its constituents,

6-gingerol (Grzanna, 2005). This same constituent is thought to be responsible for ginger's ability to reduce nausea and vomiting from chemotherapy, motion sickness or pregnancy (Ali, 2007; Lumb, 1993; Portnoi, 2003). Current evidence for its use in pain is exclusively from adult studies and includes possible reduction of severity and duration in migraine headache (Grontved, 1986), and decreased pain and swelling in patients with rheumatoid arthritis (Srivastava, 1989, 1992).

Ginger is usually well tolerated and considered safe when used in typical doses; however side effects may develop, such as abdominal discomfort, heartburn, or diarrhea, with doses greater than 5 g per day (Srivastava, 1989). It is generally recommended that doses not exceed 4 g per day in adults. Ginger can be given by brewing 0.5–1 g of dried root into 150 ml boiling water for 5–10 minutes before straining. Tinctures can be taken in doses of 0.25–3 ml depending on its concentration. Powered root in capsule form can also be used and dosed 250–500 mg 3–4 times daily up to the maximum of 4 g per day.

DEVIL'S CLAW Devil's Claw has been used traditionally to treat pain disorders such as rheumatoid arthritis, osteoarthritis, myalgia, low back pain and migraine headache. It contains iridoid glycoxide constituents that have anti-inflammatory effects through alteration of the cyclo-oxygenase and lipoxygenase inflammatory pathways and through increased synthesis of tumor necrosis factor (TNF-alpha) (Chrubasik, 2000; Grant, 2007). Adult studies have supported its effects in improving pain (back, hip, and knee), stiffness, level of function, and quality of life (Warnock, 2007) and it is comparable in safety and efficacy to a prescription NSAID when used for 1 year. (Chrubasik, 2005). Devil's Claw is generally well tolerated with only rare side effects of nausea, vomiting, diarrhea, anorexia or loss of taste. A usual dose of Devil's Claw is from 1 to 4.5 g of dried root per day.

OMEGA-3-FATTY ACIDS Omega-3 FA (DHA and EPA) are long-chained polyunsaturated fatty acids (PUFA) found in oily fish, marine mammals, fish liver oils and commercially prepared fish oil products. They have anti-inflammatory effects by competing with arachidonic acid for inclusion in the cyclo-oxygenase and lipooxygenase pathways. Significant analgesic effects have been demonstrated in several patient populations, including patients with dysmenorrhea (Harel, 1996), migraine (Harel, 2002), rheumatoid arthritis (Goldberg, 2007), and sickle cell disease (Tomer, 2001).

There are minimal safety issues associated with omega-3 FA supplementation. Although DHA alone does not seem to affect blood clotting, when used in conjunction with EPA as fish oil there may be an increased risk of bleeding with concomitant drugs or herbs that affect platelet aggregation (Nelson, 1997). The recommended dosing for pain is 1–3 g orally each day.

FEVERFEW Feverfew traditionally has been used for the prevention of migraines and treatment of headaches, arthritis, fever and menstrual irregularities. The mechanism of action of feverfew is unknown, although there is evidence that it may inhibit platelet aggregation, inhibit serotonin release from platelets and leukocytes, inhibit leukotrienes, and block prostaglandins (Sumner, 1992). It has also been suggested that it may have serotonin 5-HT receptor blocking effects (Shrivastava, 2006) which has relevance for migraine headaches as serotonin dysregulation is thought to play a key role in headache initiation. Indeed, randomized trials of feverfew in adult patients have supported its efficacy in reducing the number and severity of migraine attacks when used in isolation (Murphy, 1988) or in combination with white willow bark (Shrivastava, 2006) or ginger (Cady, 2005). There have been no trials of feverfew for pain management in any pediatric populations, although this agent does occasionally get recommended clinically for pediatric headache management. No significant adverse effects have been reported with long-term use of feverfew (Pittler, 2000). The recommended dosing is 50–125 mg of feverfew extract, or 2–3 fresh leaves daily.

BUTTERBUR   Butterbur traditionally has been used to treat headaches, migraines, allergic rhinitis, chronic cough, and as a stomach and bladder anti-spasmodic. The active ingredients are petasin and isopetasin which have anti-spasmodic effects on smooth muscle and vascular walls (Anon, 2001), inhibit leukotriene synthesis, and decrease the priming of mast cells, which in turn decreases the concentration of histamine (Lee DK, 2003). Trials have been supportive of the efficacy for using butterbur to reduce the frequency of migraine attacks in children and adolescents with no serious adverse effects (Pothman, 2005).

The major safety concern in the use of butterbur is that the unsaturated pyrolizidine alkaloid (UPA) content may be hepatotoxic, nephrotoxic, carcinogenic, and mutagenic (McGuffin, 1997). The recommend use is alkaloid-free butterbur extracts standardized to 7.5 mg petasin and isopetasin at a dose of 50–100 mg twice a day for at least 4 months.

COENZYME Q-10   CoQ10 functions as an anti-oxidant, membrane stabilizer, and as a co-factor in many metabolic pathways. It is especially necessary in the generation of ATP in oxidative respiration (Turunen, 2004). When taken as a supplement for the prophylactic treatment of migraine headaches, it is thought to improve mitochondrial oxidative phosphorylation which seems to be impaired in some patients with migraines (Welch, 1998). Studies have supported the efficacy of supplementation with CoQ10 in reducing the frequency of headaches in adult patients (Rozen, 2002; Sandor, 2005). It also improved headache frequency and related disability in children with migraine found to have abnormally low CoQ10 levels (Hershey, 2007). CoQ10 is generally well tolerated and has no significant adverse effects. The recommended dosing when used for migraine prevention is 150–300 mg daily.

VITAMIN B   In general, the B Vitamins are known to promote nerve conduction, neuromuscular transmission, tissue respiration and glycogenolysis (the breakdown of carbohydrates into glucose for energy) and have been implicated in the treatment of pain

(Sandor, 2000). Specifically, Riboflavin (B2) has been found to reduce migraine headache frequency as effectively as beta-blockers when used prophylactically. Pyridoxine (B6) can reduce symptoms of PMS related breast pain and depression at 50–100 mg per day (Wyatt, 1999). Further, supplementation improves myalgias and weakness associated with thiamine deficiency (Koike, 2006). When used orally the B-Vitamins are generally regarded as safe even in large doses as these are water soluble. Typically a B-complex mixture of eight of the B Vitamins is used rather than supplementing each single vitamin as the B Vitamins work synergistically to promote optimum functioning in the cells.

CHAMOMILE Chamomile traditionally has been used for the treatment of nausea, nervous diarrhea, gastrointestinal spasms, restlessness, and insomnia. One of the active constituents, apigenin, binds to GABA receptors, which are also the primary receptor sites of benzodiazepines in the central nervous system, to exert sedative effects (Viola, 1995). Chamomile extract can inhibit cyclo-oxygenase and lipooxygenase which thereby reduces the production of inflammatory prostaglandins and leukotrienes. In addition, constituents of chamomile also inhibit histamine release from mast cells and has antispasmodic effects on smooth muscle (Hormann, 1994). Tea may be brewed from 3 g of dried flower heads in half cup of boiling water steeped for 10 minutes, or a 1:1 liquid extract of 1–4 ml may taken before bedtime to help induce sleep or help with abdominal and/or menstrual cramps.

VALERIAN AND SEDATIVE HERBS Valerian is used for some problems that may be associated with pain including insomnia, restlessness and anxiety. Multiple constituents (e.g., valepotriates, valerinic acid, valerenone, berneol, and kessyl glycol) contribute to its pharmacological effects (Houghton, 1999). Valerian helps decrease sleep onset time and promote a deeper sleep (Gyllenhaal, 2000) though its full effects may not be evident until 2–3 weeks of continuous treatment (Wheatley, 2005). One study completed on children with intellectual deficits found valerian to be helpful in improving their sleep without harmful side-effects (Francis, 2002).

Other herbs such as lemon balm, passion flower, hops and lavender also have mild sedative effects when taken orally (Natural Medicines Database, 2005). Their essential oils used as aromatherapy have been used to improve sleep (Lewith, 2005; Goel, 2005).

MELATONIN Melatonin, as a dietary supplement, has been widely studied as a treatment for sleep disorders in individuals with primary insomnia, sleep disorders associated with ADHD, autism, or other neurodevelopment disorders (Pandi-Perumal, 2007; van der Heijden, 2007). Melatonin is naturally synthesized in the pineal gland from its precursor, tryptophan which is converted to 5-hydroxytryptophan, then to serotonin, to N-acetylserotonin and finally to melatonin (Brzezinski, 1997). Melatonin increases the binding of gamma-aminobezazoic acid (GABA) to receptors to induce sedation (Munoz-Hoyos, 1998). To treat insomnia, a dose of 0.3–5 mg is taken orally between 6 and 8 pm. Melatonin is considered safe to use long term but must be avoided in those individuals receiving immunosuppression therapy as melatonin does have immune stimulating effects (Lissoni, 1999).

Manipulation Therapies

Treatments included in the domain of manual therapies include massage, osteopathic and chiropractic manipulation, Feldenkrais, Rolfing, cranial sacral therapy and a host of other hands-on therapies, as well as interventions such as exercise or physical therapy (PT). The details of these individual therapies are extensively reviewed in other chapters of this text. These body-based therapies are very effective in the treatment of pain as they work to restore normal structure and function of the body's bones, joints, fascia, and soft tissues that may have developed abnormal patterns due to illness, trauma or stress.

OSTEOPATHIC/CRANIO-SACRAL/CHIROPRACTIC THERAPIES. Through manipulation of the cranium, spine, tissues, and joints, restrictions are released to improve blood flow and enhance central nervous system function which thereby allows the body to self regulate (Carlson, 2006). In addition to the obvious manual component to these therapies, circulatory pain biomarkers [beta endorphin, serotonin, palmitoy-ethanolamide (PEA) and arachidonoyethanolamide (AEA)] are altered and correlate with post-treatments reports of reduced pain and stress (Degenhardt, 2007). These therapies are thought to act through a central mechanism to modulate autonomic reactivity by a cortical-limbic process (Hoyt, 1979).

Research for using manipulative therapies for specific pain entities in children found benefit for the treatment of chronic headaches (Bronfort, 2001), low back pain (Hayden JA, 2003), recurrent otitis media (Mills, 2003), children with physical disabilities and discomfort (McManus, 2007), infantile colic (Hayden C, 2006), and fibromyalgia (Gamber, 2002). Each study reported improvement in both pain levels and level of functioning with no adverse effects.

MASSAGE Massage has effects on reducing restricted muscle patterns found on the body that can contribute to pain. It also has anti-nociceptive and cardiovascular effects mediated by endogenous opioids, cortisol and dopamine with stress-alleviating effects due to activation of the parasympathetic nervous system (Field, 2005). Other documented effects in addition to pain relief and stress reduction include increased alertness, diminished depression and enhanced immune function (Field, 1998).

Specific studies done in children found massage had significant effects in reducing pain behaviors and increasing muscle relaxation in those undergoing venipuncture (Garcia, 1997), in children with JIA (Field, 1997), and for children during burn treatment and dressing changes (Hernandez-Reif, 2001). Atopic dermatitis symptoms, including itching, redness, scaling, and anxiety all improved in another study in young children in which parents provided massage 20 minutes each day for 30 days (Schachner, 1998).

No adverse effects were noted in any of these studies indicating this therapy to be very safe.

PHYSICAL THERAPY (PT) AND EXERCISE PT and exercise are the mainstays for treatment of both acute and chronic pain. Rehabilitation of injured bones, muscle and fascia helps restore normal functioning, improves endurance and conditioning, and elevates mood. In prospective studies, exercise capacity and overall conditioning was lower in children with musculoskeletal pain syndromes with generalized joint hyper- and/or hypo-mobility than in age- and gender-matched controls (Englebert, 2006). It is apparent that introduction of therapies, such as low level endurance training and core-strengthening exercises, would augment function and reduce pain in these cases. In children with JIA, adherence to an exercise program combined with medication was found to result in greater reductions in pain, greater improvements in functioning, and greater improvements in parents' perception of the child's overall wellbeing compared to medication only (Feldman, 2007).

Alternative Medical Systems

Of the various integrative approaches to pediatric pain, alternative medical systems per se are perhaps the least well studied at least in the West. Nonetheless, at least some parts of alternative medical systems have been frequently borrowed and implemented in clinical pediatric pain settings in the United States. The most common pain management modalities adopted from other medical systems include acupuncture, homeopathic and naturopathic remedies, and meditative exercises such as yoga.

ACUPUNCTURE Perhaps foremost among the techniques borrowed from alternative medical system to apply to pain in children is acupuncture (and acupressure). Approximately one-third of pediatric teaching hospitals currently offer acupuncture therapy to treat pain in children (Lee AC, 1999). Although many pediatric patients may be initially reluctant to pursue a therapy involving needles, in our experience children typically become open to this treatment following an age-appropriate introduction and the opportunity to observe an actual acupuncture needle.

The mechanisms underlying acupuncture analgesia remain somewhat poorly understood. In general, the stimulation of acupuncture points appears to activate the endogenous anti-nociceptive system to inhibit pain signals (He, 1987; Lewith, 1984; Lin, 2003). The application of acupuncture needles has been found to increase endomorphin-1, beta endorphin, encephalin, and serotonin levels in plasma and brain tissue, all of which are related to analgesia, sedation, and recovery of motor functions (Cabýoglu, 2006). Functional brain imaging studies also have shown that there are in fact acupoint-specific patterns of brain activity within the pain processing network of the brain, such as the hypothalamus, limbic system, anterior cingulate cortex, and cerebellum (Chae, 2007; Yan, 2005). Further, there is some evidence that acupuncture may increase local blood perfusion, rendering it a potentially valuable treatment option for Complex Regional Pain Syndrome (Bär, 2002).

Although acupuncture is becoming increasingly used for the treatment of pain in children, including neonates (Golianu, 2007), there is almost no empirical data supporting its use for this application. Most of the published data on acupuncture treatment for pain comes from adult studies which show that approximately 50%–70% of adults with painful conditions experience at least short-term benefits from acupuncture (Lin, 2003). Children with chronic pain problems such as headaches and Complex Regional Pain Syndrome Type I have reported acupuncture to be a "definite help" for improving pain (Kemper, 2000), and acupuncture has been shown through trials in children to be effective in reducing pain from headaches (Gottschling, 2007; Pintov, 1997) and other chronic pain conditions (Zeltzer, 2002). However, many of the studies that have been done in this area have serious design flaws that significantly impede the interpretation of results. Further, several studies have failed to find "real" acupuncture to be significantly better than "sham" acupuncture for treatment of pain (Campbell, 2006). Thus, acupuncture appears to have some potential merit for certain chronic pain disorders in children, but clearly more sound research is needed.

With regard to safety, any conclusions are difficult to make given the limited amount of studies of acupuncture in children. Based primarily on adult studies, the most significant of potential side effects observed include infection, broken or retained needles, pneumothorax, and cardiac tamponade (Ernst, 1997, 1998). However, these adverse effects are rare in occurrence and are often no greater of concern than some of the adverse effects occurring with more traditional pain therapies (e.g., a nerve block). No safety issues were reported in the pediatric studies that have been conducted.

HOMEOPATHY AND NATUROPATHY Homeopathic remedies borrowed in the United States from some European medical approaches also are sometimes adopted by integrative programs for the treatment of some pain conditions in children. Again, however, there are very few studies available guiding their use or safety profiles. To date, the only published empirical evidence for a homeopathic remedy for pediatric pain has been in a sample of children with otitis media, showing superior efficacy relative to placebo (Jacobs, 2001).

Similar to homeopathy, data on the safety and efficacy of naturopathic remedies for any pediatric pain condition are rare. The only published pediatric trials on the analgesic effects of naturopathic remedies also are based on samples of children with acute otitis media (Sarrell, 2001, 2003; Wustrow, 2004). Overall, results from these studies were somewhat equivocal for demonstrating superior efficacy of this approach to more conventional approaches (anesthetic ear drop or oral amoxicillin). No adverse events associated with the extract were reported. Again, clearly more research is needed before making sound evidence-based recommendations for naturopathic or homeopathic remedies in pediatric pain.

AYURVEDIC MEDICINE To our knowledge, there have been no published studies on the application of Ayurvedic medicine to a pediatric pain condition. We nonetheless include this section here because there have been a few studies evaluating specific Ayurvedic drugs in adult arthritis populations. A review of these studies has shown largely equivocal evidence for recommending Ayurvedic medicine for adult rheumatoid arthritis (Park, 2005), though the multiplant Ayurvedic drug "RA-11" has been shown to be superior to placebo in improving pain and physical functioning in adult patients with osteoarthritis of the knee (Chopra, 2004). There have been some reports in the literature of lead poisoning and anemia associated with Ayurvedic medicines due to some of these medicines containing heavy metals (Kales, 2007). Given potential safety issues and no data on Ayurvedic medicine in a pediatric pain population, this approach cannot be recommended for pain management at this time.

MEDITATIVE EXERCISES (YOGA AND QI GONG) Meditative exercises are a component of several of the alternative medical systems and are sometimes used by chronic pain patients as a method for relaxation, analgesia, and improved physical functioning. Studies on Qi Gong in adults have yielded largely equivocal results, with one study supporting its efficacy in improving pain and functioning in patients with chronic pain from fibromyalgia (Chen KW, 2006) while another study failed to demonstrate superior effects in this population beyond what is attained with education and supportive attention (Astin, 2003). Studies on the use of yoga for adult pain management have led to the conclusion that yoga exercises are generally effective for improving pain and functional outcomes for patients with chronic low back pain (Chou, 2007) and may be effective in improving migraine frequency (John, 2007). The only published trial evaluating yoga for a pediatric pain condition was conducted in adolescents with irritable bowel syndrome, with results indicating significant positive effects on improving functional disability, anxiety, and gastrointestinal symptoms relative to a wait-list control condition (Kuttner, 2006). However, there is some indication that yoga may not be perceived by children as a useful treatment option for pain (Tsao, 2005, 2007), which has implications for whether or not children will follow through with implementing this approach on their own. In summary, yoga and Qi Gong have not been well studied for pediatric pain conditions. However, given limited likelihood of significant adverse effects of these approaches, they may be helpful for improving pain and functioning in certain chronic pain conditions, particularly if other forms of exercise are not well tolerated.

Energy Therapies

Energy medicine is a domain in CAM that deals with energy fields of two types—the bioelectromagnetic-based therapies that involve the unconventional use of electromagnetic fields, and biofield therapies that are intended to affect the energy fields that surround and penetrate the human body (Tan, 2007). The former includes pulsed electromagnetic fields, magnetic fields, or cranial electrotherapy stimulation that can readily be measured. Biofield energy, which includes Therapeutic Touch, Healing Touch, Reiki, Johrei, Intercessory Prayer and others, has defied measurement to date by reproducible methods but is based on the concept that human beings are infused with a subtle form of energy that can be manipulated to effect change in the physical body and influence health. Of the NCCAM domains, this category is most controversial and difficult to research as neither the external energy fields nor their therapeutic effects have been demonstrated convincingly by any biophysical means (NCCAM).

PULSED ELECTROMAGNETIC FIELD (PEMF) Studies using high-power PEMF in the treatment of migraine headaches in adults found a significant decrease in headache activity that was sustained over many months. Similar effects were not seen in patients with tension-type headaches. None of these studies reported negative side effects (Sherman, 1998, 1999). These generators have been shown to increase blood flow in the areas exposed to the electromagnetic fields (Ross, 1990). Increased blood flow commonly results in a reduction of migraine activity through unknown mechanisms (Freedman, 1991).

CRANIAL ELECTROTHERAPY STIMULATION (CES) Cranial electrotherapy stimulation delivers a low-level current that is usually below the threshold of sensory detection but affects electrical and neurochemical mechanisms in the brain to mediate arousal, sensory processing and pain modulation (Tan, 2007). There is evidence that indicates changes in the serotonin and norepinephrine levels as a result of this therapy (Giordano, 2006). A double-blind, placebo-controlled study of adult patients with fibromyalgia found CES reduced tender points by 28% and self-rated pain by 27% when compared to sham treatment or wait-list control (Lichtbroun, 2001).

REIKI, THERAPEUTIC TOUCH, HEALING TOUCH Reiki and therapeutic touch, as well as the other biofield energy therapies, share the goal of balancing the vital energy fields in the body, either through laying hands on or with non-touch interventions of the biofields, to restore health and healing. The proposed mechanisms of action of these interventions for pain relief are the gate theory, discussed previously, or activation of the acupuncture meridians with resultant endogenous opioid production. Data on biological markers measured before, during, and after Reiki sessions that lasted 30 minutes found a significant reduction in state anxiety and systolic blood pressure and an increase in the salivary IgA levels indicating a stress reduction response (Wardell, 2001). Other reports of qualitative data included a heightened state of awareness, feelings of safety and perceived relationship with the practitioner, liminal states of consciousness hovering between sleep and awareness, and a sense of connectedness (Miles, 2003). Any of these reported events could contribute to pain relief.

CAM IN SPECIFIC PEDIATRIC PAIN CONDITIONS

In the next section, we provide an overview of a few select pain presentations commonly encountered in children and provide suggestions for integrative approaches to these conditions based on extant efficacy and safety data.

Acute Procedural Pain

Sources of acute procedural pain are usually anticipated and as such are amenable to interventions implemented before and during the actual procedure to lessen the pain response. Studies in infants have found that inadequate treatment of procedural pain leads to heightened pain responses with each subsequent intervention (Taddio, 1997). With the many options for pain management available, the suggestions listed below should be considered with any age group for any invasive or diagnostic procedure.

Mind-body techniques used for infants might include talking or singing in a soft, low voice using repetitive tones. Music with a rhythm of less than 60 beats per minute has a very calming effect and may be helpful in this situation (Butt, 2000). For infants, toddlers, or children distraction techniques such as blowing pin wheels, singing songs, or reading pop-up books can help take the attention away from the procedure (Sinha, 2006). Having parents present to comfort their child may or may not be helpful depending on their own level of distress. Excessive parental reassurance, criticism or apology appears to increase distress, whereas humor and distraction may lessen it (Schechter, 2007). A matter-of-fact, supportive, non-apologetic approach by parents is encouraged. For children and adolescents, breathing and relaxation techniques, guided imagery, or hypnosis can be used, with the caveats previously mentioned, to reduce stress and pain perception (Olness, 1996).

VR therapy during procedures is becoming more mainstream and has proven benefits in reducing pain for some children during I.V. placement (Gold, 2006), and with dressing changes in burn patients (van Twillert, 2007).

Biological agents may offer some relief for procedural pain. In infants younger than 6 months of age, 12.5% sucrose or dextrose solution given directly into the mouth followed with a pacifier reduces evidence of distress (Akman, 2002). Breastfeeding had similar effectiveness as glucose/sucrose for reducing pain (Shah, 2006). Sucrose is relatively inexpensive and readily available for use for painful procedures, but should not be used as a general comfort technique for infants crying for other reasons unrelated to painful interventions. Aromatherapy with calming essential oils such as chamomile, lavender, or lemon balm may help reduce stress and pain in all age groups (Emslie, 2002). Bach's Rescue Remedy has good anxiolytic affects without causing sedation so may be helpful in older children and adolescents as they prepare for a procedure (Howard, 2007). No untoward side effects have been associated with use of any of these agents when used as directed.

Body-based therapies that can offer comfort include swaddling infants during and after procedures. Older infants and children can be held facing their parents or care-givers on their laps for many procedures as this way of holding is more comforting than laying on their backs. Gentle massage of the extremities or back can promote comfort as well as offer distraction during various procedures. Reflexology of the solar plexus points on the palms and soles of the feet can reduce stress and anxiety thereby lessening the discomfort related to procedures (Stephenson, 2007). Pressure applied around the site of an intramuscular injection can reduce pain as activation of the pressure nerve fibers modulates firing of the pain fibers (Barnhill, 1996; Chung, 2002).

Both auricular acupressure and acupuncture of specific meridian points have been found to decrease pain and anxiety in patients in prehospital settings provided by Emergency Medical Service (EMS) providers during ambulance transport for medical and trauma events (Kober, 2003; Lang, 2007) and may be helpful to reduce pain and anxiety prior to invasive procedures.

Studies suggest that various energy techniques have efficacy in reducing anxiety; improving muscle relaxation, aiding in stress reduction, relaxation, and sense of well-being, promoting wound healing; and reducing pain (Engebretson, 2007). Of the conventional therapies available, use of topical anesthetic agents is warranted in many of the invasive procedures with the choice of agent dependant on the procedure and the age of the child. For the more invasive or diagnostic procedures in which children need to lie quietly, conscious sedation with the use of pharmaceutical agents such as midazolam, fentanyl, ketamine, or propofol may be indicated, therefore refer to protocols outlined at your specific institution for guidance.

Primary Headaches

Chronic primary headaches are the most common pain problem in children, affecting as many as one in five children (Perquin, 2000). The most common type of primary headache in children is tension-type headache, characterized by a frequent tightness around the head and typically moderate pain localized around the back of the head and shoulders (IHS, 2004; Rothner 2001). Pain in this type of headache typically lasts for brief periods during the day, often increasing in intensity throughout the day (Labbé, 1998). The other main type of primary headache in children is migraine headache. This type of headache is typically characterized by a severe, throbbing unilateral or bilateral pain in the frontal or temporal region, often accompanied by nausea, vomiting, and sensitivity to certain lights and sounds (IHS, 2004; Rothner, 2001). Pediatric migraines last for at least 1 hour and can sometimes last up to a couple of days. Recent theories of headache etiology increasingly point to similarities between migraine and tension-type headache, with both types of headache reflecting variations of underlying heightened central nervous system sensitivity (Seshia, 2004; Peres, 2007).

The conventional medication approach to treating headaches involves targeting headache episodes (symptomatic medication) and preventing the frequency of such episodes (prophylactic medication). Of the symptomatic medications, mild pain relievers can be effective for both milder migraine and tension-type headaches presentations. Acetaminophen at a dose of 10-15 mg/kg up to every 4 hours to a maximum of 4 g per day is generally recommended in these cases (Welborn, 1997). Ibuprofen can be used at a dose of 5–10 mg/kg every 8 hours for children ages 2–12, but there are possible risks that warrant caution, including gastrointestinal bleeding, renal failure, and anaphylaxis (Levin, 2001). As another caveat, short-acting analgesics should be avoided for the symptomatic treatment of frequent headaches if a child is taking several doses per week given the risk of developing an analgesic rebound syndrome (Vasconcellos, 1998). In this case, a longer acting analgesic such as naproxen is preferred. For more intense migraine headaches, triptan agents can be considered (e.g., zolmitriptan, naratriptan, rizatriptan, sumatriptan), which act by inhibiting the transmission of pain signals in the peripheral trigeminal sensory nerves and in the brainstem (Ferrari, 1997; Hargreaves, 1999). For severe migraine attacks, intravenous ergotamine derivatives in the ED may be required. For migraine prophylaxis, beta-blockers (e.g., propranolol) and calcium channel blockers (e.g., flunarizine) are effective in some children and are frequently prescribed (Levin, 2001). Psychotropic medications such as tricyclic antidepressants (e.g., amitriptyline or trazadone) and anticonvulsant drugs (e.g., valproic acid and gabapentin) also are frequently used for migraine prophylaxis in children despite largely unknown mechanisms of action and limited outcomes data (Levin, 2001; Wasiewski, 2001). Tricyclics such as amitriptyline also can be used for tension-type headache prophylaxis (Grazzi, 2004).

Pharmocological interventions used in isolation are often not very efficacious by virtue of not addressing the multitude of biological, emotional, cognitive, and behavioral factors that interact to maintain a headache syndrome (Labbé, 1998). Lifestyle factors are often primary in initiating and maintaining headache syndromes in children and should always be addressed prior to or in conjunction with initiating medical treatments (Grazzi, 2004; Gordon, 2004). Children with chronic headaches often are highly sensitive to inconsistency in routines, such that large variability in mealtimes, sleep and wake times, and activities may initiate headache episodes. A good diet with hydration, sleep, daily exercise habits and effective stress management strategies are in fact often sufficient in and of themselves for significantly reducing or eliminating headache problems in children. There is a great deal of clinical speculation on food triggers of migraine headaches, particularly foods containing tyramine, phenylethylamine, histamine, nitrites, and sulfites (e.g., cheese, chocolate, citrus fruits, hot dogs, monosodium glutamate (MSG), aspartame, fatty foods, ice cream, caffeine, and alcoholic drinks) (Millichap, 2003). However, a universal migraine diet with simultaneous elimination of all potential food triggers is generally not advised (Millichap, 2003). Instead, a well-balanced diet should be encouraged with particular emphasis on avoiding skipped meals and keeping well hydrated with water. Headache diaries in which information on headache occurrences and potential precursors (such as "suspect" specific diet items) recorded on paper or into a personal digital assistant often can be useful in helping families identify any patterns associated with headaches that can be addressed as part of a self-management approach to treatment.

There is quite an extensive amount of data supporting the efficacy of mind-body therapies such as relaxation and stress management techniques (with or without bio-feedback assistance) for reducing headache activity and headache-related disability in children with either or both tension-type and migraine headache (Connelly, 2002: Eccleston, 2003: Holden, 1999: Trautmann, 2006). The extant data suggest that in most cases relatively comparable results can be attained from mind-body therapies for pediatric chronic headache done in a primarily self-help format without requiring ongoing professional contacts, making this form of therapy both efficacious and cost-effective (Connelly, 2006; Kroener-Hedwig, 2002) In addition to these mind-body therapies, a recent randomized trial evaluated a creative therapy (music therapy) against other methods of migraine management in primary schoolchildren (Oelkers-Ax, 2007). The results reflected a statistically significant reduction of headache frequency up to 6 months following the 4 month music therapy program. Underlying all of these efficacious mind-body therapies is the production of a relaxation response. Thus, children with chronic idiopathic headache should be instructed early on in at least one or more methods of producing a relaxation response either through in-office instruction, suggestions for resources (e.g., websites with relaxation scripts for children), or referral to a provider of mind-body treatments.

There have been several adult studies of various biological agents for the treatment of migraine and tension-type headache, although trials in children are rare. Oral magnesium over the course of 16 weeks has been shown to safely reduce migraine frequency and severity in children and can thus be recommended for use (Wang, 2003). Butterbur root extract also has been studied for use in pediatric headache and has been shown in an open trial to result in at least a 50% reduction in migraine attacks in 77% of children aged 6–17 (Pothmann, 2005). In another study, butterbur was found to have continued efficacy in reducing migraine attacks in children 6 months following a 12-week course of treatment (Oelkers-Ax, 2007). No safety issues were identified with the use of butterbur in these studies. CoQ10 also has recently been shown to safely reduce migraine frequency and associated disability in children who were found on screening to have low clinical CoQ-10 values (Hershey, 2007). Providers might therefore consider obtaining CoQ-10 levels in children presenting with chronic headache and prescribe supplementation if indicated. Although feverfew has been well-studied for migraine prophylaxis in adults (Pittler, 2004), no studies to our knowledge have yet been conducted in pediatric headache patients. However, feverfew appears safe and thus a trial of this may be warranted in children who have not responded to these other biological agent options.

Of the remaining complementary and alternative medical approaches, acupuncture has been the only other CAM approach studied in pediatric headache. In a relatively well-designed trial, acupuncture was shown to be more effective than "sham acupuncture" in reducing migraine frequency and severity (Pintov, 1997). In a subsequent study, acupuncture was shown to be effective in reducing pain in combination with self-hypnosis in a sample of chronic pain patients, about one-third of which were children with a primary headache disorder (Zeltzer, 2002). More recently, a double-blind placebo-controlled randomized trial in 43 children with migraine or tension-type headache found a significant improvement in headache-free days for children receiving "true" acupuncture with low level laser (Gottschling, 2007). No safety concerns associated with acupuncture treatment were reported in any of these studies. Thus, acupuncture is another therapeutic option to consider with established efficacy and safety for treating pediatric idiopathic headaches. Although some energy therapies such as therapeutic touch and cranial electrostimulation have shown some efficacy in adult primary headache patients (Bronfort, 2004; McCrory, 1997; Schwedt, 2007), currently there is no published evidence that these therapies have efficacy in the pediatric headache population

Complex Regional Pain Syndrome (CRPS)

Once considered rare in children, this central pain disorder, previously known as Reflex Sympathetic Dystrophy (RSD), is being recognized and treated at increasing rates. The hallmarks of this pain disorder, in contrast to nociceptive pain, are

1. Pain out of proportion to inciting events
2. Extreme sensitivity to touch (allodynia)
3. Color and/or temperature changes of the affected limb or body part
4. Pain described as burning, tingling, numbness, "pins and needles", and/or shocking/electrical in nature
5. Pain that is typically unresponsive to opioids
6. Pain and physical findings that often do not conform to known segmental dermatomes, myotomes, or peripheral nerve distributions

There are no definitive laboratory tests or radiological studies which can be used to diagnose CRPS. Typically diagnosis is made by taking an extensive history of the current problem and observing the physical findings. Knowing that this disorder is mediated within the CNS and that stress and anxiety activate the central nervous system, the goal of treatment for CRPS is to calm and balance the central nervous system both to alleviate pain and to prevent relapse. As compared to adults with the same disorder, children often have a better response rate to non-invasive treatments (Low, 2007).

Any of the self-regulation techniques used to reduce anxiety, muscle tension, and pain can be of benefit in this disorder. Coaching with cognitive-behavioral techniques to help reframe the current situation, learning pain coping strategies, or engaging patients in guided imagery with the help of a therapist may be helpful for those who state they "can't relax" or need skills to manage stress (Murray, 2000).

Though no specific dietary supplement or nutrient is consistently indicated for the treatment of CRPS, one study found Vitamin C helped reduce the incidence of CRPS in patients with isolated closed fracture of the distal radius. It was theorized that the antioxidant effects of the Vitamin C prevented lipid peroxidation at the site of the initial injury which could activate nerve dysregulation (Cazenauve, 2002). Other nutrients, such as the B vitamins or Mg^{++}, that have calming effects on nervous tissues may also be beneficial. Sedative herbs that promote restful sleep may also play a role in healing and pain reduction. Food additives such as MSG and aspartame should be avoided as these are considered nerve stimulants and neurotoxins that potentially could aggravate this disorder (Olney, 1989).

Intense PT is crucial for the treatment of CRPS to restore normal functioning of the affected limb and to prevent muscle wasting (Sherry, 1999). Desensitization therapy is also helpful to retrain the nervous system to accept normal touch again. In addition to these interventions, cranio-sacral therapy is very important in treating this disorder as it targets the nervous system directly to bring about balance to the central nervous system and therefore pain relief (McManus, 2007). The experience in our clinic has found that patients receiving this particular therapy have reported profound relaxation and reduction of pain when medication and PT have not been successful.

Acupuncture has been used successfully in the treatment of CRPS to alleviate pain with no recurrence for both adults and children (Kelly, 2004; Kho, 1995). It is felt acupuncture offers its effects by reducing sympathetic nervous system activity.

Again, various energy techniques can be utilized to lessen pain and distress from this disorder, though definite research has not been conducted using this intervention for CRPS.

Conventional therapies include pharmaceutical drugs such as the nerve stabilizing agents (Gabapentin, Tiagabine, Pregabalin), tricyclic antidepressants (Amitriptyline), or alpha adrenergic blockers (Clonidine). Though the true mechanism of action is not known for these agents, they are thought to work on calcium and sodium channels to block nerve impulses (Chen H, 2004). Often these agents are used together to lessen pain so that aggressive PT can be initiated. Typically opioids are not helpful in treating this type of central pain with the exception of Methadone. Methadone has effects on the NMDA nerve receptors which are activated in CRPS, so can be of help in reducing pain, though it can be very sedating. Doses of this should be given on a scheduled basis and increased gradually to reach the desired affect without excess sedation.

Stellate ganglion block for CRPS of the upper body, or lumbar sympathetic block for the lower body, when performed by a skilled anesthesiologist, may provide relief for patients with this disorder. In patients who are unable to ambulate due to the severe pain, placement of a lumbar epidural for 3–5 days may be indicated so that aggressive PT can be initiated. This approach often "resets" the sympathetic nervous system to provide ongoing pain relief even after the epidural is removed (Boswell, 2007).

Widespread Myofascial Pain (Fibromyalgia, Pain Amplification Syndrome)

This ailment is also considered one of the central pain syndromes with disorders of the afferent processing systems involving skin, muscles, joints, bladder, or the gastro-intestinal system and abnormal levels of serotonin, substance P, and/or norepinephrine. There may be dysregulation of the autonomic nervous system with symptoms of tachycardia at rest, a feeling of dizziness, cold hands and feet, and hypervigilence. The underlying etiology may be multifactorial with chronic stress, trauma, or infections leading to neuroendocrine dysfunction (Adler, 2002). It is also theorized that certain viruses attack nerve cells directly or set up persistent infections in muscle tissue with defective viral replication (Douche-Aourik, 2003). Still other theories involve the role of environmental toxins, genetic predisposition, food sensitivities, yeast overgrowth, weakened immune system, or a combination of these factors as contributors to this disorder (Teitelbaum, 2001).

In the patient history, patients often report pain of their joints, head, or back, achy muscles, fatigue, non-restorative sleep, problems with concentration, allergies to food or medications, frequent infections, anxiety, or depression. On further questioning, these patients often are high achievers in school or work, are overly committed in their daily responsibilities, or regularly short-change themselves on sleep. The physical examination may reveal tenderness of many muscle groups with trigger points and restricted muscle flexibility. Their hands and feet may be cool to the touch and their resting heart rate may be elevated indicating activation of the autonomic nervous system. The goal of therapy, therefore, is to employ strategies that will calm and balance the central nervous system to restore homeostasis.

Various self-regulation techniques may help patients with this disorder develop a better awareness of the abnormal patterns of muscle tension in their bodies so changes can then be made at the tissue level to promote relief (Babu, 2007). CBT may help address anxiety, stress, or depression to modify maladaptive beliefs that may be contributing to the pain experience. CBT may also promote active coping skills to help improve the overall level of functioning though they may still be experiencing pain. These techniques can also be used to help promote more restorative sleep.

Biologically based therapies for treatment include identifying any food allergies or sensitivities as these may trigger chronic histamine release that leads to ongoing pain and other symptoms. The primary foods that commonly cause sensitivities are wheat, dairy, corn, soy, and eggs. Patients with this disorder seem to do better on a diet of whole, unprocessed foods which include good quality protein, fruits, vegetables, nuts, seeds, and whole grains. These whole foods provide sources of the B vitamins and magnesium which help to stabilize nerve functioning (Donaldson, 2001) and improve symptoms of fatigue and mental confusion (Heap, 1999) Preventing episodes of hypoglycemia by eating small meals every few hours throughout the day is also important to improve overall energy and mental functioning. Food additives such as aspartame and MSG should be avoided as these aggravate nerve functioning which can augment pain. Supplementing with Vitamin D 1000–2000 IU per day can be helpful in decreasing myalgias (Shinchuk, 2007). One study in patients with fibromyalgia used L-malic acid 1200–2400 mg plus magnesium 300–600 mg daily and reported significant reductions in pain severity measures (Russell, 1995). It is felt these nutrients enhance immune function by increasing natural killer cells, and improve energy levels by supporting cellular function and metabolism.

Herbs and natural products may be helpful in promoting good quality sleep for patients with widespread myofascial pain/fibromyalgia. Valerian, Passion flower, Chamomile, and Lemon balm all have been found to have sedative effects and are considered safe for daily use (Blumenthal, 1998). L-theanine, melatonin, and 5-Hydroxytryptophan have also been helpful in promoting restorative sleep without causing habituation or morning hang-over effects (Attele, 2000).

Low-intensity daily exercise is very important in the treatment of this disorder to both prevent physical deconditioning and to restore normal functioning (Mannerkorpi, 2007). Manual therapy, such as cranio-sacral therapy, may help calm and balance the autonomic nervous system thereby reducing pain. Massage therapy can also offer benefit by promoting more restorative sleep, reducing levels of measured substance P, decreasing tender points, and lowering overall pain ratings (Field, 2002). Massage must be done with a light touch, however, so as to not induce more pain.

Classical homeopathy may offer substantial relief in those with widespread myofascial pain/fibromyalgia. Again in adult studies, patients who received individualized remedies had less tender point pain, improved quality of life, and better overall global health compared to the placebo group. (Bell, 2004). Because of the paucity of side effects and relative safety, homeopathy could be considered for use in children and adolescents in the hands of a trained classical homeopathic practitioner.

Traditional Chinese medicine also would provide holistic treatment in this disorder with use of acupuncture, herbs, massage, diet, and exercise to restore proper flow of Qi and body fluids (Zheng, 2005). A pilot study of Qigong therapy did provide significant improvement in the level of functioning, pain, and other fibromyalgia symptoms (Chen KW, 2006).

Patients who received therapeutic touch treatments in a pilot study had a statistically significant decrease in pain for each pre-therapeutic to post-therapeutic touch treatment, as well as significant improvement in quality of life from pre-first to pre-sixth treatment (Denison, 2004). Because of the known effects of energy medicine on reducing the stress response, this would be a good adjunctive therapy in the treatment of this disorder and would be considered safe to use in children.

Conventional pharmaceutical therapies are often prescribed to provide symptom relief and can be helpful on a short-term basis, but these need to be used in conjunction with the above therapies to provide long-term results. Antidepressants with dual effects on serotonin and norepinephrine (i.e., duloxetine) appear to have more consistent benefits than selective serotonin antidepressants for the treatment of persistent pain associated with fibromyalgia (Arnold, 2007). Pregabalin, at 300 and 450 mg/day, proved effective in reducing the pain and accompanying symptoms of FMS and improved quality of life domains in one short-term study. Dizziness and somnolence were the most frequent adverse events (Crofford, 2005). Gabapentin (1200–2400 mg/day) was found to be safe and effective for the treatment of pain and other symptoms associated with fibromyalgia in a 12-week, randomized, double-blind study (Arnold, Goldberg, 2007). Indexes of physical functioning, body pain, health transition, and physical component summary all improved in patient receiving Tramadol 37.5 mg/325 mg acetaminophen combination tablets compared to placebo (Bennett, 2003). These studies were done on adult patients and have not been replicated in the pediatric population so caution should be exercised in using these agents. Though claimed to have offered benefit, dextromethorophan and guaifenesin cannot be supported for use in children or adolescents at this time.

Juvenile Idiopathic Arthritis

Childhood arthritis is the fifth most common chronic disease of childhood and the most common of the pediatric rheumatic diseases, affecting as many as 300,000 American children (Cassidy, 1988). The conventional medical approach to pain management in children with arthritis typically includes non-steroidal anti-inflammatory drugs, opioids, or other analgesics (e.g., acetaminophen, amitriptyline). Some of the disease-modifying agents used in the treatment of juvenile arthritis (e.g., methotrexate and etanercept) also may have analgesic effects, although typically they are not used specifically for this purpose. Despite the use of these conventional medical therapies, persistent pain continues to be a predominant problem in children with chronic arthritis (Malleson, 2004; Schanberg, 2003). CAM therapies are thus frequently used or sought by families of these children with estimates of use ranging up to 70% of children with arthritis (Hagen, 2003; Southwood, 1990). In fact, the most predictive reason why families of children with arthritis initially seek CAM therapies appears to be a desire for better pain relief (Feldman, 2004). As such, pediatric providers should be familiar with the evidence base of these therapies for these children.

There are very few CAM interventions that been evaluated for efficacy and safety in children with chronic arthritis. Of the mind-body approaches, there is some support from very small studies showing the efficacy of CBT (Walco, 1992) and biofeedback (Lavigne, 1992) in improving adaptive functioning and reducing self-reported pain in children with arthritis. There is solid adult evidence from randomized trials showing that omega-3 and omega-6 (gamma-linolenic acid) fatty acid supplementation over several months can reduce reported joint pain intensity, number of painful and/or tender joints, and NSAID consumption in patients with rheumatoid arthritis (Christie, 2007; Goldberg, 2007; Soeken, 2004). However, there have only been two small studies of dietary supplementation in children with arthritis. One study found that omega-3 polyunsaturated fatty acid supplementation over several months can decrease consumption of non-steroidal antirheumaitc drugs (Vargová, 1998), and the other found a decrease in CRP values (Alpigiani, 1996); outcomes specific to pain were not reported in these studies.

A study in adults with RA has evaluated the effects of an anti-inflammatory diet (AID) alone or in combination with supplemental fish oil capsules on joint symptoms relative to a conventional Western diet (WD). An anti-inflammatory diet is one that is high in fresh fruits and vegetables and high quality protein (from plants and fish) that provide the best sources of dietary anti-oxidants which neutralize free-radicals involved in the inflammatory process. AID patients had a 14% reduction of tender and swollen joints during the fish oil placebo phase when compared to the WD. This change increased to 34% when fish oil was added to the AID. This study concluded that an anti-inflammatory diet augmented the beneficial effects of fish oil supplementation (Adam, 2003). This would be a safe and healthy diet for any child and should be considered in this population.

Other studies in adults investigated the use of acupuncture for pain relief in RA. In a recent pilot study, acupuncture produced statistically significant improvements in the disease activity score (DAS28), pain and global activity, swollen joint count, health-related quality of life (SF-36) and ESR. No major acupuncture-related adverse events were reported (Lee H, 2008). Because of the known affects of acupuncture in children with other pain disorders, this could be considered safe and possibly effective for children with RA.

Massage therapy also has been studied for the treatment of juvenile arthritis. In the one study evaluating efficacy of this treatment, results suggested that massage done by a parent for 15 minutes per day for a month can reduce pain and decrease anxiety in children with chronic arthritis (Field, 1997). No safety issues were reported with any of these approaches. Additionally, there is a great deal of data supporting the need to include regular exercise and/or formal PT as part of the approach to improving physical functioning and pain in children with arthritis (Kimura, 2007; Singh-Grewal, 2007).

Table 24-1 provides a therapeutic review of the CAM treatments for these five pediatric pain conditions.

Table 24-1. Therapeutic Review of CAM Treatments for Specific Pain Conditions

Type of Therapy	Procedural Pain	Headaches	CRPS	Myofascial Pain	JIA
Conventional Therapies	• Use topical analgesic agents according to specific guidelines for invasive procedures such as IV starts, blood draws, catheterizations, or spinal taps. • Consider use of conscious sedation for those invasive or diagnostic procedures that require the child to lie quietly or are considerably more painful (i.e, burn dressing changes).	• For mild and relatively infrequent headaches, consider: • acetaminophen 10–15 mg/kg up to every 4 hours; or • ibuprofen 5–10 mg/kg every 8 hours for children ages 2 and up • For mild to moderate but frequent headaches (two or more per week), • naproxen sodium 2.5–5 mg/kg twice per day in children ages 6 and up • For moderate to severe headaches, consider a triptan agent as an abortive taken as early as possible in the course of a headache (dosing dependent on type; tablets, dissolving wafers, and nasal sprays are available) • For migraine prophylaxis, consider trial of: • cyproheptadine 0.25 to 1.5 mg/kg (or 2–8 mg at bedtime for children younger than 10)	For symptomatic treatment of CRPS. • Consider use of nerve-stabilizing agents • Gabapentin (Neurontin) 1,200–2,400 mg/day • Tiagabine (Gabitril) 4–24 mg/day • Pregabalin (Lyrica) 300–450 mg/day • Tricyclic antidepressants • Amitriptyline 10–50 mg/day at bedtime • Alpha adrenergic blockers • Clonidine 2 mcg/Kg/dose po Q 6 hours or • Clonidine 0.1 mg transdermal patch every 7 days • Methadone 0.1 mg/Kg/dose every 6–12 hours up to 10 mg TID • For those who have significant disability from CRPS, referral to a pain specialist/anesthesiologist may be necessary for sympathetic nerve block or placement of epidural analgesics.	• Consider using pharmaceutical therapies short term for symptom relief: • Duloxetine (Cymbalta) 60 mg twice a day • Pregabalin (Lyrica) 300–450 mg/day • Gabapentin (Neurontin) 1,200–2,400 mg/day • Tramadol 37.5 mg/325 mg acetaminophen (Ultracette) 3–4 times daily • Target sleep disorders with sleep hygiene strategies • Regular wake/sleep schedule • Evening ritual to promote relaxation • Consider Amitriptyline 10–50 mg at bedtime.	• For mild to moderate pain, consider: • acetaminophen (10–15 mg/kg/dose every 4 hours up to 2–4 g per day) • ibuprofen (30–40 mg/kg tid up to 2400 mg) • naproxen (10–20 mg bid up to 1000 mg), • nabumetome (30 mg/kg qd up to 2000 mg), • meloxicam (0.125 mg/k qd up to 7.5 mg per day); or • celecoxib (100 mg bid for ≤25 kg, 200 mg bid for >25kg up to 200 mg per day) • For moderate to severe acute pain during disease flares, consider using hydrocodone 0.15 mg/kg every 4 hours, or oxycodone 0.05–0.2 mg/kg every 3–6 hours

	• amitriptyline 10–50 mg at bedtime, • propranolol 2–4 mg/kg daily, valproic acid 20–40 mg/kg per day; • carbamazepine 20–40 mg/kg per day; or naproxen sodium 250–500 mg twice daily • Encourage well-balanced diet, regular meals with healthy snacks in between, adequate hydration, and consistent sleep and wake times during the week and weekends (no more than 2 hour difference)			• For poorly controlled chronic pain, consider methadone 0.1 mg/kg bid up to 1 mg/kg TID • Consider amitriptyline 10–30 mg at bedtime for sleep disturbance
Mind-Body Therapies	• Use hypnotic language, music, or repetitive tones to comfort and soothe infants prior to and during procedures. • Use distraction techniques such as pinwheels, singing, or story-telling in older children. • Implement guided imagery or self-hypnosis techniques along with breathing	• Teach (or suggest resources on) self-regulation skills such as diaphragmatic breathing, self-hypnosis, autogenic relaxation, and progressive muscle relaxation and have child regularly practice inducing a relaxation response with one of these skills (at least once per day) • Refer for biofeedback if available (typically thermal biofeedback for children with migraine,	• Encourage use of self-regulation skills on a regular basis, such as diaphragmatic breathing, self-hypnosis, progressive muscle relaxation or autogenic relaxation, to promote the relaxation response and decrease sympathetic arousal. • Refer for cognitive-behavioral coping skills training and stress reduction techniques to improve overall level of functioning.	• Encourage use of self-regulation techniques to promote relaxation and comfort and to promote restorative sleep. • Consider cognitive-behavioral pain coping skills training and stress reduction techniques to improve overall level of functioning.	• Teach (or suggest resources on) basic relaxation skills such as diaphragmatic breathing and progressive muscle relaxation • Refer for biofeedback assisted relaxation training in children whose pain appears highly influenced by stress and heightened autonomic activity

Table 24-1. (Continued)

Type of Therapy	Procedural Pain	Headaches	CRPS	Myofascial Pain	JIA
	and relaxation techniques to calm and to suggest ongoing comfort. • Offer Virtual Reality therapy	and electromyographic biofeedback for children with tension-type headache) • Refer for cognitive-behavioral coping skills training for children with significant headache-related interference in functioning (e.g., frequent school absenteeism, chronic mood disturbance, withdrawal from social activities)			• Refer for cognitive-behavioral therapy for children with evidence of concerning functional impairments from pain (e.g., school absenteeism, chronic depressed or anxious mood, withdrawal from social activities)
Biologically-Based Therapies	• Offer 12.5% sucrose/dextrose or breast-feeding for infants < 6 months of age prior to painful interventions. • Aromatherapy with essential oils such as chamomile, lemon balm, or lavender may offer calming effect. • Consider Bach's Rescue Remedy prior to procedures and interventions in older children and adolescents.	• Consider a trial of any of the following biological agents as a migraine preventative: • Oral magnesium at a dose of 9 mg/kg dose given 3 times daily for at least 4 months • Butterbur root extract standardized to 7.5 mg petasin and isopetasin at a dose of 50–100 mg twice per day for a least 4 months • Feverfew at a dose of 50–125 mg daily of feverfew extract or the dried leaf daily (or about 2 fresh leaves daily)	• Consider starting Magnesium 250–500 mg twice daily for its effects on the NMDA receptors that are activated in CRPS. • Consider using Vitamin C 1,000 mg daily for its antioxidant effects • Avoid nerve-stimulating agents in the diet such as monosodium glutamate and aspartame.	• Identify food allergies/sensitivities and eliminate these from the diet • Encourage a diet of whole, unprocessed foods that include good sources of protein, fruits, vegetables, whole grains, seeds, and nuts. • Avoid food additives such as aspartame and monosodium glutamate which are considered neurotoxins	• Omega-3 fatty acids 1–3 g orally each day • Ginger 250–500 mg 3–4 times daily up to a maximum of 4 g per day • Devil's Claw 1–4.5 g of dried root per day • Promote a diet high in fruits and vegetables and low in arachadonic acid (anti-inflammatory diet)

• Consider evaluating Co-enzyme Q10 levels in children with migraine and supplementing if values areow using 1 to 3 mg/kg per day in liquid gel capsule formulation	• Consider supplementing with the following nutrients: • Vitamin B complex that provides at least 100% of the RDA • Vitamin D 1,000–2,000 IU daily • Magnesium 300–600 mg daily with L-malic acid 1,200–2,400 mg daily • Consider the use of sedative herbs such as valerian, passion flower, chamomile or lemon balm to help with sleep disorders. • Consider the use of dietary supplements listed to promote restorative sleep: • L-theanine 50–200 mg per day • Melatonin 0.1–3 mg at bedtime • 5-Hydroxytryptophan 50–300 mg at bedtime

Table 24-1. (Continued)

Type of Therapy	Procedural Pain	Headaches	CRPS	Myofascial Pain	JIA
Manipulative/ Body-Based Therapies	• Swaddling, positioning for comfort, comfort holds may be used to promote a calm environment and to prevent unwanted movements during a procedure • Consider massage of non-affected areas to provide comfort and distraction. • Reflexology of the solar plexus points of the hands and feet may help to induce relaxation and analgesia. • Apply pressure around site of injection.	• Consider referral for massage evaluation and treatment with a licensed massage therapist for children with tension-type headache • Consider referral for osteopathic evaluation for children with recurrent headaches that are observed on exam to have abnormal body mechanics or a history significant for musculoskeletal traumas • Consider referral for craniosacral physical therapy in children who have signs of autonomic dysfunction associated with their headaches (e.g., lightheadedness, palpitations, fatigue, fainting)	• Aggressive physical and desensitization therapy is imperative in the treatment of CRPS to retrain the nervous system. • Cranio-sacral therapy or osteopathic manipulation should be utilized to calm and balance the autonomic nervous system.	• Encourage daily activity with low-level endurance exercises. • Consider treatment with osteopathic manipulation or cranio-sacral therapy to calm and balance the nervous system. • Use gentle therapeutic massage to promote comfort and sleep.	• Teach (or suggest resources on) basic massage techniques and comfort holds to parents of children with chronic arthritis or refer for massage treatment with a licensed massage therapist • Physical therapy and regular exercise

Alternative Medical Systems	• Acupressure or acupuncture of specific meridian points can help to promote relaxation and comfort.	• Consider referral for at least 4 weeks of traditional or laser acupuncture treatment for children with tension-type or migraine headache • Consider teaching (or suggesting resources on) yoga for children with migraine or tension-type headache	• Consider offering acupuncture as treatment for CRPS for its effects on the autonomic nervous and endogenous opioid systems	• Classical homeopathy may offer relief through an individualized remedy prescribed for each patient. • Traditional Chinese Medicine would offer holistic treatment with use of acupuncture, herbs, massage, diet, and exercise.	• Consider teaching (or suggesting resources on) yoga and/or other meditative exercises particularly for children with evidence of soft tissue restrictions or muscle deconditioning • Consider acupuncture to decrease pain, swelling, and stiffness
Energy Therapies	• Consider biofield therapies such as Reiki or therapeutic touch to reduce anxiety and pain during and after procedures.	• Consider cranial electrotherapy stimulation or occipital nerve stimulation in cases of severe, disabling, intractable headache syndromes • Consider use of therapeutic touch or other biofield therapy	• Consider energy techniques such as Reiki or therapeutic touch to reduce pain and promote comfort	• Consider using any of the energy therapies which would provide balance to the biofield promoting comfort and pain relief • Consider Cranial Electrotherapy Stimulation (CES)	• Consider treatment with pulsed low-frequency electromagnetic fields for patients with evidence of pain amplification in addition to their arthritis • Consider use of Reiki, Healing Touch or other forms of biofield energy therapy which may help reduce pain and anxiety

Resources on Pain

American Academy of Pain Medicine http://www.painmed.org/
The medical specialty society representing physicians practicing in the field of Pain Medicine which is involved in education, training, advocacy, and research in the specialty of Pain Medicine.

Academy for Guided Imagery http://www.academyforguidedimagery.com/
Dedicated to educating and supporting practicing clinicians in their uses of imagery and imagery related approaches to therapy and healing.

American Pain Society http://www.ampainsoc.org/advocacy/pediatric.htm
Multidisciplinary organization of basic and clinical scientists, practicing clinicians, policy analysts, and others to advance pain related research, education, treatment, and professional practice.

American Pain Foundation http://www.painfoundation.org/
Provides people with practical, up-to-date, scientifically-sound information about pain and pain management.

Integrative Pain Management http://www.healingchronicpain.org
From the Continuum Center for Health and Healing at Beth Israel Medical Center, New York, this site describes an approach to pain management that includes a wide spectrum of therapies from drugs to stress reduction.

Kidshealth http://www.kidshealth.org
Doctor-approved health information about children from before birth through adolescents. Select Kids (K), Teens(T), or Parents(P), then type "pain in search.

MindBody Institute http://www.mbmi.org/home/
The Benson-Henry Institute for Mind Body Medicine at Massachusetts General Hospital is a world leader in the study, advancement, and clinical practice of mind/body medicine.

The National Pain Foundation http://www.nationalpainfoundation.org/
An on-line educational and support community for persons in pain, their families and physicians.

Pediatric Pain http://pediatric-pain.ca/, http://painsourcebook.ca/
This site has information for professionals, parents, and children designed to provide easy access to standard pediatric pain management information.

REFERENCES

Adam, O., Beringer, C., Kless, T., Lemmen C., Adam A., Wiseman M., et al. (2003). Anti-inflammatory effects of a low arachadonic acid diet and fish oil in patients with rheumatoid arthritis. *Rheumatology International, 23*(1), 27–36.

Adler, G. K. (2002). Neuroendocrine abnormalities in fibromyalgia. *Current Pain and Headache Reports, 6*(4), 289–298.

Aitken, J. C., Wilson, S., Coury, D., & Moursi, A. M. (2002). The effect of music distraction on pain, anxiety and behavior in pediatric dental patients. *Pediatric Dentistry, 24,* 114–118.

Akman, I., Ozek, E., Bilgen, H., Ozdogan T., & Cebeci D. (2002). Sweet solutions and pacifiers for pain relief in newborn infants. *The Journal of Pain, 3*(3), 199–202.

Ali, B. H., Blunden, G., Tanira, M. O., & Nemmar, A. (2007). Some phytochemical, pharmacological and toxicological properties of ginger (Zingiber officinal Roscoe): A review of recent research. *Food and Chemical Toxicology, 18;* (Epub).

Alpigiani, M. G., Ravera, G., Buzzanca, C., Devescovi, R., Fiore, P., & Iester, A. (1996). The use of n-3 fatty acids in chronic juvenile arthritis. *La Pediatria medica e chirurgica, 18*(4), 387–390.

Arnold, L. M. (2007). Duloxetine and other antidepressants in the treatment of patients with fibromyalgia. *Pain Medicine 8*(Suppl 2), S63–S74.

Arnold, L. M., Goldberg, D. L., Stanford, S. B., Lalonde, J. K., Sandhu, H. S., Keck, P. E. Jr, et al. (2007). Gabapentin in the treatment of fibromyalgia: A randomized, double-blind, placebo-controlled, multicenter trial. *Arthritis and Rheumatism, 56*(4), 1336–1344.

Arts, S. E., Abu-Saad, H. H., Champion, G. D., Crawford, M. R., Fisher, R. J., Juniper, K. H., & Ziegler, J. B. (1994). Age-related response to lidocaine–prilocaine (EMLA) emulsion and effect of music distraction on the pain of intravenous cannulation. *Pediatrics, 93,* 797–801.

Astin, J. A. (1998). Why patients use alternative medicine: Results of a national study. *JAMA, 279*(19), 1548–1553.

Astin, J. A., Berman, B. M., Bausell, B., Lee, W. L., Hochberg, M., & Forys, K. L. (2003). The efficacy of mindfulness meditation plus Qigong movement therapy in the treatment of fibromyalgia: A randomized controlled trial. *The Journal of Rheumatology, 30*(10), 2257–2262.

Attele, A. S., Xie, J. T., & Yuan, C. S. (2000). Treatment of insomnia: An alternative approach. *Alternative Medicine Review, 5*(3), 249–259.

Babu, A., Mathew, E., Danda, D., & Prakash, H. (2007). Management of patients with fibromyalgia using biofeedback: A randomized control trial. *Indian Journal of Medical Sciences, 61*(8), 455–461.

Bär, A., Li, Y., Eichlisberger, R., & Aeschlimann, A. (2002). Acupuncture improves peripheral perfusion in patients with reflex sympathetic dystrophy. *Journal of Clinical Rheumatology, 8*(1), 6–12.

Barnhill, B. J., Holbert, M. D., Jackson, N. M., & Erickson R. S. (1996). Using pressure to decrease the pain of intramuscular injections. *Journal of Pain and Symptom Management, 12*(1), 52–58.

Bausell, R. B., Lee, W. L., & Berman, B. M. (2001). Demographic and health-related correlates to visits to complementary and alternative medical providers. *Med Care, 39*(2), 190–196.

Bell, I. R., Lewis, D. A., Brooks, A. J., Schwartz, G. E., Lewis, S. E., Walsh, B. T., et al. (2004). Improved clinical status in fibromyalgia patients treated with individualized homeopathic remedies versus placebo. *Rheumatology (Oxford), 43*(5), 577–582.

Bennett, R. M., Kamin, M., Karim, R., & Rosenthal, N. (2003). Tramadol and acetaminophen combination tablets in the treatment of fibromyalgia pain: A double-blind, randomized, placebo-controlled study. *The American Journal of Medicine, 114*(7), 537–545.

Berde, C. B., & Sethna, N. F. (2002). Analgesics for the treatment of pain in children. *The New England Journal of Medicine, 347*(14), 1094–1103.

Bieri, D., Reeve, R. A., Champion, G. D., Addicoat, L., & Ziegler, J. B. (1990). The FACES pain scale for the self assessment of the severity of pain experienced by children: Development, initial validation, and preliminary investigation for ratio scale properties. *Pain, 41,* 139–150.

Birrer, R. B., Shallash, A. J., & Totten, V. (2002). Hypermagnesemia-Induced fatality following Epsom salt gargles. *The Journal of Emergency Medicine, 22,* 185–188.

Blumenthal, M. (Ed.). (1998). The complete German Commission E Monographs, *Austin, Tex: American Botanical Council; Integrative Medicine Communications,* 179–180.

Borsook, D., & Becerra, L. R. (2006). Breaking down the barriers: fMRI applications in pain, analgesia and analgesics. *Molecular Pain, 2,* 30.

Boswell, M. V., Trescot, A. M., Datta, S., Schultz, D. M., Hansen, H. C., Abdi, S., et al. (2007). Interventional techniques: Evidence based practice guidelines in the management of chronic spinal pain. *Pain Physician, 10*(1), 7–111.

Breau, L. M., McGrath, P. J., Camfield, C. S., & Finley, G. A. (2002). Psychometric properties of the non-communicating children's pain checklist-revised. *Pain, 99*(1–2), 349–357.

Brzezinski, A. (1997). Melatonin in humans. *The New England Journal of Medicine, 336,* 186–195.

Bronfort, G. (2001). Efficacy of spinal manipulation for chronic headache: A systematic review. *Journal of Manipulative and Physiological Therapeutics, 24*(7), 457–466.

Bronfort, G., Nilsson, N., Haas, M., Evans, R., Goldsmith, C. H., Assendelft, W.J., & Bouter, L. M. (2004). Noninvasive physical treatments for chronic/recurrent headache. *Cochrane Database of Systematic Reviews,* (3), CD001878.

Bursch, B., Walco, G. A., & Zeltzer, L. (1998). Clinical Assessment and Management of chronic pain and pain associated disability syndrome. *Journal of Developmental and Behavioral Pediatrics, 19,* 45–53.

Butt, M. L., & Kisilevsky, B. S. (2000). Music modulates behaviour in premature infants following heel lance. *The Canadian Journal of Nursing Research, 31*(4), 17–39.

Cabýoglu, M. T., Ergene, N., & Tan, U. (2006). The mechanism of acupuncture and clinical applications. *The International Journal of Neuroscience, 116*(2), 115–125.

Cady, R. K., Schreiber, C. P., Beach, M. E., & Hart, C. C. (2005). Gelstat Migraine (sublingually administered feverfew and ginger compound) for acute treatment of migraine when administered during the mild pain phase. *Medical Science Monitor, 11*(9), PI 65–69. Epub 2005.

Campbell, A. (2006). Point specificity of acupuncture in the light of recent clinical and imaging studies. *Acupuncture in Medicine, 24*(3), 118–122.

Carlson, M. J., & Krahn, G. (2006). Use of complementary and alternative medicine practitioners by people with physical disabilities: Estimates from a National US Survey. *Disability and Rehabilitation, 28,* 505–513.

Cassidy, J. T., & Nelson, A. M. (1988). The frequency of juvenile arthritis. *The Journal of Rheumatology, 15,* 535–536.

Cazenauve, J. F. (2002). Vitamin C and prevention of reflex sympathetic dystrophy following surgical management of distal radius fractures. *Acta Orthopaedica Belgica, 68*(5), 481–484.

Chae, Y., Park, H. J., Hahm, D. H., Hong, M., Ha, E., Park, H. K., & Lee, H. (2007). fMRI review on brain responses to acupuncture: The limitations and possibilities in traditional Korean acupuncture. *Neurological Research, 29,* S42–S48.

Chen, E., Cole, S. W., & Kato, P. M. (2004). A review of empirically supported psychosocial interventions for pain and adherence outcomes in sickle cell disease. *Journal of Pediatric Psychology, 29*(3), 197–209.

Chen, H., Lamer, T., Rho, R., Marshall, K. A., Sitzman, B. T., Ghazi, S. M., & Brewer, R. P. (2004). Contemporary Management of Neuropathic pain for the primary care physician. *Mayo clinic Proc, 79*(12), 1533–1545.

Chen, K. W., Hassett, A. L., Hou, F., Staller, J., & Lichtbroun, A. S. (2006). A pilot study of external qigong therapy for patients with fibromyalgia. *Journal of Alternative and Complementary Medicine, 12*(9), 851–856.

Chopra, A., Lavin, P., Patwardhan, B., & Chitre, D. (2004). A 32-Week Randomized, Placebo-Controlled Clinical Evaluation of RA-11, an Ayurvedic Drug, on Osteoarthritis of the Knees. *Journal of Clinical Rheumatology, 10*(5), 236–245.

Chou, R., & Huffman, L. H. (2007). Nonpharmacologic therapies for acute and chronic low back pain: A review of the evidence for an American Pain Society/American College of Physicians clinical practice guideline. *Annals of Internal Medicine, 147*(7), 492–504.

Christie, A., Jamtvedt, G., Dahm, K. T., Moe, R. H., Haavardsholm, E. A., & Hagen, K. B. (2007). Effectiveness of nonpharmacological and nonsurgical interventions for patients with rheumatoid arthritis: An overview of systematic reviews. *Physical Therapy, 87*(12), 1697–1715.

Chrubasik, S. (2000). Physicochemical properties of harpagoside and its in vitro release from Harpagophytum procumbens extract tablets. *Phytomedicine, 6,* 469–73.

Chrubasik, S. (2005). A 1-year follow-up after a pilot study with Doloteffin for low back pain. *Phytomedicine, 12*(1–2), 1–9.

Chung, J. W., Ng, W. M., & Wong, T. K. (2002). An experimental study on the use of manual pressure to reduce pain in intramuscular injections. *Journal of Clinical Nursing, 11*(4), 457–461.

Cohen, M. H., & Kemper, K. J. (2005). Complementary therapies in pediatrics: A legal perspective. *Pediatrics, 115*(3), 774–780.

Cohen, J. S. (2002). High-dose oral magnesium treatment of chronic, intractable erythromelalgia. *The Annals of Pharmacotherapy, 36*(2), 255–260.

Connelly, M. (2002). Recurrent pediatric headache: A comprehensive review. *Children's Healthcare, 32*(3), 153–89.

Connelly, M., Rapoff, M., Thompson, N., & Connelly, W. (2006). 'Headstrong': A pilot study of a CD-ROM intervention for recurrent pediatric headache. *Journal of Pediatric Psychology, 31*(7), 737–747.

Craig, A. D. (2003). A new view of pain as a homeostatic emotion. *Trends in Neurosciences, 26*(6), 303–307. Review.

Craig, A. D. (2003). Interoception: The sense of the physiological condition of the body. *Current Opinion in Neurobiology, 13*(4), 500–5. Review.

Crofford, L. J., Rowbotham, M. C., Mease, P. J., Russell, I. J., Dworkin, R. H., Corbin, A. E.,et al. (2005). Pregabalin for the treatment of fibromyalgia syndrome: Results of a randomized, double-blind, placebo controlled trial. *Arthritis and Rheumatism, 52*(4), 1264–1273.

Crosby, V., Wilcock, A., & Corcoran, R. (2000). The safety and efficiency of a single dose (500 mg or 1 g) of intravenous magnesium sulfate in neuropathic pain poorly responsive to strong opioid analgenis in patients with cancer. *Journal of Pain and Symptom Management, 19,* 35–39.

Das, D. A., Grimmer, K. A., Sparnon, A. L., McRae, S. E., & Thomas, B. H. (2005). The efficacy of playing a virtual reality game in modulating pain for children with acute burn injuries: A randomized controlled trial. *BMC Pediatrics, 5*(1), 1.

deCharms, R. C., Maeda, F., Glover G H., Ludlow, D., Pauly, J. M., Soneji, D,et al. (2005). Control over brain activation and pain learned by using real-time functional MRI. *Proceedings of the National Academy of Sciences of the United States of America, 102*(51), 18626–18631.

Degenhardt, B. F. (2007). Role of osteopathic manipulative treatment in altering pain biomarkers: A pilot study. *J The Journal of the American Osteopathic Association, 107*(9), 387–400.

Degotardi, P. J., Klass, E. S., Rosenberg, B. S., Fox, D. G., Gallelli, K. A., Gottlieb, B. S. (2006). Development and evaluation of a cognitive behavioral intervention for juvenile fibromyalgia. *Journal of Pediatric Psychology, 31*(7), 714–723.

Demirkaya, S., Dora, B., & Topcuoglu, M. A. (2000). A comparative study of magnesium, flunarizine and amitriptyline in the prophylaxis of migraine. *The Journal of Headache and Pain, 1,* 179–186.

Denison, B. (2004). Touch the pain away: New research on therapeutic touch and persons with fibromyalgia syndrome. *Holistic Nursing Practice, 18*(3), 142–151.

Donaldson, M. S., Speight, N., & Loomis, S. (2001). Fibromyalgia syndrome improved using mostly raw vegetarian diet: An observation study. *BMC Complementary and Alternative Medicine, 1, 7.* Epub 2001.

Douche-Aourik, F. (2003). Detection of enterovirus in human skeletal muscle from patients with chronic inflammatory muscle disease or fibromyalgia and healthy subjects. *Journal of Medical Virology, 71*(4), 540–547.

Eccleston, C., Morley, S., Williams, A., Yorke, L., & Mastroyannopoulou, K. (2002). Systematic review of randomized controlled trials of psychological therapy for chronic pain in children and adolescents, with a subset meta-analysis of pain relief. *Pain, 99*(1–2), 157–165.

Eccleston, C., Yorke, L., Morley, S., Williams, A. C., & Mastroyannopoulou, K. (2003). Psychological therapies for the management of chronic and recurrent pain in children and adolescents. *Cochrane Database of Systematic Reviews,* (1), CD003968.

Eisenberg, D. M., Davis, R. B., Ettner, S. L., Appel, S., Wilkey, S., Van Rompay, M., & Kessler, R. C. (1998). Trends in alternative medicine use in the United States, 1990–1997: Results of a follow-up national survey. *JAMA, 280*(18), 1569–1575.

Emslie, M. J., Campbell, M. K., & Walker, K. A. (2002). Changes in the public awareness of, attitudes to, and use of complementary therapy in North Eastern Scotland: Surveys in 1993 and 1999. *Complementary Therapies in Medicine, 10*(3), 148–153.

Engebretson, J., & Wardell, D. W. (2007). Energy-based modalities. *The Nursing Clinics of North America, 42*(2), 243–259, vi. Review.

England, J. D., Gamboni, F., & Levinson, S. R. (1991). Immunocytochemical localization of sodium channels along demyelimated axous. *Brain Research, 548,* 334–337.

Englebert, R. H. (2006). Exercise tolerance in children and adolescents with musculoskeletal pain in joint hypermobility and joint hypomobility syndrome. *Pediatrics, 118*(3), e690–e696.

Ernst, E., & White, A. (1997). Life-threatening adverse reactions after acupuncture? A systematic review. *Pain, 71,* 123–126.

Ernst, E., & White, A. R. (1998). Acupuncture for back pain: A meta-analysis of randomized controlled trials. *Archives of Internal Medicine, 158,* 2235–2241.

Feldman, D. E., DeCivita, M., Dobkin, P. L., Malleson, P. N., Meshefedjian, G., & Duffy, C. M. (2007). Effects of adherence to treatment on short-term outcomes in children with juvenile idiopathic arthritis. *Arthritis and Rheumatism, 57*(6), 905–912.

Feldman, D. E., Duffy, C., De Civita, M., Malleson, P., Philibert, L., & Gibbon, M., et al. (2004). Factors associated with the use of complementary and alternative medicine in juvenile idiopathic arthritis. *Arthritis and Rheumatism, 51*(4), 527–532.

Ferrari, M. D. (1997). 311C90: Increasing the options for therapy with effective acute antimigraine 5HT1B/1D receptor agonists. *Neurology, 48*(Suppl. 3), S21–S24.

Field, T. (1998). Massage therapy effects. *The American Psychologist, 53*(12), 1270–1281.

Field, T., Diego, M., Cullen, C., Hernandez-Reif, M., Sunshine, W., & Douglas, S. (2002). Fibromyalgia pain and substance P decrease and sleep improves after massage therapy. *Journal of Clinical Rheumatology, 8*(2), 72–76.

Field, T., Hernanadez-Reif, M., Diego, M., Schanberg, S., & Kuhn, C. (2005). Cortisol decreases and serotonin and dopamine increase following massage therapy. *The International Journal of Neuroscience, 115*(10), 1397–1413.

Field, T., Hernandez-Reif, M., Seligman, S., Krasnegor, J., Sunshine, W., Rivas-Chacon, R., et al. (1997). Juvenile rheumatoid arthritis: Benefits from massage therapy. *Journal of Pediatric Psychology, 22*(5), 607–617.

Fitzgerald, M., & Howard, R. F. (2002). The neurobiologic basis of pediatrics pain. In Schechter, Berde, & Yaster, (Eds.), *Pain in infants, children and adolescents,* (2nd ed.). Lippincott Williams & Wilkins.

Francis, A. J., & Dempster, R. J. (2002). Effect of valerian, Valeriana Edulis, on sleep difficulties in children with intellectual Deficits: Randomized trial. *Phytomedcine, 9,* 273–279.

Freedman, R. R. (1991). Physiological mechanisms of temperature biofeedback. *Biofeedback and Self-Regulation, 16*(2), 95–115.

Fowler-Kerry, S., & Lander, J. R. (1987). Management of injection pain in children. *Pain, 30,* 169–175.

Gamber, R. G., Shores, J. H., Russo, D. P., Jimenez, C., & Rubin, B. R. (2002). Osteopathic manipulative treatment in conjunction with medication relieves pain associated with fibromyalgia syndrome: Results of a randomized clinical pilot project. *The Journal of the American Osteopathic Association, 102*(6), 321–325.

Garcia, R. M., Horta, A. L., & Farias, F. (1997). The effect of massage before venipuncture on the reaction of pre-school and school children. *Revista da Escola de Enfermagem da U S P, 31*(1), 119–128.

Gatchel, R. J., Peng, Y. B., Peters, M. L., Fuchs, P. N., & Turk, D. C. (2007). The biopsychosocial approach to chronic pain: Scientific advances and future directions. *Psychological Bulletin, 133*(4), 581–624.

Gauntlett-Gilbert, J., & Eccleston, C. (2007). Disability in adolescents with chronic pain: Patterns and predictors across different domains of functioning. *Pain, 131*(1–2), 132–141.

Gershon, J., Zimand, E., Pickering, M., Rothbaum, B.O., & Hodges, L. (2004). A pilot and feasibility study of virtual reality as a distraction for children with cancer. *Journal of the American Academy of Child and Adolescent Psychiatry, 43*(10), 1243–1249.

Giordano, J. (2006). How Alpha-Stim cranial electrotherapy stimulation (CES) works. Mineral Wells, TX: Electromedical Products International, Inc.

Goel, N., Kim, H., & Lao, R. P. (2005). An olfactory stimulus modifies nighttime sleep in young men and women. *Chronobiology International, 22*(5), 889–904.

Goffaux, P., Redmond, W. J., Rainville, P., & Marchand, S. (2007). Descending analgesia—When the spine echoes what the brain expects. *Pain, 130*(1–2), 137–143.

Gold, J. I., Kim, S. H., & Kant, A. J. (2006). Effectiveness of virtual reality for pediatric pain distraction during i.v. placement. *Cyberpsychological Behavior, 9*(2), 207–212.

Goldberg, R. J., & Katz, J. (2007). A meta-analysis of the analgesic effects of omega-3 polyunsaturated fatty acid supplementation for inflammatory joint pain. *Pain, 129*(1–2), 210–223.

Golianu, B., Krane, E., Seybold, J., Almgren, C., & Anand, K. J. (2007). Non-pharmacological techniques for pain management in neonates. *Seminars in Perinatology, 31*(5), 318–322.

Gordon, K. E., Dooley, J. M., & Wood, E. P. (2004). Self-reported headache frequency and features associated with frequent headaches in Canadian young adolescents. *Headache, 44*(6), 555–561.

Gottschling, S., Meyer, S., Gribova, I., Distler, L., Berrang, J., & Gortner, L., et al. (2007). Laser acupuncture in children with headache: A double-blind, randomized, bicenter, placebo-controlled trial. *Pain* (Epub ahead of print).

Grant, L., McBeam, D. E., Fyfe, L., & Warnock, A. M. (2007). A review of the biological and potential therapeutic actions of Harpagophytum procuymbens. *Phytotherapy Research, 21*(3), 199–209.

Grazzi, L. (2004). Headache in children and adolescents: Conventional and unconventional approaches to treatment. *Neurological Sciences, 25*(Suppl 3), S223–S225.

Grontved, A., Brask, T., Kamskard, J., & Hentzer, E. (1986). Ginger root against seasickness: Controlled trial on the open sea. *Acta Otolaryngology, 48,* 282–286.

Grossman, W., & Schmidramsl, H. (2001) An extract of Petasites hybridus is effective in the prophylaxis of migraine. *Alternative Medicine Review, 6*(3):303–310.

Grzanna, R., Lindmark, L., & Frondoza, C. G. (2005). Ginger—an herbal medicinal product with broad anti-inflammatory actions. *Journal of Medicinal Food, 8*(2), 125–132.

Gyllenhaal, C., Merritt, S. L., Peterson, S.D., Block, K.I., & Gochenour, T. (2000). Efficacy and safety of herbal stimulants and sedatives in sleep disorders. *Sleep Medicine Reviews, 4*(3), 229–251.

Gutiérrez-Suárez, R., Pistorio, A., Cespedes Cruz, A., Norambuena, X., Flato, B., et al. (2007). Health-related quality of life of patients with juvenile idiopathic arthritis coming from 3 different geographic areas. The PRINTO multinational quality of life cohort study. *Rheumatology, 46*, 314–320.

Hagen, L. E., Schneider, R., Stephens, D., Modrusan, D., & Feldman, B. M. (2003). Use of complementary and alternative medicine by pediatric rheumatology patients. *Arthritis and Rheumatism, 49*(1), 3–6.

Hammond, D. C. (2007). Review of the efficacy of clinical hypnosis with headaches and migraines. *The International Journal of Clinical and Experimental Hypnosis, 55*(2), 207–219.

Harel, Z., Biro, F. M., Kottenhahn, R. K., & Rosenthal, S. L. (1996). Supplementation with omega-3 polyunsaturated fatty acids in the management of dysmenorrhea in adolescents. *American Journal of Obstetrics and Gynecology, 174*(4), 1335–1338.

Harel, Z., Gascon, G., Riggs, S., Vaz, R., Brown, W., & Exil, G. (2002). Supplementation with omega-3 polyunsaturated fatty acids in the management of recurrent migraines in adolescents. *The Journal of Adolescent Health, 31*(2), 154–161.

Hargreaves, R. J., & Shepheard, S. L. (1999). Pathophysiology of migraine—new insights. *The Canadian Journal of Neurological Sciences,* (Suppl 3), S12–S19.

Hayden, C., & Mullinger, B. (2006). A preliminary assessment of the impact of cranial osteopathy for the relief of infantile colic. *Complementary Therapies in Clinical Practice, 12*(2), 83–90.

Hayden, J. A., Mior, S. A., & Verhoef, M. J. (2003). Evaluation of chiropractic management of pediatric patients with low back pain: A prospective cohort study. *Journal of Manipulative and Physiological Therapeutics, 26*(1), 1–8.

He, L. (1987). Involvement of endogenous opioid peptides in acupuncture analgesia. *Pain, 31*, 99–121.

Heap, L., Peters, T., & Wessley, S. (1999). Vitamin B status in patients with chronic fatigue syndrome. *Journal of the Royal Society of Medicine, 92*, 1183–1185.

Hernandez-Reif, M., Field, T.,Largie, S., Hart, S., Redzepi, M., Nierenberg, B., & Peck, T. M. (2001). Childrens' distress during burn treatment is reduced by massage therapy. *The Journal of Burn Care & Rehabilitation, 22*(2), 191–195.

Hershey, A. D., Powers, S. W., Vockell, A. L., Lecates, S. L., Ellinor, P. L., & Segers, A, et al. (2007). Coenzyme Q10 deficiency and response to supplementation in pediatric and adolescent migraine. *Headache, 47*(1), 73–80.

Hicks, C. L., von Baeyer, C. L., Spafford, P. A., van Korlaar, I., & Goodenough, B. (2001). The Faces Pain Scale-Revised: Toward a common metric in pediatric pain measurement. *Pain, 93*(2), 173–183.

Hoffman, H. G., Doctor, J. N., Patterson, D. R., Carrougher, G. J., & Furness, T. A. 3rd. (2000). Virtual reality as an adjunctive pain control during burn wound care in adolescent patients. *Pain, 85*(1–2), 305–309.

Hoffman, H. G., Garcia-Palocios, A., & Patterson, D. R., (2001). The effectiveness of virtual reality for dental pain control: A case study. *Cyberpsychological Behavior, 4*, 527–535.

Holden, E. W., Deichmann, M. M., & Levy, J. D. (1999). Empirically supported treatments in pediatric psychology: recurrent pediatric headache. *Journal of Pediatric Psychology, 24*(2), 91–109.

Hormann, H. P., & Korting, H. C. (1994). Evidence for the efficacy and safety of topical herbal drugs in dermatology: Part I: Anti-inflammatory agents. *Phytomedicine, 1*, 161–171.

Houghton, P. J. (1999). The scientific basis for the reputed activity of Valerian. *The Journal of Pharmacy and Pharmacology, 51*(5), 505–512.

Howard, J. (2007). Do Bach flower remedies have a role to play in pain control? A critical analysis investigating therapeutic value beyond the placebo effect, and the potential of Bach flower remedies as a psychological method of pain relief. *Complementary Therapies in Clinical Practice, 13*(3), 174–183.

Hoyt, W. H., Shaffer, F., Bard, D., Benesler, J. S., Blankenhorn, G. D., & Gray, J. H. (1979). Osteopathic manipulation in the treatment of muscle contraction headache. *Journal of American Osteopathic Association., 78*, 322–325.

International Headache Society Classification Subcommittee. (2004). *International classification of headache disorders* (2nd ed.). *Cephalalgia, 24*(Suppl 1), 1–160.

Jacobs, J., Springer, D. A., & Crothers, D. (2001). Homeopathic treatment of acute otitis media in children: A preliminary randomized placebo-controlled trial. *The Pediatric Infectious Disease Journal, 20*, 177–183.

Janicke, D. M., & Finney, J. W. (1999). Empirically supported treatments in pediatric psychology: Recurrent abdominal pain. *Journal of Pediatric Psychology, 24*(2), 115–127.

John, P. J., Sharma, N., Sharma, C. M., & Kankane, A. (2007). Effectiveness of yoga therapy in the treatment of migraine without aura: A randomized controlled trial. *Headache, 47*(5), 654–661.

Kales, S. N., Christophi, C. A., & Saper, R. B. (2007). Hematopoietic toxicity from lead-containing Ayurvedic medications. *Med Sci Monit, 13*(7), CR295–298.

Kashikar-Zuck, S., Swain, N. F., Jones, B. A., & Graham T. B. (2005). Efficacy of cognitive-behavioral intervention for juvenile primary fibromyalgia syndrome. *The Journal of Rheumatology, 32*(8), 1594–1602.

Kelly A. C. (2004). Treatment of reflex sympathetic dystrophy in 3 pediatric patients using 7 external dragons and devils acupuncture. *Acupuncture in Medicine, 15*(3), 29–30.

Kemper, K. J., Sarah R., Silver-Highfield, E., Xiarhos, E., Barnes, L., & Berde, C. (2000). On pins and needles? Pediatric pain patients' experience with acupuncture. *Pediatrics, 105*, 941–947.

Kho, K. H. (1995). The impact of acupuncture on pain in patients with reflex sympathetic dystrophy. *Pain Clinic, 8*(1), 59–61.

Kimura, Y., & Walco, G. A. (2007). Treatment of chronic pain in pediatric rheumatic disease. *Nature Clinical Practice. Rheumatology, 3*(4), 210–218.

Kingston, J., Chadwick, P., Meron, D., & Skinner, T. C. (2007). A pilot randomized control trial investigating the effect of mindfulness practice on pain tolerance, psychological wellbeing, and physiological activity. *Journal of Psychosomatic Research, 62*(3), 297–300.

Kober, A., Scheck, T., Schubert, B., Strasser, H., Gustorff, B., & Bertalanffy, P. (2003). Auricular acupressure as a treatment for anxiety in prehospital transport settings. *Anesthesiology, 98*(6), 1328–1332.

Koike, H., Watanabe, H., Inukai, A., Iijima, M., Mori, K., Hattori, N., & Sobue, G. (2006). Myopathy in thiamine deficiency: Analysis of a case. *Journal of the Neurological Sciences, 249*(2), 175–179.

Konijnenberg, A. Y., Uiterwaal, C. S. P. M., Kimpen, J. L. L., van der Hoeven, J., Buitelaar, J. K., de Graeff-Meeder, E. R. (2005). Children with unexplained chronic pain: Substantial impairment in everyday life. *Archives of Disease in Childhood, 90*, 680–686.

Koyama, T., McHaffie, J. G., Laurienti, P. J., & Coghill, R. C. (2005). The subjective experience of pain: Where expectations become reality. *PNAS, 102*(36), 12950–12955.

Kroener-Herwig, B., & Denecke, H. (2002). Cognitive-behavioral therapy of pediatric headache: Are there differences in efficacy between a therapist-administered group training and a self-help format? *Journal of Psychosomatic Research, 53*(6), 1107–1114.

Kuttner, L., Chambers, C. T., & Hardial, J. (2006). A randomized trial of yoga for adolescents with irritable bowel syndrome. *Pain Research & Management, 11*(4), 217–223.

Labbé, E. (1998). Pediatric headaches. In T. Ollendick & M. Hersen (Eds.), *Handbook of child psychopathology* (3rd ed., pp. 381–394). New York: Plenum Press.

Lang, T., Hager, H., Funovits, V., Barker, R., Steinlechner, B., Hoerauf, K., & Kober, A. (2007). Prehospital analgesia with acupressure at the Baihui and Hegu points in patients with radial fractures: A prospective, randomized, double-blind trial. *The American Journal of Emergency Medicine, 25*(8), 887–893.

Lavigne, J. V., Ross, C. K., Berry, S. L., Hayford, J. R., & Pachman, L. M. (1992). Evaluation of a psychological treatment package for treating pain in juvenile rheumatoid arthritis. *Arthritis Care and Research, 5*(2), 101–110.

Lee, A. C., Highfield, E. S., Berde, C. B., & Kemper, K. J. (1999). Survey of acupuncturists: practice characteristics and pediatric care. *The Western Journal of Medicine, 171*, 153–157.

Lee, B. H., Scharff, L., Sethna, N. F., McCarthy, C. F., Scott-Sutherland, J., Shea, A. M., et al. (2002). Physical therapy and cognitive-behavioral treatment for complex regional pain syndromes. *The Journal of Pediatrics, 141*(1), 135–140.

Lee, D. K., Carstairs, I. J., Haggart, K., Jackson, C. M., Currie, G. P., & Lipworth, B. J. (2003). Butterbur, a herbal remedy, attenuates adenosine monophosphate induced nasal responsiveness in seasonal allergic rhinitis. *Clinical and Experimental Allergy, 33*, 882–886.

Lee, H., Lee, J. Y., Kim, Y. J., Kim, S., Yin, C., Khil, J. H., et. al. (2008). Acupuncture for symptom management of rheumatoid arthritis: A pilot study. *Clinical Rheumatologyl, 27*(5):641–645.

Lee, L. H., & Olness, K. H., (1996). Effects of self-induced mental imagery on autonomic reactivity in children. *Journal of Developmental and Behavioral Pediatrics, 17*, 323–327.

Levin, S., Drug therapies for childhood headache. In: P. McGrath & L. Hillier (Eds.), *The child with headache: Diagnosis and treatment* (pp. 109–127). Seattle: IASP Press.

Lewith, G. T., & Kenyon, J. N. (1984). Physiological and psychological explanations for the mechanism of acupuncture as a treatment for chronic pain. *Social Science & Medicine, 19*, 1367–1378.

Lewith, G. T., Godfrey, A. D., & Prescott, P. (2005). A single-blinded, randomized pilot study evaluating the aroma of *Lavandula augustifolia* as a treatment for mild insomnia. *Journal of Alternative and Complementary Medicine, 11*(4), 631–637.

Lichtbroun, A. S., Raicer, M. M., & Smith, R. B. (2001). The treatment of fibromyalgia with cranial electrotherapy stimulation. *Journal of Clinical Rheumatology, 7*(2), 72–78.

Lin, Y. (2003). Acupuncture. In N. L. Schecter, C. B. Berde, & M. Yaster (Eds.), *Pain in infants, children, and adolescents* (2nd ed., pp. 462–470). Philadelphia: Lippincott Williams & Wilkins.

Lissoni, P., Barni, S., Mandala, M., Ardizzoia, A., Paolorossi, F., Vaghi, M., et al. (1999). Decreased toxicity and increased efficacy of cancer chemotherapy using the Pineal hormone melatonin in metastatic solid tumor patients with poor clinical status. *European Journal of Cancer, 35*, 1688–1692.

Low, A. K., Ward, K., & Winer, A. P. (2007). Pediatric complex regional pain syndrome. *Journal of Pediatric Orthopedics, 27*(5), 567–572.

Lumb, A. B. (1993). Mechanism of antiemetic effect of ginger. *Anaesthesia, 48*, 1118.

Macres, S. M., & Richeimer, S. H. (1998). Understanding neuropathic pain: Pathophysiology and treatment modalities. *Current Reviews in Clinical Anesthesia, 19*(2), 14–20.

Malleson, P. N., Oen, K., Cabral, D. A., Petty, R. E., Rosenberg, A. M., & Cheang, M. (2004). Predictors of pain in children with established juvenile rheumatoid arthritis. *Archives de Rhumatologie, 51*(2), 222–227.

Malone, A. B. (1996). The effects of live music on the distress of pediatric patients receiving intravenous starts, venipunctures, injections, and heel sticks. *Journal of Music Therapy, 33*, 19–33.

Mannerkorpi, K., & Henriksson, C. (2007). Non-pharmacological treatment of chronic widespread musculoskeletal pain. *Best practice & Research. Clinical Rheumatology, 21*(3), 513–534.

Marchette, L., Main, R., Redick, E., Bagg, A., & Leatherland, J. (1991). Pain reduction interventions during neonatal circumcision. *Nursing Research, 40*, 241–244.

McCrory, D. C. (1997). Cranial electrostimulation for headache: Meta-analysis. *The Journal of Nervous and Mental Disease, 185*(12), 766–767.

McGrath, P. J., & Craig, K. D. (1989). Developmental and psychological factors in children's pain. *Pediatric Clinics of North America, 36*(4), 823–36.

McGrath, P. J., & McAlpine, L. (1993). Psychologic perspectives on pediatric pain. *The Journal of Pediatrics, 122*(5 Pt 2), S2–8.

McGrath, P. A., & Hillier, L. M. (2003). Modifying the psychological factors that intensify children's pain and prolong disability. In N. L. Schecter, C. B. Berde, & M. Yaster, (Eds.), *Pain in infants, children, and adolescents* (2nd ed., pp. 85–104). Philadelphia: Lippincott Williams & Wilkins.

McGrath, P. A., & Dade, L. A. (2004). Effective strategies to decrease pain and minimize disability. In D. D. Price & M. C. Bushnell (Eds.), *Psychological methods of pain control: Basic science and clinical perspectives, progress in pain research and management* (Vol. 29, pp. 73–96). Seattle: IASP Press.

McGuffin, M., Hobbs, C., Upton, R., & Goldberg, A. (Eds.). (1997). *American herbal products association's botanical safety handbook.* Boca Raton, FL: CRC Press.

McGuire, J. K., Kulkarni, M. S., & Baden, H. P. (2000). Fatal hypermagnesemia in a child treated with megavitamin/megamineral therapy. *Pediatrics, 105*, e18.

McManus, V., & Gliksten, M. (2007). The use of CranioSacral therapy in a physically impaired population in a disability service in Southern Ireland. *Journal of Alternative and Complementary Medicine, 13*, 929–930.

Megel, M. E., Houser, C. W., & Gleaves, L. S. (1999). Children's responses to immunizations: Lullabies as a distraction. *Issues in Comprehensive Pediatric Nursing, 21*, 129–145.

Melzack, R., & Wall, P. D. (1965). Pain mechanisms: A new theory. *Science, 150*, 971.

Melzack, R. (1999). From the gate to the neuromatrix. *Pain,* (Suppl 6) S121–S126. Review.

Melzack, R., & Katy, J. (2007). A conceptual framework for understanding pain in the human. In S. D. Waldman (Ed.), *Pain management.* Saunders: Philadelphia, PA.

Merskey, H., & Bogduk, N. (Eds.). (1994). *Classification of chronic pain: Description of chronic pain syndrome and definitions of pain terms* (2nd ed.). Seattle, WA: IASP Press.

Miles, P., & True, G. (2003). Reiki—Review of a biofield therapy. History, theory, practice, and research. *Alternative Therapies in Health and Medicine, 9*(2), 62–72.

Millichap, J. G., & Yee, M. M. (2003). The diet factor in pediatric and adolescent migraine. *Pediatric Neurology, 28*(1), 9–15.

Mills, M. V., Henley, C. E., Barnes, L. L., Carreiro, J. E., & Degenhardt, B. F. (2003). The use of manipulative treatment as adjuvant therapy in children with recurrent acute otitis media. *Archives of Pediatrics & Adolescent Medicine, 157*, 861–866.

Morone, N. E., Greco, C. M., & Weiner, D. K. (2008). Mindfulness meditation for the treatment of chronic low back pain in older adults: A randomized controlled pilot study. *Pain, 134*(3), 310–319.

Munoz-Hoyos, A., Sanchez-Forte, M., Molina-Carballo, A., Escames, G., Martin-Medina, E., Reiter, R. J., et al. (1998). Melatonins role as an anticonvulsant and neuronal protector: Experimental and clinical evidence. *Journal of Child Neurology, 13*, 501–509.

Murphy, J. J., Heptinstall, S., & Mitchell, J. R. (1988). Randomized double-blind placebo-controlled trial of feverfew in migraine prevention. *Lancet, 2*(8604), 189–192.

Murray, C. S., Cohen, A., Perkins, T., Davidson, J. E., & Sills, J. A. (2000). Morbidity in reflex sympathetic dystrophy. *Archives of Disease in Childhood, 82*, 231–233.

NCCAM. National Center on Complementary and Alternative Medicine. www.nccam.nih.gov

Natural Medicines Comprehensive Database. www.naturaldatabase.com

Nelson, G. J., Schmidt, P. S., Bartolini, G. L., Kelley, D. S., & Kyle, D. (1997). The effect of dietary docosahexaenoic acid on platelet function, platelet fatty acid composition, and blood coagulation in humans. *Lipids, 32*, 1129–1136.

NIH Technology Assessment Panel. (1996). Integration of behavioral and relaxation approaches into the treatment of chronic pain and insomnia. *JAMA, 276*(4), 313–318.

Oelkers-Ax, R., Leins, A., Parzer, P., Hillecke, T., Bolay, H. V., Fischer, J., et al. (2007). Butterbur root extract and music therapy in the prevention of childhood migraine: An explorative study. *European Journal of Pain* **12(3):301-313.**

Olness, K., & Kohen, D. P. (1996). *Hypnosis and hypnotherapy with children* (3rd ed.) The Guilford Press, New York.

Olney, J. W., (1989). Glutamate, a neurotoxic transmitter. *Journal of Child Neurology, 4*(3), 218–226.

Palermo, T. M., & Chambers, C. T. (2005). Parent and family factors in pediatric chronic pain and disability: An integrative approach. *Pain, 119*(1–3), 1–4.

Palermo, T. M., & Kisler, R. (2005). Subjective sleep disturbances in adolescents with chronic pain: Relationship to daily functioning and quality of life. *The Journal of Pain, 6*(3), 201–207.

Pandi-Perumal, S. R., Srinivasan, V., Spence, D. W., & Cardinali, D. P. (2007). Role of the melatonin system in the control of sleep: Therapeutic implications. *CNS Drugs, 21*(12), 995–1018.

Park, J., & Ernst, E. (2005). Ayurvedic medicine for rheumatoid arthritis: A systematic review. *Semin Arthritis and Rheumatism, 34*(5), 705–713.

Payne, R. (2007). Medical professionalism and responsibility in pain management. *Practical Bioethics, 3*(3), 1–6.

Pediatric Chronic Pain Task Force. (2007). Pediatric chronic pain: A position statement from the *American Pain Society.*

Peres, M. F., Gonçalves, A. L., & Krymchantowski, A. (2007). Migraine, Tension-type Headache, and Transformed Migraine. *Current Pain and Headache Reports, 11*(6), 449–453.

Perquin, C., Hazebroek-Kampschreur, A., Hunfeld, J., Bohnen, A. M., van Suijlekom-Smit, L. W., Passchier, J., & van der Wouden, J. C. (2000). Pain in children and adolescents: A common experience. *Pain, 87*, 51–58.

Petrovic, P., Kalso, E., Petersson, K. M., & Ingvar, M., (2001). Placebo and opioid analgesia—imaging a shared neuronal network. *Science, 295*, 1737–1740.

Pintov, S., Lahat, E., Alstein, M., Vogel, Z., & Barg, J. (1997). Acupuncture and the opioid system: Implications in management of migraine. *Pediatric Neurology, 17*, 129–133.

Pittler, M. H., Vogler, B. K., & Ernst, E. (2000). Feverfew for preventing migraine. *Cochrane Database of Systematic Reviews*, (3), CD002286.

Pittler, M. H., & Ernst, E. (2004). Feverfew for preventing migraine. *Cochrane Database of Systematic Reviews*, (1), CD002286.

Portnoi, G., Chng, L. A., Karimi-Tabesh, L., Koren, G., Tan, M. P., & Einarson, A. (2003). Prospective comparative study of the safety and effectiveness of ginger for the treatment of nausea and vomiting in pregnancy. *American Journal of Obstetrics and Gynecology, 189*, 1374–1377.

Pothmann, R., & Danesch, U. (2005). Migraine prevention in children and adolescents: Results of an open study with a special butterbur toot extract. *Headache, 45*(3), 196–203.

Rainville, P. (2002). Brain mechanisms of pain affect and pain modulation. *Current Opinion in Neurobiology, 12*, 195–204.

Ross, J. (1990). Biological effects of pulsed high peak power: Electromagnetic energy using Diapulse. In M. E. O'Connor, R. H. Bentall, & J. C. Monahan (Eds.), *Emerging electromagnetic medicine* (pp. 269–282). New York: Springer Verlag.

Rothner, A. (2001). Differential diagnosis of headaches in children and adolescents. In P. McGrath & L. Hillier (Eds.), *The child with headache: Diagnosis and treatment* (pp. 57–76). Seattle: IASP Press.

Rozen, T. D., Oshinski, M. L., Gebeline, C. A., Bradley, K. C., Young, W. B., Shechter, A. L., & Silberstein, S. D. (2002). Open label trial of coenzyme Q10 as a migraine preventative. *Cephalalgia, 22*(2), 137–141.

Russell, I. J., Michalek, J. E., Flechas, J. D., & Abraham, G. E. (1995). Treatment of fibromyalgia syndrome with Super Malic: A randomized, double blind, placebo controlled, crossover pilot study. *The Journal of Rheumatology, 22*, 953–958.

Sándor, P. S., Afra, J., Ambrosini, A., & Schoenen, J. (2000). Prophylactic Treatment of migraine with beta-blockers and riboflavin: Differential effects on the intensity dependence of auditory evoked cortical potentials. *Headache, 40*, 30–35.

Sándor, P. S., Di Clemente, L., Coppola, G., Saenger, U., Fumal, A., Magis, D., et. al. (2005). Efficacy of coenzyme Q10 in migraine prophylaxis: A randomized controlled trial. *Neurology, 64*(4), 713–715.

Sarrell, E. M., Cohen, H. A., & Kahan, E. (2003). Naturopathic treatment for ear pain in children. *Pediatrics, 111*, e574–579.

Sarrell, E. M., Mandelberg, A., & Cohen, H. A. (2001). Efficacy of naturopathic extracts in the management of ear pain associated with acute otitis media. *Archives of Pediatrics & Adolescent Medicine, 155*, 796–799.

Schachner, L., Field, T., Hernandez-Reif, M., Duarte, A. M., & Krasnegor, J. (1998). Atopic dermatitis symptoms decreased in children following massage therapy. *Pediatric Dermatology, 15*(5), 390–395.

Schanberg, L. E., Anthony, K. K., Gil, K. M., & Maurin, E. (2003). Daily pain and symptoms in children with polyarticular arthritis. *Arthritis and Rheumatism, 48*(5), 1390–1397.

Schechter, N. L., Zempsky, W. T., Cohen, L. L., McGrath, P. J., McMurtry, C. M., & Bright, N. S. (2007). Pain reduction during pediatric immunizations: Evidence-based review and recommendations. *Pediatrics, 119*(5), e1184–1198.

Schwedt, T. J., Dodick, D. W., Hentz, J., Trentman, T. L., & Zimmerman, R. S. (2007). Occipital nerve stimulation for chronic headache—long-term safety and efficacy. *Cephalalgia, 27*(2), 153–157.

Seshia, S. S. (2004). Mixed migraine and tension-type: A common cause of recurrent headache in children. *The Canadian Journal of Neurological Sciences, 31*(3), 315–318.

Shah, P. S., Aliwalas, L. I., & Shah, V. (2006). Breastfeeding or breast milk for procedural pain in neonates. *Cochrane Database of Systematic Reviews, 3* CD004950.

Sherman, R. A., Acosta, N. M., & Robson, L. (1999). Treatment of migraine with pulsing electromagnetic fields: A double-blind, placebo-controlled study. *Headache, 39*(8), 567–575.

Sherman, R. A., Robson, L., & Marden, L. A. (1998). Initial exploration of pulsing electromagnetic fields for treatment of migraine. *Headache, 38*(3), 208–213.

Sherry, D. D., Wallace, C. A., Kelley, C., Kidder, M., & Sapp, L. (1999). Short and long term outcomes of children with complex regional pain syndrome type 1 treated with exercise therapy. *The Clinical Journal of Pain, 15*, 218–223.

Shinchuk, L. M., & Holick, M. F. (2007). Vitamin D and rehabilitation: Improving functional outcomes. *Nutrition in Clinical Practice, 22*(3), 297–304.

Shrivastava, R., Pechadre, J. C., & John, G. W. (2006). Tanacetum parthenium and Salix alba (Mig-RL) combination in migraine. *Clinical Drug Investigation, 26*(5), 287–296.

Singh-Grewal, D., Schneiderman-Walker, J., Wright, V., Bar-Or, O., Beyene, J., Selvadurai, H., et al. (2007). The effects of vigorous exercise training on physical function in children with arthritis: A randomized, controlled, single-blinded trial. *Arthritis and Rheumatism, 57*(7), 1202–1210.

Sinha, M., Christopher, N. C., Fenn, R., & Reeves, L. (2006). Evaluation of nonpharmacologic methods of pain and anxiety management for laceration repair in the pediatric emergency department. *Pediatrics, 117*(4), 1162–1168.

Soeken, K. L. (2004). Selected CAM therapies for arthritis-related pain: The evidence from systematic reviews. *The Clinical Journal of Pain, 20*(1), 13–18.

Southwood, T. R., Malleson, P. N., Roberts-Thomson, P. J., & Mahy, M. (1990). Unconventional remedies used for patients with juvenile arthritis. *Pediatrics, 85*(2), 150–154.

Srivastava, K. C., & Mustafa, T. (1989). Ginger (Zingiber officinale) and rheumatic disorders. *Medical Hypotheses, 29*, 25–28.

Srivastava, K. C., & Mustafa, T. (1992). Ginger (Zingiber officinale) in rheumatism and musculoskeletal disorders. *Medical Hypotheses, 39*(4), 342–348.

Steele, E. B., Grimmer, K., Thomas, B., Mulley, B., Fulton, I., & Hoffman, H. (2003). Virtual reality as a pediatric pain modulation technique: A case study. *Cyberpsychological Behavior, 6*, 633–638.

Stephenson, N. L., Swanson, M., Dalton, J., Keefe, F. J., & Engelke, M. (2007). Partner-delivered reflexology: Effects on cancer pain and anxiety. *Oncology Nursing Forum, 34*(1), 127–132.

Sumner, H., Salan, U., Knight, D. W., & Hoult, J. R. (1992). Inhibition of 5-Lipoxygenase and cyclo-oxygenase in leukocytes by Feverfew. Involvement of sesquiterpene lactones and other Components. *Biochemical Pharmacology, 43*, 2313–2320.

Tan, G., Craine, M. H., Bair, M. J., Garcia, M. K., Giordano, J., Jensen, M. P., et. al. (2007). Efficacy of selected complementary and alternative medicine interventions for chronic pain. *Journal of Rehabilitation Research and Development, 44*(2), 195–222.

Taddio, A., Katy, J., Gersich, A. L., & Koren, G. (1997). Effect of neonatal circumcision on pain response during subsequent routine vaccination. *Lancet, 349*, 599–603.

Taketomo, C. K., Hodding, J. H., & Kraus, D. M. (2007). *Pediatric dosage handbook* (14th ed.). LexiComp, Inc. Hudson, Ohio.

Teitelbaum, J. (2001). *From fatigued to fantastic.* New York: Penguin Putnam Inc.

Tomer, A., Kasey, S., Connor, W. E., Clark, S., Harker, L. A., & Eckman, J. R. (2001). Reduction of pain episodes and prothrombotic activity in sickle cell disease by dietary n-3 fatty acids. *Thrombosis And Haemostasis, 85*(6), 966–974.

Trautmann, E., Lackschewitz, H., & Kröner-Herwig, B. (2006). Psychological treatment of recurrent headache in children and adolescents—a meta-analysis. *Cephalalgia, 26*(12), 1411–1426.

Tsao, J. C., Meldrum, M., Bursch, B., Jacob, M. C., Kim, S. C., & Zeltzer, L. K. (2005). Treatment expectations for CAM interventions in pediatric chronic pain patients and their parents. *Evidence-Based Complementary and Alternative Medicine, 2*(4), 521–527.

Tsao, J. C., Meldrum, M., Kim, S. C., Jacob, M. C., & Zeltzer, L. K. (2007). Treatment preferences for CAM in children with chronic pain. *Evidence-Based Complementary and Alternative Medicine, 4*(3), 367–374.

Turunen, M., Olsson, J., & Dallner, G. (2004). Metabolism and function of coenzyme Q. *Biochimica et Biophysica Acta, 1660*, 171–199.

van der Heijden, K. B., Smits, M. G., van Someren, E. J., Ridderinkhof, K. R., & Gunning, W. B. (2007). Effect of melatonin on sleep, behavior, and cognition in ADHD and chronic sleep-onset insomnia. *Journal of the American Academy of Child and Adolescent Psychiatry, 46*(2), 233–241.

van Twillert, B., Bremer, M., & Faber, A. W. (2007). Computer-generated virtual reality to control pain and anxiety in pediatric and adult burn patients during wound dressing changes. *Journal of Burn Care & Research, 28*(5), 694–702.

Vargová, V., Veselý, R., Sasinka, M., & Török, C. (1998). Will administration of omega-3 unsaturated fatty acids reduce the use of nonsteroidal antirheumatic agents in children with chronic juvenile arthritis? *Casopís Lékařů českých, 137*(21), 651–653.

Vasconcellos, E., Piña-Garza, J. E., Millan, E. J., & Warner, J. S. (1998). Analgesic rebound headache in children and adolescents. *Journal of Child Neurology, 13*, 443–447.

Viola, H., Wasowski, C., Levi de Stein, M., Wolfman, C., Silveira, R., Dajas, F., et al. (1995). Apigenin, a component of matricaria recutita flowers, is a central benzodiazepine receptors-ligand with anxiolytic effects. *Planta Medica, 61*, 213–216.

Walco, G. A., Varni, J. W., & Ilowite, N. T. (1992). Cognitive-behavioral pain management in children with juvenile rheumatoid arthritis. *Pediatrics, 89*(6 Pt 1), 1075–1079.

Wang, F., Van Den Eeden, S. K., Ackerson, L. M., Salk, S. E., Reince, R. H., & Elin, R. J. (2003). Oral magnesium oxide prophylaxis of. frequent migrainous headache in children: A randomized, double-blind, placebo controlled trial. *Headache, 43*, 601–610.

Wardell, D. W., & Engebretson, J. (2001). Biological correlates of Reiki Touch(sm) healing. *Journal of advanced Nursing, 33*(4), 439–45.

Warnock, M., McBean, D., Suter, A., Tan, J., & Whittaker, P. (2007). Effectiveness and safety of Devil's Claw tablets in patients with general rheumatic disorders. *Phytotherapy Research, 21*(12), 1228–1233.

Wasiewski, W. (2001). Preventive therapy in pediatric migraine. *Journal of Child Neurology, 16*(2), 71–78.

Watson, K., Papageorgiou, A., Jones, G., Taylor, S., Symmons, D. P., Silman, A. J., & Macfarlane, G. J. (2003). Low back pain in schoolchildren: the role of mechanical and psychosocial factors. *Archives of Disease in Childhood, 88*, 12–17.

Welborn C. A. Pediatric migraine. *Emergency Medical Clinics of North America* (1997) 15, 625–636.

Welch, K. M. (1998). Current opinions in headache pathogenesis: Introduction and synthesis. *Current Opinion in Neurobiology, 11*, 193–197.

Weydert, J. A., Shapiro, D. E., Acra, S. A., Monheim, C. J., Chambers, A. S., & Ball, T. M. (2006). Evaluation of guided imagery as treatment for recurrent abdominal pain in children: A randomized controlled trial. *BMC Pediatrics, 6*, 29.

Wheatley, D. (2005). Medicinal plants for insomnia: A review of their pharmacology, efficacy and tolerability. *Journal of Psychopharmacology, 19*(4), 414–421.

Wicksell, R. K., Dahl, J., Magnusson, B., & Olsson, G. L. (2005). Using Acceptance and Commitment Therapy in the rehabilitation of an adolescent female with chronic pain: A case example. *Cognitive and Behavioral Practice, 12*, 415–423.

Wustrow, T. P. (2005). Naturopathic therapy for acute otitis media. An alternative to the primary use of antibiotics. *HNO, 53*(8), 728–734.

Wyatt, K. M., Dimmock, P. W., Jones, P. W., & O'Brien, P. M. (1999). Efficacy of vitamin B in the treatment of premenstrual syndrome. *BMJ, 318*, 1375–1381.

Yan, B., Li, K., Xu, J., Wang, W., Li, K., Liu, H., Shan, B., & Tang, X. (2005). Acupoint-specific fMRI patterns in human brain. *Neuroscience Letters, 383*(3), 236–240.

Zeltzer, L. K., Tsao, J. C. I., Stelling, C., Powers, M., Levy, S., & Waterhouse, M. (2002). A phase I study on the feasibility of an acupuncture/hypnotherapy intervention for chronic pediatric pain. *Journal of Pain and Symptom Management, 24,* 437–446.

Zeltzer, L. K., Tsao, J. C., Bursch, B., & Myers, C. D. (2006). Introduction to the special issue on pain: From pain to pain-associated disability syndrome. *Journal of Pediatric Psychology, 31*(7), 661–666.

Zheng, L., & Faber, K. (2005). Review of the Chinese medical approach to the management of fibromyalgia. *Current Pain and Headache Reports, 9*(5), 307–312.

25

Integrative Pediatric Palliative Care

STEFAN J. FRIEDRICHSDORF, LEORA KUTTNER, KRISTA WESTENDORP, AND RUTH MCCARTY

KEY CONCEPTS

- A dying child is often highly symptomatic, and providing symptom relief is one of the most compelling domains of pediatric palliative care.
- State of the art in managing pediatric pain and other distressing symptoms at the end of life requires integrating pharmacological with integrative therapeutic interventions.
- Both published case studies and our personal experience strongly endorse integrative treatment modalities, especially imagery, hypnosis, music, aromatherapy, massage, therapeutic/healing touch, and acupuncture as effective therapies to control distressing symptoms at children's end-of-life, and improve their quality of life (QoL).

■

Having a child in palliative care is one of the most anguishing experiences for a family. For pediatric staff there is an added responsibility to provide more than standard medical care during this traumatic time. Going beyond standard medicine, hospices, hospitals and palliative home care services are drawing on complementary and alternative methods, and integrating them into their care to meet the complex physical, emotional and spiritual needs of children and teens who are "living while knowing they are dying" (Kuttner, 2003).

Palliative Care—An Introduction

While comprehensive palliative care is the expected standard of care at the end-of-life (Council on Scientific Affairs, 1996; National Quality Forum, 2006), services for the majority of children with life-limiting or terminal conditions fall significantly below those for adults. In the United States and most countries in the developed world, the vast majority of infants, children, and teenagers at end-of-life do not have access to multidisciplinary pediatric palliative care (PPC) services in their community or at their children's hospital.

PPC is for children and teenagers suffering from a life-threatening or life-limiting condition that threatens their survival into adulthood if curative treatments fail. As a result, PPC may last over many years. According to the Association for Children's Palliative Care (ACT) and the British Royal College of Pediatrics and Child Health (ACT, 2003). PPC "is an active and total approach to care, embracing physical, emotional, social and spiritual elements. It focuses on enhancement of quality of life for the child and support for the family and includes the management of distressing symptoms, provision of respite and care through [disease], death and bereavement."

Integrative approaches that address symptom management, emotional, spiritual and behavioral issues, and include parents, siblings, and school concerns provided by a multi-disciplinary team are now becoming accepted practice. This chapter will examine the current integrative therapeutic interventions for children and teens during the provision of palliative care. Clinical case examples elaborate on the implementation and impact of these approaches.

DISTRESSING SYMPTOMS AT THE END-OF-LIFE

Five studies looking at prevalence of symptoms in 473 children with malignant and non-malignant diseases reveal that the majority of dying children experience pain, vomiting, and dyspnea (Table 25-1). Wolfe et al. (2000a) show in their retrospective study among bereaved parents of 103 cancer patients, that the majority of distressing symptoms were not treated, and when treated, the therapy was commonly ineffective. A dying child is often highly symptomatic, and providing symptom relief is one of the most compelling domains of PPC. Wolfe et al. (2000b) demonstrated that an earlier recognition by both physicians and parents of no realistic chance of cure led to a stronger emphasis on treatment to lessen suffering and integrate palliative care. Consequently, proponents in the field urge that these options be provided early—at best, at diagnosis or early in treatment. As medicine advances, many children are living longer with complex conditions, and the need for ongoing care, support, pain, and symptom management increases over longer periods of time.

MYTHS

Persisting myths and misconceptions have led to inadequate symptom control in children with terminal disease. One of the most enduring is the wrongly held belief

Table 25-1. Symptom prevalence of children with malignant and non-malignant life-limiting conditions during their end-of-life period.

	Dangel, 2001 (Poland) n = 160	Drake, 2003 (Australia) n = 30	Goldman, 2000 (United Kingdom) n = 152	Hongo, 2003 (Japan) n = 28	Wolfe, 2000a (United States) n = 103	Total n = 473	Prevalence in %
Pain	134	16	140	21	84	395	**84**
Fatigue	86	21	79	20	100	297	**63**
Vomiting	101	12	87	16	58	274	**58**
Dyspnea	80	12	62	23	84	261	**55**
Constipation	94	8	58	13	51	224	**47**

that in the management of pain and dyspnea, opioids would hasten death and should only be administered as a last resort. It is a common experience of PPC teams that administering opioids and/or benzodiazepines, together with comfort care to relieve dyspnea and pain, both improves the QoL and prolongs a child's life. Education about the use of opioids and an understanding that tolerance plus physical dependence does not equal addiction, is an important principle in PPC. Furthermore PPC advocates the provision of comfort care, pain and symptom management concurrently with curative treatments. Families no longer have to opt for one or the other. They can pursue both options, and include integrative approaches to maximize the child's quality of life.

SYMPTOM MANAGEMENT

If a child is suffering from pain during the end-of-life, the team providing PPC needs to provide prompt and effective pharmacological pain management. Commonly this requires using strong opioids (e.g., morphine, fentanyl, hydromorphone, oxycodone, or methadone) by different routes of application (e.g., oral, sublingual, buccal, intranasal, transdermal, intravenous, subcutaneous, rectal, but not intramuscular, as it causes unnecessary pain). The use of adjuvant analgesia may be appropriate (e.g., anticonvulsants, tricyclic antidepressants, benzodiazepines, N-methyl-D-aspertate receptor [NMDA] antagonists, bisphosphonates, antispasmodics, low-dose general anesthetics) and anesthetic or neurosurgical options may be required (Friedrichsdorf & Kang, 2007).

Today the state-of-the-art in managing pain and other distressing symptoms at the end of life requires integrating pharmacological with integrative treatment modalities. In our experience a pharmacological approach alone will not provide optimal symptom management. Drawing on a combination of physical methods (e.g., massage, physical therapy, cuddles/rocking from family/friends, transcutaneous electrical nerve stimulation [TENS], or hot water bottle or cold pack) with cognitive-behavioral methods (e.g., guided imagery, hypnosis, biofeedback, or abdominal breathing) or modalities such as acupuncture/acupressure, music, expressive art, provides the best possible symptom management.

Integrative Therapeutic Interventions in Palliative Care

Complementary therapies aim to restore balance and harmony by working simultaneously on physical, mental, emotional, and spiritual needs (McDonald et al., 2006). In British adult hospice and palliative care units, aromatherapy, massage and reflexology are the most popular therapies and are provided in over 90% of these cases (Tavares, 2003). Furthermore, it is recognized that interventions that develop internal coping skills empower children and teens and enhance their quality of life (Sourkes BM, 2000). To date, there are no randomized controlled trials (RCTs) in PPC or RCTs evaluating pharmacological or non-pharmacological treatment strategies for pain and symptom management.

In discussing the frequently used integrative therapeutic interventions in PPC, we will report existing pediatric data and present case studies to indicate the mode of application. Since the different CAM methods are described elsewhere in this book, methodology will be briefly mentioned.

PROVIDER SURVEY ON USING INTEGRATIVE THERAPEUTIC INTERVENTIONS IN PEDIATRIC PALLIATIVE CARE

Background

There is a lack of published data about the prevalence of integrative therapeutic intervention usage in PPC yet.

Methods

The authors sent a questionnaire in November 2007 to the staff of the Pain & Palliative Care and Integrative Medicine Program at the Children's Hospitals and Clinics of Minnesota in Minneapolis, Minnesota, United States (with a daily census of 80–90 children in palliative care) and Canuck Place in Vancouver, British Columbia, Canada (a free standing, in-patient children's hospice that cared for 209 patient and outpatients in 2007).

Part 1 surveyed the usage measured by a 5-point Lickert scale of integrative therapeutic interventions: acupuncture, aromatherapy, biofeedback, culturally based healing traditions, energy medicine (Reiki, therapeutic, and healing touch), guided imagery, hypnosis, massage, music (played to child), music therapy, and relaxation. It also asked for effectiveness on a 5-point Lickert scale of those methods for the respondent's palliative patients.

Part 2 inquired, in open-ended questions, about the respondent's experience of the effectiveness of these integrative therapeutic interventions in treating pain, nausea and vomiting, fatigue, dyspnea, and anxiety in pediatric palliative and end-of-life care.

Results

Twenty-eight PPC professionals returned the survey (Vancouver $n = 8$, Minneapolis $n = 20$): 14 nurses, 4 physicians, 4 social workers/counselors, 2 psychologists, and 1 advanced nurse practitioner, chaplain, child life specialist, and teacher, respectively. Mean experience in PPC was 10.4 years (median 6.5 years).

The most commonly used integrative therapeutic interventions ("often" or "always") for children and teens in pediatric palliative or end-of-life care at the two centers in Minneapolis and Vancouver were relaxation (64%), guided imagery (46%), energy medicine (39%), and hypnosis (32%) (see Figure 25-1).

Responses to the open questions regarding integrative therapeutic modalities for specific distressing symptoms, which the respondent witnessed to be "effective" or "very effective" in palliative and end-of-life care of children, are in Table 25-2.

Discussion

The majority of surveyed PPC professionals experienced integrative therapeutic interventions as effective in managing distressing end-of-life symptoms in their patients. However, only guided imagery and relaxation are reported to be widely used techniques,

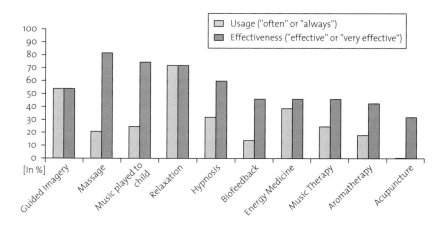

FIGURE 25-1. Responses from 28 pediatric palliative care professionals regarding the subjectively perceived effectiveness of integrative therapeutic interventions in pediatric palliative care, in daily practice.

Table 25-2. Effectiveness of integrative therapeutic interventions in pediatric palliative and end-of-life care for distressing symptoms as experienced by 24 pediatric palliative care professionals

Symptom	Integrative Modality	"Effective" or "Very effective" (%)
Pain	Guided imagery	54
	Massage	54
	Hypnosis	42
	Acupuncture	29
	Biofeedback	25
	Energy work (e.g., Reiki, healing touch)	25
Fatigue	Aromatherapy	29
	Music	29
	Energy work (Reiki, healing touch)	29
Nausea and vomiting	Aromatherapy	54
	Guided imagery	29
	Hypnosis	29
Dyspnea	Guided Imagery	38
	Relaxation	33
	Hypnosis	25
Anxiety	Guided imagery	63
	Hypnosis	46
	Relaxation	46
	Massage	42
	Music	42
	Aromatherapy	33
	Energy work (Reiki, healing touch)	25

furthermore, only a minority of children receive other integrative therapeutic interventions, despite their reported effectiveness.

Mind-Body Medicine

Mind-body medicine focuses on intervention strategies that integrate mind processes with body function and experience in order to promote health. For children and teens, these include relaxation, hypnosis, imagery, meditation, yoga, biofeedback, tai chi, qi gong, cognitive-behavioral therapies, group support, autogenic training, and spiritual practices. Mind-body interventions constitute a major portion of the overall use of CAM by the public (NCCAM, 2007). In 2002, mind-body techniques, including relaxation techniques, meditation, guided imagery, biofeedback, and hypnosis, were used for health reasons by about 17% and prayer was used by 45% of the adult US population (Barnes et al, 2002).

IMAGERY

Imagery is a non-intrusive, child-centered, gentle therapeutic modality, which can provide a meaningful alternate experience when the present reality is fraught with pain, fear, fatigue, or physical tension. Imagery can be used in many ways. Two often-used techniques include, focusing directly on the distressing symptom, engaging with it so that it begins to change, or creating a favorite or familiar image that is a more pleasant alternative to the distressing symptom. Imagery is a precursor to hypnosis, and often used as an induction to hypnotic trance in which change can more rapidly occur.

Pediatric Evidence

When used for pain control, imagery works synergistically with analgesics to reduce pain and discomfort (Kuttner & Stutzer, 1995). This modality enables a child to focus attention on a personally meaningful imagery experience and as the imagery becomes more absorbing, the child or teen may dissociate from pain, increase comfort, reduce anxiety, or alter the pain sensations and perceptions (Kuttner 1997; LeBaron & Zeltzer 1984; Zeltzer & LeBaron 1982). For general principles, the book, *Mortally Wounded* details the clinical use of imagery to ease a patient's anguish at the end of life (Kearney, 1996).

Case Example

Ian was an 8-year-old boy with endstage cancer (rhabdomyosarcoma). He experienced dyspnea during his last week of life. His parents were taught to assist him with guided imagery, which allowed Ian to review and enjoy important events in his life. Together, using a poster board they created a time line, starting with Ian's birth. Ian and his family spent hours each day on this activity. Ian visibly calmed during the sessions, his breathing becoming deeper and more regular. Focusing on his important life events, recreating images and soliciting information from his parents to round out the stories, he created a full and meaningful sense of his own life. Ian died peacefully the day after he completed his full imaginative reminiscing, bringing his own closure and giving his family the comfort of vivid memories of their life together.

HYPNOSIS

Hypnosis involves the cultivation of an altered state of awareness, leading to heightened suggestibility that allows for changes in a child's perception and experience, bypassing conscious effort. In hypnosis the clinician enters the child's world, engaging the child's imagination as the agent of change and creating alternate experiences to promote therapeutic change. In trance, the child addresses distressing symptoms utilizing suggestions by the clinician for altering sensations, perceptions, and increasing comfort (Olness & Kohen, 1996).

PEDIATRIC EVIDENCE

Hypnosis has been used over the last two decades in a number of RCT treatment studies to control pain during invasive medical procedures (e.g., Kuttner, 1988; Liossi, 2002; Zeltzer & LeBaron, 1982). Zeltzer et al. (2002) in a feasibility study successfully combined acupuncture and hypnosis for 33 children to improve chronic pain. Acupuncture, according to traditional Chinese medicine (TCM), and hypnosis comprised of muscle relaxation, the suggestion of going to a safe or favourite place, followed by imagery designed to strengthen the child's sense of mastery in which the child's brain became the cockpit of her airplane.

Case Example 1

Ann was a 17-year-old with a terminal prognosis of lung and abdominal metastases following a malignant bone tumor (osteosarcoma). She had three sessions to teach her self-hypnosis to reduce her anxiety and chronic pain before a radical pelvicectomy for palliation for unremitting bone pain. The hospice chaplain conducted a ceremony with Ann and her family before the amputation to acknowledge the impending loss of her leg.

After surgery she experienced phantom limb pain and found self-hypnosis insufficient. The therapist asked Ann for permission to talk to the part of her brain that perceives pain from her leg, and gave the suggestion that she did not need to listen to this part of the session if she did not want to. This was a confusing concept for Ann and helped to facilitate her trance. Using a hand levitation induction with the creation of a safe place image, the therapist said:

"I'm addressing the part of your brain that sends and receives messages about discomfort and pain from your right leg. You do not need to worry about **not** getting messages from the right leg anymore. The right leg is in a safe place where there is not any discomfort or pain. You can shift your attention to the rest of your body and know that the right leg is safe. It's not part of your job anymore to monitor the right leg."

This message was repeated several times interspersed with messages about how she could now allow herself to relax and be pain free. She experienced a marked decrease of phantom limb pain after this session. Four weeks later she was readmitted to remove lung metastases, and after surgery had a severe pain crisis with a return of phantom limb pain. Another hypnosis session was held. Ann was informed that her brain and neural pathways had been hyper-activated by the pain crisis, and we just needed to remind the part of the brain that had monitored the right leg that it could once again rest and not send messages to the right leg. Her phantom limb pain again subsided to mild and infrequent.

Case Example 2

Katie was a 12-year-old girl with a rare progressive neurological disease, with its onset a year earlier. Previously diagnosed with Asperger's disorder, she was cognitively intact but was losing muscle control and required assistance with her personal care. She started experiencing dyspnea and used an opioid and a benzodiazepine medication to ease this symptom. The social worker had met Katie at her home and spent time with her parents discussing their coping of Katie's terminal diagnosis and their focus on providing comfort care for her. On the next visit she found Katie terrified, lying on the couch in the den experiencing breathlessness. Her mother had given Katie morphine for the dyspnea and was on her knees talking to Katie trying to reassure her. The therapist decided to coach the mother in calming Katie, who was whispering, "I can't breathe!" The therapist knelt beside the mother and talking to both mother and child in a calm voice said:

Katie, I want to help you and your mother breathe. Katie, look into your mother's eyes, she is going to help you breath. Joan (mother), Breathe nice and easy and keep looking into Katie's eyes. Katie, you can now breathe with your mother. She can help you while your medicine starts to work. Your mother has you.

The mother had a hand on each of Katie's arms. Katie quickly slowed her respirations and started to breath with her mother. Her panic quickly subsided. There was no need for an induction, as Katie terrified, was already in a trance. The therapist became directive, and drawing upon their healthy attachment, restructured the experience for both mother and child. The mother naturally joined with her child to help her to regulate her anxiety and her breathing. With this coaching, Katie's mother was able to calm and prevent panic as Katie became weaker and approached death.

BIOFEEDBACK

Biofeedback is a self-regulatory skill that uses electronic or electromechanical equipment to measure and then return information about physiologic functions, which the child uses to gain control over these responses in a desired direction. The functions include, heartbeat, blood pressure, and muscle tension. The feedback is provided in auditory, visual, and multimedia game formats that appeal to children. There are no published adult RCT or pediatric case reports using biofeedback in palliative care.

Case Example

Ravi, a 16-year-old with terminal cancer (recurrent germ-cell tumor and myelodysplastic syndrome) with recurrent chest pain at the site of tumor, leg pain of unknown cause, and recurrent nausea associated with anxiety. He took morphine doses for chest pain, resulting in drowsiness and additional nausea. His coping pattern in the hospital consisted of withdrawal, isolation, little physical activity and keeping his room dark. Ravi denied emotional distress, and when not withdrawn, he frequently used humor. Although Ravi had met psychosocial and CAM providers in the hospital, he reported "those things do not work on me." At home, Ravi met the team psychologist, and agreed to meet again in the outpatient pain and palliative clinic.

Ravi had 13 visits over four months with the psychologist, focused on rapport, emotional support, processing medical events, and address symptoms using relaxation strategies. Initially he reported little relief with guided imagery or diaphragmatic breathing. He tried the biofeedback game on a couple of occasions, then participated in self-hypnosis and relaxation, ultimately acknowledging their benefit and initiating use on his own. The biofeedback program was based on heart rate variability, and Ravi's ability to control heart rate with breathing. It was explained that the better he became at controlling his breathing, the more likely he could control his pain. This was illustrated concretely on the computer screen with changing color patterns as well as transforming images (e.g., the higher the hot air balloon, the better the performance). Ravi said that he saw the biofeedback as a challenge and wanted to get good at it. By coupling the physical challenge with suggestion of pleasant memories or feelings, Ravi enjoyed the activity and challenged himself to evoke the relaxation response. The biofeedback program, with its technology and entertainment provided him with a personally acceptable technique suiting his age, personality and avoidant coping style.

YOGA

Yoga is a 5000-year-old practice from Ayurvedic medicine that combines breathing exercises, physical postures, and meditation. It is intended to calm the nervous system and balance the body, mind, and spirit (NCCAM, 2007). Experience suggests that yoga can be of benefit during palliation if the child or teen is already familiar with the practice, has used diaphragmatic breathing, or has favorite postures (asanas) that ease pain, reduce anxiety or discomfort, such as the "child's pose" or "cat stretch."

Pediatric Evidence

While there are no published pediatric case reports about the use of yoga in palliative care, yoga has been studied in a RCT to treat adolescents with recurrent abdominal pain and irritable bowel syndrome and found to significantly lower functional disability, reduce anxiety and hold promise for reducing GI symptoms (Kuttner et al., 2006).

MUSIC

Music has been used for centuries to soothe distress. Defined as an intentional auditory stimulus, it has organized elements including melody, rhythm, harmony, timbre, form and style (Kemper & Danhauer, 2005). Repetitive listening allows the listener to identify and predict sounds (Standley JM, 2002) and is thought to help reorganize and reregulate the nervous system, improving mood.

Pediatric Evidence

There is evidence that classical music and lullabies among premature infants decreases distressed behavior and episodes of oxygen desaturation and increase weight gain and non-nutritive sucking (Caine, 1991; Collins, 1991; Standley & Moore, 1995; Standley, 1998; Standley, 2002). The results from a recent Italian prospective RCT found that pediatric patients (4–13 years) exposed to music during venipunctures demonstrated significantly lower distress and pain intensity in the music group compared with the control group before, during, and after blood sampling (Caprilli et al., 2007). Songs and music performed by "professional" musicians, the authors concluded, have a beneficial effect in reducing distress before, during, and after blood tests and that the presence of musicians has a minor, but yet significant, effect on needle insertion pain. A Norwegian case series with four children with advanced cancer (two of them with terminal disease progression) showed that music therapy changed the children from passive recipients of care to being socially active (Aasgaard, 2001). Music therapy improves the QoL at the end-of-life and can ease communication between child and family.

Case Example 1

John was a 2-year-old with arthrogryposis and brain stem lesion resulting in muscle spasticity with extreme muscle weakness. He had poor chest wall expansion for respiration with compromised perfusion. For his first 8 months of life, he did not move his skeletal muscles at all. As he grew older he began to move tentatively with great effort. His parents played music for him from birth and sang songs to him daily. They noticed that his breathing regulated and began to go in sync with the musical rhythms. He relaxed and his color improved. By age two he had not yet moved his entire body in a coordinated fashion, but now began to move his arms and legs. One day as he lay on one end of the living room floor on a blanket, his father put a new LP on the stereo: Keith Jarrett's "The Köln Concert." The speakers were on the far end of the living room. John rolled across the floor until he reached the point exactly midway between the speakers. He stayed there listening to the entire jazz piano concert. John received music therapy from ages 3 to 5, enjoying working on pronation and supination of his wrists playing percussion instruments, and learning to direct music. Years later now 22-year-old, John plays percussion with a band, researches and catalogues music as a hobby, and shares his love of music with friends and college classmates.

Case Example 2

Three-year-old Angela was actively dying at home. Her cancer (neuroblastoma) had relapsed, and she was being treated for severe dyspnea. With parents at her side, she showed signs of restlessness and anxiety as her breathing became more difficult. Oxygen was not improving Angela's dyspnea. When the hospice chaplain arrived, he asked what Angela enjoyed most. When they told him she loved music, he suggested they sing some of her favorite songs. With the familiar music and her parents' continued closeness, Angela relaxed and her breathing calmed considerably. Music was an important part of her last hours, and her parents loved being able to provide this comfort for her.

ART

Art activities have been shown to be particularly helpful for children and teens to express their feelings and difficult experiences in a child-centred manner (Kuttner, 2003). Often children don't have the vocabulary to express their feelings, or the feelings are too painful or awkward to discuss (Devlin, 2006). Art provides a non-verbal expressive medium to convey these complex, confusing emotions and experiences in a way that is personally satisfying.

Pediatric Evidence

Case reports show the effective use of art therapy in facilitating expressive communication and coming to terms with grief both for a lost family member and for children affected with an incurable disease (Devlin, 1996). Sourkes (2007) shows the clinical value, honesty and poignancy of children's drawings, graphically depicting their psychological experience as they struggle with a life-threatening illness.

VIRTUAL REALITY

Virtual reality is a recent technology that fully absorbs and stimulates the human senses giving the feeling of being in another world. As an intervention with adult cancer patients it decreased fatigue and emesis (Oyama, 2000). With children it is a popular form of play experience.

Pediatric Evidence

Since 2005, the investigative clinical research using virtual reality has accelerated, bringing new evidence of its therapeutic potential for the alleviation of pain as a distraction technique during procedural pain (Das et al., 2005; Gold et al., 2006; Lange et al., 2006; Magora et al., 2005) As yet here are no published pediatric case reports about the use of virtual reality in palliative care, although some hospices use these devices for play and diversion with children who are still mobile.

MULTISENSORY ENVIRONMENT (SNOEZELEN)

Hospices have adopted the word "Snoezelen" from the Dutch meaning sniffling and dozing to describe a multisensory room supplied with changing colored lights across the walls, music, aroma, tactile stimulation, and taste. These sensory changes create a dusky, attractively lit room, providing a soothing environment for ailing children (Schofield, 2003). Many freestanding inpatient children's hospices incorporate a multisensory room on site. As yet, there are no published pediatric case reports about the use of a multisensory environment in palliative care.

AROMATHERAPY

Hundreds of receptor cells have been identified in the nasal passages which relay smell to the brain (Balacs, 1992). Essential oils are highly concentrated non-oily, fragrant substances extracted from plants by distillation, which evaporates readily. Aromatherapy is thought to work by promoting the release of neurotransmitters once the nasal receptor cells are stimulated by these distilled fragrances (Kyle, 2006). Sandalwood oil was effective in reducing anxiety (Kyle, 2006). In the United Kingdom, aromatherapy combined with massage is the most widely used complementary therapy in nursing practice (Macmillan Cancer Relief, 2002; Rankin-Box, 1997).

Pediatric Evidence

Styles reports that aromatherapy was beneficial in managing the distressing symptoms for 20 children with HIV disease in palliative care (Styles, 1997).

Case Example 1

Thirteen-year-old Jasmine received aggressive chemotherapy for osteosarcoma in her pelvis. Her nausea was severe, subsiding only with scheduled dosing of diphenhydramine, lorazepam, and ondansetron. Jasmine had much difficulty with the sedating effects of the antihistamine and benzodiazepine. She agreed to try aromatherapy. Essential oil of ginger, considered to have beneficial affects on the GI tract, was introduced using a diffuser in her hospital room. Jasmine responded beautifully. Dipenhydramine and lorazepam became less necessary to control nausea. Together with diffused aromatic ginger, ondansetron became Jasmine's only scheduled medication for nausea.

Case Example 2

When Marta, a 6-year-old with a retinoblastoma, was introduced to opioids for localized pain, she experienced urinary retention. Marta had become increasingly fearful as she underwent treatments and procedures. It was clear to her care providers that urinary catheterization, another invasive procedure, would be difficult for Marta to tolerate. Two drops of oil of peppermint, known to relax the urinary sphincters was dropped into the "hat" placed in the commode, and Marta was able to urinate without catheterization.

Manipulative and Body-Based Practices

Manipulative and body-based practices is a heterogeneous group of integrative interventions and therapies, which include chiropractic and osteopathic manipulation, massage therapy, Tui Na, reflexology, Rolfing, Bowen technique, Trager bodywork, Alexander technique, Feldenkrais method, and a host of others (NCCAM, 2007).

MASSAGE

Massage includes pressing, rubbing, and moving muscles and other soft body tissues primarily using the hands and fingers. The aim is to increase blood-flow and oxygen to the massaged area (NCCAM, 2007). Massage was helpful reducing anxiety and enhancing hope in cancer patients (Downer et al., 1994; Wilkinson et al., 1999). Massage Therapy in a pediatric hospice setting can have significantly unique demands, and therefore the term massage can be confusing. Hence the terminology is sometimes being changed into "Integrative Touch" or "Compassionate Touch" (Beider et al., 2007).

Pediatric Evidence

While there are no published pediatric case reports about the use of massage in palliative care, massage has been effective in ameliorating pain and distress in infants (Fields, 2002).

Case Example

Amy, a 17-year-old girl diagnosed with metastasized colon cancer, had a tumultuous psychosocial history of abandonment by her biologic mother and abuse by an adoptive parent. When she was diagnosed with terminal disease, her newly retired paternal grandparents offered their home to her. In addition to psychosocial supports and medications for pain management, home-based massage therapy was offered, which at first she shyly refused. With encouragement, Amy accepted reporting much comfort and relief from these sessions. For her, massage therapy provided added benefits. Human touch was especially helpful in view of her troubled background with few close positive human interactions. She also had opportunities to relax and talk about her concerns with the therapist. Medically, massage assisted Amy with circulatory problems that were developing because of rapid tumor growth and decreased activity. Amy reported better sleep quality and less muscle tightness and pain after she began regular massage therapy sessions and her caregivers noted an overall improvement in her anxiety level.

REFLEXOLOGY

Reflexology is the process of gentle, but firm manipulations of the feet and/or hands to stimulate specific reflex points of the body. This is based on the principle that there are reflexes running along the body, which terminate in the feet and the hands, and that the body's organs and systems are represented on the skin's surface (Hodgson, 2000; Norman & Cowan, 1989). First documents describing the use of reflexology are dated to 2300 BC in Egypt (Lockett, 1992). A Japanese study of 20 terminally ill cancer patients showed that combined modality treatment consisting of aromatherapy, footsoak, and reflexology was found effective for alleviating fatigue at end-of-life (Kohara et al., 2004). There are no pediatric case reports on the use of reflexology in palliative care.

Energy Medicine

The National Center for Complementary and Alternative Medicine describes Energy Medicine as

> …based on the concept that human beings are infused with a subtle form of energy. Vital energy is believed to flow throughout the material human body, but it has not been unequivocally measured by means of conventional instrumentation…Herbal medicine, acupuncture, acupressure, moxibustion, and cupping, for example, are all believed to act by correcting imbalances in the internal biofield, such as by restoring the flow of qi through meridians to reinstate health…Examples of practices that focus on these energy fields include:
>
> Acupuncture and acupressure
> Reiki and Johrei (both of Japanese origin)
> Qi gong (a Chinese practice)
> Healing touch/Therapeutic touch in which the therapist identifies imbalances and corrects a client's energy by passing his or her hands over the patient
> Intercessory prayer, in which a person intercedes through prayer on behalf of another
> These approaches are among the most controversial of CAM practices because neither the external energy fields nor their therapeutic effects have as yet been demonstrated convincingly by any biophysical means. (NCCAM, 2007)

Despite the controversy, world-wide acceptance of these modalities has made them increasingly accepted in Australia, Europe, and North America, and therapeutic touch practiced by nurses in North American hospitals has gained considerable credibility.

ACUPUNCTURE

Acupuncture includes a family of procedures originating in TCM. Acupuncture is the stimulation of specific point on the body by a variety of techniques, including the insertion of thin metal needles through the skin, to remove blockages in the flow of qi, and to restore and maintain health (NCCAM, 2007).

TCM approaches the child in a holistic manner, recognizing the inseparable relationship of the body mind and spirit (Flaws, 1997). TraditionalChinese medicine teaches that, when a person is in a state of health, Qi or life energy is flowing smoothly through meridians or pathways that connect all systems of the human being, physical, mental and spiritual (Kaptchuk, 1983). When a child suffers from pain, associated symptoms, such as anxiety, stress, depression, insomnia, loss of appetite are also treated. Pain is considered a symptom of the stagnation of the flow of life energy or Qi. TCM treatments aim to restore a balance of these systems and the smooth flow of life energy in a coherent approach (Maciocia, 1994). Improving QoL is the main objective of TCM treatment. There are no published adult RCTs or pediatric case reports about the use of acupuncture in palliative care.

Case Example

Eight-year-old Corey's initial complaints about back and leg pain started innocently with progressive difficulty walking. An extensive medical workup diagnosed Neuroblastoma in his spinal cord. He had multiple surgeries and was treated with multiple trials of chemotherapy, conventional spine and brain radiation, gamma knife, proton beam sterotactic radiosurgery and experimental drug protocols.

Two years later, with uncontrollable tumor spread, escalating pain and failing neurological function, his medical team met with his family to discuss discontinuation of therapies including OT and PT. Corey had lost the ability to walk and became incontinent for bowel and bladder, and his death was thought to be imminent. With a palliative treatment plan in effect, Corey was discharged home with an intravenous opioid (fentanyl) infusion pump. His neurosurgeons, having little to offer with standard Western support, referred him for TCM to salvage some quality of life

Corey's mother was skeptical that Chinese medicine offered her son any hope of relief when Western medicine had failed. But on the advice of her son's neurosurgeon, she took him to the TCM clinic. On his initial visit, Corey was sitting in the waiting room, banging his head against the wall crying and moaning that his leg pain was unbearable. His fentanyl infusion pump had been increased to deliver 975 µg per hour; he had not slept in 3 days and had been crying uncontrollably. Acupuncture began by placing two 40-gauge acupuncture needles (the width of a strand of hair) in appropriate points, with immediate effect. Corey fell asleep within 2 minutes for the first time in days and continued to sleep for 90 minutes. He awoke reporting that his pain was significantly lower, told his mom he was hungry and wanted to stop at Taco Bell. Calmed, he asked if he could return to the clinic. We scheduled Corey for treatment twice a week. Corey received acupuncture, acupressure, Tui Na medical massage, moxibustion, herbal therapy, and seed patch therapy. All were aimed at improving quality of life.

Corey's dose of opioid analgesia was not providing adequate pain relief and he had severe anxiety attacks—terrified that his pain was uncontrollable—insomnia, anorexia, and depression. Corey was treated with the National Acupuncture Detoxification Association (NADA) protocol, a five-point auricular (ear) acupuncture treatment utilized in the treatment of addiction, tolerance, and pain (Oleson, 2002). Corey was also treated with main meridian acupuncture, acupressure, and moxibustion (Scott, 1986).

Corey responded wonderfully. After 6 acupuncture treatments his fentanyl dose was reduced to less than 200 μg per hour. By week 5 he was rotated to 50 μg per hour fentanyl patches. Corey experienced significant improvement in quality of life, participating in daily activities, interacting with family and most significantly, his pain was well-controlled. At the beginning of each visit he would share these activities and joyfully recount playing games or funny episodes of a Sponge Bob cartoon. He was sleeping well and enjoying meals. With his QOL improving, the scope of his TCM treatments expanded to address his neurological deficits such as weakness and loss of bowel and bladder control. Corey improved so much that his physicians recommended that physical and occupational therapy be reinitiated. By the 4th month of treatment Corey was able to stand and walk down the hall wearing leg braces.

Corey's "wish" was to attend 3rd grade, a fantasy previously impossible. Due to his illness, he had spent little time in school with other children. He wanted to be like other 8-year-olds and go to school. He was so excited preparing for his first day that he brought his new school backpack to the clinic to share. Corey started 3rd grade. He attended school for the first half of the year until a reoccurrence of spinal tumors led to his death. Corey passed peacefully with his family and loved ones by his side.

When the parent or caregiver is also supported with treatment and their stress is addressed, the child can receive greater benefits from their own treatments (Jarret, 1998). Over the course of Corey's 17 months of treatment, his mother also received acupuncture and herbal therapy to support her through a most difficult time. Although his diagnosis never changed, he lived many months longer than expected. During this time, he enjoyed a dramatically improved QoL.

SHIATSU

Shiatsu is a Japanese body therapy, developed from an ancient form of massage, that works on the energetic pathways (meridians) and points of access (tsubos) in order to harmonize the energy flow (qi). The philosophy is rooted in the theory of TCM, which holds that energy imbalances cause ill health and that by rebalancing the qi, relief may be experienced (Cheesman et al., 2001). No pediatric case reports about the use of shiatsu in palliative care have been published.

ENERGY HEALING

Energy healing is predicated on a structured system of dynamic energy surrounding and penetrating the human body; auras and chakras (energy centers) within individuals and from the Universal Energy Field. This energy system can be impacted, influenced, balanced, and strengthened or weakened by the person or other people. People can be trained to balance, strengthen, and repair their own and others' energy systems. A well functioning energy system allows the human body's own self-healing mechanisms to function at optimal levels. At this time there are no published adult RCTs or pediatric case reports about the use of energy healing in palliative care. However, Reiki and therapeutic touch are frequently used in hospices and pediatric hospitals to alleviate pain and soothe and settle distressed children.

Case Example 1

Lulu, a young adolescent Hispanic American girl was diagnosed with leukodystrophy and global developmental delay. She was gradually losing her physical and cognitive abilities, and at the time we knew her, she was only able to speak in short sentences. She crawled around in a hopping rabbit sort of fashion. She was a physically beautiful girl with a very loving spirit, and an innocence that people often referred to as angelic. Her parents called saying that they were upset because she was "seeing things." Speaking with mom at the next visit she explained that she would walk into Lulu's room and she would be talking and playing, but there was no-one else there. This upset both parents, as they worried Lulu was losing her mind. When we asked Lulu about the experience, she said that she had two or three playmates that visited regularly, and was surprised her mom could not see them. She said they stayed a while and then would go away, but they always said they would be back to play some more. She was happy to have their visits, and seemed absolutely comfortable with it all. After several reports, we began to postulate that friends "from the other side" were indeed visiting, so that when Lulu did die, she would have playmates in the next life. Lulu's mother was further comforted when Lulu's energy system, assessed during healing touch sessions, showed an increasing brightness and openness of Lulu's spiritual chakras. This provided a new conceptual framework for her, and "normalized" the experience for the family, allowing them to continue to relate to Lulu as they always had. They were no longer afraid.

Case Example 2 (Craniosacral Therapy)

Greg was an infant with a genetically inherited terminal neuro-degenerative disease. He had a 5-year-old healthy sister and parents in their late 20's, who had previously lost a baby to the same disease. They were well-educated European Americans who were pro-environment and health-food-oriented people. Caring for Greg was a 24-hour job because of his neuroirritability. He needed to be held constantly, and even then his high-pitched cries went on for hours. Various medications were tried to soothe his hyperactive nervous system and decrease his sensitivity, but nothing worked until craniosacral therapy was provided by a trained nurse. This gentle technique, physically holding the baby's cranium and slowly "unwinding" tension, calmed him, and this effect lasted for hours, sometimes for days. It was a miracle to the family. At last they could all have some good QoL. Greg's mom became trained and was able to continue daily craniosacral therapy with Greg. He lived a much calmer and more peaceful life with his family until he died in his parents' arms.

RITUALS/PRAYER

Case Example

When Britta, a teenaged patient with metastasized osteosarcoma of the left leg was facing an above-the-knee palliative amputation, she became anxious and withdrawn. Her family was unable to comfort her with explanations about the efficacy of treatment. The team chaplain offered to do a ritual leg blessing for Britta. In the session, Britta's upcoming loss was acknowledged, and she was given the opportunity to reflect on the blessing her leg had been to her, how it had served her, and how its sacrifice was now providing her with the gift of improved quality-of-life. After this session, Britta approached surgery with greater acceptance in the face of her devastating loss.

6. Culturally Based Healing Traditions

Pediatric palliative care needs to be provided within families' spiritual-cultural boundaries. First-generation immigrants may frequently adhere to spiritual and cultural practices, and at a time of imminent loss may be hesitant to embrace Western medical practices. It is paramount for the palliative care team to learn about their beliefs and practices, and where possible include rituals and practices important to the family and their culture.

Case Example

Chue was a 10-year-old born in the United States with parents who were first-generation immigrants, highly identified with their traditional Hmong culture. Chue had a brainstem glioma and when referred to palliative care was given a prognosis of less than a few months. He was aspirating significantly with a series of secondary pneumonias. Mom was encouraged not to feed him as this posed aspiration risks as his capacity to suck/ swallow continued to deteriorate. He was fairly non-verbal when we met him, but engaged actively with his parents and three siblings through vocalizations and eye contact.

It was important to his mother to feed him orally, though this took her many hours. She reported it was not a problem, and related he did better with the special way she took care to feed him. She provided Chue with a tea or soup made of traditional herbal medicines, sent to her by a friend in Laos. She brewed/cooked these dried herbs in a large pot of water, and spooned the traditional medicine into his mouth in a painstaking way. She couldn't say what was in it, and eventually the medical care team decided not to delve further as there appeared to be no drug interactions.

Chue's condition progressed at a much slower rate than had been anticipated. He had no further pneumonias, and though he aspirated, he seemed pretty stable. Mom however, became distressed and agitated. After a few visits and with effort to understand her upset she disclosed that the family had no money to pay the shaman to perform the essential traditional rituals and she was fearful about what would happen to her son's spirit. She would not disclose what these rituals were; only that money was needed to pay the shaman to obtain the chicken and other materials for the rituals.

Through philanthropic funds in our program, the family was given the $200 for this ritual. They contracted and held the ceremony privately in accordance with their traditions. We were not given information about it. After the ritual, mom's demeanor and mood seemed lighter, and she reported that she was deeply relieved knowing they had fulfilled their obligations to their son's spirit, and whatever happened, he would be all-right. Chue outlived the original prognosis by over a year, and was comfortable and apparently happy with his mother's care. He required very little pain medicine throughout his last year of life.

Summary

Pediatric palliative care is an emerging new field of care for children and teens with life-limiting and life threatening illness. It draws on all commonly used Western-based medical treatments as well as complementary and alternative treatments to attain the best patient comfort and ease at end of life. While there are no RCTs evaluating the use of these integrative therapeutic interventions—interestingly the same holds true for pharmacologic treatments in PPC. Both published case studies and our personal experience strongly endorse integrative treatment modalities, especially imagery, hypnosis, music, aromatherapy, massage, therapeutic/healing touch, and acupuncture as effective therapies to control distressing symptoms at a child's end-of-life, and improve quality of life for them. Parents and other caregivers can be trained in some of these methods empowering their capacity to provide care. Participation in a child's end-of-life care lessens bereavement complications in families, and promotes parents' ability to come to terms with the loss of their child.

Acknowledgments

We would like to thank Llyn Bjorklund, RN, Cyndee Daughtry, LICSW, Christine Gibbon, PhD, LP, and Stacy Remke, LICSW, from the Pain & Palliative Care Program at the Children's Hospitals and Clinics of Minnesota for their contribution of case examples.

REFERENCES

Aasgaard, T. (2001). An ecology of love: Aspects of music therapy in the pediatric oncology environment. *Journal of Palliative Care, 17*(3), 177–181.

ACT: Association for Children with Life-threatening or Terminal Conditions and their Families and The Royal College of Paediatrics and Child Health. (2003). *A guide to the development of children's palliative care services* (2nd ed.). Bristol, UK: ACT.

Balacs, T. (1992). Research reports. *International Journal of Clinical Aromatherapy, 4*(1), 6–8.

Barnes, P. M., Powell-Griner, E., McFann, K., & Nahin, R. L. (2004). Complementary and alternative medicine use among adults: United States, 2002. CDC Advance Data Report #343.

Beider, S., Mahrer, N. E., & Gold, J. I. (2007). Pediatric massage therapy: An overview for clinicians. *Pediatric Clinics of North America, 54*, 1025–1041.

Caine, J. (1991). The effect of music on the selected stress behaviors, weight, caloric and formula intake, and length of hospital stay of premature and low birth weight neonates in a newborn intensive care unit. *Journal of Music Therapy, 28*, 180–192.

Caprilli, S., Anastasi, F., Grotto, R., Abeti, M., & Messeri, A. (2007). Interactive Music as a Treatment for Pain and Stress in Children During Venipuncture: A Randomized Prospective Study. *Journal of Developmental and Behavioral Pediatrics, 28*(5), 399–403.

Cheesman, S., Christian, R., & Cresswell, J. (2001). Exploring the value of shiatsu in palliative care day services. *International Journal of Palliative Nursing, 7*(5), 234–239.

Collins, S. K., & Kuck, K. (1991). Music therapy in the neonatal intensive care unit. *Neonatal Network, 9*, 23–26.

Council on Scientific Affairs, American Medical Association. (1996). Good care of the dying patient. *The journal of the American Medical Association, 275*, 474–478.

Dangel, T. (2001). *Domowa opieka paliatywna nad dziecmi w Polsce.* Department of Palliative Care—Institute for Mother and Child, Warsaw, Poland.

Das, D. A., Grimmer, K. A., Sparnon, A. L., McRae, S. E., & Thomas, B. H. (2005). The efficacy of playing a virtual reality game in modulating pain for children with acute burn injuries: A randomized controlled trial. *BMC pediatrics, 5*(1), 1.

Devlin, B. (2006). The art of healing and knowing in cancer and palliative care. *International Journal of Palliative Nursing, 12*(1), 16–19.

Devlin, B. (1996). Helping children to grieve. *International Journal of Palliative Nursing, 2*(2), 63–70.

Downer, S. M., Cody, M. M., & McCluskey, P. (1994). Pursuit and practice of complementary therapies by cancer patients receiving conventional treatments. *British Medical Journal, 309,* 86–89.

Drake, R., Frost, J., & Collins, J. J. (2003). The symptoms of dying children. *Journal of Pain and Symptom Management, 26*(1), 594–603.

Field, T. (2002). Preterm infant massage therapy studies: An American approach. *Seminars in Neonatology, 7,* 487–494.

Flaws, B. (1997). *TCM pediatrics. Key points in diagnosing children* (pp. 15–26). Boulder, CO: Blue Poppy Press.

Freeman, L., Caserta, M., Lund, D., Rossa, S., Dowdy, A., & Partenheimer, A. (2006). Music thanatology: Prescriptive harp music as palliative care for the dying patient. *The American Journal of Hospice & Palliative Care, 23*(2), 100–104.

Friedrichsdorf, S. J., & Kang, T. (2007). The management of pain in children with life-limiting illnesses. *Pediatric Clinics of North America, 54,* 645–672.

Gold, J. I., Kim, S. H., Kant, A. J., Joseph, M. H., & Rizzo, A. S. (2006). Effectiveness of virtual reality for pediatric pain distraction during IV placement. *Cyberpsychological Behavior, 9*(2), 207–212.

Goldman, A., Beardsmore, S., & Hunt, J. (1990). Palliative care for children with cancer-home, hospital, or hospice? *Archives of Disease in Childhood, 65,* 641–643.

Hodgson, H. (2000). Does reflexology impact on cancer patients' quality of life? *Nursing Standard, 14*(31), 33–38.

Hongo, T., Watanabe, C., Okada, S., Inoue, N., Yajima, S., Fujii, Y., & Ohzeki, T. (2003). Analysis of the circumstances at the end of life in children with cancer: Symptoms, suffering and acceptance. *Pediatrics International, 45*(1), 60–664.

Kaptchuk, T. (1983) *The web that has no weaver. The fundamental substances* (pp. 34–47). Chicago, Ill: Congdon & Weed, Inc.

Kearney, M. (1996) *Mortally wounded.* New York: Scribner.

Kemper, K. J., & Danhauer, S. C. (2005). Music as therapy. *The Southern Medical Journal, 98*(3), 282–288.

Kohara, H., Miyauchi, T., Suehiro, Y., Ueoka, H., Takeyama, H., & Morita, T. (2004). Combined modality treatment of aromatherapy, footsoak, and reflexology relieves fatigue in patients with cancer. *Journal of Palliative Medicine, 7*(6), 791–796.

Kuttner, L., Chambers, C. T., Hardial, J., Israel, D. M., Jacobsen, K., & Evans, K. (2006). A randomized trial of yoga for adolescents with irritable bowel syndrome. *Pain Research & Management, 11,* 217–223.

Kuttner, L. (2003). "Making Every Moment Count" documentary(38 min) on pediatric palliative care directed by Leora Kuttner, distributed by The National Film Board of Canada 800-267-7710 [Canada & International] and Fanlight 800-937-4113 (US).

Kuttner, L. (1997). Mind-body methods of pain management. In S. J. Weisman (Ed.)., *Child and Adolescent Psychiatric Clinics of North America, 6*(4), 783–795.

Kuttner, L., Bowman, M., & Teasdale, M. (1988). Psychological treatment of distress, pain and anxiety for young children with cancer. *Journal of Developmental and Behavioral Pediatrics, 9,* 374–381.

Kuttner, L., & Stutzer, C. (1995). Imagery for children in pain: Experiencing threat to life and the approach of death. In D. W. Adams & E. J. Deveau (Eds.), *Beyond the innocence of childhood* (Vol. 2, pp. 251–265). New York: Baywood Publishing Co.

Kyle, G. (2006). Evaluating the effectiveness of aromatherapy in reducing levels of anxiety in palliative care patients: Results of a pilot study. *Complementary Therapies in Clinical Practice, 12*(2), 148–155.

Lange, B., Williams, M., & Fulton, I. (2006). *Pediatric Pain Letter, 8,* 1.

LeBaron, S., & Zeltzer, L. K. (1984). Behavioral interventions for reducing chemotherapy-related nausea and vomiting in adolescents with cancer. *The Journal of Adolescent Health, 5,* 178–182.

Lockett, J. (1992). Reflexology—a nursing tool? *The Australian Nurses' Journal, 22*(1), 14–15.

Macmillan Cancer Relief. (2002). *Directory of complementary therapy services in UK cancer care: Public and voluntary services.* London: Macmillan Cancer Relief.

Magora, F., Cohen, S., Shochina, M., & Dayan, E. (2005). *IMAJ, 8,* 261.

National Center for Complementary and Alternative Medicine [NCCAM]. (2007). http://nccam. nih.gov/health/

National Quality Forum: A National Framework and Preferred Practices for Palliative and Hospice Quality. (2006). A Consensus Report.

Norman, L., & Cowan, T. (1989). *The reflexology handbook.* London, Piatkus.

Oleson, T. (2002). *Auriculotherapy manual: Chinese and Western systems of ear acupuncture. Theoretical basis of auriculotherapy* (pp. 9–20). Edinburgh, UK: Churchill Livingstone.

Olness, K., & Kohen, D. P. (1996). *Hypnosis and hypnotherapy with children,* (3rd ed.). New York, NY: Guilford Press.

Oyama, H., Kaneda, M., Katsumata, N., Akechi, T., & Ohsuga, M. (2000). Using the bedside wellness system during chemotherapy decreases fatigue and emesis in cancer patients. *Journal of Medical Systems, 24*(3), 173–182.

Rankin-Box, D. (1997). Therapies in practice: A survey assessing nurses' use of complementary therapies. *Complementary Therapies in Nursing & Midwifery, 3,* 92–99.

Schofield, P. (2003). A pilot study into the use of a multisensory environment (Snoezelen) within a palliative day-care setting. *International Journal Palliative Nursing, 9*(3), 124–130.

Schroeder-Sheker, T. (1994). Music for the dying: A personal account of the new field of music-thanatology—history, theories, and clinical narratives. *Journal of Holistic Nursing, 12*(1), 83–99.

Scott, J. (1986). *Acupuncture in the treatment of children. Using acupuncture in the treatment of children* (pp. 80–91). Seattle, Washington: Eastland Press.

Scott, J. (1986). *Acupuncture in the treatment of children. Differences between children and adults* (pp. 3–8). Seattle, Washington: Eastland Press.

Smith, M. (1979). Acupuncture & healing in drug detoxification. *American Journal of Acupuncture, 7,* 97–107.

Sourkes, B. M. (2000). Psychotherapy with the dying child. In H. Chochinov & W. Breitbart (Eds.), *Psychiatric dimensions of palliative medicine* (pp. 265–272). New York, Oxford University Press.

Sourkes, B. M. (2007). Armfuls of time: The psychological experience of the child with a life-threatening illness. *Medical Principles and Practice, 16*(suppl 1), 37–41.

Standley, J. M. (2002). A meta-analysis of the efficacy of music therapy for premature infants. *Journal of Pediatric Nursing, 17,* 107–113.

Standley, J. M. (1998). The effect of music and multimodal stimulation on responses of premature infants in neonatal intensive care. *Pediatric Nursing, 24,* 532–538.

Standley, J. M., & Moore, R. S. (1995). Therapeutic effects of music and mother's voice on premature infants. *Pediatric Nursing, 21,* 509–512.

Styles, J. L. (1997). The use of aromatherapy in hospitalized children with HIV disease. *Complementary Therapies in Nursing & Midwifery, 3,* 16–20.

Tavares, M. (2003). *National guidelines for the use of complementary therapies in supportive and palliative care*. London: Prince of Wales Foundation for Integrated Care.

Wolfe, J., Grier, H. E., Klar, N., Levin, S. B., Ellenbogen, J. M., Salem-Schatz, S., et al. (2000a). Symptoms and suffering at the end of life in children with cancer. *The New England Journal of Medicine, 342*, 326–333.

Wolfe, J., Klar, N., Grier, H. E., Duncan, J., Salem-Schatz, S., Emanuel, E. J., et al. (2000b). Understanding of prognosis among parents of children who died of cancer: Impact on treatment goals and integration of palliative care. *The Journal of the American Medical Association, 284*(19), 2469–2475.

Zeltzer, L. K., Tsao J. C., Stelling, C., Powers, M., Levy, S., & Waterhouse, M. (2002). A phase I study on the feasibility and acceptability of an acupuncture/hypnosis intervention for chronic pediatric pain. *Journal Of Pain and Symptom Management, 24*(4), 437–446.

Zeltzer, L. K., & LeBaron, S. (1982). Hypnosis and non-hypnotic technique for reduction of pain and anxiety during painful procedures in children and adolescents with cancer. *Journal of Pediatrics, 101*, 1032–1035.

26

Integrative Pediatric Primary Care

LAWRENCE D. ROSEN

KEY CONCEPTS

- Primary care is collaboration between healthcare providers and families. Communication is key to success.
- The medical home paradigm provides a framework for integrative primary care.
- Primary care should focus on the promotion of wellness.
- Common problems during infancy, like colic, atopy, and ear infections, are best addressed from an evidence-guided integrative perspective and offer opportunities to promote wellness and healing concepts.
- Immunizations should be discussed openly and honestly by all parties. Families have many concerns and questions which are best answered through respectful dialogue.
- The "primary care" of a child is shared by many: pediatricians or other healthcare practitioners, the child's family and community, and the child herself.
- It is not so much the use of any specific CAM therapy that defines someone as an integrative pediatrician but the belief that healing is inexorably bound to the connection between practitioner and patient. In no area of healing practice is this more evident and needed than in primary care.
- Individualizing a treatment plan is extremely important in the management of colic, as some approaches work quite well for some families and not at all for others.
- Randomized controlled trials have demonstrated that probiotics (Lactobacillus GG) given prenatally to women and then postnatally to either breastfeeding mothers or directly to formula-fed infants can reduce the incidence of atopic dermatitis by half in those infants at high risk for up to 7 years postnatally.

- Given the links between immune dysregulation and the development of atopic phenomena, a growing number of practitioners are concerned about the potential contribution of vaccines in a subset of children to disease expression.
- Primary care practitioners, in ideal position to adopt and advocate the medical home paradigm, should engage their patients and families in respectful, collaborative dialogue regarding the use of CAM therapies. As the number of children with special healthcare needs grows, and as more families develop an interest in a holistic model of care for prevention and treatment, integrative primary care is poised to become the standard of healthcare.

Introduction

Primary care, in the world of medicine, is conventionally defined as "the activity of a healthcare provider who acts as a first point of consultation for all patients" (Primary Care—Wikipidia, 2007). Historically, many types of healthcare practitioners have served as primary care providers for children, including pediatricians, family practice doctors, nurses, and alternative healthcare practitioners. In truth, the "primary care" of a child is shared by many: pediatricians or other healthcare practitioners, the child's family and community, and the child herself. The scope of primary care includes a focus on prevention and well-care, and implies a comprehensive, collaborative and coordinated approach exemplified by the medical home model developed by the American Academy of Pediatrics (AAP, 2002). The medical home model is holistic in the sense that it views the health of a child as intricately connected to the child's environment—her family, her community and the world around her. And holistic pediatrics—the concept of nurturing the whole child toward optimal wellness—is simply "good medicine," as noted by Dr. Kathi Kemper in her Presidential Address to the Ambulatory Pediatric Association (Kemper, 2000).

Integrative pediatrics, a holistic practice that includes an examined integration of complementary and alternative medicine (CAM) and conventional therapies, is ideally suited for primary care. In addition to supporting medical home tenets, integrative pediatrics emphasizes a collaborative and individualized approach to working with families and other healthcare practitioners, including open discussions about CAM therapies, environmental health concerns, nutrition, immunization, and parenting practices. Integrative pediatric practitioners view lifestyle issues (nutrition, fitness, mind-body-spirit connections) as cornerstones of optimal health. Perhaps most importantly, one of the central tenets of integrative primary care—the one that serves as the core—is the belief that the relationship between practitioner and patient/family is what truly provides the power in holistic practice. It is not so much the use of any specific CAM therapy that defines someone as an integrative pediatrician but the belief that healing is inexorably bound to the connection between practitioner and patient. In no area of healing practice is this more evident and needed than in primary care.

The appeal of the integrative model for pediatric primary care is indeed growing, witnessed by the anecdotal growth in office- and hospital-based integrative practices, and by the documented increased use of CAM therapies for both well and chronically-ill children (Loman, 2003; Sanders, 2003; Sawni-Sikand, 2002; Spigelblatt, 1994) Adolescent use of CAM in particular is rising (Braun, 2005; Wilson, 2002), and primary care practitioners need to engage teens in discussions about safety and efficacy concerns, as they would with any therapies. Children with special healthcare needs—those with chronic or serious acute illnesses (e.g., autism, cancer)—are seen in increasing numbers in primary care offices and a majority are likely to use CAM therapies (Cohen, 2006; Harrington, 2006; Sanders, 2003).

Pediatricians are more interested than ever in learning about CAM therapies so that they can more effectively communicate and connect with their patients and families (AAP, 2001). In order to increase awareness and knowledge of commonly used CAM therapies, this chapter will feature clinical scenarios that illustrate the potential for evidence-based integrative care as a new paradigm for primary care pediatric practice.

General Approach to the Newborn

Ideally, primary care is grounded in the concept of prevention and emphasizes regular well care visits to provide anticipatory guidance for families. We meet with families most frequently in the first months of a child's life in order to assess growth and development but also to establish a relationship so that we can, together, create a foundation for optimal health for each and every child. This nonjudgmental, two-way relationship is one of the keys to the success for pediatric primary care, especially with families of children with special healthcare needs. Liptak et al. (2006) reported that families of children with developmental disabilities were unsatisfied with their current primary care practitioners, in part because of pediatricians' perceived lack of knowledge about and unwillingness to discuss CAM therapies.

In the scope of daily practice, primary care pediatricians encounter a variety of common conditions requiring acute intervention. These acute problems offer us opportunities not simply to treat the presenting problem but to modulate the course of an infant's health for the future. The following case discussion, emphasizing prevention and evidence-guided integration of CAM and conventional therapies, will be threaded throughout this chapter to serve as a window into the actual practice of integrative primary care.

CASE (Part I): A 6-week-old baby, new to your practice, is brought in by his parents for a well visit. The family is interested in "holistic" care and has heard in the community that you are open-minded to "natural approaches." The baby was full-term and has been generally quite healthy; he is breastfed with occasional supplemental bottles of a cow's milk-based formula. The parents are concerned about how fussy their baby has become over the past month, and they are wondering if you can help them.

Colic

When the typical baby cries an average of 2.25 hours per day (Brazelton, 1962), others are excessively irritable and are said to have "colic." Surveys indicate that over one-quarter of infants are diagnosed with colic (Fireman, 2006), making the condition one of the most common reasons for infant visits to primary care practitioners today. Dr. Morris Wessel (1954), who studied infant crying behavior as part of the Yale Rooming-In Project, defined colic as paroxysmal fussing in infancy for more than 3 hours per day, at least 3 days per week, for at least 3 weeks duration. Colic is currently best understood as an extreme variant of infant irritability, perhaps related to neural regulation differences. Pediatrician Harvey Karp (2004) speculates that some babies have a more difficult time adjusting to what he terms the "fourth trimester," a 3-month period of time in which infants must cope with potentially overwhelming sensory stimuli. Just like adults, babies vary in how well they integrate external stimuli, and colic may well represent an adjustment disorder, the far end of an infant irritability syndrome, or perhaps an early sensory integration disorder. Most parents with colicky babies believe that there is some component of abdominal pain; in fact, the gastrointestinal tract may be involved in colic through neuro-gut-immune pathways. Atopic disorders, as will be discussed in more detail, have been associated with colic, perhaps through an immunomodulatory mechanism involving gastroesophageal (GE) reflux (Heine, 2006). Of greatest concern, a recently published 10-year prospective study challenges the commonly held view that there are no long term health-related issues in children who had colic in infancy (Savino, 2005). In this prospective study of one hundred children, there was an association noted between infantile colic and later recurrent abdominal pain, atopic disease, and sleep disorders. This association does not prove causation, but suggests that processes involved in the development of colic may also predispose children to subsequent health concerns. Larger prospective studies are needed for confirmation, but the theoretical impetus for colic intervention is strengthened by the trial's findings.

CONVENTIONAL APPROACH

It is often difficult to distinguish conventional from CAM approaches for managing colic, as culture and geography play such a large role in what is "conventional." The typical conventional pediatric approach to colic might include psychological support for care-givers with reassurance that the baby is physically well and that the colic will resolve by 12 weeks or so. This approach is distinguishable by intent and by intensity from the mind-body methods described below. Additionally, many parents comment that fussi-ness is often accompanied by "gas" or other gastrointestinal concerns, and practitioners frequently advise the use of simethicone-containing infant drops. This therapy has been shown to be no more effective than placebo (Garrison, 2000), and most simethicone-containing over-the-counter products contain artificial sweeteners and dyes.

CAM THERAPIES

Individualizing a treatment plan is extremely important in the management of colic, as some approaches work quite well for some families and not at all for oth-ers. Common CAM approaches for colic include the use of mind-body methods, biologically based therapies, and manipulative and body-based methods, and whole medical systems.

Mind-Body Methods

Mind-body medicine "focuses on the interactions among the brain, mind, body, and behavior, and on the powerful ways in which emotional, mental, social, spiritual, and behavioral factors can directly affect health" (Mind-Body Medicine, NCCAM, 2007), Stress can indeed modulate neurological responses, supporting the need to promote parental stress-coping mechanisms in the face of excessive infant irritability. In a chick-en-egg analogy, it is likely that both parental stress and infant colic exacerbate each other. There are established links between maternal mood states, including post-partum depression, and the development of colic in infants (Akman, 2006). Reducing parenting stress is a proven method of helping families cope with irritable infants (Keefe, 2006), and there are many strategies to do so. This study by Keefe et al. utilized a home-based nursing intervention for stress reduction, but teaching families other mind-body thera-pies may be equally helpful. Other parenting interventions, included parent-to-parent guidance, have been demonstrated to reduce crying time in colicky babies (Dihigo, 1998; Wolke, 1994). Despite the lack of randomized controlled trials proving efficacy or cost-effectiveness in colic management, practices such as guided imagery, self-hypno-sis, mindfulness-based stress reduction, or yoga might be equally helpful in reducing parental distress.

BIOLOGICALLY BASED THERAPIES

Surveys of CAM use in culturally diverse populations indicate that colic is a common reason for use of biologically based therapies (Lohse, 2006; Smitherman, 2005). The largest systematic review to date of treatments for colic found little evidence to support many routinely advocated therapies while noting that several nutritional and botani-cally based approaches were quite safe and effective (Garrison, 2000).

Botanicals

Biologically based therapies for colic have been used historically in many cultures. One of the more widely known in recent times, gripe water, dates back to the 1800s, when it was developed by William Woodward, a British pharmacy apprentice (Blumental, 2000). Woodward's formula, a mixture of dill seed oil, sodium bicarbonate and alcohol, among other substances, derived from a solution used at the time to treat babies with "fen fever," related to malaria. Babies soothed by the concoction reportedly found relief from gastrointestinal troubles ("watery gripes"). Over the years, the gripe water formula has changed and commercially available solutions may contain any number of botanicals, though alcohol has been removed from many of these products. One must ask families specifically about the use of gripe water and other herbal blends for colic treatment in order to determine which herbs are being ingested.

One natural health product database lists five separate products labeled as "gripe water," all with different constituents (Natural Medicines Comprehensive Database, 2007). Herbs most commonly found in these preparations include dill (*Anethum graveolens*), fennel (*Foeniculum vulgare*), ginger (*Zingiber officinale*) and German chamomile (*Matricaria recutita*). There have been several published studies of herbal remedies for colic. Weizman et al. (1993) evaluated an herbal tea preparation containing chamomile, vervain, licorice, fennel, and lemon balm. In this trial, 68 colicky infants aged 2–8 weeks were randomized to receive either tea or placebo for 7 days. Infants were allowed drink up to 5 ounces up to three times per day, but the average actual intake per baby was approximately 3 ounces per day. Significantly more babies in the treatment group (57%) improved than in the placebo group (26%). No significant adverse effects were reported. Unfortunately, many unknown variables in the study design make it difficult to base recommendations on the results. The amounts and types of each herb and the exact nature of the placebo are unspecified and may have had an impact on resolution of colic. Alexandrovich et al. (2003) examined the effect on colic of an emulsion of fennel seed oil in a randomized controlled trial of 125 infants. The babies were allowed 5 to 20 ml of either fennel seed oil emulsion or placebo up to four times per day for 1 week, but actually ingested an average of 2 to 3 doses per day, for a total of less than 2 ounces per day. Colic was eliminated in 65% of the treatment group versus 23.7% of the placebo group. There were no reported adverse effects in this trial. Savino et al. (2005) compared a standardized extract of three herbs (chamomile, fennel, and lemon balm) with a placebo in 93 breastfed colicky infants. Each infant received a standardized dose of extract or placebo at 2 ml/kg per day twice daily prior to breastfeeding for a 7 day trial period. A significant reduction in crying time was observed in 85.4% of patients receiving the treatment extract and in 48.9% of infants receiving the placebo. Interestingly, crying time was still reduced 2 weeks after the end of the trial in the intervention group. There were no reported adverse side effects in either group.

Nutritional Modulation

Modulating the diets of babies, whether breastfed or formula-fed, is often attempted to reduce infant fussiness. While breastfeeding exclusively does not seem to prevent colic (Clifford, 2002), nursing mothers may have success in reducing infant irritability by altering their nutritional intake. Hill et al. (2005) found that elimination from maternal diet of common allergenic foods (cow's milk, soy, wheat, eggs, peanuts, tree nuts, and fish) was associated with a reduction in colic in breastfed infants. Both cruciferous vegetables (e.g., broccoli, cauliflower) and chocolate in the maternal diet have been linked to colic in breastfed babies (Lust, 1996). Some food constituents, like essential fatty acids, may actually be desirable in higher amounts; though not directly connected to colic, maternal docosahexaenoic acid (DHA) levels have been associated with positive infant sleep patterning (Cheruku, 2002).

Certain formulas have been shown to reduce colic symptoms though no prospective studies evaluating prevention of colic have been published. Extensively hydrolyzed casein and whey formulas are both more effective than non-hydrolyzed cow's milk formulas in reducing crying times in colicky babies (Jakobsson, 2000; Lucassen, 2000) Studies do not support either soy and partially hydrolyzed formulas as options for colic reduction (AAP, 1998, 2000).

Probiotics and Prebiotics

Probiotics are "viable, defined microorganisms in sufficient numbers, which alter the microflora (by implantation or colonization) in a compartment of the host and by that exert beneficial health effects in this host" (Schrezenmeier, 2001). Prebiotics are biological substances that increase the growth and activity of probiotic organisms. There are differences in the types and number of probiotic microorganisms colonizing the intestinal tracts of infants with colic versus those without (Savino, 2004, 2005).

Savino et al. (2007) have evaluated the effect of probiotics and prebiotics on colic. In one trial, they compared a probiotic (*Lactobacillus reuteri*) with simethicone in a randomized controlled trial in 90 exclusively breastfed colicky infants. Simethicone, a conventional non-prescription medication, has been previously shown to be ineffective for colic treatment (Garrison, 2000). After the 1 month trial, 95% of the probiotic treatment group responded (no longer met Wessel criteria for colic) versus only 7% of the simethicone group. The second study randomized 267 formula-fed infants to one of two arms (Savino, 2006). The treatment group was fed a novel partially hydrolyzed whey protein formula supplemented with prebiotic oligosaccharides and the control group received the standard formula (without prebiotics) and simethicone. The treatment group, after both 1 and 2 weeks, had a significant reduction in crying episodes when compared with the control group.

MANIPULATIVE AND BODY-BASED METHODS

Infant Massage

A Cochrane Database Systematic Review of infant massage acknowledged "evidence of benefits on mother–infant interaction, sleeping and crying, and on hormones influencing stress levels" (Underdown, 2006). Infant massage is effective in reducing excessive crying in even the most vulnerable of infants, including premature babies and cocaine-exposed neonates (Field, 1995; Wheeden, 1993). Self-care is a important part of the healing power for many CAM modalities, including massage, and families can learn infant massage techniques for safe and effective use at home. This positive effect for soothing infants seems to be superior to simple vibration devices (Huhtala, 2000) and may be enhanced by the use of essential oils such as sesame seed oil (Agarwal, 2000). Whether this latter effect is related to the oil as aromatherapy or simply adds to the physical massage technique, or both, is unknown.

Osteopathy

Hayden and Mullinger (2006) evaluated cranial osteopathy for the treatment of infant colic in an open, controlled, prospective study. Twenty-eight infants received weekly OMT for 4 weeks, and parents reported a significant reduction in crying time and improvement in sleeping time in treated infants versus controls (no intervention). Authors concluded that "this preliminary study suggests that cranial osteopathic treatment can benefit infants with colic; a larger, double-blind study is warranted."

Chiropractic

Hewitt, in a 2004 publication, notes that the rationale for chiropractic treatment in colic is "that an 'infant irritability continuum' exists with contentment on one end and colic on the other. In between are various degrees of irritability, many of which may be the result of discomfort secondary to mechanical lesions in the infant's spine and cranium… the fussiness may be due to discomfort arising from mechanical lesions, also termed subluxations, in the infant's spine and/or cranium. Subluxations may arise from in utero malposi-tion or from subtle trauma to the spine or cranium during the birth process" (Hewitt, 2004). A review of the chiropractic literature with respect to colic treatment includes two controlled single-blinded clinical trials, one uncontrolled prospective study and several case studies (Klougart, 1989; Wiberg, 1999). All but one published study suggest that there seems to be a positive effect of chiropractic spinal manipulation for infantile colic. The one negative trial (Olaffsdottir, 2001) was a randomized, single-blinded, controlled study with a tremendous intention response. While nearly 70% of the treatment group improved, 60% of the control group similarly improved; this difference was not statistically significant.

WHOLE MEDICAL SYSTEMS

Homeopathy

According to a general practice homeopathy survey from Scotland, "The most frequently prescribed medicines were for common self-limiting infantile conditions such as colic…" (Ekins-Daukes, 2005). There are multiple homeopathic remedies used for newborn colic, including single remedies and pre-packaged combinations, and while frequently used by parents, there are no published research trials regarding the safety or efficacy of homeopathy for colic treatment available for review at the present time.

Case (Part 2): The parents return for a visit several weeks later. They have been using chamomile tea and gripe water with some success, and find that the infant massage lessons they took are helping to calm their baby as well. While he is less fussy, he is now spitting up most of his feedings, though his mother is trying to avoid dairy and other common food allergens in her diet; they are still occasionally supplementing with an "easier-to-digest" cow's milk formula. Furthermore, he is covered by a patchy, dry, red rash and has noticeable nasal congestion with a frequent nighttime cough.

Atopic Disorders

Atopic disorders, including asthma and food allergies, are widely considered to be rising in prevalence at epidemic rates (Asher, 2006). Practitioners report they are seeing many more infants today suffering from early atopic signs (dermatitis, gastroesophageal reflux, chronic rhinorrhea, and recurrent wheezing) than ever before. Some infants with colic develop signs and symptoms of atopy, including eczema, chronic rhinitis, and gastroesophageal reflux. Research supports the finding that atopy may be responsible for symptoms of colic(Heine, 2006), although infants with colic do not necessarily develop atopy at higher rates than other babies later in life (Castro-Rodriguez, 2001). The atopic march, as it has come to be known, represents the natural tendency of children with early signs of allergic reaction to environmental stimuli (e.g., atopic dermatitis) to progress to more severe manifestations of allergic disease (e.g., asthma) (Spergel, 2003).

What predisposes certain infants to develop atopic symptoms? While it has long been appreciated that some are at higher risk for atopic disorders based on family history, we are only now recognizing how complicated the nature-nurture equation might be. Even single nucleotide polymorphisms (SNP's, or very small DNA shifts) may not only account for the presence or absence of atopy in a given person, but may also affect the severity of disease, the likelihood of other atopic conditions developing, and the success of various therapies (Negoro, 2006). A baby with a given genomic predisposition, under certain environmental conditions, will manifest immune dysregulation, resulting in an imbalance between Th1 dominant and Th2 dominant responses (Kidd, 2003). Th2 dominance leads to immune dysregulation marked by a proliferation of inflammatory cellular mediators (e.g., cytokines, interleukins, leukotrienes). Inflammation involves excess mucous production and other clinically observable phenomena we call "allergies."

The "hygiene hypothesis" is a popular current theory to explain why we are experiencing a surge in atopic disease prevalence (Noverr, 2005). According to this theory, our environments are now too "clean"—we are not exposed to as many antigens (bacteria, fungal, viral) as previous generations. With a reduction in infectious exposure, certain individuals over time may produce altered gastrointestinal, immunologically active microorganisms, leading to a Th2 immune shift (Duramad, 2006). Numerous studies also have supported a correlation between early life antibiotic exposure and atopy (particularly wheezing) in children (Johnson, 2005; Kozyrskyj, 2007; Kummeling, 2007; Marra, 2006; Noverr, 2004; Thomas, 2006). Other environmental factors, too, have been implicated in triggering allergic responses. These include immune and endocrine disrupting agents in air, water, food, and industrial products (Bornehag, 2004; Chalubinski, 2006; Sherriff, 2005).

CONVENTIONAL APPROACHES

The assessment of atopy in conventional pediatric practice may include measuring blood IgE response to common dietary allergens or prick skin testing. If testing reveals documented allergy, parents are advised to avoid the offending food(s). Environmental modulation including household control of dust mites and discussion of pet exposure is sometimes employed. Classically, pharmaceutical agents including immunomodulators (e.g., steroids) and antihistamines are used for symptom management of atopic conditions.

CAM THERAPIES

Many families turn to CAM therapies for their children suffering atopic disorders (Bielroy, 2004; Braganza, 2003; Johnston, 2003; Ko, 2006; Reznick, 2002). Parents may be wary of potential adverse effects of conventional pharmaceuticals or may be interested in a more preventative approach. The most well-studied CAM therapies for both prevention and treatment of infant atopy are those that are biologically based. Other CAM approaches integrated include mind-body methods, manipulative and body-based methods, and whole medical systems.

Mind-Body Methods

The stress connection to atopic expression is well documented. On a clinical level, psychological stress has been demonstrated to exacerbate asthma in children (Bloomberg, 2005; Wright, 2005). On a molecular level, anxiety is associated with an acceleration of the pro-atopic Th2 response in patients with atopic dermatitis (Hashizume, 2005). These findings provide a rationale for the use of mind-body medicine therapies for atopic disorders. Self-hypnosis has been demonstrated by Anbar (2001, 2005) to be effective for the management of pulmonary conditions such as asthma, probably through the reduction of stress mechanisms. Similar results have been shown for children with eczema as well (Mantle, 1999).

BIOLOGICALLY BASED THERAPIES

Nutritional Modulation

For those infants at risk, exposure to certain foods in- and ex-utero may contribute to the development of atopy. We will focus on the following key areas: maternal pre- and post-natal antigen avoidance, breastfeeding, choice of infant formula supplementation, timing of solid food introduction, and fatty acid intake (both in breastfeeding mothers and in infants). General antigen avoidance (milk, soy, eggs, tree nuts, peanuts, shellfish) for the population as a whole is not supported by current data (Kramer, 2006). In families at highest risk (parents and/or siblings with significant atopic history), avoidance of most highly-allergenic foods, especially peanuts and tree nuts, should be considered during pregnancy and during duration of breastfeeding. The AAP advises avoiding peanuts and tree nuts for nursing mothers for maximal atopy prevention (Zeiger, 2003). If avoiding specific food groups, one must take great care to ensure proper compensatory intake of vitamins, minerals, and amino acids.

The AAP also supports breastfeeding as a means to reduce allergic disorders. Exclusive breastfeeding for 4 to 6 months is associated with a lower risk of developing atopic dermatitis, food allergy, allergic rhinitis, and asthma (Friedman, 2005; Kull, 2005a, 2005b) If exclusive breastfeeding is not possible, the AAP recommends hydrolyzed protein formulas for high-risk babies (Zeiger, 2003). A Cochrane database systematic review supports this recommendation (Osborn, 2006a). These formulas may contain extensively or partially hydrolyzed cow's milk proteins (casein or whey), and there is debate about whether they are both equivalently effective in preventing atopic expression (Hays, 2005). Most experts currently recommend extensively hydrolyzed products, but cost and availability issues are factors. The AAP recommends against using soy formulas for atopic prevention in high risk infants (Zeiger, 2003); again, this contention is supported by a Cochrane database systematic review (Osborn, 2006b).

There is no clear consensus guideline for treating infants who develop atopic symptoms, even in the absence of family history. Common practice includes advising exclusive breastfeeding with maternal antigen avoidance, or, if not possible, using extensively hydrolyzed formulas.

When is the optimal time to introduce solid foods to infants for both the general population and those at high risk? Prevention of atopy seems to be the key focus in published trials. With increasing prevalence of allergic disorders, some experts are advocating for delayed solid food introduction in all babies until 6 months, with the introduction of highly allergenic foods as follows: dairy products at 12 months, eggs at 24 months, and peanuts, tree nuts and shellfish until 36 months. (80) These guidelines are supported by other major US and European groups, but only for infants at high risk (Zeiger, 2003). Early solid feeding (prior to 4 months of age), particularly of gluten-containing products, is associated with atopic disease as well as celiac disease (Norris, 2005; Tarini, 2006). There have also been several encouraging studies looking at the treatment of atopic disorders with nutritional modulation (avoiding specific food allergens) (Fiocchi, 2004; Johnston, 2004; Lothian, 2006).

Recent studies have looked at the role of essential fatty acids in both preventing and reducing allergic disease. Atopy can be prevented when mothers ingest higher amounts of omega-3 polyunsaturated fatty acids (Puffs) (Denburg, 2005). It also appears that babies who ingest breast milk relatively rich in omega-3 are less likely to develop allergic symptoms (Oddly, 2006; Wigan, 2006). This effect is most evident in those babies at highest risk genetically. The results of directly feeding infants PUFAs are not as clear. Some studies of dietary modification with omega-3s PUFAs in children at high risk demonstrated reduction in atopy (Mihrshahi, 2004; Peat, 2004), and another study showed improvement with supplementation of evening primrose oil, an omega-6 PUFA (Biagi, 1988). Perhaps it is the balance of the two that is most important, and one must also take into account pre-existing dietary deficiencies and genomic factors. More research is clearly needed in this realm before universal recommendations can be made.

Probiotics

Randomized controlled trials have demonstrated that probiotics (Lactobacillus GG) given prenatally to women and then postnatally to either breastfeeding mothers or directly to formula-fed infants can reduce the incidence of atopic dermatitis by half in those infants at high risk for up to 7 years postnatally (Kalliomaki, 2001, 2003, 2007). Prebiotics have also been shown to prevent eczema in a vulnerable infant population (Moro, 2006). Several randomized controlled trials have pointed towards a positive effect of probiotics and prebiotics on the course of atopic dermatitis (Passeron, 2006; Rosenfeldt, 2003; Viljanen, 2005; Weston, 2005), though one publication reported no such effect (Brouwer, 2006). More research is needed to determine the ideal doses and types of pre- and probiotics for atopy prevention and treatment.

MANIPULATIVE AND BODY-BASED METHODS

Most of the studies of manual therapies for atopic disorders are for the treatment of asthma. A 2005 Cochrane Database Systematic Review of all manual therapies for asthma identified only three trials with acceptable methodology for review, including two on chiropractic and one on massage (Hondras, 2005). The authors concluded that "there is insufficient evidence to support or refute the use of manual therapy for patients with asthma."

Therapeutic Massage

One published trial of massage for asthma demonstrated that children in the intervention group had less anxiety and improved pulmonary function testing compared with a relaxation therapy control group (Field, 1998). A small, controlled trial of massage for atopic dermatitis yielded positive results, too, as treated children's clinical skin measures, affect and activity level significantly improved (Schachner, 1998).

Osteopathy

Guiney, Chou, Vianna, and Lovenheim (2005) conducted a randomized controlled trial demonstrating the effect of OMT for pediatric asthma. The treatment group showed a statistically significant improvement in peak expiratory flow rates. In another small controlled trial of OMT for childhood asthma, Bockenhauer, Julliard, Lo, Huang, and Sheth (2002) found that some measures of pulmonary function in the intervention group (compared with control) improved while others did not.

Chiropractic

Published trials of chiropractic for pediatric asthma treatment are few and generally negative. One study reported that children in the intervention group noted improved quality of life and decreased asthma severity but also demonstrated "no important changes in lung function or hyperresponsiveness at any time" (Bronfort, 2002). Two other randomized trials of chiropractic for asthma demonstrated no statistically or clinically relevant effect compared with control measures (Balon, 1998; Nilsson, 1995).

WHOLE MEDICAL SYSTEMS

Homeopathy

According to Colin (2006), "Allergies, especially respiratory allergies, are one of the indications for which homeopathic treatment is most frequently sought." The author presents a summary of 147 cases of respiratory allergy treated in a private homeopathic practice as evidence of success with the treatment. He notes that only seven patients did not improve with treatment in this case series. He comments that "Lycopodium, Pulsatilla and Sulphur were most frequently prescribed for ENT allergies and that there was no predominantly prescribed remedy in the pulmonary allergy group." White et al. (2003) published a randomized, double-blinded, placebo-controlled study of individualized homeopathy combined with conventional therapy for the treatment of childhood asthma. The authors concluded that there was no evidence in this group of a superior effect of homeopathy versus placebo in the integrative treatment of asthma.

Case (Part 3): With the careful elimination of dairy from Mom's diet and the introduction of probiotics and essential fatty acids, the baby returns for his four-month visit with reduced eczema and GE reflux, no coughing, and only occasional rhinorrhea. However, given his continued symptoms and a reportedly "bad reaction" (high fever, severe irritability, poor feeding) after his first set of immunizations, his parents wonder whether it's prudent to delay further vaccination at this point in time.

IMMUNIZATION

Perhaps no subject in primary care practice today draws more attention and debate than vaccination. Historically, some holistic groups have always questioned immunization, but public health agencies and conventional pediatric associations in many countries today include the development of herd immunity as a cornerstone of preventative health policies. Almost all public educational institutions (based on state laws) require specific immunizations for entry, though all states allow for medical exemption, most (48) allow for religious exemption, and some (20) allow for philosophical exemption (parent and patient choice) (VaccineEthics.org, 2007). Furthermore, third-party payors (health insurers) are starting to expand "pay-for-performance" models based in part by a practice's vaccine coverage (percent of patients "appropriately" vaccinated).

There are several issues informing the vaccine debate. There are biological questions about the influence of immunization on infant immune/neuroimmune regulation. These questions center on both particular vaccine antigens and other biological substances used as preservatives (Offit, 2003). Vaccine antigens and their additional components do in fact induce immune modulation. This is, of course, the intended effect of immunization—to stimulate a strong enough immune response to a given antigen to induce immunity so the child does not develop the targeted infectious disease upon exposure. Following logically, given a specific genomic predisposition and environmental circumstances, vaccine antigens can also induce undesirable immune and other biological effects. All studies used for vaccine licensing include lists of adverse effects, though rare, and noted adverse reactions include seizures (Geier, 2004), wheezing (Belshe, 2007), and arthritis (Asakawa, 2005). Vaccine additives, which include 2-phenoxyethanol, phenol, thimerosal (ethyl mercury), various aluminum compounds, formaldehyde, antibiotics, egg and yeast proteins, gelatin and albumin, are included to either enhance immune response or preserve the product from contamination (Offit, 2003). Some of the preservative compounds also stimulate the immune response in animal models, including heavy metal-based compounds such as thimerosal and aluminum that have known immune and neuroimmune dysregulation properties (Havarinasab, 2006; Hornig, 2005; Petrovsky, 2004). The difficulty has been in conclusively demonstrating these effects in children. Given the links between immune dysregulation and the development of atopic phenomena, a growing number of practitioners are concerned about the potential contribution of vaccines in a subset of children to disease expression. Clearly, much more research is needed in this area.

Ethically, the immunization issue involves the principles of human rights and the common good (individual rights versus state/societal rights) and of informed consent (risk-benefit decisions, exemptions, and waivers). Integrative practice is in part grounded in the tenets of individualizing care and in supporting a relationship-centered, open approach to child wellness care. Practitioners even in conventional circles are urged not to dismiss families who wish to alter standard vaccine practice and are encouraged to discuss risk and benefits in an open-minded manner (Diekema, 2005). But prevention is a key concept, too, and most integrative pediatricians concur that vaccines effectively prevent disease. In fact, it is in part the near-disappearance of vaccine-preventable diseases like polio and measles that have led some parents to conclude that the risks of their children developing the disease are outweighed by the perceived risks of developing vaccine-related illnesses. How does one reconcile the scientific and ethical principles noted above when there is so much uncertainty? In the "real-world" practice of integrative primary care, parents and practitioners communicate and debate risks and benefits, and we develop a plan that best serves each individual child.

> **Case (Part 4):** The now 6-month-old baby has developed a series of acute ear infections with persistent middle ear fluid, which seem to be associated with the onset of teething and frequent upper respiratory infections. Both you and his parents would like to avoid antibiotic use and surgical intervention if possible. What are your other options?

Otitis Media

One of the most common reasons parents visit pediatricians is for the evaluation and treatment of ear infections (acute otitis media or AOM). AOM is the most common infection for which antibacterial agents are prescribed for children in the United States. There are billions of dollars spent yearly on prescriptions medications for AOM, and there is great concern about the appropriate use of antibiotics for the condition in an age when we are witnessing increasing rates of microbial resistance to anti-infectives (AAP, 2004).

There is a known association of AOM with URIs; less certain is the connection to teething. Anecdotally, many parents will report that teething seems to trigger ear infections in their infants. It is unclear whether teething simply causes ear pain or actually predisposes to Eustachian tube dysfunction. The main concern in these families regarding AOM is the need, regardless of cause, for quick and effective pain relief as well as prevention of chronic serous otitis media (CSOM), or persistent middle ear fluid. The latter is the most common reason for elective surgery in children (other than circumcision) in the United States (Kogan, 2000).

CONVENTIONAL APPROACH

Although widely debated, the use of antibiotics for AOM is currently the standard of care for children under 2 years old in the United States. Indeed, for many older children, antibiotics are often prescribed for acute otitis media. These practices are less certain in other parts of the world. Concern regarding the development of antibiotic resistance has led more practitioners to develop an interest in integrating CAM therapies for the treatment of AOM (MacKay, 2003). Additionally, many parents use and practitioners recommend over-the-counter remedies for URI and teething symptoms. The use of these products in infants is not recommended due to concerns about lack of efficacy and potential for harm (Public Health Advisory, 2007), so that safe and effective alternatives for pain management are desirable. The conventional management of CSOM includes a wait-and-see approach, and if fluid persists for some length of time, myringotomy and pressure-equalizing tube placement is advised (American Academy of Family Physicians, 2004). Even this approach, however, is under scrutiny as to when and whether benefits outweigh risks (Lous, 2005).

CAM THERAPIES

In integrative care, the goal is primarily prevention of otitis media, and secondarily the use of naturally based methods for symptom management to optimize children's inherent healing mechanisms. Effective preventative measures include breastfeeding (Duncan, 1993) and avoiding environmental triggers like second-hand smoke and air pollution (Adair-Bischoff, 1998; Brauer, 2006). Regarding symptom management, we encourage parents to view URI and AOM symptoms (fever, congestion, rhinorrhea, cough) as the body's way of fighting infection. Natural viral infections theoretically allow for natural immune system development. Of course, one must consider the degree of symptoms and the possibility of overwhelming bacterial infection requiring the use of pharmaceutical agents including antibiotics. Pain relief—alleviating the suffering of children with AOM—is paramount as well and not to be dismissed lightly. Commonly used CAM therapies for otitis media management include biologically-based therapies, manipulative and body-based methods, and whole medical systems.

BIOLOGICAL-BASED THERAPIES

Botanical

Botanically based naturopathic topical ear drops have been shown to be effective and safe in prospective, randomized, and controlled trials (Sarrell 2001, 2003). The specific product tested included the following extracts: allium sativum, verbascum thapsus, calendula flores, hypericum perfoliatum, lavender and vitamin E, in an olive oil base. These components have anti-viral, anti-bacterial, anti-fungal, and anti-inflammatory properties. This topical botanical combination appears to be as effective for acute otitis media pain relief as prescription anesthetic ear drops with or without concurrent antibiotic use. No adverse effects were reported in these two trials. This approach seems to be a reasonable complement for AOM management during a time of observation without antibiotic use if clinically warranted.

Nutritional

Cod liver oil, which contains omega-3 essentially fatty acids as well as vitamins A and D, was studied in combination with selenium (an antioxidant mineral), in a small pilot trial for prevention of AOM (Linday, 2002). Eight children, serving as their own historical controls, received this combination of nutritional supplements for one "OM season" and were noted to receive antibiotics for significantly fewer days than in the prior "OM season." Larger, controlled trials are needed before general recommendations can be made.

Larch arabinogalactans, polysaccharides made up of galactan backbones with side-chains of galactose and arabinose sugars, have been linked in one report to decreased frequency and severity of pediatric AOM (D'Adamo, 1996). Larch arabinogalactan is a source of dietary fiber and also serves as a prebiotic, or substrate for growth of probiotic organisms. Whether its immune stimulating effects are via this mechanism or others is unclear.

Probiotics

When used, antibiotics cause significant gastrointestinal morbidity in children. Antibiotic-associated diarrhea (AAD) has been clearly demonstrated to be lessened by the preventive use of probiotics (Johnston, 2007). Whether this is particularly true or not with respect to AOM treatment has not been studied, but there is no reason to believe probiotics would not be helpful in this scenario. Which strain(s) and what dose(s) are safe and effective for AAD in children is debatable and worthy of further research.

MANIPULATIVE AND BODY-BASED METHODS

Osteopathy

Osteopathic manipulative treatment (OMT) has been studied in two published trials for preventing recurrent otitis media, with the goal of decreasing the need for surgical intervention for CSOM and recurrent AOM. Degenhardt and Kuchera (2006) treated eight children with recurrent AOM in an uncontrolled, pilot study. Patients received weekly OMT for 3 weeks; intervention was performed in a complementary manner, concurrently with traditional medical management. Five children had no recurrence of symptoms, and only one required myringotomy and tube placement surgery at 1-year follow-up.

Mills, Henley, Barnes, Carreiro, and Degenhardt (2003) performed a prospective, controlled trial of OMT in 57 children with recurrent AOM. The control group received routine pediatric care and the intervention group OMT plus routine care for nine visits over a 6 month study period. Children receiving OMT has significantly fewer episodes of AOM, surgical procedures and "surgery-free months." No adverse reactions were reported.

Chiropractic

Although prevention of recurrent AOM and treatment of CSOM are both frequent reasons for pediatric chiropractic visits, there is little published data regarding the safety and efficacy of this practice. Most reported trials demonstrating success are uncontrolled, non-randomized case-studies (Froehle, 1996; Fysh, 1996). Sawyer, Evans, Boline, Branson, and Spicer (1999) demonstrated the feasibility of performing a randomized study of active chiropractic spinal manipulative therapy (SMT) or placebo chiropractic SMT. There are no RCT trials of chiropractic SMT for otitis media available for review on NCBI PubMed.

WHOLE MEDICAL SYSTEMS

Homeopathy

Two published studies evaluated the use of individualized homeopathic remedies for treatment of AOM in children. A group from Switzerland found that pain resolution was significantly faster in homeopathically-treated children than in controls (Frei, 2001). A US study reported that children receiving individualized homeopathic remedies had more significant reductions in symptoms (pain) at 24 and 64 hours than in placebo-controls (Jacobs, 2001). There is difficulty, of course, in extrapolating the importance of these positive findings of individualized treatments to a larger, generalized pediatric population. However, the study design mechanism does take into account the actual practice of homeopathy, which is based on individualizing remedies.

> **Case (Part 5/Conclusion):** Now approaching his first birthday, our young patient and his family are thriving. With continued dietary vigilance and judicious use of topical herbals, homeopathy and manipulative therapy, the baby is growing and developing as expected, and everyone is looking forward to an exciting second year.

Conclusion

The integration of CAM therapies into primary care pediatric practice is well illustrated by the case discussion threaded throughout this chapter. CAM therapies are being more frequently utilized in the pediatric population, and primary care pediatricians are in an ideal position to work with families to explore all safe and effective remedies. Evidence supporting the use of CAM therapies for common pediatric conditions has steadily increased in volume and improved in quality. While we clearly need additional research examining the safety and efficacy of all therapies for these common childhood conditions, evidence to date supports the judicious use of specific CAM therapies. Primary care practitioners, in ideal position to adopt and advocate the medical home paradigm, should engage their patients and families in respectful, collaborative dialogue regarding the use of CAM therapies. As the number of children with special healthcare needs grows, and as more families develop an interest in a holistic model of care for prevention and treatment, integrative primary care is poised to become the standard of children's healthcare.

Internet Resources

AAP Provisional Section on Complementary, Holistic and Integrative Medicine: http://www.aap.org/sections/CHIM

AAP National Center of Medical Home Initiatives for Children with Special Needs: http://www.medicalhomeinfo.org

Center for Medical Home Improvement: http://www.medicalhomeimprovement.org

The Collaborative on Health and the Environment: http://healthandenvironment.org

Commonweal: http://www.commonweal.org

Environmental Working Group: http://www.ewg.org

Environmental Health News: http://www.environmentalhealthnews.org

The Green Guide (National Geographic): http://www.thegreenguide.com

Healthy Child Healthy World: http://healthychild.org

Institute for Children's Environmental Health: http://www.iceh.org

Integrative Pediatrics Council: http://www.integrativepeds.org

The National Environmental Education & Training Foundation: http://www.neetf.org

Teleosis Institute: Green Health Care—Ecologically Sustainable Medicine: http://www.teleosis.org

The Whole Child Center http://www.wholechildcenter.org

REFERENCES

Adair-Bischoff, C. E., & Sauve, R. S. (1998). Environmental tobacco smoke and middle ear disease in preschool-age children. *Archives of Pediatrics & Adolescent Medicine, 152*(2), 127–133.

American Academy of Family Physicians; American Academy of Otolaryngology-Head and Neck Surgery; American Academy of Pediatrics Subcommittee on Otitis Media With Effusion. (2004). Otitis media with effusion. *Pediatrics, 113*(5), 1412–1429.

AAP Committee on Nutrition. (1998). Soy protein-based formulas: recommendations for use in infant feeding. *Pediatrics, 101,* 148–153.

AAP Committee on Nutrition. (2000). Hypoallergenic infant formulas. *Pediatrics, 106,* 346–349.

AAP Division of Health Policy Research. Periodic Survey of Fellows #49: Complementary and Alternative Medicine (CAM) Therapies in Pediatric Practices (2001). Retrieved November 6, 2007, from http://www.aap.org/research/periodicsurvey/ps49bexs.htm

AAP Medical Home Initiatives for Children with Special Needs Project Advisory Committee. (2002). The medical home. *Pediatrics, 110*(1), 184–186.

AAP Subcommittee on Management of Acute Otitis Media. (2004). Diagnosis and management of acute otitis media. *Pediatrics, 113*(5), 1451–1465.

Agawam, K. N., Gupta, A., Pushkin, R., et al. (2000). Effects of massage & use of oil on growth, blood flow & sleep pattern in infants. *The Indian Journal of Medical Research, 112,* 212–217.

Kaman, I., Kusch, K., Ozdemir, N., et al. (2006). Mothers' postpartum psychological adjustment and infantile colic. *Archives of Disease in Childhood, 91,* 417–419.

Alexandrovich, I., Rakovitskaya, O., Kolmo, E., et al. (2003). The effect of fennel (foeniculum vulgare) seed oil emulsion in infantile colic: A randomized, placebo-controlled study. *Alternative Therapies in Health and Medicine, 9,* 58–61.

Anbar. R. D. (2001). Self-hypnosis for management of chronic dyspnea in pediatric patients. *Pediatrics, 107,* e21.

Anbar, R. D., & Geisler, S. C. (2005). Identification of children who may benefit from self-hypnosis at a pediatric pulmonary center. *BMC Pediatrics, 5,* 6.

Asakawa, J., Kobayashi, S., Kaneda, K., Ogasawara, H., Sugawara, M., Yasuda, M., et al. (2005). Reactive arthritis after influenza vaccination: Report of a case. *Modern Rheumatology, 15*(4), 283–285.

Asher, M. I., Montefort, S., Bjorksten, B., et al. (2006). Worldwide time trends in the prevalence of symptoms of asthma, allergic rhinoconjunctivitis, and eczema in childhood: ISAAC Phases One and Three repeat multicountry cross-sectional surveys. *Lancet, 368,* 733–743.

Balon, J., Aker, P. D., Crowther, E. R., Danielson, C., Cox, P. G., O'Shaugnessy, D., et al. (1998). A comparison of active and simulated chiropractic manipulation as adjunctive treatment for childhood asthma. *New England Journal of Medicine, 339*(15), 1013–1020.

Belshe, R. B., Edwards, K.M., Vesikari, T., Black, S. V., Walker, R. E., Hultquist, M, et al. (2007). CAIV-T Comparative Efficacy Study Group. Live attenuated versus inactivated influenza vaccine in infants and young children. *The New England Journal of Medicine, 356*(7), 685–696.

Biagi, P. L., Bordoni, A., Masi, M., et al. (1988). A long-term study on the use of evening primrose oil (Efamol) in atopic children. *Drugs Under Experimental and Clinical Research, 14,* 285–290.

Bielroy, L. (2004). Complementary and alternative interventions in asthma, allergy, and immunology. *Annals of allergy, Asthma and Immunology, 93*(Suppl 1), S45–S54.

Bloomberg, G. R., & Chen, E. (2005).The relationship of psychological stress with childhood asthma. *Immunology and Allergy Clinics of North America, 25,* 83–105.

Blumental, I. (2000). The gripe water story. *Journal of the Royal Society of Medicine, 93,* 172–174.

Bockenhauer, Se., Julliard, K. N., Lo, K. S., Huang, K. E., & Sheth, A. M. (2002). Quantifiable effects of osteopathic manipulative techniques on patients with chronic asthma. *Journal of the American Osteopathic Association, 102*(7), 371–375.

Bornehag, C. G., Sundell, J., Weschler, C. J., et al. (2004). The association between asthma and allergic symptoms in children and phthalates in house dust: A nested case-control study. *Environmental Health Perspectives, 112,* 1393–1397.

Braganza, S., Ozuah, P. O., & Sharif, I. (2003). The use of complementary therapies in inner-city asthmatic children. *The Journal of Asthma, 40,* 823–827.

Brauer, M., Gehring, U., Brunekreef, B., de Jongste, J., Gerritsen, J., Rovers, M., et al. (2006). Traffic-related air pollution and otitis media. *Environmental Health Perspectives, 114*(9), 1414–1418.

Braun, C. A., Bearinger, L. H., Halcon, L. L., et al. (2005). Adolescent use of complementary therapies. *The Journal of Adolescent Health, 37,* 76e.1–76e.9.

Brazelton, T. B. (1962).Crying in infancy. *Pediatrics, 29,* 579–588.

Bronfort, G., Evans, R. L., Kubic, P., & Filkin, P. (2002). Chronic pediatric asthma and chiropractic spinal manipulation: A prospective clinical series and randomized clinical pilot study. *Journal of Manipulative and Physiological Therapeutics, 24*(6), 369–377.

Brouwer, M. L., Wolt-Plompen, S. A., Dubois, S. E., et al. (2006). No effects of probiotics on atopic dermatitis in infancy: A randomized placebo-controlled trial. *Clinical and Experimental Allergy, 36,* 899–906.

Castro-Rodriguez, J, A., Stern, D.A,, Halonen, M., Wright, A. L., Holberg, C. J., Taussig, L. M., et al. (2001). Relation between infantile colic and asthma/atopy: a prospective study in an unselected population. *Pediatrics, 108*(4), 878–882.

Chalubinski, M., & Kowalski, M. L. (2006). Endocrine disrupters—potential modulators of the immune system and allergic response. *Allergy, 61,* 1326–1335.

Cheruku, S. R., Montgomery-Downs, H. E., Farkas, S. L., et al. (2002). Higher maternal plasma docosahexanoic acid during pregnancy is associated with more mature neonatal sleep-state patterning. *The American Journal of Clinical Nutrition, 76,* 608–613.

Clifford, T. J., Campbell, M. K., Speechley, K. N., et al. (2002). Infant colic: empirical evidence of the absence of an association with source of early infant nutrition. *Archives of Pediatrics & Adolescent Medicine, 156,* 1123–1128.

Cohen, M. H. (2006). Legal and ethical issues relating to use of complementary therapies in pediatric hematology/oncology. *Journal of Pediatric Hematology/Oncology, 28,* 190–193.

Colin, P. (2006). Homeopathy and respiratory allergies. *Homeopathy, 95,* 68–72.

D'Adamo, P. (1996). Larch arabinogalactan. *Journal of Naturopathic Medicine, 6,* 33–37.

Degenhardt, B. F., & Kuchera M. L. (2006). Osteopathic evaluation and manipulative treatment in reducing the morbidity of otitis media: A pilot study. *The Journal of the American Osteopathic Association, 106*(6), 327–334.

Denburg, J. A., Hatfield, H. M., Cyr, M. M., et al. (2005). Fish oil supplementation in pregnancy modifies neonatal progenitors at birth in infants at risk of atopy. *The Journal of the American Osteopathic Association, 57,* 276–281.

Diekema, D. S.; American Academy of Pediatrics Committee on Bioethics. (2005). Responding to parental refusals of immunization of children. *Pediatrics, 115*(5), 1428–1431.

Dihigo, S. K. (1998). New strategies for the treatment of colic: Modifying the parent/infant interaction. *Environmental Health Perspectives, 12,* 256–262.

Duncan, B., Ey, J., Holberg, C. J., Wright, A. L., Martinez, F. D., & Taussig L. M. (1993). Exclusive breast-feeding for at least 4 months protects against otitis media. *Pediatrics, 91*(5), 867–872.

Duramad, P., Harley, K., Lipsett, M., et al. (2006). Early environmental exposures and intracellular Th1/Th2 cytokine profiles in 24-month-old children living in an agricultural area. *Environmental Health Perspectives, 114*, 1916–1922.

Ekins-Daukes, S., Helms, P. J., Taylor, M. W., Simpson, C. R., & McLay J. S. (2005). Paediatric homoeopathy in general practice: Where, when and why? *British Journal of Clinical Pharmacology, 59*(6), 743–749.

Fallon J. M. (1997). The role of the chiropractic adjustment in the care and treatment of 332 children with otitis media. *Journal of Clinical Chiropractic Pediatrics, 2*(2), 167–183.

Field, T. (1995). Massage therapy for infants and children. *Journal of Developmental & Behavioral Pediatrics*, 105–111.

Field, T., Henteleff, T., Hernandez-Reif, M., Martinez, E., Mavunda, K., Kuhn, C., et al. (1998). Children with asthma have improved pulmonary function after massage. *The Journal of Pediatrics, 132*(5), 854–858.

Fiocchi, A., Bouygue, G. R., Martelli, A., et al. (2004). Dietary treatment of childhood atopic eczema/dermatitis syndrome (AEDS). *Allergy, 59*(Suppl. 78), 78–85.

Fiocchi, A., Assa'ad, A, Bahna, S., et al. (2006). Food allergy and the introduction of solid foods to infants: A consensus document. Adverse Reactions to Foods Committee, American College of Allergy, Asthma and Immunology. *Annals of Allergy, Asthma and Immunology, 97*, 10–20.

Fireman, L. (2006). Colic. *Pediatr Review, 27*, 357–358.

Frei, H., & Thurneysen, A. (2001). Homeopathy in acute otitis media in children: Treatment effect or spontaneous resolution? *The British Homoeopathic Journal, 90*, 178–179.

Friedman, N. J., & Zieger, R. S. (2005). The role of breast-feeding in the development of allergies and asthma. *The Journal of Allergy and Clinical Immunology, 115*, 1238–1248.

Froehle R. M. (1996). Ear infection: A retrospective study examining improvement from chiropractic care and analyzing for influencing factors. *Journal of Manipulative and Physiological Therapeutics, 19*(3), 169–177.

Fysh P. N. (1996). Chronic recurrent otitis media: Case series of five patients with recommendations for case management. *Journal of Clinical Chiropractic Pediatrics, 1*, 66–178.

Garrison, M. M., & Christakis, D. A. (2000). A systematic review of treatments for infant colic. *Pediatrics, 106*, 184–190.

Geier, D. A., & Geier M. R. (2004). An evaluation of serious neurological disorders following immunization: A comparison of whole-cell pertussis and acellular pertussis vaccines. *Brain and Development, 26*(5), 296–300.

Guiney, P. A., Chou, R., Vianna, A., & Lovenheim, J. (2005). Effects of osteopathic manipulative treatment on pediatric patients with asthma: A randomized controlled trial. *Journal of the American Osteopathic Association, 105*, 7–12.

Harrington, J. W., Rosen, L., Garnecho, A., & Patrick, P. A. (2006). Parental perceptions and use of complementary and alternative medicine practices for children with autistic spectrum disorders in private practice. *Journal of Developmental and Behavioral Pediatrics, 27*(2 Suppl), S156–S161.

Hashizume, H., et al. (2005). Anxiety accelerates T-helper 2-tilted immune responses in patients with atopic dermatitis. *The British Journal of Dermatology, 152*, 1161–1164.

Havarinasab, S., & Hultman, P. (2006). Alteration of the spontaneous systemic autoimmune disease in (NZB x NZW)F1 mice by treatment with thimerosal (ethyl mercury). *Toxicology and Applied Pharmacology, 214*(1), 43–54.

Hayden, C., Mullinger, B. (2006). A preliminary assessment of the impact of cranial osteopathy for the relief of infantile colic. *Complementary Therapies in Clinical Practice, 12*(2), 83–90.

Hays, T., & Wood, R. A. (2005). A systematic review of the role of hydrolyzed infant formulas in allergy prevention. *Archives of Pediatrics & Adolescent Medicine, 159*, 810–816.

Heine, R. G. (2006). Gastroesophageal reflux disease, colic and constipation in infants with food allergy. *Current Opinion in Allergy and Clinical Immunology, 6*, 220–225.

Hewitt, E. G. (2004). Chiropractic care and the irritable infant. *Journal of Clinical Chiropractic Pediatrics, 6*(2), 394–397.

Hill, D. J., Roy, N., Heine, R. G., et al. (2005). Effect of a low-allergen maternal diet on colic among breastfed infants: a randomized, controlled trial. *Pediatrics, 116*, e709–e715.

Hondras, M. A., Linde, K., & Jones, A. P. (2005). Manual therapy for asthma. *Cochrane Database of Systematic Reviews, 18*(2), CD001002.

Hornig, M., Chian, D., & Lipkin W. I. (2004). Neurotoxic effects of postnatal thimerosal are mouse strain dependent. *Molecular Psychiatry, 9*(9), 833–845.

Huhtala, V., Lehtonen, L., Heinonen, R., et al. (2000). Infant massage compared with crib vibrator in the treatment of colicky infants. *Pediatrics, 105*, e84–e89.

Jacobs, J., et al. (2001). Homeopathic treatment of acute otitis media in children: A preliminary randomized placebo-controlled trial. *The Pediatric Infectious Disease Journal, 20*, 177–183.

Jakobsson, I., Lothe, L., Ley, D., et al. (2000). Effectiveness of casein hydrolysate feedings in infants with colic. *Acta Paediatrica, 89*, 18–21.

Johnson, C. C., Ownby, D. R., Alford, S. H., et al. (2005). Antibiotic exposure in early infancy and risk for childhood atopy. *The Journal of Allergy and Clinical Immunology, 115*, 1218–1224.

Johnston, G. A., Bilbao, R. M., & Graham-Brown, R. A. (2003). The use of complementary medicine in children with atopic dermatitis in secondary care in Leicester. *British Journal of Dermatology, 149*, 566–571.

Johnston, G. A., Bilbao, R. M., & Graham-Brown, R. A. (2004). The use of dietary manipulation by parents of children with atopic dermatitis. British Journal of Dermatology, *150*, 1186–1189.

Johnston, B. C., Supina, A. L., Ospina, M., & Vohra, S. (2007). Probiotics for the prevention of pediatric antibiotic-associated diarrhea. *Cochrane Database of Systematic Reviews, 18*(2), CD004827.

Kalliomaki, M., Salminen, S., Arvilommi, H., et al. (2001). Probiotics in primary prevention of atopic disease: A randomized placebo-controlled trial. *Lancet, 357*, 1076–1079.

Kalliomaki, M., Salminen, S., Poussa, T., et al. (2003). Probiotics and prevention of atopic disease: 4-year follow-up of randomised placebo-controlled trial. *Lancet, 361*, 1869–1871.

Kalliomaki, M., Salminen, S., Poussa, T., & Isolauri, E. (2007). Probiotics during the first 7 years of life: A cumulative risk reduction of eczema in a randomized, placebo-controlled trial. *The Journal of Allergy and Clinical Immunology, 119*(4), 1019–1021.

Karp, H. (2004). The "fourth trimester": A framework and strategy for understanding and resolving colic. *Contemporary Pediatrics, 21*, 94–116.

Keefe, M. R., Kajrlsen, K. A., Lobo, M. L., et al. (2006). Reducing parenting stress in families with irritable infants. *Nursing Research, 55*, 198–205.

Kemper K. J. (2000). Holistic pediatrics = good medicine. *Pediatrics, 105*(1 Pt 3), 214–218.

Kidd, P. (2003). Th1/Th2 balance: The hypothesis, its limitations, and implications for health and disease. *Alternative Medicine Review, 8*, 223–246.

Klougart, N., Nilsson, N., & Jacobsen, J. (1989). Infantile colic treated by chiropractors: A prospective study of 316 cases. *Journal of Manipulative and Physiological Therapeutics, 12*(4), 281–288.

Ko, J., Lee, J. I., Munoz-Furlong, A., et al. (2006). Use of complementary and alternative medicine by food-allergic patients. *Annals of Allergy, Asthma and Immunology, 97*, 365–369.

Kogan, M. D., Overpeck, M. D., Hoffman, H. J., & Casselbrant, M. L. (2000). Factors associated with tympanostomy tube insertion among preschool-aged children in the United States. *American Journal of Public Health, 90*(2), 245–250.

Kozyrskyj, A. L., Ernst, P., & Becker, A. B. (2007). Increased risk of childhood asthma from antibiotic use in early life. *Chest, 131*(6), 1753–1759

Kramer, M. S., & Kakuma, R. (2006). Maternal antigen avoidance during pregnancy or lactation, or both, for preventing or treating atopic disease in the child. *Cochrane Database of Systematic Reviews, 19*, 3, CD000133.

Kull, I., Wickman, M., Lilja, G., et al. (2002). Breast feeding and allergic disease in infants—a prospective birth cohort study. *Archives of Disease in Childhood, 87*, 478–481.

Kull, I., Almqvist, C., Lilja, G., et al. (2005a). Breast-feeding reduces the risk of asthma during the first 4 years of life. *The Journal of Allergy and Clinical Immunology, 114*, 755–760.

Kull, I., Bohme, M., Wahlgren, C. F., et al. (2005b). Breast-feeding reduces the risk for childhood eczema. *The Journal of Allergy and Clinical Immunology, 116*, 657–661.

Kummeling, I., Stelma, F. F., Dagnelie, P. C., Snijders, B. E., Penders, J., Huber, M., et al. (2007). Early life exposure to antibiotics and the subsequent development of eczema, wheeze, and allergic sensitization in the first 2 years of life: The KOALA Birth Cohort Study. *Pediatrics, 119*(1), e225–231.

Linday, L. A., Dolitsky, J. N., Shindledecker, R. D., & Pippenger C. E. (2002). Lemon-flavored cod liver oil and a multivitamin-mineral supplement for the secondary prevention of otitis media in young children: Pilot research. *The Annals of Otology, Rhinology, and Laryngology, 111*(7 Pt 1), 642–652.

Liptak, G. S., Orlando, M., Yingling, J. T., Theurer-Kaufman, K. L., Malay, D. P., Tompkins, L. A., et al. (2006). Satisfaction with primary healthcare received by families of children with developmental disabilities. *Journal of Pediatric Health Care, 20*(4), 245–252.

Lohse, B., Stotts, J. L., & Priebe, J. R. (2006). Survey of herbal use by Kansas and Wisconsin WIC participants reveals moderate, appropriate use and identifies herbal education needs. *Journal of the American Dietetic Association, 106*, 227–237.

Loman, D. G. (2003). The use of complementary and alternative healthcare practices among children. *Journal of Pediatric Health Care, 17*, 58–63.

Lothian, J. B., Grey, V., & Lands, L. C. (2006). Effect of whey protein to modulate immune response in children with atopic asthma. *International Journal of Food Sciences and Nutrition, 57*, 204–211.

Lous, J., Burton, M. J., Felding, J. U., Ovesen, T., Rovers, M. M., & Williamson I. (2005). Grommets (ventilation tubes) for hearing loss associated with otitis media with effusion in children. *Cochrane Database of Systematic Reviews, 25*(1), CD001801.

Lucassen, P. L., Assendelft, W. J., Gubbels, J. W., et al. (2000). Infantile colic: Crying time reduction with a whey hydrolysate: A double-blind, randomized, placebo-controlled trial. *Pediatrics, 106*, 1349–1354.

Lust, K. D., Brown, J. E., & Thomas, W. (1996). Maternal intake of cruciferous vegetables and other foods and colic symptoms in exclusively breast-fed infants. *Journal of the American Dietetic Association, 96*, 46–48.

Mantle, F. (1999). Hypnosis in the management of eczema in children. *Paediatric Nursing, 11*, 24–26.

Marra, F., Lynd, L., Coombes, M., et al. (2006). Does antibiotic exposure during infancy lead to development of asthma? A systematic review and metaanalysis. *Chest, 129*, 610–618.

Mihrshahi, S., Peat, J. K., Webb, K., et al. (2004). Effect of omega-3 fatty acid concentrations in plasma on symptoms of asthma at 18 months of age. *Pediatric Allergy and Immunology, 15,* 517–522.

Mills, M. V., Henley, C. E., Barnes, L. L. B., Carreiro, J. E., & Degenhardt B. F. (2003). The use of osteopathic manipulative treatment as adjuvant therapy in children with recurrent acute otitis media. *Archives of Pediatrics and Adolescent Medicine, 157*(9), 861–866.

Mind-Body Medicine: An Overview (NCCAM). Retrieved November 6, 2007, from http://nccam.nih.gov/health/backgrounds/mindbody.htm#intro

Moro, G., Arslanaglu, S., Stahl, B., et al. (2006). A mixture of prebiotic oligosaccharides reduces the incidence of atopic dermatitis during the first six months of age. *Archives of Disease in Childhood, 91,* 814–819.

Natural Medicines Comprehensive Database. Retrieved November 6, 2007, from http://www.naturaldatabase.com

Negoro, T., Orihara, K., Irahara, T., et al. (2006). Influence of SNP's in cytokine-related genes on the severity of food allergy and atopic eczema in children. *Pediatric Allergy and Immunology, 17,* 583–590.

Nilsson, N. H., Bronfort, G., Bendix, T., Madsen, F., & Weeke, B. (1995). Chronic asthma and chiropractic spinal manipulation: A randomized clinical trial. *Journal of Clinical and Experimental Allergy, 25*(1), 80–88.

Norris, J. M., Barriga, K., Hoffenberg, E. J., et al. (2005). Risk of celiac disease autoimmunity and timing of gluten introduction in the diet of infants at increased risk of disease. *The Journal of the American Medical Association, 293,* 2343–2351.

Noverr, M. C., Noggle, R. M., Toews, G. B., et al. (2004). Role of antibiotics and fungal microbiota in driving pulmonary allergic responses. *Infection and Immunity, 72,* 4996–5003.

Noverr, M. C., & Huffnagle, G. B. (2005). The 'microflora hypothesis' of allergic diseases. *Clinical and Experimental Allergy, 35,* 1511–1520.

Oddy, W. H., Pal, S., Kusel, M. M., et al. (2006). Atopy, eczema and breast milk fatty acids in a high-risk cohort of children followed from birth to 5 yr. *Pediatric Allergy and Immunology, 17,* 4–10.

Offit, P. A., & Jew, R. K. (2003). Addressing parents' concerns: Do vaccines contain harmful preservatives, adjuvants, additives, or residuals? *Pediatrics, 112*(6 Pt 1), 1394–1397.

Olafsdottir, E., Forshei, S., Fluge, G., & Markestad, T. (2001). Randomised controlled trial of infantile colic treated with chiropractic spinal manipulation. *Archives of Disease in Childhood, 84*(2), 138–141.

Osborn, D. A., & Sinn, J. (2006a). Formulas containing hydrolysed protein for prevention of allergy and foodx intolerance in infants. *Cochrane Database of Systematic Reviews, 18*(4), CD003664.

Osborn, D. A., & Sinn, J. (2006b). Soy formula for prevention of allergy and food intolerance in infants. *Cochrane Database of Systematic Reviews, 18*(4), CD003741.

Passeron, T., Lacour, J. P., Fontas, E., et al. (2006). Probiotics and synbiotics: Two promising approaches for the treatment of atopic dermatitis in children above 2 years. *Allergy, 61,* 431–437.

Peat, J. K., Mihrshahi, S., Kemp, A. S., et al. (2004). Three-year outcomes of dietary fatty acid modification and house dust mite reduction in the Childhood Asthma Prevention Study. *The Journal of Allergy and Clinical Immunology, 114,* 807–813.

Petrovsky, N., & Aguilar J. C. (2004). Vaccine adjuvants: Current state and future trends. *Immunology and Cell Biology, 82*(5), 488–496.

Primary Care—Wikipedia. Retrieved November 6, 2007, from http://en.wikipedia.org/wiki/Primary_care

Public Health Advisory: Nonprescription Cough and Cold Medicine Use in Children. Retrieved November 6, 2007, from http://www.fda.gov/cder/drug/advisory/cough_cold.htm

Reznick, M., Ozuah, P. O., Franco, K., et al. (2002). Use of complementary therapy by adolescents with asthma. *Archives of Pediatrics & Adolescent Medicine, 156*, 1042–1044.

Rosenfeldt, V., Benfeldt, E., Nielsen, S. D., et al. (2003). Effect of probiotic Lactobacillus strains in children with atopic dermatitis. *The Journal of Allergy and Clinical Immunology, 111*, 389–395.

Sanders, H., Davis, M. F., Duncan, B., et al. (2003). Use of complementary and alternative medical therapies among children with special healthcare needs in southern Arizona. *Pediatrics, 111*, 584–587.

Sarrell, E. M., Mandelberg, A., Cohen, H. A. (2001). Efficacy of naturopathic extracts in the management of ear pain associated with acute otitis media. *Archives of Pediatrics & Adolescent Medicine, 155*(7), 796–799.

Sarrell, E. M., Cohen, H. A., & Kahan, E. (2003). Naturopathic treatment for ear pain in children. *Pediatrics, 111*(5 Pt 1), e574–e579.

Savino, F., Cresi, F., Pautasso, S., et al. (2004). Intestinal microflora in breastfed colicky and non-colicky infants. *Acta Paediatrica, 93*, 825–829.

Savino, F., Castagno, E., Bretto, R., et al. (2005). A prospective 10-year study on children who had severe infantile colic. *Acta Paediatrica, 94*(Suppl), 129–132.

Savino, F., Cresi, F., Castagno, E., et al. (2005). A randomized double-blind placebo-controlled trial of a standardized extract of Matricariae recutita, Foeniculum vulgare and Melissa officinalis (ColiMil) in the treatment of breastfed colicky infants. *Phytotherapy Research, 19*, 335–340.

Savino, F., Bailo, E., Oggero, R., et al. (2005). Bacterial counts of intestinal Lactobacillus species in infants with colic. *Pediatric Allergy and Immunology, 16*, 72–75.

Savino, F., Palumeri, E., Castagno, E., et al. (2006). Reduction of crying episodes owing to infantile colic: A randomized controlled study on the efficacy of a new infant formula. *European Journal of Clinical Nutrition, 60*, 1304–1310.

Savino, F., Pelle, E., Palumeri, E., et al. (2007). *Lactobacillus reuteri* (American Type Culture Collection Strain 55730) versus simethicone in the treatment of infantile colic: A prospective randomized study. *Pediatrics, 119*, e124–e130.

Sawni-Sikand, A., Schubiner, H., & Thomas, R. L. (2002). Use of complementary/alternative therapies among children in primary care pediatrics. *Ambulatory Pediatrics, 2*, 99–103.

Sawyer, C. E., Evans, R. L., Boline, P. D., Branson, R., & Spicer, A. (1999). A feasibility study of chiropractic spinal manipulation versus sham spinal manipulation for chronic otitis media with effusion in children. *Journal of Manipulative and Physiological Therapeutics, 22*(5), 292–298.

Schachner, L., Field, T., Hernandez-Reif, M., Duarte, A. M., & Krasnegor, J. (1998). Atopic dermatitis symptoms decreased in children following massage therapy. *Pediatric Dermatology, 15*(5), 390–395.

Schrezenmeir, J., & de Vrese, M. (2001). Probiotics, prebiotics, and synbiotics—approaching a definition. *The American Journal of Clinical Nutrition, 73*, 361S–364S.

Sherriff, A., Farrow, A., Golding, J., et al. (2005). Frequent use of chemical household products is associated with persistent wheezing in pre-school age children. *Thorax, 60*, 45–49.

Smitherman, L. C., Janisse, J., & Mathur, A. (2005). The use of folk remedies among children in an urban black community: Remedies for fever, colic, and teething. *Pediatrics, 115*, e297–e304.

Spergel, J. M., & Palier, A. S. (2003). Atopic dermatitis and the atopic march. *The Journal of Allergy and Clinical Immunology, 112*, 118–127.

Spigelblatt, L., Laine-Ammara, G., Pless, I. B., et al. (1994). The use of alternative medicine by children. *Pediatrics, 94*, 811–814.

Tarini, B. A., Carroll, A. E., Sox, C. M., et al. (2006). Systematic review of the relationship between early introduction of solid foods to infants and the development of allergic disease. *Archives of Pediatrics & Adolescent Medicine, 160,* 502–507.

Thomas, M., Custovic, A., Woodcock, A., et al. (2006). Atopic wheezing and early life antibiotic exposure: A nested case-control study. *Pediatric Allergy and Immunology, 17,* 184–188.

Underdown, A., Barlow, J., Chung, V., et al. (2006). Massage intervention for promoting mental and physical health in infants aged under six months. *Cochrane Database of Systematic Reviews, 18*(4), CD005038.

VaccineEthics.org: Vaccination Requirements and Exemptions. Retrieved November 6, 2007, from http://www.vaccineethics.org/issue_briefs/requirements.php

Viljanen, M., Savilahti, E., Haahtela, T., et al. (2005). Probiotics in the treatment of atopic eczema/dermatitis syndrome in infants: a double-blind placebo-controlled trial. *Allergy, 60,* 494–500.

Weizman, Z., Alkrinawi, S., Goldfard, D., et al. (1993). Efficacy of herbal tea preparation in infantile colic. *The Journal of Pediatrics, 122,* 650–652.

Wessel, M. A., Cobb, J. C., Jackson, E. B., et al. (1954). Paroxysmal fussing in infancy, sometimes called "colic." *Pediatrics, 14,* 421–435.

Weston, S., Halbert, A., Richmond, P., et al. (2005). Effects of probiotics on atopic dermatitis: A randomized controlled trial. *Archives of Disease in Childhood, 90,* 892–897

Wheeden, A. (1993). Massage effects on cocaine-exposed preterm neonates. *Journal of Developmental and Behavioral Pediatric, 14*(5), 318–322.

White, A., Slade, P., Hunt, C., Hart, A., & Ernst. E. (2003). Individualized homeopathy as an adjunct in the treatment of childhood asthma: A randomised placebo controlled trial. *Thorax, 58*(4), 317–321.

Wiberg, J. M. M., Nordsteen, J., Nilsson, N. (1999). The short-term effect of spinal manipulation in the treatment of infantile colic: A randomized controlled trial with a blinded observer. *Journal of Manipulative and Physiological Therapeutics, 22*(8), 517–522.

Wijga, A. H., van Houwelingen, A. C., Kerkhof, M., et al. (2006). Breast milk fatty acids and allergic disease in preschool children: The Prevention and Incidence of Asthma and Mite Allergy birth cohort study. *The Journal of Allergy and Clinical Immunology, 117,* 440–447.

Wilson, K. M., & Klein, J. D. (2002). Adolescents' use of complementary and alternative medicine. *Ambulatory Pediatrics, 2,* 104–110.

Wolke, D., Gray, P., & Meyer, R. (1994). Excessive infant crying: A controlled study of mothers helping mothers. *Pediatrics, 94,* 322–332.

Wright, R. J., Cohen, R. T., & Cohen, S. (2005). The impact of stress on the development and expression of atopy. *Current Opinion in Allergy and Clinical Immunology, 5*(1), 23–29.

Zeiger, R. S. (2003). Food allergen avoidance in the prevention of food allergy in infants and children. *Pediatrics, 111,* 1662–1671.

27

Integrative Pediatric Pulmonology

JOHN D. MARK

KEY CONCEPTS

- Pediatric lung disorders such as asthma are common in children and most pediatric health care practitioners will care for children with lung problems.
- Pediatric lung disorders have both an acute and chronic components, thus making an "integrative approach" ideal since conventional therapies (such as medication) as well as complementary and alternative therapies (such as diet and mind-body therapies) are helpful in the management of these disorders.
- Often treating pediatric pulmonary problems with complementary and alternative therapies will result in the decrease or discontinuation of conventional medications (decreasing the does or need for inhaled corticosteroids [ICS] in children with asthma as an example).
- There is a growing body of scientific literature in pediatric pulmonary disorders that support the use of mind-body medicine, dietary supplements, nutrition, and life style changes that improve these conditions by reducing symptoms and decreasing the possible side effects of conventional medications.
- Therapeutic suggestions for two common pediatric pulmonary disorders, asthma and cystic fibrosis, are presented at the end of this chapter illustrating how an integrative approach could be utilized.

■

Overview

Integrative medicine combines treatments from conventional medicine and CAM for which there is evidence of safety and effectiveness. These various treatments including conventional medications along with dietary supplements, mind-body therapies, manipulative therapies, and acupuncture are commonly used in children with pulmonary problems. As an example, in a review of surveys of children with asthma, the most common chronic pediatric pulmonary disorder with an incidence of 5.8% (Elder et al., 2006), it was found that 33%–89% of the children used CAM therapies (Slader, Reddel, Jenkins, Armour, & Bosnic-Anticevich, 2006). Since childhood asthma is not one disease but a spectrum of symptoms and clinical presentations and the diagnosis is made based on history, physical exam, and assessment of airway reversibility, many children who may have asthma like symptoms may be given various CAM therapies as well. The treatment of asthma and other chronic pulmonary problems (including cystic fibrosis, chronic lung disease of the newborn, sleep disordered breathing and chronic or recurrent pneumonia/bronchitis) begins with developing therapies for the child by the health care provider, the family, and the child as a team. The primary goal is to reduce symptoms and exacerbations by using a variety of therapies.

Pediatric pulmonary disorders in children are thought to have multiple causes including infection, nutritional deficiencies (or excess such as in obesity), environmental exposures, and the child's genetic predisposition. Therefore the therapies may include conventional medications, environmental controls, life style modification such as exercise and weight control, with the goal to reduce symptoms, promote health and minimize potential for adverse effects of medications. CAM may also assist the patient, the family and the health care team in obtaining this goal by adding non-medical therapies such as dietary supplements, mind-body therapies, homeopathic medicines, and traditional Chinese medicine. By using conventional and CAM therapies in an "integrative medicine" approach, the management and improvement of many pediatric pulmonary disorders may be obtained in a safe and efficacious manner.

> Integrative medicine is using both conventional and non-conventional therapies in which there is evidence of safety and effectiveness.

Pathophysiology of Pediatric Pulmonary Disorders

Pediatric pulmonary disorders as mentioned above are common. These disorders include problems in lung growth, development, and repair such as bronchopulmonary dysplasia primarily seen in babies born prematurely. Respiratory infections (pneumonia, bronchiolitis, croup, etc.) are the number one cause of pediatric hospitalizations and are the second leading cause of death in children under 5 years. Asthma is the most common chronic pediatric pulmonary disorder and the number one reason for school absenteeism. In addition, factors including environmental exposure and air pollution may exacerbate and play a role in asthma and other chronic lung disorders. Finally, the care and impact of the child with chronic lung disease such as cystic fibrosis, asthma, and sickle cell disease make pediatric pulmonary disorders an area where practitioners will have frequent exposure whether in a pediatric primary practice setting or tertiary medical facility. Asthma, in particular, may cause many respiratory symptoms found in other pulmonary disorders. One may find acute respiratory distress, dyspnea (shortness of breath), exercise difficulties, disruptive sleep, chronic cough, acute and recurrent pneumonia, atelectasis (airway collapse), poor growth, need for acute and chronic medications and significant socioeconomic expense in children with asthma depending on the severity and the age of the patient. In the following sections, therapies for asthma will be outlined since many of the same integrative (conventional and CAM) therapies may be applicable to other pediatric pulmonary disorders with similar symptoms and aspects of disease. These signs and symptoms include chronic cough, congestion, exercise limitation, and nutrition limitations (allergies and sensitivities).

Asthma Mechanism

Asthma is a complex and heterogeneous disease with many phenotypic expressions; often it is difficult to even make the diagnosis especially in young children since some children who wheeze as infants, may no longer wheeze after age 6 years (Martinez et al., 1995). Since asthma is a multi-factorial disease, it is likely to be the result of interactions between a genetically determined predisposition to allergic diseases and environmental factors that serve to enhance inflammation of the lower airway. Genetic factors include regulation of cytokines that control the production of IgE, along with polymorphisms in genes that regulate airway tone and repair mechanisms for acute injuries (Gern & Lemanske, 2003). It has been shown (Bisgaard, 2004) that environmental factors, especially exposures in early infancy, may play a major role in the development of the immune system. Such exposures include microbial products, food and aeroallergens, stress, and infections such as RSV and rhinovirus. These exposures may help the immune system to mature so that allergies are less likely to occur. However, if asthma or allergies are already present, then a respiratory infection may actually cause damage to the lungs and increase inflammatory responses in the lower airway, which then may promote the development of asthma.

Asthma was once thought to be primarily a problem with excessive mucus production and bronchial smooth muscle contraction causing swelling and airway obstruction. It is now believed to be caused by inflammation and its resultant effects on airway structure leading to the development and persistence of asthma. Airway plugs found at post mortem exams consist of mucus, serum proteins, inflammatory cells, and cellular debris. The airways are infiltrated with various inflammatory cells including eosinophils and mononuclear cells. The other findings include damage done at the epithelial cell level with cellular leakage in the microvascular space. The increase mucus production is due to increased number of goblet cells. The smooth muscle is hypertrophied and is characterized by new formation of vessels, and an increase of interstitial collagen. These findings are important in the theory that this chronic inflammation may ultimately lead to irreversible changes in the airway. This remodelling and fibrosis of the airway has lead medical practitioners to advocate the use of medications early in the treatment of asthma, however, it is not known which children will go on to develop the irreversible changes even with anti-inflammatory medications such as ICS.

Asthma-Conventional Therapies

There are now evidence based guide lines for the pharmacological treatments for infants, pre-school children, and older children with asthma. These recently updated guide-lines and classifications of asthma severity along with suggested therapies are from the National Asthma and Education Program through the National Institutes of Health (NIH, 2007). The individual therapies will not be discussed but may be found in a recent review (Milgrom, 2006). The use of controller medications, such as ICS, are the main-stay of chronic asthma in children and adults, and have made a significant impact in the care of children with chronic asthma. Their clinical effects include reduction in severity of symptoms; improvement in asthma control and quality of life; improvement in lung function (such as peak flow and spirometry); diminished airway hyperresponsiveness; prevention of exacerbations; reduction in systemic corticosteroid courses, emergency department care, hospitalizations, and deaths due to asthma; and possibly the attenuation of loss of lung function in adults.

However, patients and families are aware of the potential side effects and complications of chronic steroids use, even if only given by inhalation. Patients and families will often withhold this type of medication in favor of non-pharmacological treatments. This reluctance, in addition to the potential overuse of short acting inhaled β_2-agonists (SABA), may lead to the under-treatment of children with asthma. By using both conventional and CAM therapies, the integrative approach may actually lead to better adherence and control of asthma in children, but this has yet to be studied.

Acute or chronic respiratory problems should always be evaluated by medically trained health care provider before any CAM therapies be started.

Asthma-Integrative Approaches

MIND-BODY THERAPIES

Mind-body therapies have been used in the treatment of asthma in various ways. They are at times referred to as cognitive behavioral therapies and encompass several approaches. Research in this area started in the early 1960s, and approaches have included relaxation therapy, breathing exercises, biofeedback, and hypnosis/guided imagery. The theory behind using mind-body therapies is based on the inflammatory process that can be triggered by the autonomic nervous system through emotions. It has been reported that stress, particularly in children with asthma from lower socio-economic levels, is associated with higher morbidity and cytokine levels attributed to airway inflammation (Chen et al., 2006). In addition to anxiety, stress has been shown to influence the immune response and may promote an increase sympathetic activity,

----

Prior to relaxation therapies, belly breathing is often taught

- Explain to child that there are two ways of breathing.
- One way is to breathe from the chest; the other way is to breathe from the diaphragm.
- Many people use a combination of chest and diaphragm breathing throughout the day.
- "When we use our chest to breathe our body can cause uncomfortable bodily sensations and make it difficult to breath. Belly breathing, on the other hand, helps us become relaxed. So, one way to help us breath is to breathe from the belly rather than from the chest."
- Instruct the child to sit comfortably and model for the child how to breathe with the diaphragm. Take a deep abdominal breath (inhale for a count of 4) and release the air slowly (exhale for a count of 4).
- Place your hand on your belly and direct the child's attention to the expansion of your belly as you inhale and the falling of the abdomen as you exhale. Instruct the child to try several deep abdominal breaths, noticing the difference in the way the breathing and the body feels.
- Identify feelings associated with relaxation—sleepy, warm, tingly—after the breathing exercise.

Ask child if he/she had any difficulties with this breathing. When the child is comfortable with belly breathing, you may proceed to relaxation techniques.

----

augment IgE production, shift from a TH1 to TH2 allergic type response and promote airway inflammation without overt symptoms (Marshall, 2004). Studies have also shown that using different types of cognitive behavioral therapies such as relaxation, story telling, and self-hypnosis may decrease symptoms and medication use (Kohen & Wynne, 1997). This can be accomplished by a team approach as well as referring to specialist such as a psychologist. During a 3-year period, one pediatric pulmonary center reported instructing 72 children (average age 11.6 years) in self-hypnosis and 82% reported improvement or resolution in symptoms such as anxiety, asthma, chest pain, dyspnea, habit cough, sighing, and vocal cord dysfunction (Anbar & Hummell, 2005).

The use of breathing exercises may be considered a type of mind-body therapy. It has been known that dysfunctional breathing has been associated with asthma symptoms since the 1960s. The use of breathing exercises in controlling asthma symptoms has been taught and promoted by the American Lung Association and the Centers for Disease and Prevention through the Open Airways for Schools (OAS) where belly breathing (diaphragmatic breathing) is taught as one of the lessons for doing well at school. Other types of breathing exercises and breathing retraining have been used in the management of asthma. One specific form of breathing therapy, known as the Buteyko breathing technique, has been thought to help asthma my decreasing the respiratory rate, allowing carbon dioxide to increase resulting in bronchodilation. A Cochrane review concluded that breathing exercises for asthma, such as Buteyko, yoga, and diaphragmatic breathing, led to decreased use of SABA and a trend towards improvement in quality of life, but not in decreasing the amount of anti-inflammatory medications, reducing airway reactivity or improving lung function (Holloway & Ram, 2004). The use of mind-body therapies has also included prayer in many CAM questionnaire studies. Prayer, at this time, has not been studied in asthma in children or adults with pulmonary disorders as a CAM therapy. In conclusion, if used with conventional therapies, various mind-body modalities appear to be safe and possibly efficacious in treating chronic asthma and possibly other chronic pulmonary disorders such as habit cough, dyspnea, and chronic lung disease such as cystic fibrosis.

BIOLOGICAL THERAPIES
(NUTRITION AND HERBAL SUPPLEMENTS)

Nutrition

The role of nutrition in the development of asthma is thought to be important. Since the diet is the major source of antioxidants, suboptimal intake during airway growth may lead to airway damage and reduced airway compliance. It has been hypothesized that in industrialized countries there had been an increase in atmospheric pollution and exposure to cigarette smoke, and a decrease in vegetable and fruit consumption. This could then lead to a dietary deficient in antioxidants and increase susceptibility to oxidant damage (Devereux & Seaton, 2005). This reduced consumption of foods rich in antioxidants has been accompanied by the decrease in dietary intake of oily fish (tuna, herring, mackerel, trout, and salmon) and fish oil (cod liver oil) which are high in n-3 polyunsaturated fatty acids (PUFAs), mainly eicosapentaenoic acid (EPA) and docosahexaenoic acid (DHA). This reduction in n-3 PUFAs was also observed at the same time as an increase in the intake of n-6 polyunsaturated fatty acids which are present in margarine and vegetable oils. It has been hypothesized that the consequence of increasing n-6 and decreasing n-3 PUFA intakes may result in increase arachidonic acid and prostaglandin E-2 production with consequent increase in atopic TH2 sensitization, asthma and atopic disease (Black et al., 1997).

There have been epidemiological studies showing the beneficial association between fruits, vegetables and other antioxidant rich foods. One study investigated 690 children taking in a traditional Mediterranean diet characterized by in increase in plant foods such as fruits and vegetables, bread and cereals, legume and nuts (all sources of dietary antioxidants) and where the primary oil was olive oil. Eighty percent of these children were eating fresh fruit and 68% were eating vegetables twice and day. This diet was found a to be protective for wheezing and atopy (Chatzi et al., 2007). The Children's Health Study (10 year longitudinal study of respiratory health in over 2000 schoolchildren around Los Angeles, CA) used a cross sectional analysis of dietary intake data to look at the effect of antioxidant vitamin intake on lung function comparing low intake with a high intake (Gilliland et al., 2003). Fruit and vegetable intake was monitored using servings per day. This study showed that low intake of antioxidant vitamins had adverse effects on lung function among both boys and girls. The effects of vitamins A, C, and E appeared to be independent of asthma status. The deficits found in this study were felt to be clinically significant.

Another study (Burns et al., 2007) examined the association of dietary factors (fruit, vegetables, vitamin C, vitamin E, beta-carotene, retinol, and n-3 PUFA) in 2112 high school students in the United States and Canada. It as hypothesized that fruits, antioxidants, and other micronutrients may prevent or limit the inflammatory response of the respiratory system by reducing reactive oxygen species and inhibiting lipid peroxidation. Since adolescents often have poor dietary habits, this group of children may have lower lung function and decreased pulmonary function. In reviewing completed questionnaires, it was found that dietary fruit and vegetables, vitamin E, vitamin A, beta carotene, and n-3 PUFA were low in one third or more of the students. Low fruit intake was associated with lower lung function measuring the forced expiratory volume in one second (FEV1) compared with higher intake as well as increased report of chronic bronchitis type symptoms and asthma. Low vitamin E intake was also associated with increased report of asthma and low dietary n-3 PUFA also had increase report in chronic bronchitis type symptoms, wheeze and asthma compared to higher intake. The authors conclude that lower pulmonary function, chronic cough and wheeze were found more often in adolescents with low dietary micronutrient intake. The promoting of fruit and fish consumption in addition to vitamin supplementation may be important to ensure adequate intake of antioxidants and n-3 PUFA in this group of rapidly growing children.

However, dietary antioxidant deficiency influencing lung health through immunomodulatory and decreased antioxidant mechanism using interventional studies in established disease (such as asthma) have been not shown significant improvement. In a Cochrane meta-analysis of nine randomized controlled trials conducted in adults and children with established asthma, concluded that there was no consistent effect of n-3 PUFA supplementation on asthma symptoms, asthma medication use, lung function or bronchial hyperresponsiveness (Woods, Thien, & Abramson, 2002). There has been some evidence that fish oil supplementation has a protective effect on exercise induced bronchoconstriction (EIB) which may be attributed to its anti-inflammatory properties. In a study of 16 young adult asthmatic patients with documented EIB where one group ($n = 8$) received fish oil supplementation (EPA and DHA) and the other group ($n = 8$) were given placebo. Pre-exercise and post-exercise measurements were assessed and it was found that the fish oil diet improved pulmonary function to below the diagnostic EIB threshold with a concurrent reduction in bronchodilator use. Biomarkers of inflammation using induced sputum and activated polymorphonuclear leukocytes for eicosanoid metabolites, prostaglandin D2, and cytokines were reduced in the subjects on the fish oil diet. It was felt that fish oil supplementation may represent a potentially beneficial intervention to asthmatic subjects with EIB (Mickleborough, Lindley, Ionescu, & Fly, 2006).

It may be that dietary intervention such as increased antioxidant intake might be particularly important during pregnancy and early childhood. However, this has yet to been shown in a published study. In the Childhood Asthma Prevention Study (CAPS) 616 children were randomized to an active diet intervention and received fish oil supplements high in n-3 PUFA and minimized n-6 PUFA intake. Of the 189 children who completed all parts of the study, there was no association between plasma levels of n-3 or n-6 PUFA at 10 months, 3 years, and 5 years and the prevalence of asthma or wheezing illness, eczema, or atopy at 5 years even though the active dietary intervention group had high levels of n-3 PUFA and lower levels of n-6 PUFA at 5 years of age (Almqvist et al., 2007). Further research in to dietary manipulation as a public health measure is needed to evaluate its role in reducing the risk of asthma. Nutritional and dietary interventions may also be important in combination with other therapies (breast feeding, avoidance environmental tobacco smoke and air pollution) in improving overall lung health but the evidence is not clear in children as to what ones are most efficacious.

Fruits-High in antioxidants:
Prunes Raisins Blueberries Blackberries Strawberries Raspberries Plums
Oranges Red grapes Cherries Kiwi fruit Grapefruit, pink
Vegetables-High in antioxidants:
Kale Spinach Brussels sprout Alfalfa sprouts Broccoli Flowers Beets Red bell
Onion Corn Eggplant

Herbal Supplements

Herbal supplements are a type of dietary supplement that contain parts of plants such as the flowers, leaves, stems, bark, berries, seeds, and roots. This various plant parts may be taken orally as pills, freeze dried capsules, or powders. They may also be given as tinctures, syrups or brewed in teas and decoction. Herbal supplements can also be "applied" as salves, ointments, or poultices to the skin or mucous membranes They are commonly used for the treatment of asthma and in survey studies are often the most common CAM therapy utilized. In a review of 17 studies including seven in pediatric populations, one in adolescents and two including both adults and children, the use of herbal supplements (including herbal medicines, minerals, vitamins, honey, teas, quail eggs, naturopathy, and Ayurvedic therapies) ranged from 12% to 53% of patients surveyed (Slader et al., 2006).

This has caused concern since herbs may have interactions with conventional medications and even other herbal supplements. Also, in many herbal supplements the active ingredients are not known and there may be dozen or more compounds. This, along with the possibility of not always knowing the exact ingredients (may be different then what is listed on the supplement container), makes understanding how herbal supplements affect the body in such conditions as asthma difficult. There has also been a question of safety in herbal supplements due to the reporting of some being contaminated with metals, unlabeled prescription drugs, microorganisms, and other substances (Woolf, 2006). In the United States, herbal and other dietary supplements are regulated by the US Food and Drug Administration (FDA) as foods. This means that they do not have to meet the same standards as drugs and over-the-counter medications for proof of safety, effectiveness. In June 2007, the FDA announced new regulations requiring rules for previously not well enforced good manufacturing practices (cGMEP). These new rules ensure that dietary supplements are produced in a quality manner, do not contain contaminants or impurities, and are accurately labeled.

This is important since there has been research regarding herbal supplements in the treatment of asthma, including several in children. One study investigated the use of butterbur (*Petasites hybridus*) in children and adults with asthma. Butterbur is a perennial shrub that has traditionally been used for such things as urinary problems, back pain, wound healing, and asthma. In this study, 64 adults and 16 children were studied in a prospective nonrandomized open trial in subjects who had mild to moderate asthma. The subjects took butterbur for 8 weeks in addition to their regular asthma medications and by the end of the study, the number and duration of asthma exacerbations had decreased by 48% and 75% respectively. There was also reported reduction in the dose of ICS (42.9%), reduction in the use of SABA (48.3%) and improvement in lung function measuring FEV_1 and peak flow (70.6 and 83.9% respectively). The butterbur was generally well tolerated but seven subjects reported 11 adverse events with such complaints as abdominal pain, allergic type symptoms (sneezing, rhinitis) and halitosis (Danesch, 2004). Although this appears promising, the study was limited by the lack of blinding and small sample size.

There have been recent attempts to improve the study design for herbal supplements and asthma in children. In a randomized, placebo controlled, double-blind study involving 60 subjects ages 6–18 years, Pycnogenol (a proprietary mixture of water-soluble bioflavonoids extracted from French maritime pine) was studied in mild to moderate asthma (Lau et al., 2004). Using peak flow monitoring, symptoms diaries, medication use, changes in oral medications (zafirlukast) along with urine samples for leukotriene $C_4/D_4/E_4$, the group who took Pycnogenol for three months had significant improvement in pulmonary function and asthma scores along with reduction in urinary leukotrienes. The Pycnogenol group also was able to reduce or discontinue their use of rescue inhalers (SABA) more often then the placebo group. This included 18 of 30 subjects in the Pycnogenol group who did not use their SABA inhaler during the third month. It is possible that this herbal supplement which is felt to have potent anti-inflammatory properties may be helpful in treating children with asthma. Another small study in 40 adults with asthma using *Boswellia serrata* gum (felt to inhibit leukotriene synthesis), a double-blind, placebo controlled 6-week study showed that in the group taking the gum resin 70% had decrease in physical symptoms (dyspnea and number of attacks) and improvement in lung function. They also demonstrated decrease in eosinophilia in peripheral blood and lower erythrocyte sedimentation rate (Gupta et al., 1998).

Many of the studies for herbal supplementation include antioxidants such as vitamin C and selenium. Antioxidants may help limit oxidative stress which is thought to play a role in the pathogenesis of asthma. These studies are primarily in adults with asthma but since many children are given these types of supplements, they will be briefly discussed. Vitamin C is an antioxidant vitamin that has been promoted as a supplement that may help asthma control and even decrease asthma attacks. It has been shown to be low in children and adults with asthma particularly subjects with a low intake of fruits and vegetables as previously discussed. In a Cochrane review of vitamin C supplementation for asthma (Ram, Rowe, & Kaur, 2004), 71 abstracts and titles were analyzed and 8 studies were selected for inclusion. Of the eight studies, one involved children and one involved both children and adults. All studies were placebo controlled and randomized. The conclusion was that from these randomized controlled trials there was insufficient evidence to recommend a specific role for vitamin C in the treatment of asthma. Another anti-oxidant that may suppress asthma inflammation by increasing glutathione peroxidase in the airway epithelial lining fluid is selenium (Kelly, Mudway, Blomberg, Frew, & Sandstrom, 1999). In a randomized, double-blind, placebo-controlled trial of 197 adult with asthma there was not a significant improvement in asthma-related quality of life scores or secondary outcomes measures of lung function, asthma symptom scores, peak flow measurements or bronchodilator usage (Shaheen et al., 2007). At this time there is insufficient evidence to suggest the routine addition of vitamin C and selenium will improve asthma or prevent exacerbations.

Magnesium is a supplement that has long been known to be a potent bronchodilator. It is found in the diet in whole seeds, grains, nuts, and vegetables and the United States Department of Agriculture (USDA) survey in 1990 showed that children's mean intakes of some vitamins and minerals including magnesium were below the Recommended Daily Allowance (RDA). It has also been shown through epidemiological data that low magnesium intake is associated with airway hyper-reactivity and self-reported wheez-ing (Soutar, Seaton, & Brown, 1997). Magnesium is often promoted as a routine sup-plement for asthma by alternative health care providers and is an ingredient of many herbal supplements for improving lung health. A study (Gontijo-Amaral, Ribeiro, Gontijo, Condinoo-Neto, & Ribeiro, 2007) investigating the effects of oral magnesium supplementation on clinical symptoms, bronchial reactivity, lung function and aller-gen-induced skin responses in children with moderate persistent asthma. This random-ized placebo-controlled study in 37 subjects aged 7–19 years which both groups were taking ICS (fluticasone) showed that after 2 months of therapy, the magnesium group had decrease in airway reactivity using methacholine challenge, had decrease in skin responses to known allergens and had fewer asthma exacerbations along with using less rescue medication (salbutamol) compared to the control group. The pulmonary lung function was similar in both groups. The role of magnesium in the general treatment of asthma in children needs to be further studied since this study did show a potential beneficial effect of a low cost mineral supplement.

Another area where herbal supplements are commonly used for asthma is the use of herbal remedies in traditional Chinese medicine (TCM). TCM is a major compo-nent of CAM therapies used in the United States and both acupuncture and herbal remedies are the major TCM modalities of treatment. Asthma has been recognized in Chinese medicine for centuries and there are traditional formulas used in TCM prac-tice. The classic Chinese herbal remedy used for breathing disorders such as asthma was ephedra (known as Ma huang or *Ephedra sinica*). The pharmaceutical ephedrine derived from Ma huang was used in asthma therapy until the advent of more specific beta-agonist medications. Ma huang may be present in many combinations of other botanicals for respiratory problems including licorice which is felt to enhance airway clearance through its mucilaginous properties. Most recently, Ma Huang has been avail-able in combinations with other stimulant herbal supplements such as caffeine and caf-feine related products (primarily promoted for weight loss and energy), and there have been reported deaths associated with its use. Central nervous system problems such as nausea, vomiting, sweating, and nervousness along with heart palpitations, tachycardia, hypertension, anxiety, and myocardial infarction have all been reported (Haller & Benowitz, 2000). For this reason, ephedra is not recommended in the treatment of asthma due to the warnings from the FDA and reports of serious side effects.

In TCM, herbal supplements are commonly prepared as a combination of many herbs tailored for the individual patient. The herbal combination is then decocted (to concentrate by boiling) in the preparation the patient it to use. There are usually one or two main herbal supplements that target the asthma symptoms particular to that patient and there are several others added to adjust the formula to achieve balance (yin/yang) for the patient's condition. The balance and interaction of the ingredients are felt to be as important as the effect of the individual ingredient. It is believed that the complex interaction between the various herbs in the formulation produce synergistic effects and reduce possible side effects of some of the individual herbs. In the last several years, there have been several double-blind, placebo-controlled clinical studies investigating both the safety and efficacy of Chinese herbal supplements in both the treatment and the mechanism of asthma. Although few studies have been reported in using the various herbal supplements in children with asthma, a recent review presented an update on some of the more promising Chinese herbal remedies for asthma (Li, 2007).

STA-1 is a Chinese herbal mix that was studied in 120 children age 5–20 years with mild to moderate asthma and who had frequent respiratory symptoms seen in a clinic in the Chinese Medical Center in Taiwan. In this randomized double-blind placebo-controlled study that took place over 6 months using two different formulations, it was shown that pulmonary function (FEV1) and clinical symptoms improved in the STA-1 group over placebo especially in those children with dust mite allergy and asthma (Chang, Huan, & Hsu, 2006). The role of these various Chinese herbal mixtures in the control of asthma is still to be determined in children but the results in the few adult studies are promising.

> Traditional Chinese herbal remedies may contain mixtures of several herbs. They should only be prescribed by someone trained in their use with children.

Other herbal supplements that are commonly used for asthma and pediatric pulmonary disorders but have not been studied in detail, especially in children, include tylophora (*Tylophora indica or asthmatica*). It is a climbing perennial plant indigenous to India, where it grows wild in the southern and eastern regions and has a reputation as a remedy for asthma. Another herb sometimes recommended for asthma also comes from India and is called coleus (*Coleus forskohlii*). The active ingredient is Forskolin and my work in asthma by stabilizing cells that release histamine and other inflammatory compounds as well as relaxing smooth muscle. Other supplements include the antioxidants lycopene and beta-carotene for exercise induced asthma. Vitamins B6 and B12 have been proposed as asthma therapies but there are no well controlled studies to support its use. If one peruses the Internet, herbs such as gingko, aloe, chamomile, garlic, ginger, horehound, licorice, marshmallow, mullein, onion, lobelia, yerba santa and hundreds more have been used by traditional herbalist for respiratory problems in children and adults. None of these treatments have any scientific supporting evidence for use in children under age 18 for chronic pulmonary disorders.

MANIPULATIVE THERAPIES

Manipulative therapies encompass a variety of techniques that are commonly used as part of CAM in the treatment of asthma and other pulmonary conditions. These include massage therapy, chiropractic manipulation, osteopathic manipulation (cranio-sacral as an example), chest percussion, and vibrational therapy. Chiropractic physicians have used chiropractic spinal manipulation as a standard of care for asthma for many years. A randomized controlled trial of chiropractic manipulation for 91 children with mild to moderate asthma did not show any significant difference in peak flow monitoring and there was no difference between quality of life scores and use of rescue medications (Balon et al., 1998). In a smaller study, 36 subjects ages 6–17 with mild to moderate asthma were given chiropractic spinal manipulative therapy (SMT) in addition to their medical management. Outcome measure included pulmonary function tests, quality of life questionnaires, asthma severity, peak flow measurements, and symptom diaries. The subjects received 3 months of either active SMT or sham SMT. At the end of the study, the quality of life measurements improved and asthma severity was lower in the treatment group (Bonfort, Evans, Kubic, & Filkin, 2001).

A Cochrane review of a variety of manual therapies in the treatment of asthma was undertaken since a similar biologic mechanism of action has been postulated. From over 473 citations, 3 randomized control trials met inclusion criteria. Two were chiropractic manipulation studies and one was massage therapy compared to relaxation. In the conclusion there was insufficient evidence to support the use of manual therapies in the treatment of asthma. As in common in other areas of CAM research, the majority of the studies are small in number of subjects, and have poor methodology in regard to controls and blinding. Future trials need to be designed to account for these weaknesses in study designs (Hondras, Linde, & Jones, 2005).

Alternative Health Systems

TRADITIONAL CHINESE MEDICINE

Traditional Chinese medicine (TCM) has been practiced for several thousand years and has many forms. The basis is the understanding of the connections between body, mind, and spirit in health and disease. The belief in an unseen vital energy that affects the patient's health and how this energy or qi (chi) flows through the appropriate channels is the basis of this practice. The practitioner can affect this flow or intensity by manipulating the balance using acupuncture, Chinese herbs, diet, and physical therapy. The use of Chinese herbal supplements has been previously discussed. The other modality that is commonly used as a TCM therapy for asthma is acupuncture. Although the National Institutes of Health 1997 Consensus Development Conference on Acupuncture did recommend acupuncture for many conditions, including asthma, the studies have not supported the use of acupuncture in children or adults for either chronic or acute therapy. A review by the Cochrane collaboration 11 studies for acupuncture and asthma concluded that there is not enough evidence to make recommendations about the value of acupuncture in asthma treatment. The review goes on to recommend further research considering the complexities and different types of acupuncture (McCarney, Brinkhaus, Lasserson, & Linde, 2004). Until recently, most studies were small, uncontrolled and there were methodological problems with blinding, lack of standardization and developing controls such as sham acupuncture. Recently using such techniques as laser acupuncture, some of these methodological problems have been addressed. In a double-blind, placebo-controlled crossover study, laser acupuncture was studied in 44 children with known exercise induced asthma. The laser acupuncture was performed on real and placebo points and lung function was measured before and after cold air challenge using isocapnic hyperventilation. There was no significant difference in the FEV1 between the two groups (Gruber et al., 2002). Another study in 17 children with asthma investigated whether a 10-week course of laser acupuncture and 7 weeks of probiotic treatment (*Enterococcus faecalis*) offered better asthma control then did a control group. This pilot study was randomized, placebo-controlled, and double-blinded but the numbers were small (8 and 9 patients in each group). Measurement of asthma control included peak flow variability, FEV1, and quality of life using a standard questionnaire. The laser acupuncture and probiotics significantly decreased peak flow variability and there was no significant effect on FEV1, quality of life criteria or need for additional medication (Stockert et al., 2007).

Even though the research methods are improving for evaluating acupuncture and asthma, there is insufficient evidence at this time to recommend acupuncture in the treatment of acute or chronic asthma. With that being said, there has been some research suggesting that the lack of positive findings in acupuncture and asthma studies is in part due to model of research being used (Paterson & Britten, 2004). Attempts to isolate the effect of a specific therapy, or "needling" may interfere with the positive outcomes that are not part of the study design since TCM is an holistic approach to a chronic problem and acupuncture is but one part of the therapeutic relationship.

HOMEOPATHY

Homeopathy has become popular in the treatment of both acute and chronic health problems and globally is among the five most widely used CAM therapies. In India there are over 200,000 registered practitioners, 182 colleges and over 300 homeopathic hospitals (Vickers & Zollman, 1999). It is classified as a drug therapy in the United States by the FDA and in some countries has been integrated into the national health care systems. In the United States the qualifications of practitioners vary; some are trained exclusively in homeopathy, others are trained in homeopathy following professional qualification as a medical doctor, dentist, naturopath or osteopathy.

Homeopathy is a therapeutic method using specific preparations of substances whose effects, when administered to healthy subjects, correspond to the manifestations of the disorder (symptoms, clinical signs, and pathological states) in the individual patient. It is believed that the effect is to stimulate a healing response in the patient. A second principle in homeopathy is individualization of patient. This may be at the "whole person" level, or at a more clinical level, especially in the treatment of acute conditions. The doses used in homeopathy range from those that are similar in concentration to some conventional medicines to very high dilutions containing no material trace of the starting substance. There is no currently understood way that substances no material trace could have a specific physiological effect and this is undoubtedly one of the sources of scepticism about the claimed results of clinical trials in homeopathy.

Homeopathy has become an increasingly popular CAM modality used to treat asthma. A Cochrane review looked at six trials that were all placebo-controlled and double-blinded but noted they had variable quality in the treatment of chronic asthma. Since homeopathy treatments tend to be individualized, no quantitative pooling of results was possible. There was no significant effect when measuring lung function and the authors concluded that there is further need for observational data to document the different methods of homeopathic prescribing and patient response since, like TCM, this individualistic type of therapy is difficult to monitor using conventional randomized control trial (McCarney, Linde, & Lasserson, 2004).

In a randomized double-blind placebo-controlled trial of individualized homeopathic remedies compared to placebo medication in 96 children with mild to moderate asthma, the role of homeopathic remedies as an adjunct to conventional therapies were studied. The study used childhood asthma questionnaire as the primary outcome measure in addition to peak flow measurement, medication use, symptoms scores, day missed from school, asthma events, and adverse reactions. The study found no evidence that even using classical homeopathic remedies (individualized for each subject) that there was no evidence of improving the quality of life of the children ad no evidence of changes in other measurement such as rate of exacerbations (White, Slade, Hunt, Hart, & Ernst, 2003).

The safety profile for homeopathic remedies is felt to be wide since the manufacturers of these products are aware of the potential for manufacturing errors and adheres to international guidelines on production monitoring, as do pharmaceutical producers. Homeopathic medications in the United States (and Europe) are regulated as drugs according to section 201(g)(l) of the Food, Drug, and Cosmetic Act and also must comply with the labeling provisions of the FDA for OTC drugs. Homeopathic drugs must be manufactured according to good manufacturing practices (GMP) that are regulated by the FDA. Even though homeopathic medications are well regulated, with the rapidly growing use of homeopathic products and the increasing practice of self-medication, there should be raised awareness and continued vigilance to ensure the continued quality and safety of these products (Kirby, 2002).

What are the laws and principles of Homeopathy?

1. The Law of Similars

The principle that like shall be cured by like, that is the proper remedy for a patient's disease is that substance that is capable of producing, in a healthy person, symptoms similar to those from which the patient suffers.

2. The Principle of Minimum Dose

This principle states that extreme dilution enhances the curative properties of a substance, while eliminating any possible side effects. This is just the reverse of conventional drug philosophy where a minimum dose is required for effect.

3. Whole Person Prescribing

A homeopath studies the whole person using characteristics such as their temperament, personality, emotional, and physical responses when prescribing a remedy. So, a homeopath may treat different persons exhibiting the same symptom differently.

4. Laws of Cure

a. A remedy starts at the top of the body and works downward

b. A remedy works from within the body outward and from major to minor organs

c. Symptoms clear in reverse order of appearance.

EXERCISE

Exercise is both a conventional and CAM therapy that does not fit easily in any one category. It could be considered an "energy" medicine or even a mind-body therapy since exercise has been longed used for depression and anxiety. It also should be prescribed with caution since exercise in itself can induce symptoms in patients with asthma. However, there have been numerous studies to show that asthma can be better controlled in patients that regularly exercise. As to what type of exercise, there is no study illustrating the superiority of one type of exercise over another. It had long been assumed that swimming may be beneficial since the environment is more moist and cold dry air may actually exacerbate asthma symptoms. Studies have not supported this and it is recommended that any exercise that the patient will do on a regular basis and doesn't cause increase symptoms should be encouraged.

In particular, older patients may do better with their asthma or underlying chronic pulmonary problem if they follow a routine exercise regimen. This probably is in part to due to a better self-image and overall improved health associated with regular exercise in adults. Yoga could also be considered as a form of exercise that embodies many of the above therapies for improving the health of patients with asthma. It is a form of exercise, so there is a cardiovascular component; it involves using regulated breathing exercises (pranayama) and is a mind-body method by the use of relaxation and meditation as a part of many yoga practices. It was shown in a study in adults to help decrease medication use and decreased anxiety (Cooper et al., 2003).

Exercise and Chronic Lung Problems-Be careful:
Exercise to consider if your child has a lung problem:
Pool swimming (ensure good ventilation)
Outdoor swimming
Walking
Cycling
Treadmill running
Outdoor running
Exercising in warmer moister air accompanied by warm-ups may help with breathing problems.
In cold weather, wearing breathing masks which helps store the heat and moisture from the air may help decrease or avoid exercise-induced asthma
Good control of your asthma can tremendously help decrease exercise-induced asthma.
Reliever inhalers (such as albuterol) can also be helpful if used just before exercise.

SAFETY ISSUES

The mind-body therapies (Grade B) have no real safety issues when dealing with pediatric pulmonary disorders. Cognitive therapies including relaxation, biofeedback, and imagery have been used as standard to care in many pediatric disorders including irritable bowel syndrome, migraine headaches, and atopic dermatitis.

Nutrition (Grade B), unless one is taking a severely restrictive diet, also is considered safe. The area with the most risk for side effects and the area where safety is more concerning is using *herbal supplements*. The reasons for this have been previously

> Cognitive therapies should not be used in place of medications, especially if symptoms are moderate or severe. If the patient is using a peak flow meter, then these therapies can be used if peak flows are in a certain range.

discussed (see above). In general, the herbal supplements studied for pediatric asthma are generally thought to be safe at the recommended doses.

Butterbur (Petasites hybridus), Grade C: Studies have reported safety and good tolerability of commercially available butterbur products when used in recommended doses. There have been some reports of headache, drowsiness, fatigue, breathing difficulties, and pruritis. Even less common side effects include constipation, difficulty swallowing, nausea, and stomach upset. Raw, unprocessed butterbur plant should not be ingested to potential hepatotoxicity of pyrrolizidine alkaloids. This included teas, capsules of raw herb or unprocessed tinctures (This information is based on a systematic review of scientific literature edited and peer-reviewed by contributors to the Natural Standard Research Collaboration (www.naturalstandard.com).

Pycnogenol, Grade B: There has been some confusion in the United States market regarding products containing Pycnogenol or grape seed extract (GSE), because one of the generic terms for chemical constituents ("pycnogenols") is the same as the patented trade name. Scientific literature regarding this product should not be referenced as a basis for the safety or effectiveness of GSE. Pycnogenol is reported to be well-tolerated with occasional report of minor stomach discomfort. In theory, it may alter blood sugar levels and increase the risk of bleeding so caution would be advised in patients with bleeding disorders (www.naturalstandard.com).

Vitamin C, Grade C: Vitamin C is generally thought to be safe, especially in recommended doses. However, rare side effects include nausea, vomiting, heartburn, and abdominal cramps. High doses of vitamin C (greater then 1–2 gm/day) are associated with multiple adverse effects such as kidney stones, diarrhea, and gastritis. Large doses have been reported to precipitate hemolysis in patients with glucose 6-phosphate dehydrogenase deficiency (www.naturalstandard.com).

Magnesium, Grade C: A problem with using oral magnesium is the tendency of the preparations to cause diarrhea. This is usually minimal if the total daily dose is less then 400 mg per day using the magnesium gluconate formulation.

Selenium, Grade C: Selenium is generally safe and well tolerated if given at the US Recommended Dietary Allowance (RDA). Allergies and hypersensitivity are unlikely since it is a trace mineral. If taken at very high doses (4–5 times RDA), there have been reported gastrointestinal symptoms such as nausea, vomiting, abdominal pain, and diarrhea. Neuromuscular disturbances such as hyperreflexia, muscle tenderness and irritability, and weakness/fatigue have rarely been noted (www.naturalstandard.com).

Traditional Chinese medicine, herbal supplement, Grade C: There have been some promising studies using herbal supplements from TCM sources. However, there are safety issues as discussed above regarding *Ma huang* which is a common herb used in some TCM formulations. Another herbal supplement in many TCM regimens is *licorice* (*Glycyrrhiza glabra*). There is not enough scientific evidence to promote the use of licorice in children but it is commonly used in over the counter products. Licorice contains glycyrrhizic acid which is responsible for the many reported side effects. There is a deglycyrrhizinated licorice (DGL) form that is considered safer for use in adults. The adverse side effects result from electrolyte disturbances including sodium and fluid retention, low potassium levels and metabolic alkalosis. It should especially be used with caution if there is a history of congestive heart disease, kidney, liver disease or those taking diuretic type medications. Acute pseudoaldosteronism syndrome has been reported as has high blood pressure. There has also been reported interactions with various herbs and dietary supplements (www.naturalstandard.com). At the usual doses found in some TCM formulations for short term use in the child with no underlying cardiovascular or endocrine problem, the use of licorice (especially the DGL) is probably safe but has not been sufficiently studied.

Coleus (*Coleus forskohlii*), Grade C: Coleus has only been studied in adults and currently there is no proven safe or effective dose in children. Some individuals have allergy or hypersensitivity to coleus and there have been reported cases of contact dermatitis. It is generally regarded as safe but this has only been assessed in short term trials with small sample sized groups (www.naturalstandard.com).

Other herbal supplements (not sufficiently studied to provide evidence grade) used for pediatric pulmonary disorders include *tylophora* which has been reported to cause nausea, vomiting, mouth soreness, and alterations in taste sensation. *Gingko*, another commonly used herbal supplement, has been reported to interact with warfarin, aspirin, and other anticogulant therapy and should be avoided or carefully monitored for bleeding potential in susceptible individuals. Vitamin B6 if taken in high doses (usually over 500 mg/day) and with prolonged use have been associated with peripheral neuropathy.

Manipulative therapies, Grade C: Manipulative therapies are generally thought to be safe if performed by care providers with training in pediatrics. There have been reported complication of chiropractic manual treatments but none in the treatment of asthma. There is often the repeated use of radiographs in chiropractic evaluations making repeated radiation exposure an issue to some patients and their families.

Traditional Chinese medicine, Grade C: TCM, especially the use of acupuncture, have reported the rare incidence of adverse reaction including pneumothoraces. In a review of multiple reports (over a million treatments), the most common were pneumothorax and central nervous system injuries. There were also reported infections, primarily hepatitis B, but this has dramatically decreased over the last decade. The risk of serious adverse events with acupuncture was estimated to be 0.05 per 10,000 treatments and 0.55 per 10,000 individual patients (White, 2004).

Homeopathy, Grade C: Homeopathy is thought to be safe owing to the extreme dilution, and the treatments are inexpensive. In a study which only used subcutaneous administration of homeopathic remedies, there were rarely any adverse reactions noted. The most common reaction was local pain and tenderness at the injection site. In over 35 million patient encounters there was one asthma reaction noted (Baars, Adriaansen-Tennekes, & Eikmans, 2005).

Corticosteroids (conventional therapies), Grade A: The steroidal medications (especially the oral preparations) may cause problems with height velocity (in children), immune suppression, hypertension, cataracts, and hirsutism (if taken long term). The inhaled forms have rarer side effects and have been followed long term in children but may cause hoarseness, cough, temporary decrease in height velocity and oral candidiasis unless a spacer is utilized and/or good mouth rinsing is done.

Short-acting beta agonists (conventional therapies) Grade A: Beta agonists, especially the newer SABA are effective in reversing acute airway obstruction and are primarily used in asthma. However, they may cause rapid or irregular heartbeat, insomnia, and nervousness.

Case Study

During a first time evaluation for chronic asthma, a 12-year-old young girl and her family informed the physician that they did not want to take chronic conventional medications primarily ICS. She had the diagnosis of asthma since 3 years of age, had never been hospitalized, but did have frequent symptoms (cough) both at night and with exercise. She also had problems with recurrent colds and "bronchitis" during the winter months. She had been prescribed a leukotriene inhibitor (montelukast) as a control medication in addition to an inhaled corticosteroid (budesonide). She took neither regularly but did use her short acting inhaled β_2-agonist (rescue medicine, albuterol) 1–2 times per day; most days per week. Her lung function testing showed moderate airway obstruction that completely reversed to normal values after 4 puffs of albuterol medication.

Further history revealed she slept with her two cats and had exposure to both dogs and a bird. She had no exposure to tobacco smoke and she did not have any known food allergies. Her diet included some daily fruits and vegetables, but she also enjoyed snack foods and regular soda, usually drinking 1–2 "cokes" per day. The mother also had asthma but did not take medications regularly. The family lived in a large metropolitan city and the patient did well in school but was not able to participate physical activity (PE) or in after school activities

The regimen that the family, the patient and the health care provider developed included:

1. Conventional medication: budesonide dry powder inhaler (1 actuation), every morning and montelukast (5 mg) at night.

2. Diet: started eating fruits and vegetables daily, both in the morning and the evening (she helped her family shop for ones she enjoyed). In addition, her family tried to include salmon and other fish in the diet 2–3 times per week. She increased her water intake to 5–6 eight oz glasses a day and drank soda only on the weekends (1 per day max).
3. Environmental: enclosed her pillow cases and bed coverings in dust mite proof material and avoided down filled comforters during the winter. The pets were removed from her bedroom.
4. Herbal supplements: started on a once a day vitamin with RDA amounts of Vitamin C, Vitamin E, caretonoids, magnesium, zinc, and selenium. In addition she was placed on supplemental Pcynogenol.
5. Traditional Chinese Medicine: arranged to see a TCM practitioner who was trained in the care of children who would assess her for acupuncture, herbal medicine and martial arts such as Tai Chi. In addition, she would also began yoga with pranayama breathing.

She returned to the pediatric pulmonary clinic 4 months after the above therapies were started and her lung function was now normal. She had not used her rescue inhaler for 6 weeks (except pre-exercise) and she was sleeping through the night. Her budesonide dose at that time was reduced by half and was to be stopped in 4 months if she continued to do well.

Summary

Complementary and alternative medicine (CAM) and conventional medicine in combination are often used in the treatment of asthma and pediatric pulmonary disorders in children. This "integrative medicine" approach may have success in reaching the objectives of therapy: reducing symptoms, preventing exacerbations, and promoting a healthy life style with minimal adverse side effects of the various therapies used. However, there is no consensus on which type of CAM therapies should be combined with conventional ones, which CAM therapies have advantages over others and which CAM therapies may actually cause harm either using with conventional asthma treatments or alone. With the multiple and complex interaction of genetic influences and environmental exposures playing a role in asthma and other chronic lung disorders, further studies using CAM therapies with conventional treatments in the treatment of children is warranted.

SUMMARY AND THERAPEUTIC REVIEW: ASTHMA

Below is a summary of therapeutic options for treating asthma. Many of these therapies could also be used in other acute and chronic pulmonary disorders. If a patient is having persistent symptoms (daily wheezing, shortness of breath, difficulty sleeping or exercising) or severe symptoms (even if intermittent), it would be best to prescribe therapies such as short acting inhaled β_2-agonist and anti-inflammatory medications. For the patient who has mild to moderate symptoms, this step-wise approach might be considered.

- Lifestyle: Like many chronic illnesses, asthma would be best treated through prevention. Unfortunately, changing people's lifestyle including their environment is difficult. There are cultural and regional differences just in the United States that makes patient populations differ on how they approach a chronic illness and even how they used medical care. For the most part, exercise is something that once acute symptoms are controlled, helps most children with respiratory symptoms. Routine exercise will help most children and young adults with asthma (3–5 periods of exercise lasting a minimum of 20 minutes per week). It will also help will self-esteem, weight loss, and cardiovascular health.

- Conventional medications: For patients with mild to moderate symptoms that are long standing or intermittent symptoms that are severe (requiring emergency room evaluation, oral steroid use or hospitalization), using a controller medication such as an anti-inflammatory like fluticasone (Flovent), budesonide (Pulmocort) or memetasone (Asmanex) among others, may provide improvement of symptoms more rapidly while the other interventions mentioned above can be started. A patient with any history of respiratory distress should also have a short acting inhaled β2-agonist such as albuterol (Proventil, Ventolin, ProAir) available for use since this medication can be life saving. These types of medication should be considered first line if a patient has persistent or severe symptoms and should be under the care of a trained medical professional.

- Environmental: Reducing exposure to asthma triggers can be therapeutic in itself. Such things as house dust mite reduction, frequent cleaning, avoiding second hand smoke and removing all pets from the home will help decrease the "irritability" of the airways.

- Nutrition: One should consider increasing fruits and vegetables for their antioxidant contribution as well as those rich in omega-3 fatty acids while decreasing omega-6 fatty acid containing ones (vegetable oils).

- Supplements: Adding antioxidants such as vitamin C (if not adequately supplied in the diet), selenium (100 mcg a day) and fish oil capsules would be therapy to consider. Magnesium, especially with vitamin C may also be helpful. Pycnogenol and butterbur are two herbal supplements that may help in decreasing chronic asthma medications and providing better asthma control.

- Mind-body methods: These techniques can be very rewarding to use in the treatment of asthma and starting with breathing and relaxation is an excellent start.
  - The use of guided imagery and hypnosis is readily available in most communities and will also help decrease symptoms, medication use and physician/urgent care visits. Usually these methods should be used regularly (1–2 times daily) until familiar to the patient, they can then be used as needed for the asthma symptoms.
  - Breathing exercises and yoga also have been shown to help reduce stress, help with lung expansion and maybe decrease the "allergic" response of the body.
- Manipulative therapies: As adjuncts to the mentioned modalities and depending on the patient's preferences, using massage, osteopathic manipulation and chiropractic therapies may be beneficial. All three have different approaches and regimens and finding a practitioner that is familiar treating patients with asthma is the key.
- Alternative medical systems such as traditional Chinese medicine and homeopathy: It is difficult to know where to put these various modalities in the step-wise approach pediatric pulmonary problems such as asthma care. They could really fit anywhere in the treatment plan from the most mild to the most severe patient with asthma. It is important to use them in conjunction with the above therapies if the patient has moderate or severe symptoms, but would be appropriate as first line treatment in the interested patient with mild or intermittent asthma.

SUMMARY AND THERAPEUTIC REVIEW: CYSTIC FIBROSIS

Below is a summary of therapeutic options for treating cystic fibrosis. Many of these therapies could also be used in other chronic pulmonary disorders such as recurrent pneumonia, non-cystic fibrosis bronchiectasis and bronchiolitis obliterans. It is known that 50%–70% of children with cystic fibrosis use complementary and alternative therapies, the most common being herbal remedies/dietary supplements. Conventional care recommendations are well established in cystic fibrosis and there are national guidelines promoted by such groups as the Cystic Fibrosis Foundation. Most patients with cystic fibrosis (including infants) require routine airway clearance therapies and chronic medications including periodic antibiotics (both oral and inhaled). These therapies depend on the stage of the disease and which organs are involved. Cystic fibrosis (CF) may affect many organ systems the most common being the lungs and the gastrointestinal tract. Below is a common regimen for a cystic fibrosis patient to be following from a conventional care standpoint assuming that both lung and gastrointestinal systems are involved (the most common scenario):

1. Airway clearance using chest physiotherapy (CPT) which is usually done by vigorous percussion (using cupped hands) on the back and chest to "loosen" mucus from the lungs. This can also be done by various devices such as the high frequency chest wall oscillator which vibrates the lung areas using a vest type apparatus. This is usually done 2–4 times per day.

2. Often with this airway clearance, bronchodilator medications are given to help "open the airways" allowing the mobilized secretions to be expectorated.

3. Dornase alpha and hypertonic saline are two other inhaled medications that are part of the routine care for CF. Both have separate mechanisms of action but assist in keeping the airways open and clear of tenuous secretions which is part of the disease process in CF. The use of azithromycin and ibuprofen (both medications taken by mouth) for their "anti-inflammatory" properties may also be recommended even before there is significant lung disease as determined by lung function testing or on chest radiograph.

4. Inhaled antibiotics (such as tobramycin) are commonly used both routinely as well as oral or even intravenous antibiotics if there are certain organisms in the sputum or if there is a pulmonary exacerbation.

5. Multiple medications for nutritional support are prescribed and included fat soluble vitamins (E, A, and D), vitamin K, multi-vitamins, and pancreatic enzyme replacement which are taken with meals and snacks.

6. High calorie, high protein nutritional diet is also recommended along with dietary supplements such as high calorie shakes and drinks. Some CF patients require enteral feeds in addition to support their increased nutritional needs.

For the patient who has mild to moderate disease, this step-wise approach in addition to the above mentioned conventional care might be considered.

- Lifestyle: Like many chronic illnesses, CF is best treated early in an attempt to delay or decrease the progression of the disease. At times, changing people's lifestyle including their environment is difficult, especially when the child or adolescent with CF has so many regular treatments on daily basis. Exercise is an activity that not only improves self-esteem but has also been shown to improve such things as oxygen consumption and cardiopulmonary fitness.

- Environmental: Reducing exposure to any type of environmental irritants or allergic triggers is important. If the CF patient has allergic tendencies or even asthma as a co-morbidity, reducing house dust mite exposure and avoiding second hand smoke is important. Exposure to tobacco smoke has been shown to hasten the decline in lung function in patient with CF.

- Nutrition: Along with a high calorie, high protein diet, patients with cystic fibrosis should increase their consumption of fruits and vegetables. Like in asthma, increase diet in these foods has been correlated with better lung function most likely due to their antioxidant properties. Also, foods rich in omega-3 fatty acids while decreasing omega-6 fatty acid containing ones (vegetable oils) may decrease the inflammatory cascade in chronic lung disease.

- Supplements: In addition to fruits and vegetables in the diet, adding certain antioxidants such as vitamin C, selenium (100 mcg a day) and fish oil capsules would be therapy to consider. Taurine, an essential amino acid may improve fat absorption and *N*-acetylcysteine (NAC) may soon be recommended to the diet for the anti-oxidant properties it provides. Creatine is another supplement that has been studied in CF and shown to improve muscle strength, at least short term.

- Mind-body methods: Many of the techniques have been used with CF patients with positive results. Guided imagery and/or self-hypnosis has been shown to decrease shortness of breath or dyspnoea. Often as mentioned in the asthma section these services are available in most communities and may also help decrease chronic symptoms such as cough and decrease the use of certain medications such as beta agonists (asthma medication). Again, like in asthma, stress reduction is important since stress has been shown to increase airway inflammation and using such things as yoga, may help with lung expansion.

- Manipulative therapies: Children with CF and their parents have reported a positive response to massage therapy. Reduction in anxiety, improved mood and increase in peak flow measurements have been shown in small studies. The reduction in anxiety my facilitate breathing.

- Alternative Medical Systems such as Traditional Chinese Medicine and Homeopathy: As in asthma, it is difficult to know where to suggest such therapies as acupuncture, homeopathy, and Chinese herbal remedies. They may be used at any stage of disease in CF since it is a life long illness that has a natural progression that one is trying to slow. Acupuncture has been shown to decrease pain in children with CF and homeopathic remedies used to ward off early cold-like illnesses have been suggested to decrease the need for antibiotics for a full blown pulmonary exacerbation.

Integrative Medicine and Chronic Lung Problems in Children

In summary, when children with chronic lung problems such as asthma or cystic fibrosis present for medical care, using an integrative approach provides an opportunity to decrease their symptoms such as cough or shortness of breath and improve their lives.

This integrative approach may not "cure" asthma or cystic fibrosis, but by using these various therapies and lifestyle modalities, one may improve breathing, increase exercise capability and decrease the use of conventional medications (and the possibility of side effects). In cystic fibrosis, these therapies may further slow the decline in lung function even prolong life expectancy.

The integrative approach of using conventional therapies along with CAM would ideally start at a young age or when the illness is first diagnosed. Since there is a significant inflammatory component to the majority of chronic respiratory illnesses, conventional medications and therapies can often rapidly improve symptoms. Then additional therapies such as exercise, nutritional changes, environmental control and other CAM therapies may address the underlying triggers and help decrease or slow the progression of the chronic respiratory illness. These various approaches would optimize the goals of therapy—having a normal active life with normal or near normal lung function. In the case of CF, the goal would also be to slow the progression of lung disease as long as possible.

The role of some CAM therapies such as dietary supplements, alternative health medical systems (traditional Chinese medicine, Homeopathy, etc.) is not yet clear as to the degree of impact they may play over a prolonged period of time. However, studies to assess their safety and efficacy are being conducted and will hopefully assist health care providers in counselling patients and families as to which ones may best be suited to the child's particular illness and symptoms. Integrative Medicine uses all aspects of health care: preventive, psycho-social, mind-body, natural substances, energy and conventional medications and techniques (such as airway clearance therapies) in reaching the ultimate goal of improving health and well being.

Recommended Resources

NHLBI Asthma Guidelines: http://www.nhlbi.nih.gov/guidelines/asthma/asthgdln.htm

CDC Asthma Information: http://www.cdc.gov/health/asthma.htm

NCCAM herbal guide: http://www.nccam.nih.gov/health/supplement-safety/; http://nccam.nih.gov/health/herbsataglance.htm

National Library of Medicine, link to herbal supplements: http://sis.nlm.nih.gov/enviro/dietarysupplements.html

Consumer Laboratory website for analysis (subscription required): http://www.consumerlab.com/results/flaxseed.asp

Natural Standard Database, Integrative Medicine: http://www.naturalstandard.com/index.asp

American Library Association, CAM Resources: http://www.ala.org/ala/acrl/acrlpubs/crlnews/backissues2002/september/complementary.cfm

Grading system used (from Natural Standards):
http://www.naturalstandard.com/grading.html?printversion=true

Level of Evidence Grade	Criteria
A (Strong Scientific Evidence)	Statistically significant evidence of benefit from >2 properly randomized trials (RCTs), OR evidence from one properly conducted RCT AND one properly conducted meta-analysis, OR evidence from multiple RCTs with a clear majority of the properly conducted trials showing statistically significant evidence of benefit AND with supporting evidence in basic science, animal studies, or theory.
B (Good Scientific Evidence)	Statistically significant evidence of benefit from 1-2 properly randomized trials, OR evidence of benefit from ≥1 properly conducted meta-analysis OR evidence of benefit from >1 cohort/case-control/non-randomized trials AND with supporting evidence in basic science, animal studies, or theory. *This grade applies to situations in which a well designed randomized controlled trial reports negative results but stands in contrast to the positive efficacy results of multiple other less well designed trials or a well designed meta-analysis, while awaiting confirmatory evidence from an additional well designed randomized controlled trial.*
C (Unclear or conflicting scientific evidence)	Evidence of benefit from ≥1 small RCT(s) without adequate size, power, statistical significance, or quality of design by objective criteria,* OR conflicting evidence from multiple RCTs without a clear majority of the properly conducted trials showing evidence of benefit or ineffectiveness, OR evidence of benefit from ≥1 cohort/case-control/non-randomized trials AND without supporting evidence in basic science, animal studies, or theory, OR evidence of efficacy only from basic science, animal studies, or theory.
D (Fair Negative Scientific Evidence)	Statistically significant negative evidence (i.e., lack of evidence of benefit) from cohort/case-control/non-randomized trials, AND evidence in basic science, animal studies, or theory suggesting a lack of benefit. *This grade also applies to situations in which >1 well designed randomized controlled trial reports negative results, notwithstanding the existence of positive efficacy results reported from other less well designed trials or a meta-analysis. (Note: if there is ≥1 negative randomized controlled trials that are well designed and highly compelling, this will result in a grade of "F" notwithstanding positive results from other less well designed studies.)*
F (Strong Negative Scientific Evidence)	Statistically significant negative evidence (i.e. lack of evidence of benefit) from ≥1 properly randomized adequately powered trial(s) of high-quality design by objective criteria.*
Lack of Evidence†	Unable to evaluate efficacy due to lack of adequate available human data.

REFERENCES

Almqvist, C., Garden, F., Xuan, W., Mihrshai, S., Leeder, S., Oddy, W., et al. (2007). Omega-3 and omega-6 fatty acid exposure from early life does not affect atopy and asthma at age 5 years. *Journal of Allergy and Clinical Immunology, 119,* 1438–1444.

Anbar, R., & Hummell, K. (2005). Teamwork approach to clinical hypnosis at a pediatric pulmonary center. *American Journal of Clinical Hypnosis, 48,* 45–49.

Baars, E., Adriaansen-Tennekes, R., & Eikmans, K. (2005). Safety of homeopathic injectables for subcutaneous administration: A documentation of the experience of prescribing practitioners. *The Journal of Alternative and Complementary Medicine, 11,* 609–616.

Balon, J., Aker, P., Crowther, E., Danielson, C., Cox, P., O'Shaughnessy, D., et al. (1998). A comparison of active and simulated chiropractic manipulation as adjunctive treatment for childhood asthma. *New England Journal of Medicine, 339,* 1013–1020.

Black, P., & Sharpe, S. (1997). Dietary fat and asthma: Is there a connection? *European Respiratory Journal, 10,* 6–12.

Bonfort, G., Evans, R., Kubic, P., & Filkin, P. (2001). Chronic pediatric asthma and chiropractic spinal manipulation: A prospective clinical series and randomized clinical pilot study. *Journal of Manipulative and Physiological Therapeutics, 24,* 369–377.

Elder, W., Ege, M. J., & von Mutius, E. (2006). The asthma epidemic. *The New England Journal of Medicine, 355,* 2226–2235.

Bisgaard, H. (2004). The Copenhagen Prospective Study on Asthma in Childhood (COPSAC): Design, rationale, and baseline data from a longitudinal birth cohort study. *Annals of Allergy, Asthma and Immunology, 93,* 381–389.

Burns, J., Dockery, D., Neas, L., Schwartz, J., Coull, B., Raizenne, M., et al. (2007). Low dietary nutrient intakes and respiratory health in adolescents. *Chest, 132,* 238–245.

Chang, T., Huan, C., & Hsu, C. (2006). Clinical evaluation of the Chinese herbal medicine formula STA-1 in the treatment of allergic asthma. *Phytotherapy Research, 20,* 342–347.

Chatzi, L., Apostolaki, G., Bibakis, I., Skypala, I., Bibaki-Liakou, V., Tzanakis, N., et al. (2007). Protective effect of fruits, vegetables and the Mediterranean diet on asthma and allergies among children in Crete. *Thorax, 62,* 677–683.

Chen, E., Hanson, M., Paterson, L., Griffin, M., Walker, H., & Miller, G. (2006). Socioeconomic status and inflammatory processes in childhood asthma: The role of psychological stress. *Journal of Allergy and Clinical Immunology, 117,* 1014–1020.

Cooper, S., Oborne, J., Newton, S., Harrison, V., Coon, J., Lewis, S., et al. (2003). Effect of two breathing exercises (Buteyko and pranayama) in asthma: A randomised controlled trial. *Thorax, 58,* 674–679.

Danesch, U. (2004). Petasites hybridus (Butterbur root) extract in the treatment of asthma-an open trial. *Alternative Medicine Review, 9,* 54–62.

Devereux, G., & Seaton, A. (2005). Diet as a risk factor for atopy and asthma. *Journal of Allergy and Clinical Immunology, 115,* 1107–1117.

Gern, J., & Lemanske, R. (2003). Infectious triggers of pediatric asthma. *Pediatric Clinics of North America, 50,* 555–575.

Gilliland, F., Berhane, K., Li, Y., Gauderman, W., McConnell, R., & Peters, J. (2003). Children's lung function and antioxidant vitamin, fruit, juice, and vegetable intake. *American Journal of Epidemiology, 158,* 576–584.

Gontijo-Amaral, C., Ribeiro, M., Gontijo, L., Condinoo-Neto, A., & Ribeiro, J. (2007). Oral magnesium supplementation in asthmatic children: A double-blind randomized placebo-controlled trial. *European Journal of Clinical Nutrition, 61,* 54–60.

Gruber, W., Eber, E., Malle-Scheid, D., Pfleger, A., Weinhandl, E., Dorfer, L., et al. (2002). Laser acupuncture in children and adolescents with exercise induced asthma. *Thorax, 57,* 222–225.

Gupta, I., Gupta, V., Parihar, A., Ludtke, R., Safayhi, H., & Ammon, H. (1998). Effects of Boswellia serrata gum resin in patients with bronchial asthma: Results of a double-blind, placebo-controlled, 6-week clinical study. *European Journal of Medical Research, 3,* 511–514.

Haller, C., & Benowitz, N. (2000). Adverse cardiovascular and central nervous system events associated with dietary supplements containing ephedra alkaloids. *New England Journal of Medicine, 343,* 1833–1838.

Holloway, E., & Ram, F. (2004). Breathing exercises for asthma. *Cochrane Database Systematic Review,* (1), CD001277.

Hondras, M., Linde, K., Jones, A. (2005). Manual therapy for asthma. *Cochrane Database Systematic Review,* (2), CD001002.

Kelly, F., Mudway, I., Blomberg, A., Frew, A., & Sandstrom, T. (1999). Altered lung antioxidant status in patients with mild asthma. *Lancet, 354,* 482–483.

Kirby, B. (2002). Safety of homeopathic products. *Journal of the Royal Society of Medicine, 95,* 464–465.

Kohen, D., & Wynne, E. (1997). Applying hypnosis in a preschool family asthma education program: Uses of storytelling, imagery and relaxation. *American Journal of Clinical Hypnosis, 39,* 169–181.

Lau, B., Riesen, S., Truong, K., Lau, E., Rohdewald, P., & Barreta, R. (2004). Pycnogenol as an adjunct in the management of childhood asthma. *Journal of Asthma, 41,* 825–832.

Li, X. (2007). Traditional Chinese herbal remedies for asthma and food allergy. *Journal of Allergy and Clinical Immunology, 120,* 25–31.

Marshal, G. (2004). Neuroendocrine mechanisms of immune dysregulation: Applications to allergy and asthma. *Annals of Allergy, Asthma and Immunology, 93,* S11–17.

Martinez, F., Wright, A., Taussig, L., Holberg, C. J., Halonen, M., & Morgan, W. J. (1995). Asthma and wheezing in the first six years of life. The Group Health Medical Associates. *New England Journal of Medicine, 332,* 133–138.

McCarney, R., Brinkhaus, B., Lasserson, T., & Linde, K. (2004). Acupuncture for chronic asthma. *Cochrane Database Systematic Review,* (1), CD000008.

McCarney, R., Linde, K., & Lasserson, T. (2004). Homeopathy for chronic asthma. *Cochrane Database Systematic Review,* (1), CD000353.

Mickleborough, T., Lindley, M., Ionescu, A., & Fly, A. (2006). Protective effect of fish oil supplementation on exercise-induced bronchoconstriction in asthma. *Chest, 129,* 39–49.

Milgrom, H. (2006). Childhood asthma: Breakthroughs and challenges. *Advances in Pediatrics, 53,* 55–100.

National Institutes of Health (NIH), National Heart, Lung, and Blood Institute. (2007). Expert Panel Report 3 (EPR 3): Guidelines for the Diagnosis and Management of Asthma. http://www.nhlbi.nih.gov/guidelines/asthma/asthgdln.htm

Paterson, C., & Britten, N. (2004). Acupuncture as a complex intervention: A holistic model. *Journal of Alternative and Complementary Medicine, 10,* 791–801.

Ram, F., Rowe, B., & Kaur, B. (2004). Vitamin, C. supplementation for asthma. *Cochrane Database Systematic Review,* (3), CD00093.

Shaheen, S., Newson, R., Rayman, M., Wong, A., Tumilty, M., Phillips, J., et al. (2007). Randomised, double blind, placebo-controlled trial of selenium supplementation in adult asthma. *Thorax, 62,* 483–490.

Slader, C., Reddel, H., Jenkins, C., Armour, C., & Bosnic-Anticevich, S. (2006). Complementary and alternative medicine use in asthma: Who is using what? *Respirology, 11,* 373–387.

Soutar, A., Seaton, A., & Brown, D. (1997). Bronchial reactivity and dietary antioxidants. *Thorax, 52,* 166–170.

Stockert, K., Schneider, B., Porenta, G., Rath, R., Nissel, H., & Eichler, I. (2007). Laser acupuncture and probiotics in school age children with asthma: A randomized placebo-controlled pilot study of therapy guided by principles of Traditional Chinese Medicine. *Pediatric Allergy and Immunology, 18,* 160–166.

Vickers, A., & Zollman, C. (1999). ABC of complementary medicine: Homeopathy. *British Medical Journal, 319,* 1115–1118.

White, A. (2004) A cumulative review of the range and incidence of significant adverse events associated with acupuncture. *Acupuncture Medicine, 22,* 122–133.

White, A., Slade, P., Hunt, C., Hart, A., & Ernst, E. (2003). Individualised homeopathy as an adjunct in the treatment of childhood asthma: A randomised placebo controlled trial. *Thorax, 58,* 317–321.

Woods, R., Thien, F., & Abramson, J. (2002). Dietary marine fatty acids (fish oil) for asthma in adults and children. *Cochrane Database Systematic Review,* CD001283.

Woolf, A. (2003). Herbal remedies and children: Do they work? Are they harmful? *Pediatrics, 112,* 240–246.

IV

The Future of Integrative Pediatrics: Looking Ahead

28

The Future of Integrative Pediatrics

TIMOTHY P. CULBERT, KATHI J. KEMPER, AND LAWRENCE D. ROSEN

KEY CONCEPTS

- The spread of the integrative care model within pediatrics will depend upon the co-creative efforts of the authors and readers of this volume.
- Healthcare must shift from a focus on "pathogenesis" to "salutogenesis" (creating health) and include consideration of all physical and non-physical factors in the etiology and resolution of disease.
- Integrative Medicine is not only the kind of medicine most patients want, it is the kind of medicine most physicians want to practice.
- Designing optimal, customized environments (or "healing habitats") to support each child's learning, emotional, physical, and spiritual needs will become a core skill for pediatric healthcare providers.
- As current medical business and reimbursement models fail, Philanthropy will continue on as an important force in mediating healthcare change over the next few decades.
- Integrative principles and methods of care will eventually be considered core curricula in all healthcare fields.
- The medicine of the future will recognize that a whole, perfect, harmonious pattern exists within each person. Integrative Pediatrics offers the most promising solution for shifting the paradigm of healthcare toward a preventative/wellness model and away from the current focus on disease treatment.

Futures for Children

In a sense, medicine is burning, as old ideas and methods are fading on every hand. But medicine's fires are purifying: new life is emerging from the ashes as it always does. The reinventors are stepping forward and healing is in the wind. The rebirth has begun.

—L. Dossey, Reinventing Medicine 1999

Whether the future of integrative pediatrics develops slowly, evolves gradually or burns in a mighty revolution depends on the co-creative efforts of the authors and readers of this volume in the context of our changing world. Change itself is inevitable; the speed and direction can be modified. As we conclude this volume, we will consider the context in which change will occur, and the multiple frameworks for viewing our goals and strategies within this context. In this final chapter, we are honored to invite leaders from integrative medicine to help us to visualize the transformation of pediatric health care as a definitive shift (with one definition of shift being "continuously varying") occurs to a more fully integrative model.

Karen Olness, MD, Director emeritus of Behavioral Pediatrics at Rainbow Babies and Children's Hospital in Cleveland, Ohio, recalls early experiences with introducing mind/body therapies such as hypnosis and biofeedback into the field of pediatric practice some 40 years ago. These techniques which are largely considered "mainstream" at this point, were cutting-edge and controversial then. She points out that

> It is not easy to steer the ponderous ship of pediatric practice in a new direction. Western society will need some major shifting of health care values before the wonderful benefits of integrating CAM with allopathic medicine will be widely and easily available to our children. (Olness, K., Personal Communication 2008)

Dr. Gregory Plotnikoff, medical director for the Penny George Institute for Health and Healing at Abbott Northwestern Hospital in Minneapolis Minnesota, who has just returned to the USA after nearly 6 years in Japan, offers this insight:

> The predominant medical culture in the United States is blind to the qualitative, subjective and intuitive aspects of care. The concerns so important to the work we do, which include trust, compassion, empathy, hope, and healing in its broadest sense, are not quantifiable and therefore neither understandable nor fundable in the current system. Without valuing the qualitative aspects of care, we

undervalue meaningful relationships and see no problem with 'interchangeable players.' We focus on the content of a single visit but may be blinded by the larger narrative. We are tyrannized by 'relative value units' that overvalue procedures and undervalue transformations and outcomes. We measure pain and anxiety but not the capacity to tolerate or manage such symptoms. We are at risk for undervaluing the meanings, beliefs, and interpretations that patients bring to their experience of illness. When I returned to the US, I found that this drive to quantify has increased in intensity with no complementary recognition of the shortcomings. Especially in pediatrics, these elements of care must be preserved and even enhanced.

In brief, integrative pediatrics means more than incorporation of complementary therapies into conventional practice. It means integration of the subjective, qualitative, and intuitive aspects of care to counter-balance the predominant

---

Reframing the Field: From Pathogenesis to Salutogenesis

(David Rakel)

The evolution of integrative medicine has been a rapid transition from a healthcare model that has focused on the individual aspects of the physical body. This resulted in many groundbreaking discoveries that brought better treatment of disease. This success resulted in education and research directed towards understanding pathogenesis, the creation of disease and suffering. The success of this approach clouded the importance of its polar opposite, salutogenesis. The term, salutogenesis was introduced in the 1950s by the American-Israeli medical sociologist, Aaron Antonovsky, meaning the creation of health.

The high cost and inefficiency of our current healthcare model will demand change that addresses both the physical and non-physical. The pathogenesis of disease can be viewed (and often is), as purely a physical process. But when the focus becomes creating health for our patients and their communities, we cannot do this without looking at both physical and non-physical factors. An integrative approach will warrant addressing all influences of health, including but not limited to the bio-psycho-social-communal and spiritual. Imagine a healthcare system that first focused on what is needed for the creation of health in hopes of reducing our growing disease burden. This will require a better balance of economic resources and a change in our medical philosophy. (D. Rakel, personal communication, 2008)

---

quantitative approaches. It means incorporating nutritional fundamentals as the foundation for medical care. And it means integration of health psychology and mind-body skills development for wellness and prevention in all phases of chronic illness. (Plotnikoff, G., Personal communication 2008)

Andrew Weil, MD, a key figure in the Integrative medicine movement, had this to say about moving forward with integrative models of pediatric care

The future of the field is very bright...Consumer demand for integrative pediatricians is very high. A major reason is that parents are increasingly suspicious of giving pharmaceutical drugs to their children. Alternatives exist—from dietary change to botanical remedies—but these are not taught in conventional training programs. Many of these non-drug interventions work especially well in pediatric patients.

As in other specialties, Integrative Medicine can restore the core values of medicine that have so eroded in the era of managed care. Not only is it the kind of medicine that patients want, it is the kind of medicine most physicians want to practice. In pediatrics, opportunities for health promotion and disease prevention are many. Integrative pediatrics emphasizes these goals. It can better serve patients, families, and society and make clinical practice more effective and more rewarding. (Weil, A., Personal communication 2008)

Change in Environmental/Contextual Factors

In the future, integrative pediatricians will be actively involved in promoting healthy habitats for children on a variety of scales—global, national, regional, community, within healthcare settings and within individual homes.

Pediatrics, like the rest of medicine, which is part of our larger culture, is changing rapidly. Global changes impact healthcare. For example, climate change is likely to lead to drought and famine in some areas; flooding in others; population migration increasing the risk of epidemics and violence; and increases in vector-borne diseases.

The environmental news is not all gloomy. Leland Kaiser notes that in the future, we must "give as much attention to the child's environment as we give to the child. A healthy child in a sick environment becomes a sick child. Conversely, a sick child often recovers in a healing environment." Global climate change has prompted increased attention to environmental factors that affect health. This is reflected in the new Nexus on Environmental Health within the American Academy of Pediatrics, nonprofit groups such as to Healthcare Without Harm, and the Collaborative on Health and the Environment, and for-profit enterprises promoting products that are environmentally safer for babies. There is also an increasing body of research to enhance our understanding of the toxic effects of pollution and increasing political support for the precautionary principle when creating public policies. See Dr. Mark Miller's discussion of environmental medicine in Chapter 32 of this volume.

Designing healthcare environments to promote optimal healing for patients has been a passion of Dr. Wayne Jonas and is well described in Chapter 29 in this volume. As he reflects on the future, he describes social and financial influences that will shape healthcare for children:

> When asked to speculate on the future of CAM in pediatrics I find that looking historically and at current major financial and social forces provides us with the most realistic view. For those interested in the leeching lessons from history for the purpose of divining the future, I would recommend the recent book *Alternative Medicine: A History* by Roberta Bivins (Oxford University Press, 2007). It discusses many of the major forces in the past that will also likely drive the future color of CAM. Highlights of these forces include: the struggle for control of the body through the relative value given to subjective vs. objective data and the recent rise of 'patient-centered' care; the influence of women in health care now that over 50% of medical students are female; the fluctuating use of use of science and evidence in maneuvers for domination of one system or another; the public's attraction to both 'heroic' and 'humanistic' practices encapsulated by 'high-tech, high-touch' medicine; and how failure to successfully 'integrate' various practices often slows down delivery on their public benefit. These themes provide important lessons for the future for those who want to place patient benefit at the center of our health care systems.
>
> Unfortunately, few of these forces are driving the financial train in medicine. Neither policy nor public opinion have marshaled significant investment in CAM-related areas. Given this and the aging of our populations, it is unlikely that integrative pediatrics will become "top-of-mind" in the near future. The ethical triumph of pediatric integrative health care can only come when we decide to pay for prevention and healing. By prevention, I mean a true 21st century prevention that detects and modulates risk factors and early disease processes in order to maintain wellness and compress morbidity. By healing, I mean the processes of repair, recovery, and reintegration for wellness in both individual and society. Investments in research to build the science of healing and in practices that support and stimulate healing should be the focus of the future. What is needed is a wellness initiative for the nation (and world) that rallies research, education and advocacy for prevention and healing. Such an initiative would serve CAM, conventional medicine, pediatrics and people with a new value-based model of health care. (Jonas, W., Personal communication 2008)

Another important, frequent, and distressing circumstance for many children worldwide has been that of war. War and conflicts are also more apparent due to media coverage. Violence is ubiquitous in the news, sports, and electronic games. In the future, pediatricians will join physicians such as Dr. James Gordon, who has taken the use of integrative mind-body therapies directly into the care of children and adults in war-torn areas around the world. Dr Gordon had this say about the future for children of the world:

> As far as I'm concerned, the greatest contribution of an integrative approach to pediatrics will be promotion of health and wellness in the world's children.
>
> Fundamental to the understanding of Integrative Pediatrics, is the powerful role that self-awareness and self-care can play in the treatment and prevention of chronic illness, and in facilitating the promotion of health and wellness, as well as promoting a sense of self-efficacy and optimism. The primary modalities are those of stress management and mind-body medicine, nutrition, and physical exercise and movement. These need to become as central to the education of all of our children as the three R's, and they need as well to be integrated into the teaching of standard subjects, like the R's. Why not have kids take a few deep breaths before a challenging reading assignment or math problem? What about making the teaching of science personal and experiential as well as cognitive: learning about heart rate and blood pressure and seeing that you can affect them by how you breathe or what you see in your mind's eye?
>
> All of us who work professionally with children—and indeed all of us who have children—need to make integrating 'integrative pediatrics' into the education of our children our first priority. It will help stem the tide of pediatric illnesses, prevent the development of chronic adult conditions, and make life much more interesting and fun for our kids, and us too, and in the bargain, save all of us a great deal of money as well as grief. (Gordon, J., Personal communication 2008)

We end this section with healthcare futurist and change leader Leland Kaiser, who argues forcefully for adapting the context or "habitat" to the child instead of attempting to force children-each with unique talents, attributes, learning styles—all into the same environments—academic or otherwise. He feels passionately that "habitat redesign" should be a therapeutic intervention employed by all integrative pediatricians. He reviews:

> The future of pediatric integrative medicine requires that we give as much attention to the child's environment as we give to the child. The child and its environment should be seen as one interactive, holistic unit. You can't understand the dynamic of one without understanding the dynamics of the other. A healthy child in an unhealthy environment becomes a sick child. Conversely, a sick child often recovers in a healing environment.

In a case of misplaced emphasis, we have concentrated on the organic systems within the child to the exclusion of the person-environment interactions of the child. In an integrative systems approach to child health, we must consider both. In fact, the two are isomorphic.

The child's clinical profile should match the habitat's topography. We should build a supportive environment around the child rather than expect the child to adapt to a hostile environment. In Integrative Pediatrics, we need to assure a unique habitat for each child. This means we need to become familiar with the set of general design principles for healthy child environments as well as special design requirements of unique therapeutic environments.

Habitat design philosophy is built on a very simple idea—a child is the accumulation of his or her life experiences. All of these experiences are gained in habitats (life environments). Therefore, a design for life spaces is a design for consciousness. You design into the space what you want to see in the child. The child's habitat is viewed as an incubator. The home environment, the school environment, and the neighborhood environment are viewed as major incubators.

Habitat re-design plays a key role in child potentiation by asking what kind of habitat best fits the child and will invoke latent growth potentials. This concern goes well beyond traditional wellness care and prevention into the new arena of potentiation. A scan of the child's latent abilities and interests is converted in a design profile. The design profile is then used to build-out the matching habitat.

Habitat redesign for Children

(Leland kaiser)

The child's habitat should be viewed as evocative, not as a passive container. A good habitat turns on the child's DNA, stimulates brain development, excites soul potentials, and readies the child for social interaction. A well designed habitat does six things:

1. Compensates for any deficiencies in the child, so these disabilities do not become a handicap.
2. Facilitates expression of the child's existing abilities and interests.
3. Potentiates development of new abilities and interests.
4. Provides a rich opportunity structure for the child's growth.
5. Provides encouragement and coaching.
6. Provides positive reinforcement for growth. (L. Kaiser, personal communication, 2008)

Pediatric integrative medicine is concerned not only with the sick or injured child. It also focuses upon the well child. It seeks to release the child's unrealized health potentials. It seeks to accelerate normal soul unfoldment. It seeks to help each child become what it already is at the level of potential, but has not yet experienced at the level of realization. (Kaiser, L., personal communication 2008)

Change in Healthcare Delivery Models

The increased percentage of the economy devoted to medical costs with its subsequent hobbling of business productivity and profitability, combined with the lack of access to healthcare by millions in the United States, will create a tinderbox of unrest and substantial popular support for radical reforms in healthcare. It will become easier and more popular to support prevention and low cost health promotion; effective leadership, strategies and models will be sought more eagerly. Among medical specialties, pediatrics already has an impressive track record in promoting health and preventing illness. Integrative pediatricians must be prepared to show the next steps beyond immunizations, car seats and safe temperatures for hot water. We must be able to provide evidence-based information about the importance of stress management, and the importance of community planning and public policies that support optimal nutrition and fitness.

Being aware of broad societal/contextual factors helps as we consider changing what we do to help children heal, but the hard work of change lies in examining and redesigning models of care. Changing these models can be expensive. In a time of limited resources, philanthropy can be an energy source in fueling healthcare change.

The experience of the Bravewell Collaborative (see below) is a great example of how committed philanthropy can be a driving force in groundbreaking innovations that move us closer to fully realized integrative care models all over the USA. Penny George, PsyD founding member of the Bravewell Collaborative offers this:

Philanthropy has long been the engine of social change in America. In the early years of the 20th Century, it created the Flexner Report that changed medicine from a cottage industry to a science-based profession. Through the efforts of the Bravewell Collaborative and others in recent years, philanthropy is again trying to change medicine: this time to bring it back to its roots in healing.

Integrative medicine began as a consumer movement, with patients who were dissatisfied with being seen as diseases and body parts, who were already taking responsibility for making choices and demanding to be treated in a more respectful fashion by their health professionals. There was no desire to abandon conventional medicine, but to ask that it change so that they could partner more effectively with it.

Given the misalignment of financial incentives to promote health as opposed to medical procedures following diagnosis of disease, it will be some years before integrative medicine becomes simply Medicine—the prevailing standard of care. Nevertheless, the trend we see is favorable. As the healthcare system in the US is not succeeding in providing the quality of care that the dollars invested should have brought, new remedies to the approaching disaster are being sought. As philanthropists, we are optimistic that once there is a body of research demonstrating the value and cost-effectiveness of integrative approaches to care, the tipping point will be near.

In the meantime, we believe we will continue to see the following shifts occurring:

- Health institutions will increasingly be hearing—and responding to—demands from their constituents for more attention to health promotion, more effective chronic illness care, and end-of-life care that is truly caring. This is where integrative medicine approaches are especially effective.
- Healthcare systems will offer a range of healing modalities in outpatient facilities as well as at the bedside, often offered by specially trained nurses. Physician support will grow as patient satisfaction increases, as the length of stay decreases and fewer medications are required, and as intractable problems (such as costly in-hospital falls) are solved through collaboration with the resident integrative medicine teams.
- In an organic, evolving way, new care models for such expensive chronic illnesses as congestive heart failure and diabetes will emerge. These models will have more active involvement of patients (and future patients who seek to delay or avoid their parents' complicated conditions) and will provide individualized choices as well as health coaches to empower people for this enhanced involvement in their own care. Care will be much more effectively coordinated and care teams will include both integrative medicine practitioners and conventionally trained health professionals.
- In conclusion, we believe that integrative medicine should become the standard of care not only across the continuum of patient care but also across the lifespan. What if we were to take full advantage of the incredible imagination of children to teach mind-body skills to use not just when facing difficult medical procedures, but as part of prevention? We vaccinate for diseases but not for stress, yet the mind-body connection is the key to managing stress effectively, and we know how to do this. Pediatrics has much to teach us about how integrative medicine can contribute to health and to the care of very sick children.
- There may be no single model of care that is best for anything, but we believe the accumulated wisdom and experience that is underway will result in

improved health, and greater satisfaction with medicine on the parts of both patients and health professionals.

My hope is that we have the wisdom, generosity, and courage to do the work that needs to be done to finally create a fully integrative healthcare system. (P. George, personal communication, 2008)

We need successful clinical models of Integrative Pediatric Care in both inpatient and outpatient settings. In web-based chapter 31 of this volume, Dr. Richtsmeier Cyr describes the largest and longest running pediatric model in the USA at Children's Hospitals and Clinics of Minnesota. The executive responsible for creating, funding, and protecting this program for 8 years was Julie Morath, former Chief Operating Officer of Children's Hospitals and Clinics of Minnesota. A world-renowned expert on pediatric patient safety-Ms. Morath offers this perspective as the leadership "champion" for this unique service over 8 years:

The child and family has always been a unit, however our care delivery models have often fragmented, and reduced care to technical body system interventions. While the technical knowledge and expertise is essential, it is insufficient to create the holistic experience that supports the inherent healing powers of the individual and the family and identifies sources of resilience, self-reliance, locus of control and success in times of crisis.

Integrative medicine protects human dignity; promotes optimal health and well being; and develops the strengths and resources of the individual child and family. Through identifying and amplifying strengths to promote self-care, providing a co-management response to symptoms of disease and illness, and promoting peaceful, comfortable, and compassionate palliative and end of life care, integrative medicine brings to life the mission of pediatrics.

Integrative Medicine is the discipline that orchestrates and brings to the child and family a deep understanding of the individual restorative and self-regulatory capacity and the collective strength of the family unit to participate in achieving maximum function and wellness. In this manner, integrative medicine taps into the deepest motivations of healthcare providers, care givers, and parents: protecting life, learning and developing through challenges, thinking about future generations, focusing on relationships, building community, and enabling the direction of energy to maximum achievement of health—by bringing awareness, science, skills and tools to physical, mental, emotional, and energetic selves.

The evidentiary base of integrative medicine is increasing. As children are surviving childhood conditions into young adulthood and beyond, skills of self awareness are increasingly important in managing chronic conditions; among them are diabetes, cardiovascular conditions, conditions of prematurity, and cystic fibrosis.

Our current healthcare system reimburses procedural care. Integrative medicine provides preventative, effective and non-invasive solutions to healthcare conditions, thus reducing the burden of illness over the individual life span and continuum of care.

As payers and policy makers become more enlightened to the role of integrative medicine to enhance self-care, self-reliance, and improve function and quality of life for children and families; integrative medicine will become an essential and demanded component of care in mainstream medicine. Mainstream medicine will concurrently evolve to embrace the potentiating value of integrative medicine to successfully clinical outcomes.

As self-regulation and reliance is enhanced, the demand for healthcare services will be reduced thus the burdens of illness.

The meaning and joy in providing healthcare is at risk. The focus on production, technology, and regulatory compliance, has dispirited the healthcare workforce. Integrative medicine models are a pathway to rekindle and sustain meaning and joy in the work of healthcare, through the focus of the whole child, the strength of the family, focus on wellness and prevention, interdisciplinary respect and collaboration. These areas of focus are the basis of highly intimate, compassionate care processes. Care providers are reinforced for the very values and motivations that caused them to dedicate their lives to the health and care of children.

A greater distributed model of care is a consideration for the future, with assessment, and consultation, training, and evaluation as a model to prepare care givers in the basics of integrative medicine, such as skill transfer in massage therapy, healing touch, pain and symptom management to frontline care givers. The time and attention of leadership to the value of integrative medicine is essential. This includes a disciplined approach to growth and financial performance as well as, cultivation of medical-specialists and consumers. Champions for "mainstream" advocacy, nurturing philanthropic support, and research to establish an evidentiary-base is key in the leadership role to advance integrative medicine. (J. Morath, personal communication, 2008)

The "flattening" of the global marketplace due to the advent of information and communication technologies empowers those who traditionally had little access to health information to network with others; now even those without medical degrees can develop substantial expertise and access to the latest research. Families are already bringing pediatricians computer printouts from Google searches, challenging us to help patients sort through fact from fiction on the information highway. Some pediatricians have already begun to provide reliable, evidence-based information about natural therapies via the internet and family-oriented publications. The need for unbiased, thoughtful, clear information will increase in the future.

Technology and the Evolution of Pediatric Care

(Scott Shannon)

The most significant change will involve the public and the internet. Patients will begin to have access to increasingly sophisticated outcome data from the care of all providers. This will come as online data bases that summarize an individual's experience with a specific provider. The first step will be consumer driver but the response will be so dramatic that healthcare institutions will be forced to follow suit and provide this information with sophisticated outcome measures. Finally, we will have the ultimate measure of provider's behavior: patient oriented response and satisfaction.

This trend will enhance the drive towards more integrative care in all specialties. These data bases will endorse the preventative and cost- effective measures employed in integrative medicine. High levels of patient interest and a more cautious approach toward pharmaceutical interventions will speed the process further.

As more and more patients have complete access to real measures of a practitioner's clinical effectiveness, the pervasive trend towards individual empowerment unleashed by the internet will continue. Healthcare will soon consume 20% of our massive GNP and yet we have no measure of how well doctors do what they do. We have witnessed a recent trend for hospitals to be measured and compared to each other. Doctors are next. (S. Shannon, personal communication, 2008)

Furthermore, the advent of the internet and communication technologies such as cell phones and PDAs will usher in a new era of communication, promoting effective behavior changes to promote healthy lifestyles. Integrative pediatricians will be able to help patients set goals, monitor their progress and make adjustments to their strategies with fewer office visits. Lifestyle coaching will be feasible over long distances, combining electronic technology with group support via webinars and other low cost conferencing options.

Within the healthcare system, interdisciplinary approaches will be increasingly important. Dr. David Rakel, medical director for integrative medicine at University of Wisconsin Madison, points out that

No one profession will be able to facilitate healthy change alone. The future will require that we create teams that work together to empower patients and their families to find health for themselves. These teams will be different than those focused on treating chronic disease. For example, a child with renal failure will have a disease-focused team that includes a nephrologist, a dialysis technician, a pharmacist and a pediatrician among others. But a team that focuses on health may be completely different as professionals come together to address what is needed for self-healing mechanisms to unfold. For example, a team to facilitate optimal weight in kids may include a pediatrician, a nutritionist, an exercise physiologist, a psychologist, a mindfulness instructor and a spiritual guide. As these professionals come together the team learns from each other to create a transformation in health care delivery. A trans-disciplinary team transforms the traditional model that results in new insights towards solving challenging problems. The future of integrative pediatrics will require the pediatrician to be a leader in organizing these teams towards new and innovative ideas. (D. Rakel, personal Communication, 2008)

Changing healthcare models must include change within its cornerstone providers-nurses. The nursing profession in many ways, has led the way into integrative care for both adults and pediatrics. Maura Fitzgerald, RN, CNS a pioneer in pediatric integrative nursing clinical practice, education and research had this to say about the importance and evolution of holistic nursing

The profession of nursing is, by its nature and history, holistic and integrative. Although the American Association of Holistic Nursing was founded in 1981 they note that the first holistic nurse was Florence Nightingale who 'believed in care that focused on unity, wellness and the interrelationship of human beings' (AHNA, 2008). Massage therapy was once taught in all nursing programs and it was considered part of normal care to have a soothing back rub to help the hospitalized patient get a good night's sleep. Nursing education has traditionally incorporated concepts key to integrative practice such as communication, cooperation, and understanding of family, culture and environment. Pediatric nursing as a specialty has focused on the child within the context of family and community. (M. Fitzgerald, Personal communication, 2008)

In recent decades nurses have perceived a change in emphasis away from patient contact and toward the operation of sophisticated technology and electronic documentation. Many have found this in conflict with core values. Nurses, like their physician colleagues, express frustration that the heart of the profession is disappearing.

For a growing number of nurses integrative medicine is the path to reclaiming the profession. After a 2-day training on infant massage, a neonatal intensive care nurse said it was the "best thing she had done in years and made her feel like a nurse again." Nurses are requesting education and training so that they can provide therapies, consult with families, or use them for self-care. In our pediatric facility, nurses from pre/post operative care to the oncology unit have expressed interest in learning integrative medicine techniques.

Many hospitals are offering courses in holistic and integrative therapies. In Minneapolis, Abbott Northwestern Hospital (ANW) has created a comprehensive 6-day holistic nursing course for staff nurses. Children's Hospitals & Clinics of Minnesota has developed inpatient unit-based training on complementary strategies. Additionally it has partnered with ANW to send staff to the holistic nursing course at ANW and then provided additional on-site education with specific pediatric content.

In a survey of University of Minnesota School of Nursing faculty and students over 95% agreed that clinical practice should integrate the best of CAM and conventional care (Halcon, Chala, Kreitzer, & Leonard, 2003). As of 2003, 77% of nursing schools in the United States included content or experiential learning on complementary health and healing in their curriculum (Richardson, 2003). Professional nursing organizations have responded to interest from members by offering content in integrative medicine as workshops and sessions at annual conferences. The American Nurses Association recognized Holistic Nursing as a specialty in 2006.

Nurses are reclaiming the heart and soul of the profession as they seek knowledge and apply the principles of integrative medicine to their practice. They are creating a new balance between technology and care by relegating technology to its support role and, with the aid of integrative concepts, advancing nursing care. Nurses have been and will continue to be a driving force in seeking out and incorporating integrative strategies for care of patients in all settings.

Changes in Research and Training

In the future, the best elements from all realms of healing–complementary, traditional, alternative, and conventional–will all play a designated role. Integrative practitioners can demonstrate that public policy-making, education, and individual clinical encounters can all be an opportunities for facilitating the balance of the "whole child" (mind-body-emotions-spirit within the context of family and community) to promote health across a lifetime. Determining which therapies are truly "the best" is based on scientific evidence and measuring specific outcomes. Once the most relevant and clinically valid treatments are identified, they must then be incorporated into the education/training of healthcare professionals. Translating research into clinical practice is challenging as the real world of pediatric clinical practice may be less "black and white" than the careful design of a clinical research trial.

A key concept that the real-life clinical practice of integrative pediatrics brings to the transformation of medicine, is the focus on individualized care. Research studies must reflect this and therefore "standardization" of CAM interventions for research purposes may not represent what happens in the field. Not only are children not just small adults; they are not all interchangeable, and they do not all respond the same way to a cookie cutter approach to therapy. Dr. Karen Olness, a pioneer of pediatric mind/body medicine notes that

> when the National Institutes of Health began funding research in complementary medicine, many researchers saw this as a potential source of funding, and entered the field with inadequate background. Mind body interventions, such as hypnosis and guided imagery, that required individual modifications, depending on the interests, personalities and preferences of a child, were organized into "one size fits all" techniques, with results that were disappointing. (K. Olness, personal communication, 2008)

Mary Jo Kreitzer, PhD, who directs the Center for Spirituality and Healing-a leading academic CAM program at the University of Minnesota, had this to say about training the next generation of health professions students in CAM:

> As the evidence base supporting the use of integrative health continues to grow and consumer demand for access to services shows no signs of wavering, health professional education programs are increasingly incorporating content on CAM or integrative health/medicine into both required curricula and optional learning experiences. This trend is evident in undergraduate, graduate and post-graduate training.
>
> Curricular efforts were both stimulated and enhanced when the NIH National Center for Complementary and Alternative Medicine announced a grant initiative in 1999 called the 'Complementary and Alternative Medicine (CAM) Education Project Grant'. The goal of this initiative was to encourage and support the incorporation of CAM information into medical, dental, nursing and allied health professions schools' curricula, into residency training programs, and into continuing education courses. Under this initiative, 15 grants were awarded, 14 to universities and one to the American Medical Student Association. While the majority of the university grant awards went to medical schools, two were awarded to schools of nursing and several grant awards went to institutions that were launching curricular efforts that reached beyond one discipline. The hope and expectation was that these programs would widely disseminate their findings thus helping other institutions launch similar efforts. (Pearson & Chesney, 2007).
>
> In 2000, the Consortium of Academic Health Centers for Integrative Medicine was formed to advance integrative medicine overall and in particular, to stimulate changes in medical education that would facilitate the adoption of integrative medicine curricula. In less than a decade, this organization has grown from 8 to 41 highly esteemed academic health centers. The Consortium has disseminated

a curriculum guide and is a resource to medical schools initiating integrative medicine initiatives (www.imconsortium.org). Although the AAMC has not published any statement related to teaching CAM or integrative medicine or identified essential competencies, questions about CAM have been added to the annual Medical School Graduation Questionnaire. Graduates are asked whether they are confident that they have the appropriate knowledge and skills to assess the health practices of a patient using alternative therapies and whether the time devoted to teaching CAM was inadequate, appropriate or excessive. Several articles have been published that describe relevant CAM competencies for medical education (Kligler et al., 2004; Torkelson et al., 2006). Additionally, curriculum materials on CAM have been peer reviewed by the AAMC and are published on the AAMC MedEd portal (Kreitzer, M. J., Personal communication 2008).

David Steinhorn, MD, Director of Integrative Medicine and a pediatric intensivist at Memorial Children's Hospital in Chicago has been very involved in CAM research for children in intensive care settings, offers this perspective:

> There are few children who find joy and comfort in their stay in the hospital. Most of the contact hospitalized children receive from the medical staff is task oriented, short-lived, and not intended to comfort or re-assure. Conceptually, the child is always in a state of "threat" while in the hospital in spite of our attempts to make hospitals 'child friendly' and 'pain free zones.' Integrative approaches to healthcare for the hospitalized child attempt to create comfort and safety for the child and to calm the parents, making them better able to be a source of comfort for their child. The simplest of low-tech approaches such as massage, energy healing techniques and mind-body approaches provide avenues for promoting comfort for the scared and agitated hospitalized child that might otherwise be treated with escalating doses of sedatives or even manual restraints.
>
> It is unfortunate that so many academic departments of pediatrics have not embraced the potential for integrative medicine to enhance pediatric trainees' appreciation for the human needs of their patients and to provide the comfort that patients and families seek. Integrative medicine says to families and the community that a hospital genuinely cares about the overall well-being of its patients by providing services that do not generate revenue. It reminds the medical staff to consider the impact of a harsh tone of voice or the hurried touch of a tired resident on perceptions of the patient and family. It provides an algorithm by which clinicians can expand and deepen their interaction with the patient by shifting their attention and intention ever-so-slightly during their interactions with patients. In a fast-paced environment, the presence of the integrative medicine practitioner affirms the institution's positive aspirations without dwelling

on any negatives. Therefore, in its most essential form, integrative medicine has the power to communicate non-verbally our genuine concern and desire to nurture and comfort fragile patients whose potential to recover is unknown.

Future medical systems will need to find means for re-uniting the care of the body with the care of the spirit both in in-patient and out-patient medicine. New algorithms will need to be developed to demonstrate the benefits and efficacy of such holistic care because conventional western approaches to establish a scientific basis for efficacy are often inappropriate or inadequate to discern the impact of integrative therapies on patients. Such care will not necessarily rely upon any single discipline such as hospital chaplains to address the spiritual needs of patients any more than we rely solely upon psychiatrists to deal with their psycho-emotional concerns. I anticipate that boundaries between specialties will shift and become less distinct as the in-patient care team takes on a more horizontal, transdisciplinary structure which acknowledges the potential contributions of many practitioners to the healing process. While physicians will likely continue to be the ultimate decision makers in hospital-based practice, it will become clear to all sensible clinicians that other disciplines have much wisdom and insight to contribute on a case-by-case basis. Ultimately, we must work for a process where multiple practitioners evaluate the patients' and families' needs from multiple points of view and create a multifaceted plan of therapy which can truly provide an optimum healing environment for the child. (D. Steinhorn, personal communication, 2008)

Larry Dossey, MD, pioneer in CAM highlights controversies over quality of research:

Many individuals have discovered the value of complementary/alternative medicine (CAM) not through a careful weighing of the available evidence, but through personal experience when conventional therapies fail. This was true for me.

The burden of proof is on the advocates of any therapy, whether CAM or conventional, to establish evidence for the efficacy and safety of the therapy in question. In practice, however, a double standard often seems to operate, in which critics rightly demand proof of efficacy and safety for CAM, yet are lenient in these demands where conventional therapies are concerned. I raise this issue not to be churlish or to point blame, but because this double standard helps explain the massive sociological shift toward CAM that has occurred over the past four decades in nearly every industrialized nation.

The public has become increasingly aware of the spotty record and dubious claims of conventional medicine about safety and efficacy. It seems that every few months some drug or medical device, initially highly touted, is tarnished with new revelations of side effects or industry malfeasance. To add to the public's dismay, our citadels of healthcare—our modern hospitals—no longer command unqualified respect. Epidemiologist Barbara Starfield, of the Johns Hopkins School of Medicine, reported in 2000 that around 225,000 deaths occur annually in American hospitals due to the adverse effects of medications, infections, and errors, making hospital care the third leading cause of death in the United States, behind heart disease and cancer (Starfield, 2000). These findings have become part of the national conversation in the United States, particularly after the Institute of Medicine's startling report in 2000, "To Err is Human" (Kohn, Corrigan, & Donaldson, 2000).

Dr. Kenneth Pelletier, a pioneer in CAM, observed in 2002, At the root of this debate [about complementary/alternative or integrative medicine (CAM)] is a ubiquitous assertion that conventional medicine is grounded in evidence-based research and integrative medicine is not. That is grossly inaccurate.... [We should challenge] both conventional and integrative medicine to a higher standard. To provide a baseline against which to measure CAM, it is important to point out that as much as 20% to 50% of conventional care, and virtually all surgery, has not been evaluated by RCTs [randomized clinical trials]. (Pelletier, 2002)

In 2006, the British Medical Journal published their assessment of 2,404 treatments currently used in medical practice. Of these, 360 (15%) were rated as beneficial, 538 (22%) likely to be beneficial, 180 (7%) as trade-off between benefits and harms, 115 (5%) unlikely to be beneficial, 89 (4%) likely to be ineffective or harmful, and 1,122 (47%), the largest proportion, as unknown effectiveness.

These findings, extending across three decades, are troubling. They raise serious questions about the efficacy and safety of Western medicine, and help explain the socio-cultural shift toward CAM in nearly every industrialized nation over this period of time. People are understandably less trustful and more fearful of conventional therapies, and they are seeking options.

Proving efficacy for some CAM therapies is challenging, however. Some of these therapies, such as Traditional Chinese Medicine, involve a knowledge system and lexicon that are foreign to western science. Moreover, they have arisen over millennia in different social contexts. Can they be wrenched from their milieu and retain their efficacy? Will they yield to the double-blind methods of proof favored in the West?

In summary, CAM may render a service to healthcare by exposing the double standards for efficacy and safety that prevail throughout conventional medicine. CAM also raises questions that are often ignored in conventional medicine, such as the role of intentionality in experimental outcomes and the importance of preserving the socio-cultural context of certain therapies. If these questions are squarely faced, CAM may provide not merely an increase in the therapeutic options that are available for healing, but also a greater understanding of the operations of science itself. (L. Dossey, personal communication, 2008)

Creating Wholeness

The future offers us both great challenges and great opportunities to transform children's healthcare. It is of course our greatest hope that children are valued to the degree they deserve—there is no future without them. How do we value them today? What is the state of children's health as you read this text?

- Cancer continues to be the leading cause of death by disease in children. *The age-adjusted annual incidence of cancer in children increased from 129 to 166 cases per million children between 1975 and 2002.*
- One in eight babies is born prematurely, an increase of nearly 31 percent since 1981. A lack of prenatal care and poor nutrition may account for 40% of premature births in developed countries. Preterm birth contributes to more than one-third of all infant deaths and costs the US more than $26 billion per year.
- Asthma is the most prevalent chronic disease affecting American children, leading to 15 million missed days of school per year. From 1980 to 2004, the percentage of children with asthma has more than doubled, from 3.6 percent to 8.5%.
- One in three adolescents are overweight or at risk of becoming overweight. One in six youths ages 6–19 years are overweight, a 45 percent increase in the past 10 years alone. Type 2 diabetes rates, directly related to the obesity epidemic, are rapidly increasing in US youth. Of those children newly diagnosed with diabetes, the percentage with type-2 has risen from less than 5% to nearly 50% in a 10-year period. This disease disproportionately affects American Indian, African American, Mexican American, and Pacific Islander youth.
- Neurodevelopmental disorders affect one in six American children today, with autism and attention deficit hyperactivity disorder (ADHD) reported at all-time high rates. Autism spectrum disorders are most recently estimated at 1 in 150 children, a 20-fold increase since the 1980s. Most recent national surveys estimate that approximately 1 in 12 children have been diagnosed with ADHD.
- Children and adolescents are suffering from mental health disorders at alarming rates. Nearly 20% of young adolescents report symptoms of depression, with even higher rates in Native American youth. Suicide is the third leading cause of death in youth ages 10–19, and suicide rates in Native American adolescents are three times greater than the national average (Rosen & Imus, 2007).

How can we best address these challenges? Integrative medicine offers us the most promising solution for shifting the paradigm of healthcare towards a wellness-based model rather than a disease-treatment system. We must advocate for substantive change for a wholesale transformation of our current healthcare system or we will continue to lose generations of children to chronic diseases that are preventable. How does integrative medicine answer this charge? Not simply as a mixture of CAM therapies, but as the container of a holistic philosophy of care that includes tenets of the AAP's "Medical Home" and "Bright Futures" models American Academy of Pediatrics (AAP). Furthermore, the impact of the environment on our children's health and the corresponding impact of healthcare on our environment must be addressed in a serious and immediate way consistent with the precautionary principle and other principles of ecologically-sustainable medicine. It is our hope that someday we speak not of a separate integrative medicine but of a single "good medicine," one that values and promotes wellness and health for our children (Kemper, 2000).

The Emergence of Integrative pediatrics

(David Riley)

Perhaps the first step in the emergence of integrative pediatric care will be based on the integration of some complementary and alternative therapies with conventional medical care. The future also lies at least as importantly in the area of prevention through the promotion of health and wellness. It is clear that we are often creatures of habit, habits which are laid down early in life and put all of us on a life-long path over which we have some influence. Nutrition, yoga and meditation, exercise and rest, massage, how we chose to prevent and treat illnesses are important not only because of their immediate benefits but also because they have long-term effects.
I believe that the most sought after pediatricians of the future will practice integrative pediatric care and work a variety of other licensed healthcare providers to optimize health and wellness. (D. Riley, personal Communication, 2008)

The future of medicine will recognize that wholeness, a whole, perfect, harmonious pattern already exists within each person, and that it is the healer's privilege to sing the songs that celebrate and call forth (evoke) that wholeness, supporting a milieu, an environment, in which that wholeness can be expressed easily and sustainably. So, we will facilitate the expression and realization of a whole, healthy planet, culture, buildings, transportation, education, nutrition, politics; and our specific practices will be respectful and sustainable expressions of the recognition of our oneness. Not everyone in the orchestra plays every instrument simultaneously. Not every healer will use every technique, but we will rejoice that there are those whose practices complement our own, and give each a seat in the symphony.

REFERENCES

American Holistic Nurses Association. (AHNA). What is holistic nursing? Retrieved May 13, 2008, from http://www.ahna.org/AboutUs/WhatisHolisticNursing/tabid/1165/Default.aspx

Center for Spirituality and Healing at the University of Minnesota. Retrieved May 23, 2008, from www.csh.umn.edu/csh/educ/home.html.

Clinical evidence: How much do we know? *British Medical Journal* online. (2006). Retrieved May 5, 2008, from http://www.clinicalevidence.com/ceweb/about/knowledge.jsp

Halcon, L. L., Chalan, L. L, Kreitzer, M. J., & Leonard, B. J. (2003). Complementary therapies and healing practices: Faculty/student beliefs and attitudes and the implications for nursing education. *Journal of Professional Nursing, 19*(6), 387–397.

Kemper, K. J. (2000). Holistic pediatrics = good medicine. *Pediatrics, 105*(1 Pt 3), 214–218.

Kohn, L. T., Corrigan, J. M., & Donaldson, M. S. (2000). *To err is human: Building a safer health system.* Washington, DC: National Academies Press.

Pelletier, K. (2002). Mind as healer, mind as slayer: Mind-body medicine comes of age. *Advances, 18*(1), 4–15.

Richardson, S. (2003). Complementary health and healing in nursing education. *Journal of Holistic Nursing, 21*(1), 20–35.

Rosen, L. D., & Imus, D. (2007). Environmental injustice: Children's health disparities and the role of the environment. *Explore (NY), 3*(5), 524–528.

Starfield, B. (2000). Is U.S. health really the best in the world? *Journal of the American Medical Association, 284*(4), 483–485.

INDEX

Page numbers in *italics* refer to figures and tables.

AAD. *See* Antibiotic-associated diarrhea
    (AAD)
"Acceptance-based therapy," for adolescents
    with chronic pain disorders, 527
Acetaminophen, 540
Achilles tendonitis, 166
Acupressure, 105
Acupuncture
    analgesic effect of, *107,* 108
    application for treatment of
        allergy rhinitis, 118
        asthma, 111–112
        constipation, 440–441
        FAP, 431
        headache, 112–113
        nausea and vomiting, 494
        nocturnal enuresis, 114–115
        pain, 534–535
        postextubation stridor, 117
        postoperative nausea and vomiting,
            115–117
        smoking cessation, 114
    beneficial effects in adolescent patients,
        379–380
    with bloodletting, 117
    clinical evidence of pediatric, 110–111
    as complementary medicine, 211
    effectiveness in various clinical
        conditions, 110
    history of, 104–105
    and related techniques, 105–106
    for relieving nerve pain, 27
    safety issues for use in adults, 76
    scientific research for, 107–110
    theories of, 106–107
    use in
        pain management, 117–118
        palliative care, 585
Acupuncture needle, 109
    insertion of, *110*
Acupuncture points
    unit of measurement, 119
    used for migraine prophylaxis, *114*
Acute diarrheal illness, 323
Acute lymphoblastic leukemia (ALL), 488
Acute myelogenous leukemia (AML), 488
Acute otitis media (AOM), 608. *See also*
    Otitis media
Acute pseudoaldosteronism
    syndrome, 639
AD. *See* Atopic dermatitis (AD)
Additive-free diet, 333
Adenysine triphosphate (ATP)
    synthesis, 498

ADHD. *See* Attention deficit hyperactivity disorder (ADHD)
ADHD rating scale, 27
Adolescents
  beneficial effects of
    acupuncture, 379–380
    chiropractic care, 381–382
    homeopathic medicine, 380–381
    massage therapy, 380
    mind-body therapies, 382
    reiki/therapeutic touch, 384
    spirituality, 382–384
    yoga, 384–385
  and CAM therapies, 368–372
  sleep disorders in, 415
  stages of psychological growth and development in, 369
  use herbal therapies and supplements
    caffeine, 372–373
    chamomile, 376
    creatine, 378–379
    Echinacea, 377–378
    ephedra or *ma huang*, 372
    feverfew, 378
    garlic, 378
    ginseng *(Panax Ginseng)*, 374–375
    green tea *(Camellia sinensis)*, 373–374
    guaraná *(Paullinia cupana)*, 374
    hoodia gordonii, 374
    kava, 375–376
    melatonin, 376–377
    St. John's wort, 375
    valerian, 376
    yerba mate *(Ilex Paraguariensis)*, 374
Adult health care, 7
AEA. *See* Arachidonoyethanolamide (AEA)
Aerobic exercise, 206, 207
AFCAs. *See* Artificial food coloring and additives (AFCAs)
Aggressive Comfort Care (ACT), in pediatric palliative care, 63
AHG. *See* American Herbalist Guild (AHG)
AID. *See* Anti-inflammatory diet (AID)
Alcohol, abuse of, 58

ALE. *See* Artichoke leaf extract (ALE)
ALL. *See* Acute lymphoblastic leukemia (ALL)
American Herbalist Guild (AHG), 225
American Journal of Clinical Nutrition, 400
AML. *See* Acute myelogenous leukemia (AML)
Animal magnetism, 270
Antibiotic-associated diarrhea (AAD), 610
Anti-coagulant medication, 378
Anti-depressant medications, 479
Anti-inflammatory diet (AID), 547
Anti-psychotic medications, 464
Anxiety disorders, 460
AOM. *See* Acute otitis media (AOM)
Arachidonoyethanolamide (AEA), 533
Aromatherapy
  application in treatment of
    anxiety, 137
    childhood cancer, 135–136
    dermatology and skin infections, 132–134
    infant apnea, 136–137
    insomnia, 134–135, 417
    nausea, 134
  certification for, 141
  definition of, 123–124
  safety concerns and risks of, 137–141
Aromatherapy massage, 251. *See also* Massage therapy (MT)
Aromatic plant oils, 124
Artemisia vulgaris, 105
Artichoke leaf extract (ALE), 432
Artificial food coloring and additives (AFCAs), 410
Artificial sweetener, 333
ASD. *See* Autistic spectrum disorder (ASD)
Asian bodywork, 251
Asperger's syndrome, 396
Association of Healing Health Care Projects, 65
Asthma
  acupuncture for treatment of, 111–112
  effect of subluxation on, 161
  conventional therapies for treatment of, 624

and food allergies, 333–334
herbal supplements in treatment of, 629–633
integrative approaches for treatment of
  alternative health systems, 633–640
  biological therapies for, 626–633
  manipulative therapies, 633
  mind-body therapies, 625–626
  mechanism, 623–624
role of nutrition in development of, 626
Atherosclerosis, 207
Atopic dermatitis (AD), 324, 330–332
  symptoms of, 533
Atopic diseases, 305
Atopic disorders
  conventional approaches for assessment of, 603
  signs and symptoms of, 602
  treatment of
    biologically based therapies for, 604–605
    CAM therapies for, 603–604
    manipulative and body-based methods for, 605–606
ATP synthesis. *See* Adenysine triphosphate (ATP) synthesis
Attention deficit hyperactivity disorder (ADHD), 217, 225, 332
  botanical products for treatment of, 414
  conventional approach for treatment of, 407–408
  dietary modifications and food sensitivities for treatment of, 409–411
  electroencephalographic biofeedback for treatment of, 412–413
  homeopathy for treatment of, 413
  integrative approach for treatment of, 408–409
  nutritional supplements for treatment of
    omega-3 fatty acids, 411
    zinc and ferritin, 412
  traditional Chinese medicine for treatment of, 413
  trials of EEG neurofeedback in, 413
Autism, 356, 396

CAM therapies for, 397–398
etiology of, 397
integrative therapies for
  alternative behavioral approaches, 404
  conventional behavioral approaches, 403–404
  metabolic interventions for treatment of, 406–407
  nutritional supplements for treatment of
    omega-3 fatty acids, 405–406
    probiotics, 406
    zinc, 406
Autistic spectrum disorder (ASD), 396
Autoimmune abnormalities, 398, 400
Autonomic nervous system, 346, 522
Ayurveda, 30
  for treatment of
    constipation, 435
    pain, 536

Bayley Scales of Infant Development (BSID), 321
Behavior Rating Scale, 321
Beta endorphin, 533
Beta-hydroxy-beta-methylglutaryl-CoA (HMG-CoA), 378
Bifidobacterium infantis, 441
Biofeedback
  development of, 283
  as mechanism for reducing stress, 210
  in palliative care, 578
  strategies for, 286–287
  training/accreditation/licensure for, 290
  for treatment of
    FAP, 428
    pediatric pain, 528
Biofeedback-assisted relaxation training, for pain management, 528
Biofield, 182
Biological markers, 190
Bipolar disorder, 460
Blocked Atlantal Nerve Syndrome, 153
Blood-oxygenation-level-dependent (BOLD) signals, 109
Bone marrow transplantation, 497
Botanical medicines, 124

"Bowel detoxification" protocol, 399
Breastfeeding, benefits of, 317
Bronchopulmonary dysplasia, 623
BSID. *See* Bayley Scales of Infant
    Development (BSID)
Burnout
    prevention of, 59
    and risk of death by suicide, 58
    signs of, 59
Butterbur *(Petasites hybridus),* 531, 541,
    630

Caffeine, 372–373
CAHC. *See* Complementary and alternative
    healthcare (CAHC)
CAM practitioners, professional training
    of, 87
CAM product
    pediatric use of, 83
    safety issues for use in children, 76
    use and safety of, 88
CAM therapies. *See* Complementary/
    alternative medicine (CAM)
    therapies
Canadian Journal of Psychiatry, 403
Cancer, childhood
    effect of electromagnetic field on
        development of, 490
    challenges of survivorship in, 500–501
    direct anti-cancer effects, 502–503
    influence of nutrition in development
        of, 491–492
    mind-body medicine for
        treatment of, 493
    palliative care for treatment of, 501–502
    side effects of cancer therapy in
        anxiety-insomnia, 499–500
        constipation, 495–496
        diarrhea, 496
        fatigue, 498
        malnutrition, 495
        mucositis, 496–497
        nausea and vomiting, 493–494
        neuropathy, 497
        pain, 498–499
    supportive care for, 492–493

Cancer therapy, use of antioxidants
    during, 505
CAPS. *See* Childhood Asthma Prevention
    Study (CAPS)
Carnitine, 498
Carrier oils, 126
Castor oil *(Ricinus communis),* 436
CC. *See* Community care (CC)
CCK-8. *See* Cholecystokinin octapeptide
    (CCK-8)
CDI. *See* Children's Depression Inventory
    (CDI)
CDRS. *See* Children's Depression Rating
    Scale (CDRS)
Cellular pathology, 459
Central nervous system (CNS), 128
Cerebral palsy, 356
Certified HT practitioner (CHTP), 194
Certified massage therapist (CMT), 253
Cervical lordosis, 154
Cervical subluxation, 154
Cervicogenic headaches, 163
CGI. *See* Clinical Global Impression (CGI)
Chamomile, 376, 416, 532
Chemotherapy, 495
Chest physiotherapy (CPT), 644
Child
    clinical caring for, 36
    death due to malnutrition or infectious
        diseases, 34
    impact of life-threatening illness on, 451
    mental health of, 459
    spiritual beliefs and practices, 36
    use of herbal medicines and prescription
        medicine in, 83
Childhood Asthma Prevention Study
    (CAPS), 628
Children's Depression Inventory (CDI),
    322
Children's Depression Rating Scale
    (CDRS), 322
Children's Oncology Group
    (COG), 487, 488
Chinese medicine. *See* Traditional Chinese
    medicine (TCM)
Chiropractic adjusting, safety of, 149

Chiropractic care
  for adolescent patients, 381–382
  for conditions of neonate and infant,
      156–158
  for conditions of school-aged child,
      161–162
    neck and shoulder pain, 162–163
    pediatric headache, 163
    temporomandibular dysfunction and
        pediatric headaches, 163
  for injuries and sports-related condi-
      tions, 165–166
    head injuries, 166
    lower extremity conditions, 166–167
    upper extremity musculo-tendonous
        strains, 166
  to patients and their families, 167
  for pediatric asthma treatment, 606
  pediatric conditions that respond to, *157*
  for prevention of recurrent AOM, 611
  in treatment of colic, 601
Chiropractic manipulative therapy, 147
Cholecystokinin octapeptide (CCK-8), 108
Cholesterol biosynthesis, 378
Chronic congestion, 354
Chronic disease management, 80
Chronic inflammation, 357
Chronic serous otitis media (CSOM), 609
CHTP. *See* Certified HT practitioner
      (CHTP)
Citrus aurantium, 124
Clinical aromatherapy. *See* Aromatherapy
Clinical Global Impression (CGI), 322
Clinical Pastoral Education (CPE), 42
CMT. *See* Certified massage therapist
      (CMT)
CNME. *See* Council on Naturopathic
      Medical Education (CNME)
CNS. *See* Central nervous system (CNS)
Cochrane Database Systematic Review, 601
Cod liver oil, 317, 610
Coenzyme Q-10, 531
COG. *See* Children's Oncology Group
      (COG)
Cognitive-behavioral therapy (CBT), 471
  for chronic pain, 526

Cognitive development, Piaget's theory
      of, 40
Coleus *(Coleus forskohlii),* 632, 639
Colic
  biologically based therapies for
      management of, 598–600
  CAM therapies for management of, 598
  conventional approach for managing,
      597–598
  effect of probiotics and prebiotics on,
      600
  homeopathic medicine for treatment
      of, 602
  manipulative and body-based methods
      for management of, 601
Colostrum, 496
Community care (CC), 407
Compassionate Touch‧, 252
Complementary/alternative medicine
      (CAM) therapies, 3
  for adolescents, 368–372
  American Academy of Pediatrics (AAP)
      policy statement on, 87
  associated with tumor regression, 77
  for autism, 397–398
  competencies in undergraduate medical
      education, *91–92*
  digital learning repositories for, 90
  effectiveness as healthcare intervention
      for children, 84
  ethics of pediatric, 81–82
  for FAP and constipation/encopresis in
      children and adolescents, 426
  institutional readiness in, 86
  and integrative care models, 8
  for irritable bowel syndrome, 131
  lifetime use of in adolescents, 8
  major domains of, 4
  for management of colic
    biologically based therapies, 598–600
    manipulative and body-based
        methods, 601
    mind-body methods, 598
  N-of-1 trials
    inclusion and exclusion criteria
        for, *79*

Complementary/alternative medicine
(CAM) therapies *(continued)*
recommended resources about, *79*
in pediatrics, 7–8
practice in North America, 75
quality of, 81
rates of utilization in asthma populations, 9
referring pediatric patient to, 25–26
research design, ethics, and funding,
issues in
education, 83
ethics, 81–82
funding, 82
research in pediatric, 8–9
in specific pediatric pain conditions
acute procedural pain, 538–539
complex regional pain syndrome
(CRPS), 542–544
in primary headaches, 539–542
widespread myofascial
pain, 544–546
and treatments for specific pain
conditions, *548–553*
usage rates in pediatric cancer
patients, 9
utilization in children and teenagers, 8
Complementary and alternative healthcare
(CAHC), 90
Complementary medicine, imagery as,
209–210
Complex regional pain syndrome (CRPS),
535, 542–544
Congenital heart disease, 447
Congenital plagiocephaly, 159
Congenital torticollis, 354
Constipation, 432–433
biologically based practices for treatment of
fiber, 435
food, 436
herbs, 436
lactobacillus, 437
energy medicine for treatment of
acupuncture, 440–441
reflexology, 441

manipulative and body-based practices
for treatment of, 439–440
medical system for treatment of
Ayurveda, 435
Chinese herbal medicine, 434
homeopathy, 433–434
mind-body medicine for treatment of
behavioral therapies, 437–438
biofeedback, 439
group behavioral treatment, 438
health visitor teams, 439
play therapy, 439
self-hypnosis, 438
as side-effect in treatment of cancer,
495–496
vincristine-induced, 495
Coronary artery disease, 207
Corticosteroids, 640
Council on Naturopathic Medical
Education (CNME), 306
Counterstrain (CS), 349
COX. *See* Cyclo-oxygenase (COX)
CPE. *See* Clinical Pastoral
Education (CPE)
CPT. *See* Chest physiotherapy (CPT)
Cranial base distortion, 353
Cranial electrotherapy stimulation (CES),
for pain management, 537
Cranial osteopathy, 340, 349–352
as applied to infants, 352–353
Cranial-sacral therapy (CST),
benefits of, 349
Cranial scoliosis, 353
Cranio-Sacral system, 251
Creatine, 378–379
Crohn's disease, 321–322
CS. *See* Counterstrain (CS)
CSOM. *See* Chronic serous otitis
media (CSOM)
Cultural competence and humility, 37
Cupping, for treating respiratory
disease and musculoskeletal
pain, 105
Cyclo-oxygenase (COX), 529
Cystic fibrosis (CF), therapeutic options for
treating, 643

Dacryostenosis, 354
Dai-kenchu-to (DKT), 434
DBT. *See* Dialetical behavior therapy
    (DBT)
DCD. *See* Developmental coordination
    disorder (DCD)
Deep tissue massage therapy, 251
Deglycyrrhizinated licorice (DGL), 639
Delayed-onset muscle soreness
    (DOMS), 211
Depression, 322
  and risk of death by suicide, 58
Developmental coordination disorder
    (DCD), 405
Devil's Claw, 530
DGL. *See* Deglycyrrhizinated licorice
    (DGL)
Diabetes Prevention Program, 207
Dialetical behavior therapy (DBT), 475
Diarrhea
  antibiotic-associated, 324
  prevention of, 323–324
  as side-effect in treatment of, 496
Diarthrodial joints, range of movement
    in, *149*
Dietary Supplement and Health Education
    Act (DSHEA), 224
Digital learning repositories, for CAM, 90
Dill *(Anethum graveolens),* 599
Dimethylglycine (DMG), 407
Disability Adjusted Life Years
    (DALY), 461
Disease activity score (DAS$_{28}$), 547
DKT. *See* Dai-kenchu-to (DKT)
Docosahexaenoic acid (DHA), 411, 600,
    627
"Doctoring to Heal" program, 61
Doctors of Osteopathy (DOs), 439
DOMS. *See* Delayed-onset muscle soreness
    (DOMS)
Dopamine, 407
Down syndrome, 490
Drug–herb interactions, 27
Drugs, abuse of, 58
DSHEA. *See* Dietary Supplement and
    Health Education Act (DSHEA)

DSM-based diagnostic system, 458
Dysbiosis, 399
Dysmenorrhea, 530
Dyssomnia, 416

Eating disorders, 382
EBM. *See* Evidence-based
    medicine (EBM)
Echinacea, 377–378
Eczema, 331
EFS. *See* Event free survival (EFS)
EGCG. *See* Epigallacatechin gallate
    (EGCG)
EIB. *See* Exercise induced
    bronchoconstriction (EIB)
Eicosapentaenoic acid (EPA), 411, 627
Electroacupuncture, development of, 108
Electrocardiogram (ECG) biofeedback, 428
Electrodermograph (EDG)
    biofeedback, 429
Electroencephalographic biofeedback, for
    treatment of ADHD, 412–413
Electromagnetic fields (EMF), and
    development of childhood
    cancer, 490
Electromyography (EMG), 429
Elimination diet, 324, 325
Emergency Medical Service (EMS), 539
Encopresis, 433
End-of-life care, 61, 62, 573, *574*, 590, 661
Energy healing, effectiveness of, 187
Energy medicine therapy. *See* Energy
    therapies
Energy therapies
  biological mechanisms involved in, 182
  referrals for all three types of, 196
  safety and risks associated with, 195–196
  use of, 181
EPA. *See* Eicosapentaenoic acid (EPA)
Ephedra, 223, 372, 374, 481, 631
Epigallacatechin gallate (EGCG), 503
ERP. *See* Exposure response prevention
    (ERP)
Erythrocyte superoxide dismutase, 401
Essential fatty acids (EFA), 315, 411, 473, 495
    metabolic pathways of, 322

Essential oils
  application in pain management,
    130–132
  chemical composition of, 124
  dilution chart for, *128*
  emotional and cognitive reactions
    to, 128
  extraction of, 125
  healing properties of, 123
  history of, 124
  ingestion of, 126
  mechanisms of biologic effect of, 126–129
  methods of administration of, 125–126
  review of clinical applications of,
    129–130
  use against pathogenic
    microorganisms, 134
ET. *See* Eustachian tubes (ET)
Eustachian tube dysfunction, 608
Eustachian tubes (ET), 352, 355
Event free survival (EFS), 488
Evidence-based medicine (EBM), 240, 360
Exercise induced bronchoconstriction
    (EIB), 628
Exposure response prevention (ERP), 476
Eye movement desensitization and
    reprocessing (EMDR), 476

Family Adaptability and Cohesion Scale
    (FACES), 22
Family Assessment Device (FAD), 23
Family characteristics, influencing child
    outcomes
  family assessment, 22
  family environment
    adaptability, 21
    cohesion, 21–22
    communication, 22
  family resources
    education, 21
    income, 21
  family structure
    birth patterns, 20–21
    family size, 20
    single *vs.* two-parent households, 20

Family functioning and adjustment
    to illness, measures of
  dimensions of, 23
  Family Adaptability and Cohesion Scale
    (FACES), 22
  Family Assessment Device (FAD), 23
  Psychosocial Adjustment to Illness Scale
    (PAIS), 23
FAP. *See* Functional abdominal
    pain (FAP)
FDCA. *See* Food, Drug, and Cosmetic Act
    (FDCA)
Federal Food Drug and Cosmetic Act
    (FFDCA), 239
Feingold diet, 333, 409
Feingold program. *See* Feingold diet
Fen fever, 599
Fennel *(Foeniculum vulgare),* 599
Feverfew, 378, 530
FFDCA. *See* Federal Food Drug and
    Cosmetic Act (FFDCA)
FGIDs. *See* Functional gastrointestinal
    disorders (FGIDs)
Fish oil, 314
  applications in children, 321
Five phases
  cycles associated with, 106
  theory of, 106
Food additives, 333
Food allergy, 331, 333
Food, Drug, and Cosmetic Act (FDCA),
    234
Force expiratory volume in 1 second
    (FEV_1), 112, 627
Friends of Complementary and Alternative
    Therapies Society, 93
Functional abdominal pain (FAP), 425
  in children and adolescents, 426
  medical systems for treatment of
    biologically based practices, 431–432
    Chinese herbal medicine, 427–428
    energy medicine, 431
    mind-body medicine, 428–431
  symptom-based classification of, 427
Functional dyspepsia (FD), 431

Functional gastrointestinal disorders (FGIDs), 425
  characteristics of, 426
Functional magnetic resonance imaging (fMRI), 109
Furanocoumarin-free (FCF), 140

GALT. *See* Gut-associated lymphoid tissue (GALT)
Galvanic skin response (GSR), 190
Gamma-aminobezazoic acid, 532
Gamma-amino butyric acid (GABA), 520
Garlic, 378
Gas chromatography, 321
Gastroesophageal (GE) reflux, 354, 597
Gastroesophageal reflux disease (GERD), *157*
Gastrointestinal (GI) symptoms, 375
Gastrointestinal microflora, 399
Gastrointestinal system, 398–399
Generally regarded as safe (GRAS), 529
Genetic idiosyncrasies, 472
German chamomile *(Matricaria recutita)*, 125
Germ cell tumors, 488
Ginger *(Zingiber officinalis)*, 129, 131, 494, 529–530
Ginkgo *(Ginkgo biloba)*, 218, 639
Ginseng *(Panax Ginseng)*, 374–375
GI pathology, 398
Gluten-free casein-free (GFCF) diet, 404
Good manufacturing practices (GMPs), 224, 636
Grape seed extract (GSE), 638
GRAS. *See* Generally regarded as safe (GRAS)
Green tea *(Camellia sinensis)*
  metabolic effects of, 373
  side effects of, 373–374
Gripe water, 599
GSR. *See* Galvanic skin response (GSR)
Guaraná *(Paullinia cupana)*, 374
Gut-associated lymphoid tissue (GALT), 325
Gwa sha, 105

Headache
  acupuncture for treatment of, 112–113
  hypnosis for treatment of, 274–278
Head lice *(Pediculus humanus capitis)*, 133
HEADSS (Home, Education, Activities, Drugs, Sexuality and Suicide), 370
Healing touch (HT), 180
  adult literature on, 193–194
  clinical process involved in, 192–193
  definition of, 192
  history of, 192
  for pain management, 537
  pediatric literature on, 194
  training in, 194–195
Health care
  for adult, 7
  burnout in, 56–57
  challenges associated with, 48
  changes in delivery models for, 660–666
  changes in research and training for, 667–670
  guiding principles for, 65–68
  happiness in workplace and, 53–55
  hospital-based, 454
  integrative approach to, 49
  lifestyle-based personal responsibility and, 67
  pediatric medicine in, 3
  practitioner-patient relationship in, 49
  quality of, 55
Healthcare providers, personality traits of, *51*
Health education, 56
Heart rate variability (HRV), 284
Heavy metal toxicity, 401–402
Herbal medicines, 31. *See also* Phytotherapy
  definitions of, 219
  description of, 218–219
  dosing of, 225
  history of, 219
  trends in pediatric use of, 217–218
Herbal products, types of, *220*
Herb-drug interactions, 76
Herbs. *See* Pediatric herbs

High velocity low amplitude (HVLA)
  treatments, 148, 348
Hirschsprung's disease, 433, 434
Homeopathic medicines, 85
  beneficial effects on adolescent patients,
    380–381
  categories of, 236
  interactions with conventional medicine,
    243–245
  pharmacology of, 236–237
  preparation of, 234
  principles of, 235–236
  remedies for treatment of AOM, 611
  for treatment of
    ADHD, 413
    allergies, 606
    asthma, 634–636
    constipation/encopresis, 433–434
  for treatment of colic, 602
Homeopathic Pharmacopoeia of the United
  States (HPUS), 236
Homeopathy
  classical and clinical, 237
  clinical trials in, 241–242
  global use of, 237–238
  and other CAM therapies, 237
  regulation of, 238–239
  research challenges in
    funding and skepticism, 243
    individualization, 243
    patient preference, 242
    specific and non-specific effects,
      242–243
  research in, 240
  safety considerations in, 237
  training in, 239
Hoodia gordonii, 374
HPUS. See Homeopathic Pharmacopoeia
  of the United States (HPUS)
HRV. See Heart rate variability (HRV)
HT. See Healing touch (HT)
HT Certificate Program (HTCP), 194
Human faith development, stages of, 40
Hyperkinesis, 416
Hypertension, in children, 206
Hypertonic muscles, 259

Hypno-anesthesia, 273
Hypnosis
  applications in health care of adults
    and children, 274
  and biofeedback, 287–288
  clinical applications of, 271
  definition of, 272
  history of, 270–272
  key ingredients in effectiveness of, 281
  mechanism for biologic effects of,
    280–281
  safety and risks concerns associated
    with, 281
  training/accreditation/licensure
    for, 282
  for treatment of
    childhood cancer, 494
    FAP, 429–430
Hypnotherapy, 271
Hypothalamus-limbic system, 109

IBS. See Irritable bowel syndrome (IBS)
ICU syndrome, 451
Idiopathic headache, 541
IgG antibrain antibodies, 400
IM. See Integrative medicine (IM)
Immunization
  effect of, 607
  influence on infant immune/
    neuroimmune regulation, 607
  for vaccine-preventable diseases, 608
Immunocal, 495
Immunostimulants, use in cancer
  patients, 505
Infant immunizations, 401
Infant irritability syndrome, 597
Inflammatory cytokines, 400
Inhaled corticosteroids (ICS), in children
  with asthma, 621
Institutional review boards (IRBs), 81, 506
Integrative health treatment plan, 24
Integrative medicine (IM)
  challenges of pediatric oncology in
    research of, 505–506
  and chronic lung problems in children,
    645–646

definition of, 49
difference with CAM, 3
education in, 73, 89
innovative educational strategies in, 90
teaching at all levels of medical
    education, 92
therapies in use by children with
    cancer, 506
in treating injuries in sport and exercise
    acupuncture, 211
    biofeedback, 210
    imagery, 209–210
    massage, 211
    yoga, 211
Integrative nutrition, 324
Integrative oncologist, role of, 489–490
Integrative oncology, 489
    practicing of, 506–507
Integrative pediatric care
    foundations of, 6–7
    power of personal narrative of physician
        in, 60–61
    on specific therapeutic approaches, 7
Integrative pediatric education, 83
    future of, 94
Integrative pediatric medicine-specific
    networks, 89
Integrative pediatrics, 3
    assessment in family context
        biopsychosocial sensitivity, 20
        family characteristics influencing
            child outcomes, 20–22
    assessment of spirituality in, 37–40
        common errors in, 40–43
        five common signs of unmet spiritual
            needs for, 43–44
        responses to spiritual concerns in, 45
    and body's natural healing response, 4
    clinical applications in, 7
    culture and spirituality in, 30
        North American, 31–32
    development of safety research agenda
        in, 88
    different models and processes in, 10
    elements in assessment of
        conventional elements, 16

developmental progress and behav-
    ioral differences as, 16–17
environmental factors as, 18
history of using CAM, 16
lifestyle, 17–18
spirituality, 18
evolution of, 8
implementation of Cohen and Kemper's
    model on clinical decision-making
    in, 87
interdisciplinary collaboration in, 9–10
interventions for cultural and spiritual
    concerns, 36–37
learning objects and modules in, 92
research and educational
    initiatives in, 74
    cost-effectiveness, 80
    efficacy, 77–80
    safety research, 75–77
treatment planning in, 23–24
    balancing of risks and benefits for, 25
    counseling of patients and families
        for, 27
    prioritizing and sequencing, 26–27
    referral of patient to CAM Provider,
        25–26
    summarizing of patient's story and
        creation of partnership, 24–25
Integrative Touch™, 252
Intensive medication management, 407
Intensive multicomponent behavior
    therapy, 407
Intercessory Prayer, for pain
    management, 537
International Symposium on
    Back Pain, 343
Interprofessional education (IPE), 92
    best practices in implementation of, 93
    definition of, 93
Intracranial scoliosis, 353
Irritable bowel syndrome (IBS), 131, 425
Isocapnic hyperventilation, 634
Isopathy, 237. *See also* Homeopathy

Jacobsonian relaxation, 293
Japanese star anise *(Illicium anisatum)*, 223

Johrei, for pain management, 537
Joint aberration, 147
"Just-in-time" educational
    opportunities, 94
Juvenile idiopathic arthritis, 546–547

Kava, 375–376
"Ke" cycle, 106
KISS syndrome, 152–153

Lactobacillus acidophilus, 330
Lactobacillus fermentum, 324
Lactobacillus rhamnosus GG (LGG), 431
Larch arabinogalactans, 610
Laryngospasm, 117
Laser acupuncture, 112
Lavender *(Lavandula angustifolia),* 129, 135
Lavender oil, for aromatherapy, 123
"Leaky gut" phenomena, 399
Lemon *(Citrus limon),* 129
Licensed massage practitioner (LMP), 253
Licensed massage therapist (LMT), 253
Lifestyle exercise, 206
Li-Fraumeni syndrome, 491
LMP. *See* Licensed massage practitioner
    (LMP)
LMT. *See* Licensed massage therapist (LMT)
Low-velocity, low-amplitude manoeuvre
    (LVLA), 148
Lumbar lordosis, 154

Magnesium, as pain reliever, 529
Ma huang. See Ephedra
Maslach Burnout Inventory, 56
Massage therapists, categories of, 254
Massage therapy (MT), 85, 211
    beneficial effects on adolescent patients,
        380
    categories of contraindication for, 262
    clinical applications of, 257
    effects on
        cardiovascular system, 260
        digestive and urinary systems, 261
        lymphatic and immune systems, 260
        musculoskeletal system, 258–259
        nervous and endocrine systems, 259

respiratory system, 260–261
    skin, 258
health benefits in child, 257–258
history of, 249–251
as mode of symptom management, 255
professional standards, training, and
    licensure for, 253–254
and relaxation therapy, 257
safety considerations for use of, 261–262
for treatment of
    constipation, 440
    pain, 533
usage in hospitals, 249
McMaster Model of Family Functioning
    (MMFF), 23
Medical care
    effects of personal spirituality
        and practices on, 64
    to patients affecting patient wellbeing, 51
Medical culture
    role of, *51*
    stressors inherent in, *52–53*
Medical licensing, 58
Medical practice, model of, 50–53
Medical service models, 3
Medical training, pediatric health care in, 7
Medicine
    based on relationship-centered care, 58
    benefits of spirituality in, 61–62
    evidence-based, 23
    healing-oriented, 3
    integrative, 3
    preventative, 56
Meditation, 290–292
Melatonin, 376–377
    for treatment of
        pain, 532–533
        sleep disorders in children, 417
Mental health
    biochemical therapies for treatment of,
        477–478
    biomechanical modalities for treatment
        of, 478–479
    of child, 459
    diagnosis of, 470–471
    ecological perspective of, 465–466

energy-based modalities for treatment
of, 478
environmental issues affecting, 474–475
etiology of, 459
facets of integrative treatment for,
471–474
mind-body therapies for treatment
of, 476–477
non-traditional therapies for treatment
of, 476
safety issues in treatment of, 481–482
symptom oriented treatment for, 479–481
traditional modalities for
treatment of, 479
treatment plan for, 468–470
treatment system for, 464–465
Mental illness. *See* Mental health
Mental imagery, 209
Mental Processing Composite, 317
Mercury toxicity, 315, 402
Metabolic disorders, 400–401
Metabolic syndrome, 501
Metallothionein, 406
Methadone, 543
Methylenetetrahydrofolate reductase
(MTHFR), 407
Migraines, 539
Milk thistle *(Silybum marianum),* 218
Mind-body medicine, 367
for treatment of FAP, 428–431
Mind-body techniques, 296
Mind-body therapy, for treatment of pain,
525–529
Mindfulness meditation, 382
Misrakasneham, 435
MMFF. *See* McMaster Model of Family
Functioning (MMFF)
Monosodium glutamate (MSG), 540
Monosymptomatic nocturnal enuresis, 115
Moral development, Kohlberg's theory of,
40
Moxibustion, 105
MSG. *See* Monosodium glutamate (MSG)
MT. *See* Massage therapy (MT)
MTHFR. *See* Methylenetetrahydrofolate
reductase (MTHFR)

Mucositis, as side effect from cancer
therapy, 496–497
Multisystem integration (MSI), 255
Muscle energy (ME), 348–349
Muscle spasm, 347
Musculoskeletal disorders, 381
Musculoskeletal system, 345
Music therapy, for solving sleep problem in
children, 416
Myotherapy, 252

N-acetylcysteine (NAC), 645
National Certification Board for
Therapeutic Massage and
Bodywork (NCBTMB), 254
National Certification in Therapeutic
Massage and Bodywork (NCTMB),
253
National Certification in Therapeutic
Massage (NCTM), 253
Natural health products, and interactions
with prescription drugs, 75
Naturopathic medicine, 85
history of, 303–305
principles of, 305–306
for treatment of children, 309–312
Naturopathic Physician Licensing
Examinations (NPLEX), 307
Naturopathy
characteristics of medical care in, 308–309
history of, 303–305
licensing for, 307–308
referral to naturopathic physicians, 312
training and accreditation for, 306–307
NCTM. *See* National Certification in
Therapeutic Massage (NCTM)
Neurodevelopmental disorders, 332–333
autism, 356, 396
autoimmune abnormalities, 400
food sensitivities or allergies, 399–400
gastrointestinal system, 398–399
heavy metal toxicity, 401–402
metabolic disorders, 400–401
nutritional deficiencies and, 402–403
omega-3 fatty acids, 403
regressive autism, 396–397

Neuroendocrine dysfunction, 544
Neuromuscular therapy, 252
Neuropathic pain, 521
New Age Healing, 31
NHP-drug interactions, 76
N-methyl-D-aspartate (NMDA) receptor,
    521, 571
Nocturnal enuresis
    acupuncture for treatment of, 114–115
    hypnosis for treatment of, 278–280
Non-Communicating Children's Pain
        Checklist, 522
Non-Hodgkin's lymphoma, 488
Non-steroidal anti-inflammatory drugs
        (NSAIDS), 524
Non-steroidal antirheumaitc drugs, 546, 547
Norepinephrine, 407
North America
    culture, spirituality and clinician self-
        awareness in, 32–34
    influence of culture and spiritualism on
        integrative pediatrics in, 31–32
    medical professionalism in, 33
    patient desire for spiritual interaction
        in, 32
    religious and spiritual concerns of
        patients in, 34–36
    spiritual resources on loss of child in, 35
    use of prayer as health practice in, 31
North American Board of Naturopathic
        Examiners (NABNE), 307
NPLEX. See Naturopathic Physician
        Licensing Examinations (NPLEX)
Nursing dysfunction, 156
Nutritional deficiencies, 332
Nutritional medicine, 334
Nutritional therapeutics
    diets for
        elimination diet, 324–326
        gluten-and casein-free diet, 326–327
        specific carbohydrate diet, 327–329
    early nutrition stage
        breastfeeding, 317
        organic vs. conventional foods,
            318–320
        starting solids, 318

at prenatal nutrition stage, 315–317
    use of supplements in infancy and early
        childhood in, 320–321

Obesity
    childhood, 501
    exercises for treatment of, 205–206
Obsessive–compulsive disorder, 463
Occipito-attlantoaxial subluxation, 440
Omega-3 fatty acids, 495
    deficiency of, 403
    treatment of
        ADHD, 411–412
        autism, 405–406
        pain, 530
OMT. See Osteopathic manipulative
        treatments (OMT)
Opioid analgesics, 524
Opioid peptides, 108
Organic foods, 320
Organophosphate chlorpyrifos, 319
Osteopathic cranial manipulation, 479
Osteopathic manipulative treatments
        (OMT), 340
    benefits of, 345
    clinical effect of, 353
    for colic and feeding problems in infants,
        354–355
    neuroendocrine-immune connection
        with, 346
    for neurologic diseases, 356–358
    for preventing recurrent otitis media,
        610–611
    somato-visceral connections with, 345
    for treatment of atopic disorders, 606
    treatment principles and modalities for,
        347–348
    for upper respiratory infections, 355
    used for asthmatic patients, 346
Osteopathic medicine, 340, 341
    tenets of, 343–344
Osteopathy. See also Cranial osteopathy
    application of, 350
    approach for finding pediatric practi-
        tioner of, 358–359
    history of, 342–343

indirect techniques for, 349
medical education in, 359
training in manipulative medicine of,
      359
for treatment of
   colic and feeding problems in infants,
      354–355
   neurologic diseases, 356–358
   upper respiratory infections, 355
Otitis media. *See also* Acute otitis media
      (AOM)
   treatment of
      biological-based therapies for,
         609–610
      CAM therapies for, 609
      conventional approach for, 609
   treatment using osteopathy, 355
   use of antibiotics for, 608

Pain
   amplification, 521
   chronic, 519
   definition of, 519
   integrative assessment of, 521–524
   medication for, 27
   "neuromatrix" theory of, 520
   neuropathic, 521
   pathophysiology of, 519–521
   processing system, 520
   somato-visceral, 520
Pain amplification disorders, 382
Pain management
   alternative medical systems for
      acupuncture, 534–535
      ayurvedic medicine, 536
      homeopathy and naturopathy, 535
      meditative exercises, 536
   biologically-based therapies for
      butterbur, 531
      chamomile, 532
      coenzyme Q-10, 531
      Devil's Claw, 530
      feverfew, 530–531
      ginger, 529–530
      magnesium, 529
      melatonin, 532–533

omega-3-fatty acids, 530
valerian and sedative herbs, 532
vitamin B, 531–532
conventional approach to, 524–525
energy therapies for, 536–537
integrative approach using mind-body
   therapies, 525–529
manipulation therapies for
   massage, 533–534
   osteopathic/cranio-sacral/chiropractic
      therapies, 533
   physical therapy (PT) and exercise, 534
Pain modulation, "gate control" theory of,
      520
PAIS. *See* Psychosocial Adjustment to
      Illness Scale (PAIS)
Palmitoy-ethanolamide (PEA), 533
Parent–child fit, 473
Patellofemoral pain syndromes (PFPS), 166
Patient care
   healthy diet and exercise patterns in, 56
   provider wellness and impact on, 55
PDD. *See* Pervasive Developmental
      Disorder (PDD)
Pediatric CAM, ethics of, 81–82
Pediatric chiropractic
   curative care, 150–151
   physiological therapies, nutritional
      supplementation, exercise and
      lifestyle advice in, 150
   preventive care, 151
   rationale and therapeutic interventions,
      147
   for toddler and preschool-aged patient
      asthma, 161
      chronic upper respiratory infection,
         160–161
      enuresis, 161
      otitis media, 159–160
   variety of adjustment techniques
      employed in, 148–149
Pediatric exercise
   as form of medicine for treatment of
      bone density, 208
      cardiovascular disease, 206–207
      depression, 208

Pediatric exercise *(continued)*
 insulin resistance, 207–208
 obesity, 205–206
 recommendations for, 205
Pediatric health care
 biopsychosocial factors in assessment
  and treatment of problem, 8
 integrative assessment in, 14–15
  active listening in patient's problem,
   15–16
  mediating factors/co-morbid diagnoses
   in, 14–15
 in medical training, 7
 resources for, *57–58*
 spiritual issues in, 41–42
 spirituality in, 62–63
Pediatric herbs
 brief review of common, *219–222*
 commonly used, *221–222*
 safety considerations in use of, 222–223
  contamination and misidentification,
   223–224
  prescription medications, 224–229
Pediatric integrative medicine, 6
 programs in, 9
Pediatric intensive care units (PICU), 446
 assessment of risk *vs.* anticipated
  benefit, 454
 benefiting from CAM interventions, 452
 daily routines on, 448–449
 family-centered care in, 448
 integrative practitioner in, 454–455
 specific modalities applied in, 452–453
Pediatric lung disorders, acute and chronic
 components of, 621
Pediatric nutrition, 315
Pediatric oncologists, 62
Pediatric Osteopathic Manipulative
 Treatment (POMT), 343
Pediatric palliative care (PPC)
 Aggressive Comfort Care (ACT) in, 63
 biofeedback in, 578
 in culturally based healing traditions, 588
 for distressing symptoms at end-of-life of
  child, 570

 energy healing in, 586–587
 integrative therapeutic interventions in
  effectiveness of, *574*
  mind-body medicine, 574–575
  provider survey on using, 572–574
 manipulative and body-based
  practices in
  acupuncture, 584–585
  energy medicine, 584
  massage, 582–583
  reflexology, 583
  myths and misconceptions, 570–571
  shiatsu in, 586
  symptom management in, 571–572
  yoga in, 579
Pediatric pulmonary disorders
 herbal supplements used for, 639
 pathophysiology of, 622–623
 safety issues when dealing with,
  637–640
Peppermint *(Mentha piperita)*, 129, 131
Peppermint oil, for treatment of FAP, 425
Pervasive Developmental Disorder (PDD),
 165, 396
Pharmacologic analgesics, 524
Phototoxicity, 139–140
Physical therapy (PT), 533
Physician health programs, 59
Phytopharmaceuticals, 218
Phytotherapy, 218. *See also* Herbal
 medicines
PICU. *See* Pediatric intensive care units
 (PICU)
Pitcher's shoulder, 166
Plagiocephaly, 353–354
Pneumograph (PNG) biofeedback, 428
Polypharmacy, 8
Polyunsaturated fatty acids
 (PUFAs), 530, 627
POMT. *See* Pediatric Osteopathic
 Manipulative Treatment (POMT)
Positional plagiocephaly, 159
Positron emission tomography (PET), 109
Post-traumatic stress disorder (PTSD),
 462

PPC. *See* Pediatric palliative care (PPC)
Practitioner-patient relationship, in
 healthcare, 49
Prebiotics, effect on colic, 600
Prescription drug, abuse of, 58
Prescription medications, 224–225
Primary care
 general approach to newborn in
  treatment of
  atopic disorders, 602–608
  colic, 597–602
  otitis media, 608–611
 integrative model for, 596
 providers for children, 595
Primary respiratory mechanism
 (PRM), 350
"Principles to Transform Healthcare," 65
PRM. *See* Primary respiratory mechanism
 (PRM)
Probiotics
 definition of, 323
 effect on colic, 600
 safety and effectiveness for AAD
  in children, 610
 for treatment of
  atopic disorders, 605
  autism, 406
  childhood cancer, 496
Progressive relaxation, 292
 mechanism of biological effect for, 296
 pediatric applications of, 295–296
 training/accreditation/licensure for, 296
Provider discontent, 51
Psychiatric medications, 464, 477
 integrative approach to use of, 477
Psychoimmunology, theory of, 182
Psychomotor Development Index, 321
Psychoneuroimmune (PNI) model, for
 managing symptoms in cancer, 492
Psychoneuroimmunology (PNI), 255
Psychopharmacologypractice, 458
Psychosocial Adjustment to Illness Scale
 (PAIS), 23
Psychosocial development, Erik Erickson's
 theory of, 40

Psychosocial spiritual care (PSS), 62
PUFAs. *See* Polyunsaturated fatty acids
 (PUFAs)
Pulmonary hypertension, 465
Pulsed electromagnetic field (PEMF), for
 pain management, 537
Pycnogenol, 630

"Qi" energy, 106, 112
Qi Gong meditative exercises, for treatment
 of pain, 536
Quality of life (QoL), 569

Radiation therapy, 495
Randomized controlled trials (RCTs), 23,
 77, 240, 345, 572
RB. *See* Retinoblastoma (RB)
Recurrent otitis, development of, 329
Reflexology, 251
 for treatment of constipation, 441
Reflex Sympathetic Dystrophy (RSD), 542
Regressive autism, 396–397
Reiki, 180, 182
 adult literature in, 190–191
 beneficial effects on adolescent patients,
  384
 clinical process involved in, 189
 history of, 188
 pediatric literature on, 191
 training, 191–192
 for treatment of pain and depression,
  191, 537
Relationship-centered care, 49
Relaxation-mental imagery (RMI), 438
Relaxation skills, biofeedback-based, 26
Research curricula for CAM school,
 challenges and opportunities in
 developing, 87
Retinoblastoma (RB), 490
Riboflavin, 532
RMI. *See* Relaxation-mental imagery (RMI)
Roman chamomile *(Chamaemelum
 nobilis),* 125, 131
RSD. *See* Reflex Sympathetic Dystrophy
 (RSD)

Sacral chiropractic subluxation
complex, 439–440
Sacro-iliac subluxation, *155*
S-adenosylhomocysteine (SAH), 400
S-adenosylmethionine (SAM), 400
Sanicula aqua, 433
Saw palmetto *(Serenoa repens),* 218
Scoliosis, 164
SCORAD index, 324
Self-hypnosis
for management of pediatric pain, 526
training, effects of, 269
Serotonin, 533
Serotonin reuptake inhibitors (SSRI), 375
Sham acupuncture, 542
"Sheng" cycle, 106
Shiatsu (Japanese body therapy), 586
Short acting inhaled β₂-agonists (SABA),
624
Sick Kids Foundation, 90
Single nucleotide polymorphisms (SNPs),
472, 602
Single-proton emission computer
tomography (SPECT), 109
SJW. *See* St. John's wort (SJW)
Sleep medication, 27
Sleep-phase syndrome, 377
Sleep problem in children
integrative approach for solving
behavioral methods, 415–416
botanicals, 416–417
melatonin, 417
mind-body interventions, 416
SMT. *See* Spinal manipulative therapy
(SMT)
Social rhythms therapy, 471
Somatic dysfunction (SD), 352
characteristics of, 344
Somato-visceral pain, 520
Spearmint *(Mentha spicata),* 129
Specific carbohydrate diet (SCD), 324,
327–329
Spike lavender *(Lavandula spica),* 125
Spinal cord, 345
Spinal curvature, development
of, 154

Spinal manipulative therapy
(SMT), 147, 611, 633
Spinal subluxation, clues indicating
presence of, *158*
Spiritual assessment mnemonics, 45
Spiritual belief system, 39
Spirituality
benefits of, 61
on adolescents, 382–384
differences with religion, 61
and healing *vs.* curing, 63
in pediatrics, 62–63
and wellness, 63–64
Sports massage, 252
Sprain strain, 347
SSRI. *See* Serotonin reuptake inhibitors
(SSRI)
Standard Hypnotic Susceptibility Scale for
Children, 273
Staphylococcus aureus, 399
Static encephalopathy, 397
Steam inhalation, 126
St. John's wort (SJW), 375, 470
Subluxation
at atlanto-occipital junction, 164
development of spinal curvatures and
stages of locomotion, 154–155
etiology in children
birth trauma, 151–153
intrauterine constraint, 151
local and systemic effects of, 147–148
symptoms of infant/toddler indicating
presence of, *155*
Suicide, risk of death by, 58
Swedish massage, 252
Sweet fennel *(Foeniculum vulgaris),* 131
Sweet orange *(Citrus sinensis),* 129
Symptoms of disease, classification of, 103

Team-based objectively structured
clinical examinations
(TOSCEs), 94
Tea tree *(Melaleuca alternifolia),* 133
Temporomandibular dysfunction
(TMD), 163
Tennis elbow, 166

Therapeutic touch (TT), 182
adult literature on, 184–186
clinical process in, 183–184
development of, 182
for pain management, 537
pediatric literature on, 186–187
training for, 188
Thoracic subluxation, 154
Tibetan medicine, 30
TMG. *See* Trimethylglycine (TMG)
Torticollis, 156
Touch therapies, 181
Traditional Chinese medicine
(TCM), 85, 103
for treatment of
ADHD, 413
asthma, 631, 633–634
constipation, 434
FAP, 427–428
Transpersonal caring, 181
Trigger point therapy, 252
Trimethylglycine (TMG), 407
True lavender *(Lavandula offinialis)*, 125
Tui na, 105–106
Tumor necrosis factor (TNF-alpha), 530
Tympanograms, 341

Universal life energy. *See* Reiki
Unsaturated pyrolizidine alkaloid (UPA),
531
Upper respiratory infections (URI), 377

Vaccine antigens, 607
Valerian
lemon-balm, 416
sedative effects of, 376
side effects of, 376

Vasomotor instability, in infants, 353
VCUG radiographic procedures, 273–274
Vegetable oils, 126
Vertebral subluxations, 161
Virtual reality (VR) therapy, for treatment
of burn pain in children, 528–529
Vitamin B, for treatment of pain, 531

Wellness
components of, *50*
contributing factors for provider, *60*
definition of, 49
provider's pratices for, 59–60
spirituality and, 63–64
Western diet (WD), 547
White House Commission on
Complementary and Alternative
Health Care Policy, *84*
"Whole child care," 48
Wilms tumors, 490

Yerba Mate *(Ilex Paraguariensis)*, 374
Yin and Yang, concept of, 106
Ylang ylang *(Cananga odorata)*, 135
Yoga, 211
beneficial effects on adolescent patients,
384–385
in palliative care, 579
for treatment of
FAP, 430
pain, 536

Zinc
for treatment of
ADHD, 412
autism, 406
Zygapophyseal joints, 149